Promoting Mental Health

in Children and Adolescents

PRIMARY CARE PRACTICE AND ADVOCACY

Editor

Jane Meschan Foy, MD, FAAP

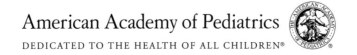

American Academy of Pediatrics

DEDICATED TO THE HEALTH OF ALL CHILDREN®

American Academy of Pediatrics Publishing Staff

Mary Lou White, *Chief Product and Services Officer/SVP, Membership, Marketing, and Publishing*

Mark Grimes, *Vice President, Publishing*

Carrie Peters, *Editor, Professional/Clinical Publishing*

Theresa Wiener, *Production Manager, Clinical and Professional Publications*

Amanda Helmholz, *Medical Copy Editor*

Linda Diamond, *Manager, Art Direction and Production*

Linda Smessaert, MSIMC, *Senior Marketing Manager, Professional Resources*

Mary Louise Carr, MBA, *Marketing Manager, Clinical Publications*

Published by the American Academy of Pediatrics
345 Park Blvd
Itasca, IL 60143
Telephone: 630/626-6000
Facsimile: 847/434-8000

www.aap.org

The American Academy of Pediatrics is an organization of 67,000 primary care pediatricians, pediatric medical subspecialists, and pediatric surgical specialists dedicated to the health, safety, and well-being of infants, children, adolescents, and young adults.

The recommendations in this publication do not indicate an exclusive course of treatment or serve as a standard of care. Variations, taking into account individual circumstances, may be appropriate.

Every effort has been made to ensure that the drug selection and dosages set forth in this text are in accordance with the current recommendations and practice at the time of publication. It is the responsibility of the health care professional to check the package insert of each drug for any change in indications and dosages and for added warnings and precautions.

The American Academy of Pediatrics is not responsible for the content of any of the resources mentioned in this publication. Web site addresses are as current as possible but may change at any time.

Brand names are furnished for identification purposes only. No endorsement of the manufacturers or products mentioned is implied.

The publishers have made every effort to trace the copyright holders for borrowed materials. If they have inadvertently overlooked any, they will be pleased to make the necessary arrangements at the first opportunity.

This publication has been developed by the American Academy of Pediatrics. The authors, editors, and contributors are expert authorities in the field of pediatrics. No commercial involvement of any kind has been solicited or accepted in the development of the content of this publication.

Disclosures: Dr Coyne-Beasley has indicated a relationship with Pfizer.

Every effort is made to keep *Promoting Mental Health in Children and Adolescents: Primary Care Practice and Advocacy* consistent with the most recent advice and information available from the American Academy of Pediatrics.

Special discounts are available for bulk purchases of this publication. E-mail Special Sales at aapsales@aap.org for more information.

Printed in the United States of America

9-414/0918   1 2 3 4 5 6 7 8 9 10

MA0886

ISBN: 978-1-61002-227-9
eBook: 978-1-61002-228-6

Library of Congress Control Number: 2018936484

Contributors

Rhonda Graves Acholonu, MD, FAAP
Associate Dean for Diversity and
   Academic Affairs
Director of Medical Education in the
   Clinical Sciences
Assistant Professor of Pediatrics
New York University School of Medicine
New York, New York
18: *Children of Divorce*

Sheryl Allen, MD, MS, FAAP
Associate Professor of Clinical
   Emergency Medicine and Pediatrics
Department of Emergency Medicine
Indiana University School of Medicine
Indianapolis, Indiana
17: *Children in Poverty*

Keli Beck, MD
Assistant Professor of Family and
   Community Medicine
Director, Maternal Child Health
Wake Forest School of Medicine
Winston-Salem, North Carolina
27: *Adolescents Who Are Pregnant or
   Parenting*

Robert J. Bidwell, MD
Associate Clinical Professor of Pediatrics
John A. Burns School of Medicine
University of Hawaii
Honolulu, Hawaii
20: *Lesbian, Gay, and Bisexual Youths*
21: *Children With Gender Expression and
   Identity Issues*

**Yolanda (Linda) Reid Chassiakos, MD,
FAAP**
Clinical Assistant Professor of Pediatrics
David Geffen School of Medicine
University of California, Los Angeles
Los Angeles, California
9: *Healthy Use of Media*

Tamera Coyne-Beasley, MD, MPH
Professor of Pediatrics and Internal
   Medicine
Department of Pediatrics
Director, North Carolina
   Multidisciplinary Adolescent
   Research Consortium for Health

University of North Carolina
Chapel Hill, North Carolina
12: *Healthy Sexual Development and
   Sexuality*

Stephanie Daniel, PhD
Professor and Vice Chair for Research
Department of Family and Community
   Medicine
Wake Forest School of Medicine
Winston-Salem, North Carolina
31: *Promoting Mental Health in Schools*

**Beth Ellen Davis, MD, MPH, FAAP
(COL, MC, USA, Retired)**
Professor of Pediatrics
Division of Developmental Pediatrics
University of Virginia
Charlottesville, Virginia
19: *Children in Military Families*

Paula M. Duncan, MD
Burlington, Vermont
30: *Promoting the Health of Adolescents*

Marian Earls, MD, MTS, FAAP
Clinical Professor of Pediatrics
University of North Carolina Medical
   School
Chapel Hill, North Carolina
Director of Pediatric Programs
Deputy Chief Medical Officer
Community Care of North Carolina
Raleigh, North Carolina
1: *Healthy Child Development*

Glenn Flores, MD, FAAP
Chief Research Officer
Director, Health Services Research
   Institute
Connecticut Children's Medical Center
Associate Chair of Research
Professor of Pediatrics
UConn School of Medicine
Hartford, Connecticut
14: *Families New to the United States*

**Barbara L. Frankowski, MD, MPH,
FAAP**
Professor of Pediatrics
University of Vermont Children's
   Hospital
Burlington, Vermont
31: *Promoting Mental Health in Schools*

Andrew Garner, MD, PhD, FAAP
Clinical Professor of Pediatrics
Case Western Reserve University School
of Medicine
Cleveland, Ohio
13: *Children Exposed to Adverse
Childhood Experiences*

Sarah Garwood, MD, FAAP
Associate Professor of Pediatrics
Division of Adolescent Medicine
Washington University
St Louis, Missouri
12: *Healthy Sexual Development and
Sexuality*

Paul L. Geltman, MD, MPH, FAAP
Medical Director for Refugee and
Immigrant Health, Division of
Global Populations and Infectious
Disease Prevention, Massachusetts
Department of Public Health
Medical Director of Ambulatory Care
Services, Franciscan Children's
Associate Professor of Health Policy and
Health Services Research, Henry M.
Goldman School of Dental Medicine,
Boston University
Brighton, MA
14: *Families New to the United States*

Melanie A. Gold, DO, DMQ
Professor of Pediatrics, Columbia
University Medical Center (CUMC)
and Professor of Population & Family
Health, Mailman School of Public
Health, CUMC
Medical Director, School Based Health
Centers, New York-Presbyterian
Hospital
New York, New York
4: *Interviewing Adolescents*
22: *Children in Gay- and
Lesbian-Parented Families*

Gary S. Goldfield, PhD
Senior Scientist, Healthy Active Living
and Obesity Research Group,
Children's Hospital of Eastern
Ontario Research Institute
Ottawa, Ontario, Canada
10: *Healthy Active Living*

Sandra G. Hassink, MD, MS, FAAP
Medical Director, American Academy of
Pediatrics
Institute for Healthy Childhood Weight
Wilmington, Delaware
8: *Healthy Weight*

Breena Welch Holmes, MD, FAAP
Director, Maternal and Child Health
Division
Vermont Department of Health
Burlington, Vermont
30: *Promoting the Health of Adolescents*

Evalyn Horowitz, MD
Physician and Surgeon
California Department of Corrections
and Rehabilitation
Mule Creek State Prison
Ione, California
28: *Children in the Juvenile Justice System*

Sandra H. Jee, MD, MPH, FAAP
Associate Professor of Pediatrics
Division of General Pediatrics
University of Rochester
Rochester, New York
15: *Children in Foster or Kinship Care or
Involved With Child Welfare*

Renée R. Jenkins, MD, FAAP
Professor and Chair Emerita
Department of Pediatrics and Child
Health
Howard University College of Medicine
Washington, DC
17: *Children in Poverty*

Sebastian G. Kaplan, PhD
Associate Professor
Department of Psychiatry and
Behavioral Medicine
Department of Family and Community
Medicine
Wake Forest University School of
Medicine
Winston-Salem, North Carolina
2: *Family-Centered Care: Applying
Behavior Change Science*

Jill Kerr, DNP, MPH
Family Nurse Practitioner (Retired)
Chapel Hill Carrboro City Schools Head
Start
Carrboro, North Carolina
29: *Promoting the Mental Health of
Young Children*

Jonathan D. Klein, MD, MPH, FAAP
Professor of Pediatrics
University of Illinois at Chicago
Chicago, Illinois
5: *Counseling Parents of Adolescents*

Jonathan Kotch, MD, MPH, FAAP
Emeritus Professor
Department of Maternal and Child
    Health
UNC Gillings School of Global Public
    Health
Chapel Hill, North Carolina
29: *Promoting the Mental Health of Young
    Children*

Daniel P. Krowchuk, MD, FAAP
Professor of Pediatrics and Dermatology
Wake Forest University School of
    Medicine
Winston-Salem, North Carolina
27: *Adolescents Who Are Pregnant or
    Parenting*

Danielle Laraque-Arena, MD, FAAP
Chair, Department of Pediatrics,
    Maimonides Medical Center
Vice President, Maimonides Infants and
    Children's Hospital of Brooklyn
Professor of Pediatrics
Albert Einstein College of Medicine
Yeshiva University
Brooklyn, New York
25: *Children Affected by Racism*

**Claire M. A. LeBlanc, MD, FAAP,
Diploma in Sport Medicine**
Associate Professor of Pediatrics
Division of Rheumatology
McGill University
Montreal, Quebec, Canada
10: *Healthy Active Living*

Lori Legano, MD, FAAP
Assistant Professor of Pediatrics
Division of General Pediatrics
New York University School of Medicine
New York, New York
18: *Children of Divorce*

Julie M. Linton, MD, FAAP
Assistant Professor of Pediatrics
Wake Forest School of Medicine
Associate Director, Integrating
    Special Populations

Maya Angelou Center for Health Equity
Winston-Salem, North Carolina
27: *Adolescents Who Are Pregnant or
    Parenting*

Anne May, MD, FAAP
Assistant Professor of Pediatrics
The Ohio State University School of
    Medicine
Columbus, Ohio
7: *Healthy Sleep*

Patricia McQuilkin, MD, MS, FAAP
Associate Professor of Pediatrics
University of Massachusetts Medical
    School
Worcester, Massachusetts
24: *Homeless Children*

Marlene D. Melzer-Lange, MD, FAAP
Professor of Pediatrics
Division of Pediatric Emergency
    Medicine
Medical College of Wisconsin
Milwaukee, Wisconsin
11: *Violence Prevention*

Robert E. Morris, MD, FAAP
Professor Emeritus
Division of Adolescent Medicine
Department of Pediatrics
David Geffen School of Medicine
University of California, Los Angeles
Los Angeles, California
28: *Children in the Juvenile Justice System*

Robert D. Needlman, MD, FAAP
Professor of Pediatrics
Case Western Reserve University School
    of Medicine
MetroHealth Medical Center
Cleveland, Ohio
23: *Children in Self-care*

Linda Nicolotti, PhD
Director of Pediatric Psychology
Assistant Professor of Pediatrics
Wake Forest Baptist Health
Winston-Salem, North Carolina
2: *Family-Centered Care: Applying
    Behavior Change Science*

Karen Olness, MD, FAAP
Professor Emerita of Pediatrics, Global
   Health and Diseases
Case Western Reserve University School
   of Medicine
Cleveland, Ohio
3: *Culturally Effective Care*

James M. Perrin, MD, FAAP
Professor of Pediatrics
John C. Robinson Chair in Pediatrics
Harvard Medical School
Associate Chair, MassGeneral Hospital
   for Children
Boston, Massachusetts
6: *Family Support*

Amy Pirretti, MS
Chandler, Arizona
6: *Family Support*

Jason Rafferty, MD, MPH, EdM, FAAP
Pediatrician and Psychiatrist
Thundermist Health Centers
Emma Pendleton Bradley Hospital
Providence, Rhode Island
24: *Homeless Children*

Cindy Schorzman, MD
Medical Director
Student Health and Counseling Services
University of California, Davis
Davis, California
22: *Children in Gay- and
   Lesbian-Parented Families*

Rashmi Shetgiri, MD, MSHS, MSCS
Assistant Professor of Pediatrics
Division of General Pediatrics
Harbor-UCLA Medical Center
David Geffen School of Medicine
Los Angeles Biomedical Research
   Institute at Harbor—UCLA Medical
   Center
Torrance, California
14: *Families New to the United States*

Mark L. Splaingard, MD
Director of Pediatric Sleep Medicine
Nationwide Children's Hospital
Professor of Pediatrics
Ohio State University School of
   Medicine
Columbus, Ohio
7: *Healthy Sleep*

Sarah H. Springer, MD, FAAP
Kids Plus Pediatrics
Pittsburgh, Pennsylvania
16: *Adopted Children*

David P. Steffen, DrPH, MSN
Director, Leadership MPH Track
Public Health Leadership Program
Gillings School of Global Public Health
University of North Carolina
Chapel Hill, North Carolina
29: *Promoting the Mental Health of Young
   Children*

Ruth E. K. Stein, MD, FAAP
Professor of Pediatrics
Albert Einstein College of Medicine
The Children's Hospital at Montefiore
Bronx, New York
26: *Children With Chronic Medical
   Conditions*

Moira Szilagyi, MD, PhD, FAAP
Professor, Department of Pediatrics
Section Chief, Developmental Behavioral
   Studies
University of California, Los Angeles
Los Angeles, California
15: *Children in Foster or Kinship Care or
   Involved With Child Welfare*

Howard Taras, MD, FAAP
Professor of Pediatrics
University of California, San Diego
La Jolla, California
31: *Promoting Mental Health in Schools*

Angelica Terepka, PsyD
Clinical Psychologist
New York-Presbyterian Hospital
Columbia University Medical Center
School Based Health Center
New York, New York
4: *Interviewing Adolescents*

Kristine Torjesen, MD, MPH, FAAP
Scientist II
FHI 360
Durham, North Carolina
3: *Culturally Effective Care*

Mark S. Tremblay, PhD, DLitt(Hon), FACSM, CSEP-CEP
Director, Healthy Active Living and
  Obesity Research Group
Children's Hospital of Eastern Ontario
  Research Institute
University of Ottawa
Ottawa, Ontario, Canada
10: *Healthy Active Living*

Timothy Wilks, MD, MHA, FAAP
Naval Medical Center Camp Lejeune
Camp Lejeune, North Carolina
19: *Children in Military Families*

Earnestine Willis, MD, MPH
Kellner Professor in Pediatrics
Vice Chair for Diversity and Inclusion in
  Pediatrics
Director, Center for the Advancement of
  Underserved Children
Medical College of Wisconsin
Milwaukee, Wisconsin
17: *Children in Poverty*

Virginia P. Young, MLS
SUNY Upstate Medical University
Syracuse, New York
25: *Children Affected by Racism*

American Academy of Pediatrics Reviewers

Committee on Communications and Media

Committee on Nutrition

Committee on Psychosocial Aspects of Child and Family Health

Committee on School Health

Medical Home Implementation Project Advisory Committee

Mental Health Leadership Work Group

Poverty and Child Health Leadership Work Group

Section on Pediatric Pulmonology and Sleep Medicine

Task Force on Diversity and Inclusion, Provisional Section on Minority Health, Equity, and Inclusion

Contents

Care of Special Populations

Part 2: Promoting Mental Health Beyond the Medical Home

Appendixes

Acknowledgements

I am grateful to the many authors and mentors who have contributed to this work, to the colleagues who served with me on the American Academy of Pediatrics (AAP) Task Force on Mental Health and the Mental Health Leadership Work Group, to the AAP staff who supported and inspired the work of those 2 groups, and to the staff and my fellow coeditors of the *American Academy of Pediatrics Textbook of Pediatric Care,* 2nd Edition, who recognized the need for *Promoting Mental Health in Children and Adolescents: Primary Care Practice and Advocacy.* I am indebted to Carrie Peters for her patient and diligent collaboration in bringing this book to publication, along with its companion book, *Mental Health Care of Children and Adolescents: A Guide for Primary Care Clinicians.*

In the spirit of this book, I also want to acknowledge the contributions of my family: Isadore and Rachel Farrer Meschan, who were physician-educators as well as loving parents; my husband, Miles Foy, whose support and encouragement made this book and all my life's work possible; and my children and grandchildren, who have been my inspiration to make the world a kinder, better place for children.

Jane Meschan Foy, MD, FAAP

Introduction

Jane Meschan Foy, MD

"Readers are invited to draw from the expertise
of the book's authors to transform their
practice and community in ways that will
promote mental health in all the children
and adolescents they serve."

This book is for pediatric primary care clinicians (PCCs)—pediatricians, family physicians, internists, nurse practitioners, physician assistants— and other health care professionals who have the great privilege and responsibility of longitudinal, trusting relationships with children, adolescents, and their families. The book aims to help PCCs (1) integrate anticipatory guidance on healthy social-emotional development with other aspects of routine health supervision; (2) identify emerging symptoms and early signs of impaired functioning that precede development of a mental disorder; and (3) apply brief evidence-based interventions to the first-line care of children, adolescents, and their families who manifest mental health risks and emerging problems. Mindful of the rapid pace of primary care practice, the book offers tools that make early identification feasible and brief interventions that can be readily incorporated into workflow. The book also describes ways PCCs can draw on their pediatric expertise to enhance the programs and services that support the mental health of children and adolescents in schools and the community more broadly.

In a policy statement published in 2009, the American Academy of Pediatrics (AAP) articulated the competencies—that is, the knowledge and skills—PCCs need to provide children and adolescents with mental health care.[1] These competencies include the capacity to

▶ Promote healthy emotional development and resilience.
▶ Provide anticipatory guidance to families.
▶ Reinforce strengths in both the child or adolescent and the family.
▶ Identify occult mental health problems.
▶ Apply evidence-based communication methods and interventions appropriate to the initial care of children, adolescents, and their families with identified risks and problems.

▶ Contribute to development of public health and other community initiatives that promote healthy development and resilience and reduce the precipitants of toxic stress.

This book includes information and tools that will help readers achieve these pediatric mental health competencies.

The book has 2 parts.

Part 1, Promoting Mental Health in the Pediatric Medical Home, describes opportunities inherent in the primary care setting for primary and secondary prevention of mental health problems. Chapters in the first section of Part 1 cover principles of health promotion: the strength-based approach, family-centered care, culturally effective care, and ways to communicate with adolescents and their parents. The next section of Part 1 describes interconnected pathways toward improving mental health and resilience: family support, healthy sleep, healthy weight, healthy use of media, healthy active living, violence prevention, and healthy sexual development and sexuality. In response to needs identified in the psychosocial assessment and the health issues a patient and family are motivated to address, PCCs can draw guidance from these chapters to customize the preventive counseling they offer to a particular patient and family. The third section of Part 1 describes the needs of special populations that, by virtue of their increased risks for mental health problems, require heightened surveillance, more-frequent psychosocial screening, focused anticipatory guidance, additional resources, or any combination of these services. Chapters in this section focus on children and adolescents (here collectively called simply *children* unless otherwise specified or, for those older than 6 years, *youths*) exposed to adverse childhood experiences, families new to the United States, children in foster or kinship care, adopted children, children in poverty, children of divorce, children in military families, LGB (lesbian, gay, and bisexual) youths, children with gender expression and identity issues, children in gay- and lesbian-parented families, children in self-care, homeless children, children affected by racism, children with chronic medical conditions, adolescents who are pregnant or parenting, and youths in the juvenile justice system.

Part 2 of the book, **Promoting Mental Health Beyond the Medical Home,** describes community-level programs and strategies to promote mental health in the entire population of children. The first 2 chapters focus on young children and adolescents, respectively. The final chapter describes programs and strategies for promoting mental health in schools, which are communities unto themselves, providing nurture as well as educational programs to their students and often serving as the default provider of mental health services to those with limited access to pediatric and mental health specialty services.

Augmenting chapter narratives are Web resources, AAP policies, and references. The book's appendixes summarize concepts and tools that are useful across multiple chapters.

This book is published as a companion to a previous AAP publication, also developed in response to the AAP-recommended mental health competencies: *Mental Health Care of Children and Adolescents: A Guide for Primary Care Clinicians*. This earlier publication provides in-depth guidance on practice enhancements and on the clinical care of children with commonly occurring problems. In contrast to psychiatry textbooks, which typically organize chapters around diagnoses, *Mental Health Care of Children and Adolescents* includes chapters organized around presenting signs and symptoms. They take the reader through a step-by-step process that begins with primary care findings (eg, positive psychosocial screening test results, parental concerns, teacher referrals, clinician observations) and offer guidance in differentiating normal variations in behavior and development from findings that suggest a need for further assessment. They go on to describe initial interventions appropriate to pediatric practice (and not necessarily dependent on a diagnosis!) and highlight indications for full diagnostic assessment, specific treatment, mental health specialty involvement, or some combination of these steps. *Mental Health Care of Children and Adolescents* includes, for example, chapters on family dysfunction, learning difficulty, nonadherence to medical treatment, medically unexplained symptoms, sleep disturbances, gender expression and identity issues, anxiety and trauma-related distress, disruptive behavior, eating abnormalities, inattention, and substance use. Together, these 2 books offer PCCs comprehensive guidance on incorporating mental health care, realistically, into the full range of primary care activities.

Pediatric PCCs benefit from the extraordinary advantage of longitudinal, trusting relationships with children, adolescents, and their families—relationships that extend beyond the medical home and empower PCCs to make meaningful changes in their communities and schools. Readers are invited to draw from the expertise of the book's authors to transform their practice and community in ways that will promote mental health in all the children and adolescents they serve.

Reference

1. American Academy of Pediatrics Committee on Psychosocial Aspects of Child and Family Health and Task Force on Mental Health. The future of pediatrics: mental health competencies for pediatric primary care. *Pediatrics.* 2009;124(1):410–421

Promoting Mental Health in the Pediatric Medical Home

General Principles

Interconnected Pathways to Resilience and Mental Health

Care of Special Populations

Healthy Child Development

Marian Earls, MD, MTS

"In addition to facilitating early identification
and referral for intervention..., screening is
an excellent health promotional strategy:
screening results, both negative and positive,
provide a discussion template for anticipatory
guidance and asset building."

Primary care clinicians (PCCs) (ie, pediatricians, family physicians, internists, nurse practitioners, physician assistants) who provide longitudinal, frontline care to children and adolescents have the opportunity at every encounter with the family to promote *healthy development*—a term used in this chapter to mean growth in motor, language, cognitive, and social-emotional competence over the course of childhood and adolescence. Recent understanding of the brain's structural development highlights the importance of social-emotional influences[1,2]: PCCs know from brain research that social-emotional experiences affect brain development, both prenatally and postnatally. The implications for prevention and intervention are profound because physical growth, development, and behavior are inextricably linked, as are physical health, mental health, and resilience—the desired outcomes of healthy development. Here and throughout this book, the term *mental health* does not mean simply the absence of a mental disorder: it is "the effective practice of

► Confidence and courage
► Adaptability
► Cheerfulness
► Attention/concentration
► Harmony
► Hardiness [resilience]
► Social connectedness."[3]

This chapter describes the PCC's role in promoting healthy child and adolescent development, identifying strengths in the patient and family, identifying risks to the patient's healthy development, intervening as early as possible to address risks and emerging concerns, and involving other professionals in care of the patient and support of the family when needed.

Background

Approximately 15% of children and adolescents (collectively called simply *children* in this chapter unless otherwise specified) have developmental or behavioral disabilities, including speech and language delays, attention-deficit/hyperactivity disorder (ADHD), intellectual disability, learning disabilities, cerebral palsy, autism spectrum disorder (ASD), hearing loss, blindness, and emotional problems.[4] Even at preschool age, 13% of children have mental health problems.[4] In 2005, the Centers for Disease Control and Prevention reported that 5% of 4- to 17-year-olds in the United States (2.7 million children and adolescents) were described by their parents in the National Health Interview Survey as having severe emotional or behavioral difficulties.[5]

These rates of disability and emotional and behavioral difficulties increase with the co-occurrence of risk factors such as poverty, maternal depression, substance use, and domestic violence. According to the National Center for Children in Poverty, in 2015 approximately 44% of children in the United States lived in low-income families. This number has been increasing since 2000, after a decade of decline. Children in poverty have an increased risk for language, learning, and behavioral problems. An infant living with a depressed mother can show disordered attachment as early as 2 months of age and is at risk for failure to thrive, impaired social interaction, and delays in language and cognitive development. For the school-aged child and adolescent of a depressed mother, there is increased likelihood of depression, anxiety, behavioral problems, or conduct disorder.[6-9] Many preterm infants, especially those of extremely low birth weight ($<$1,000 g), are at risk for visual and hearing impairment, language delays and learning problems, and problems with motor development. For infants who have had a prolonged neonatal intensive care unit course, bonding with the mother can be a challenge, particularly if ongoing medical or feeding issues exist; since maternal-infant bonding is critical to healthy emotional development, these infants are at risk for emotional problems. A number of other circumstances may also be associated with increased risk of mental and emotional problems in children: immigration, foster care, adoption, divorce, a chronic medical condition, military service of a parent, lesbian-gay-bisexual-transgender identity, homelessness, and racism. Chapters in the section of this book titled Care of Special Populations describe these risks (as well as approaches to the care of children who experience them).

Early identification of young children with developmental delays and psychosocial risks and symptoms allows for early intervention (EI) and, when needed, referral for specialty services and social supports. Even for children with significant developmental diagnoses that cannot be cured or completely remediated, EI improves function for the child and family and allows for linking families with community supports. Early intervention can also save up to $100,000 per student in special education costs over the course of the child's education.[10]

Yet, despite the medical community's knowledge of prevalence and risk, detection of developmental and behavioral problems before school age is less than 50%.[11] Also concerning is that, although 15% of children have a developmental disability in childhood, only 2% to 3% receive services of the public EI Program by 3 years of age.[12,13] These circumstances limit the possibility of EI. By contrast, 70% to 80% of children with developmental disabilities are correctly identified when standardized screening tests are used.[14]

Until recently, use of standardized screening tools to identify developmental and behavioral problems, maternal depression, and family risk or protective factors has been infrequent in primary care practice. The American Academy of Pediatrics (AAP) Periodic Survey of Fellows No. 53 in 2002 revealed that 71% of fellows used only clinical observation without a screening instrument to identify children with a developmental delay. Only 23% reported using a standardized tool. Reasons given for not screening included that screening took too long, tools were difficult to administer, children may not cooperate, and reimbursement was limited. Perceived barriers were time, cost, and staff required.[15]

Despite these perceived barriers, during the past several years, national efforts such as the Commonwealth Fund ABCD (Assuring Better Child Health and Development) initiative have increased implementation of developmental and behavioral screening, referral, and coordination of care in practices across many states.[16] Since 2000, there have been many successful models of screening in primary care practices, including developmental and behavioral screening, maternal depression screening, and family and psychosocial (social determinants of health) screening. In these projects, strategies have been implemented to integrate screening into office flow, to improve payment, and to assist practices in identifying and collaborating with community resources, including mental health resources. The ABCD initiative, funded by the Commonwealth Fund and administered by the National Academy for State Health Policy, has involved 28 states and their AAP chapters.[16] The AAP, in addition to publishing policy statements on screening, promotes screening through continuing education and quality improvement activities (eg, Bright Futures PreSIP [Preventive Services Improvement Project], Don't Just Wait and See learning collaborative). According to the National Survey of Children's Health, 2011, the use of standardized, parent-completed developmental screening in primary care has been increasing. Parents reported completing a standardized developmental screening tool in the past 12 months at a health care visit for an infant or a child between 10 months and 5 years of age 30.8% of the time in 2011, up from 19.5% of the time in 2007.[17] Likewise, in 2009 the AAP Periodic Survey of Fellows No. 74 revealed that 47.7% of pediatricians reported using a standardized tool (double the percentage in 2002).[18] Those using only clinical observation decreased to 60.5%. On survey No. 93, in 2016, 63% of pediatricians reported using a standardized tool.[19]

Office-Based Health Promotion: A Strengths-Based Approach

Bright Futures: Guidelines for Health Supervision of Infants, Children, and Adolescents, 4th Edition, recommends that, in addition to discussing with parents the developmental progress of young children (aged 0–5 years) at health supervision visits, clinicians discuss developmental and educational accomplishments of older children and strengths as well as risks in adolescents.[20] The *Bright Futures*–recommended risk assessment for substance use (annually beginning at 11 years of age) and depression screening (annually beginning at 12 years of age), when negative, offer additional opportunities to reinforce healthy choices and strengths, respectively. *Bright Futures* places emphases on promoting parental strengths and protective factors and identifying social determinants of health, which may confer either protection or risk: it includes recommendations for maternal depression screening at infant visits and routinely identifying social determinants of health as part of a behavioral/psychosocial assessment at each visit. Healthy development in childhood and, ultimately, physical and mental health in adulthood depend on caregivers' nurturing the intrinsic strengths of the child, beginning in infancy, and on reinforcement of those strengths by teachers, PCCs, other trusted adults, and peers as the child develops.

In the care of the child or adolescent, it is necessary to consider the whole child, including social-emotional development, in the context of family, school, and community. Routinely assessing risks and strengths allows for early implementation of preventive strategies. For example, a PCC recognizes that her adolescent patient Michael is socially isolated and his family is struggling financially, without transportation to youth activities; the PCC learns that Michael has strengths in school—regular attendance and good relationships with several teachers—and she knows that his high school has a late bus home for students who participate in after-school activities. The PCC can encourage (and address any barriers to) Michael's participation in sports, volunteer activities, or band, depending on his interests.

An understanding of the eco-bio-developmental model makes it clear that social determinants of health affecting the family also affect the development of the child. As noted earlier in this chapter, there are social determinants that confer risk and social determinants that are protective. Box 1-1 lists examples of each.

Box 1-1. Social Determinants of Health

<u>**Social Determinants That Confer Risk**</u>
- Food insecurity
- Poor housing
- Homelessness
- Unemployment
- Social exclusion (eg, racism, discrimination)
- Substance use
- Environmental toxins (eg, mold, lead, tobacco smoke)
- Unsafe or violent neighborhood

<u>**Social Determinants That Are Protective**</u>
- Parental knowledge and skills about child development and caregiving
- Positive father involvement
- Strong emotional bond or attachment between infant/child and parent/caregiver
- Social supports
- Safe and good housing
- Stable/secure home life
- High school or higher education level for parents/caregivers
- Opportunities for stable income/employment for household
- Food security for household
- Safe neighborhood and school
- Community resources for fresh produce, exercise, and social interactions

The primary care medical home provides the perfect setting for reinforcing strengths as well as identifying threats to healthy development. Discussing the patient's and family's assets and encouraging supportive social connections can be part of early and ongoing conversations with families, along with open discussion regarding risk factors.

Among the *Bright Futures* health promotion themes that are intertwined with healthy development are family support, healthy sleep, healthy weight, healthy use of media, healthy active living, violence prevention, and healthy sexual development and sexuality—topics that follow in this book. Primary care clinicians have "the primary care advantage" in their health promotion role, including longitudinal relationships that are foundational in building rapport and trust with patients and families. This advantage, originally described in the AAP policy statement recommending mental health competencies for pediatric primary care,[21] is outlined in Box 1-2.

Promotion of healthy development begins with the prenatal visit.[22] At that visit, the longitudinal relationship begins, and the discussion of family assets and supports as well as stressors occurs. Early identification of risk

Box 1-2. The Primary Care Advantage

- Longitudinal, trusting, and empowering therapeutic relationships with children and family members
- Patient and family centeredness of pediatric practice
- Unique opportunities to prevent future mental health problems through promoting healthy lifestyles, "purposeful" and positive parenting, and play; identifying and addressing toxic stress and social adversities; anticipatory guidance; and timely intervention for common behavioral, emotional, educational, and social problems encountered in pediatric practice
- Understanding of common social, emotional, and educational problems in the context of a child's or an adolescent's development and environment
- Comfort and capacity to care for children and adolescents with uncertain diagnoses
- Experience coordinating general care and specialty care
- Familiarity with chronic care principles and practice-improvement methods
- Greater accessibility to children, adolescents, and families than that of mental health specialty care
- Potential effectiveness in countering stigma and mental health racial and ethnic disparities

Adapted from American Academy of Pediatrics Committee on Psychosocial Aspects of Child and Family Health and Task Force on Mental Health. The future of pediatrics: mental health competencies for pediatric primary care. *Pediatrics.* 2009;124(1):410–421.

factors, such as maternal depression, allows for early strategies to support the mother and family so that the newborn is born into a nurturing environment. Reach Out and Read is an excellent example of health promotion. By reading to the infant, toddler, or preschooler, in a single activity the parent encourages healthy social-emotional development (cuddling to read), language development (imitating and pointing), and fine motor development (reaching and turning pages). Encouraging the sharing of age-appropriate books together from an early age has benefits for the relationship, for language skills, and for early reading skills.

Asking the child or adolescent about his or her best and favorite subjects at school is as important as discussing where he or she has difficulty. Primary care clinicians partner with parents in encouraging the child's efforts in school (eg, participation in class, completing homework) as well as in advocating for assessment of students who may have learning or attention difficulties and for intervention, when indicated. Showing interest in and encouraging the prosocial activities of children and adolescents are powerful tools for the PCC; such activities help young people explore their talents and promote belonging. Examples include clubs, sports teams, dance, band, and choir. Particularly for adolescents, encouraging volunteerism and community activities is positive for building self-esteem and reducing risk behaviors. For adolescents, a useful model to promote such protective factors is the Circle of Courage mnemonic GIMB: generosity, independence, mastery, and belonging.[23]

As part of routine care, the clinician can engage the family in discussion regarding social determinants of health, parental strengths, parental well-being, family supports, and information about child care or school. Primary care clinicians who care for children and adolescents have long recognized the importance of developmental and behavioral screening and surveillance in helping families optimize their children's acquisition of skills, understand behavior, and facilitate learning. In addition to facilitating early identification and referral for intervention (discussed later in this chapter), screening is an excellent health promotional strategy: screening results, both negative and positive, provide a discussion template for anticipatory guidance and asset building.

From an early age, a child should participate in reporting his or her strengths and concerns. This participation builds the PCC's relationship with the child and helps the child prepare to communicate when he or she becomes an adolescent. The Search Institute documented the protective effect of assets when a child or an adolescent is exposed to risk. The asset categories include external assets (support, empowerment, boundaries, and expectations, as well as constructive use of time) and internal assets (commitment to learning, positive values, social competencies, and positive identity).[24]

Implementation in Practice

The PCC does not need to become an expert at diagnosing and managing developmental and mental disorders, nor a mental health professional. However, the clinician has the primary care advantage noted earlier in this chapter, with the opportunity for surveillance and screening; for discussion of findings with the family (and child or adolescent); for engagement of the patient and family in addressing concerns; for trial of primary care interventions, when appropriate; for referral for further assessment and intervention, when needed; and for monitoring of the patient and family's progress over time. The PCC has multiple roles: a partner with the family in finding information and community resources, a sounding board, a trusted health care professional, a facilitator in negotiating the system, and a comanager of care with specialists.

Assessment of Development, Behavior, and Learning in Primary Care

Surveillance, Screening, and Psychosocial Assessment

Surveillance is the routine elicitation of family and patient concerns; it is generally accomplished by conversation and observation, which is assisted by questionnaires and mnemonic devices (eg, Bright Futures supplemental questionnaires and HEADSSS mnemonic [home/environment, education and employment, activities, drugs, sexuality, suicide/depression, and safety], respectively; for additional examples, see Appendix 2, Mental Health Tools for Pediatrics) or prompts within the health record. It is part of the longitudinal relationship and occurs at every visit.

Screening—that is, systematically testing with a validated instrument for an undiagnosed condition in people who do not have signs or symptoms of that condition—can be used at important intervals to understand and document development and to detect problems that are not observable through surveillance alone. Screening tests can be interwoven into the schedule of health supervision visits and into the growing relationship with the family. Screening may involve the family social environment and caregivers, as well as the child or adolescent. Screening tests can be included in the routine health supervision schedule in anticipation of critical turning points; however, they can also be used flexibly to respond to individual patient and family concerns.

Psychosocial and behavioral assessment is part of the *Bright Futures/ AAP Recommendations for Preventive Pediatric Health Care* (periodicity schedule) for every routine health supervision visit. This assessment may involve surveillance and screening, as well as observations of the patient, the family, and their interactions. It includes child social-emotional development, caregiver health, and social determinants of health. The clinician gathers information about family relationships and strengths, as well as maternal depression, domestic violence, substance use, and food insecurity (all social determinants of health). Other important questions regarding stable housing, financial resources, and insurance coverage are also pertinent. Particularly for young children, social determinants of health may indicate risk for the child and family and may identify need for action, even before developmental and behavioral screening is scheduled and before a developmental delay is identified. The psychosocial and behavioral assessment begins at the first visit with the family and is part of the history-taking process. Questionnaires to assist in data gathering and specific psychosocial screening tests, ideally gathered and reviewed in advance of the visit, can be incorporated into this assessment at health supervision visits, and their results can be woven into conversations between the clinician and parents. Psychosocial and behavioral assessment should be routine for all families, not targeted because of assumptions about risk.

Table 1-1 offers examples of conversational prompts that elicit important concerns by age-group.

American Academy of Pediatrics policy recommends universally screening general development and behavior at the 9-month, 18-month, and 30-month health supervision visits and careful surveillance or screening at 48 months. Autism spectrum disorder screening is recommended at 18 months and 24 months; maternal depression (postpartum depression) screening, at the 1-, 2-, 4-, and 6-month visits; adolescent depression screening, at ages 12 and older; and substance use risk assessment, followed by screening if positive, at ages 11 and older. Informal checklists are not a substitute for screening: they have no validated criteria for referral and result in missed intervention opportunities.

Boxes 1-3 and 1-4 summarize recommended psychosocial surveillance and screening in primary care. If a problem is already observable, a screening is unnecessary, and the PCC can proceed directly to discussion, intervention, and referral if needed.

Table 1-1. Eliciting Common Developmental Concerns

Concern	Possible Prompts
Newborn Period and Infancy (Birth–11 Months)	
Poor attachment	(Observe parent-child interactions.) Since the baby was born, have you been feeling down, depressed, irritable, or hopeless? Who is helping/supporting you?
Difficult temperament (eg, irritable, hard to console, unpredictable needs, difficulty feeding)	Are you able to comfort and care for your baby? Do you have people to call if you feel frustrated?
Child abuse/domestic violence or substance use	Do you feel safe in your home? Has your partner ever hurt you or your baby? Have you ever experienced abuse? Have you ever been afraid you might hurt your baby?
Toddlerhood and Preschool (11 Months–5 Years)	
Delayed development	Do you have any concerns about your child's development, learning, or behavior?
Poor attachment	Do you have any difficulty understanding or responding to your child's needs? What kinds of activities do you do with your child and as a family?
Difficulty forming relationships	How comfortable is your child around other people?
Behavioral problem (impulsivity/tantrums/aggression)	Do you reward your child for good behavior? What circumstances tend to lead to your child's misbehavior? How do you correct your child for misbehavior? Has your child ever had a very frightening or painful experience or an extended separation from you or another loved one?
School-aged (5–12 Years)	
Poor success at school, learning difficulties, inattention	How is your child learning and doing in school?
Bullying/violence at school	Does your child feel safe and happy at school?
Anxiety, worries	How does your child sleep? Does your child have more fears or worries than most children his or her age? Has your child ever had a very frightening or painful experience or an extended separation from you or another loved one?
Behavioral problems (impulsivity/tantrums/aggression/oppositional behavior)	Do you reward your child for good behavior? What circumstances tend to lead to your child's misbehavior? How do you correct your child for misbehavior? Has your child ever had a very frightening or painful experience or an extended separation from you or another loved one?
Depression	Does your child often seem irritable, sad, or depressed?

Table 1-1. Eliciting Common Developmental Concerns (*continued*)

Concern	Possible Prompts
Adolescence (13–18 Years)	
School problems	How are you doing in school? What do you plan to do after high school?
Depression/suicide	During the past 2 wk, how often have you felt down, depressed, irritable, or hopeless? How often have you felt little interest or pleasure in doing things? Have you had trouble falling asleep, staying asleep, or sleeping too much? Have you ever tried to kill yourself or thought about trying to kill yourself?
Anxiety	Do you worry a lot or feel overly stressed? How do you sleep?
Substance use or substance use disorder	During the past 12 mo, have you drunk any alcohol (more than a few sips), smoked any marijuana or hashish, or used anything else to get high? Have you ever ridden in a car driven by someone (including yourself) who was high or had been using alcohol or drugs? Have you talked with your adolescent about alcohol, drugs, and misuse of medications?
Sexual abuse/dating violence	Have you ever felt forced to touch someone or be touched by someone in ways that made you uncomfortable?

Adapted from Swanson JT, Foy JM. Integrating preventive mental health care into pediatric practice. In: Foy JM, ed. *Mental Health Care of Children and Adolescents: A Guide for Primary Care Clinicians.* Itasca, IL: American Academy of Pediatrics; 2018:10–11.

Box 1-3. Surveillance and Screening of Family and Social Environment for Strengths and Risk Factors

❶ Use questionnaires or prompts to systematically update family psychosocial history (including family mental health, social adversities, disruptions, strengths, and protective factors) at each health supervision visit and when symptoms or signs suggest possible psychosocial issues in the child.

❷ Use a validated instrument to screen for maternal depression at ages 1, 2, 4, and 6 months and when psychosocial history indicates.

❸ If maternal depression or any other risk factors are identified, flag child's health record and proceed to Box 1-4, step 3.

From Swanson JT, Foy JM. Integrating preventive mental health care into pediatric practice. In: Foy JM, ed. *Mental Health Care of Children and Adolescents: A Guide for Primary Care Clinicians.* Itasca, IL: American Academy of Pediatrics; 2018:26.

Box 1-4. Mental Health Screening and Surveillance of Children and Adolescents in Primary Care

❶ Perform family-centered psychosocial and behavioral assessment (including child social-emotional health, caregiver depression, and social determinants of health) at every health supervision visit to identify both risks and strengths.

❷ Use validated instruments to screen for social-emotional development in newborns, infants, and children 0–5 years of age as part of routine developmental screening (typically performed at 9 mo, 18 mo, and 24 or 30 mo) and in the following circumstances:

- Abnormal developmental screening test results
- Abnormal ASD screening test results (typically performed at 18 mo and 24 mo)
- Poor growth
- Poor attachment
- Symptoms such as excessive crying, irritability, clinginess, or fearfulness for developmental stage
- Regression to earlier behavior
- Psychosocial concerns of family

❸ Use a validated instrument to screen child for psychosocial symptoms and impaired psychosocial functioning in the following circumstances, at any age:

- Risk factors are identified in family history (Box 1-3), psychosocial and behavioral assessment, or developmental surveillance of child
- Exposure to violence, racism, homophobia, or bullying
- Family disruption
- Poor functioning in child care or school
- Behavioral difficulties reported by parent, school, or other authorities
- Symptoms or signs of mental health problems
- Recurrent somatic concerns
- Involvement of a social service or juvenile justice agency
- Psychosocial concerns of child or family or both

❹ Use a validated instrument to screen all adolescents for substance use (including tobacco) at each health supervision visit and whenever circumstances such as an injury, a car crash, or a decrease in school performance suggest the possibility of substance use. If an adolescent reports using one or more substances, assess extent of use.

❺ Use a validated instrument to screen all adolescents for depression at routine health supervision visits and whenever symptoms suggest the possibility of depression.

Abbreviation: ASD, autism spectrum disorder.

From Swanson JT, Foy JM. Integrating preventive mental health care into pediatric practice. In: Foy JM, ed. *Mental Health Care of Children and Adolescents: A Guide for Primary Care Clinicians.* Itasca, IL: American Academy of Pediatrics; 2018:26–27.

Discussion of Screening Results

Developmental and behavioral/social-emotional screening allows early identification of potential problems or delays. Of equal importance, screening also reviews appropriate expectations at a given developmental age, facilitating parents' understanding of the child's behavior and potentially facilitating their appropriate use of discipline. A conversation about the screening identifies the child's strengths and weaknesses, gives a template for anticipatory guidance, and elicits and respects parental concerns. In this way, the clinician promotes parental self-efficacy and confidence. The clinician should review and discuss the screening result, whether negative or positive, with the parents (and child or adolescent) at the time of the visit. The screening result provides a template for anticipatory guidance, facilitates patient flow (by reducing "doorknob concerns" [ie, those expressed as the clinician leaves the examination room]), and improves patient and clinician satisfaction.

Observations and Physical Examination

Each office visit provides the clinician with the opportunity to augment the developmental assessment with observations about the child's or adolescent's physical growth, mood and behavior, attachment to caregivers, and (frequently) relationships with siblings. In addition, the medical history and physical examination may offer important information about the patient's psychosocial well-being. See Box 1-5.

Interpretation of Developmental Assessment Results

Table 1-2 lists significant motor, language, cognitive, and social-emotional milestones by developmental domain. Box 1-6 lists concerning social-emotional symptoms and clinical observations by age.

If the parent has concerns about the child that are, in fact, normal variations, the clinician can offer reassurance. If, however, the parent persists in the concerns, despite reassurance, this discrepancy poses a risk to the child's development and becomes a significant concern.

Primary Care Interventions

When a concern is identified, the PCC can initiate brief primary care interventions, even if there is a plan to refer for specialty care, other interventions, or school assessment. The goal of primary care interventions is to improve the patient's functioning, to reduce distress (for both patient and parent), and to prevent or ameliorate a later disorder.

Box 1-5. Physical Symptoms and Signs Suggestive of Mental Health and Substance Abuse Concerns

Sleep Problems
- Excessive sleep
- Significant change in sleep pattern
- Difficulty falling or staying asleep
- Nightmares

Somatic Complaints
- Chronic, recurrent, or unexplained physical symptoms
- Abdominal pain
- Joint pain
- Headache
- Fatigue or low energy
- Loss of appetite
- Epigastric pain or gastritis (alcohol use)
- Chest pain or difficulty breathing (panic/anxiety attacks)
- Oligomenorrhea or amenorrhea, especially in women of low weight (anorexia, teen pregnancy)
- Irregular menses (anorexia, bulimia)

Neurologic Symptoms
- Leg weakness
- Limb paralysis (conversion reaction)
- Pseudoseizures
- Nonphysiologic neurologic symptoms
- Difficulty concentrating, inattention in school
- Irritability, restlessness

Physical Findings
- Excess weight gain or loss
- Parotid gland enlargement, dental enamel erosion, calluses or erosions on knuckles (purging)
- Cigarette burns, multiple linear cuts or patterns (self-harm, maltreatment)
- Metabolic abnormalities such as hypochloremic metabolic alkalosis, low potassium, or elevated amylase (purging)
- Recurrent injuries (maltreatment, self-harm)
- Isolated systolic hypertension (alcohol use)
- Chronic nasal congestion (cocaine use)
- Chronic red eyes (marijuana use)

Other
- Worsening symptoms of previously well-managed chronic illness
- School absences

From Appendix S13: symptoms and signs suggestive of mental health and substance abuse concerns. *Pediatrics*. 2010;125(suppl 3):S193–S194.

Table 1-2. Significant Developmental Milestones by Domain and Age

Age	Gross Motor	Fine Motor	Language and Communication	Problem-solving	Social-Emotional
Infancy (0–1 y)	Crawling, sitting, walking	Early: visual tracking, reaching Later: pointing, pincer grasp	Early: responsive vocalizing Later: gestures, first words, responses to name	Transferring object hand to hand, poking with index finger	Social smile, state regulation, parallel play
Early childhood (1–5 y)	Mastery of walking, coordination, ability to jump, running	Stacking, pencil grasp; fine motor control	Joint attention, pointing, expansion of vocabulary, forming sentences, ability to tell a story in sequence	Imaginary play; functional use of objects	Gradual increase in self-control, ability to share, cooperative play
School age (5–10 y) and adolescence (11–21 y)	Coordination, control	Handwriting, completion of written work, note-taking	Reading, phonics, written language; language organization	Homework organization; increase in attention, concentration	Healthy peer relationships, supportive family relationships, participation in prosocial activities, motivation, positive and stable affect

Box 1-6. Social-Emotional Concerns by Age

Infants and Young Children

- Excessive crying
- Feeding problems or poor weight gain
- Dysregulation (eg, difficulty organizing feelings and emotions, difficulty being soothed or comforted, difficulty falling or staying asleep)
- Irritability
- Excessive clinginess for developmental stage
- Excessive fearfulness for developmental stage
- Poor eye contact or engagement with caregiver
- Behavioral problems in child care

School-aged Children

- Anger
- Bullying
- Fighting
- Irritability
- Fear of separation
- Fluctuating moods
- Sleep disturbance
- Academic decline
- Sadness
- Isolation

Adolescents

- Numbness or avoidance of feelings
- Anger
- Fearfulness
- Aggression, fighting, or rule breaking or lawbreaking
- Self-injury
- Poor school attendance, disciplinary problems, or suspension or expulsion
- Appetite change or weight loss or gain
- Difficulty sleeping or excessive sleeping
- Exaggerated mood swings
- Academic decline
- Isolation, withdrawal from friends, or loss of interest in usual activities
- Substance use, sexual promiscuity, or other risky behaviors

All Age-groups

- Chronic, recurrent, or unexplained physical symptoms
- Very disruptive or persistent nightmares
- Regression to earlier behavior
- Change in sleep pattern
- Exacerbation of chronic mental condition

Adapted from Appendix S13: symptoms and signs suggestive of mental health and substance abuse concerns. *Pediatrics*. 2010;125(suppl 3):S193–S194.

Engagement

If findings of the assessment suggest that a developmental or emotional-behavioral problem may be present, the PCC's role is to explain those findings and seek agreement with the child or adolescent and the family on next steps, which may include further evaluation, further intervention, or both. Families are in varied stages of readiness for this conversation. For this reason, the clinician should always begin by engaging the patient and family in care.

An evidence-based approach to engagement is the use of "common factors." Common factors communication skills, discussed in Chapter 2, Family-Centered Care: Applying Behavior Change Science, help the clinician build a therapeutic relationship with the patient and family and address barriers such as denial, resistance, and conflict that may impede follow-through with seeking and accepting help. These skills include motivational interviewing and other evidence-based approaches to involve the family in developing a plan for addressing the issue together and also for following up and referring to mental health specialty care if necessary.[25] The HELP mnemonic outlines steps for implementing common factors in conversation with the family. See Box 1-7.

Expanded Assessment

If a developmental and behavioral or social-emotional screening test results in an at-risk score, the PCC (with permission of the family, in accordance with common factors principles) expands the assessment. Tools used in primary care for secondary screening (to assist in evaluation of patients who have screened positive on a general screening) include the Ages & Stages Questionnaires (ASQ): Social-Emotional, Second Edition (ASQ:SE-2); Screen for Child Anxiety Related Disorders (SCARED); CDI (Children's Depression Inventory; Center for Epidemiological Studies Depression Scale for Children (CES-DC); Patient Health Questionnaire (PHQ), specifically the PHQ-9 Modified for Adolescents; NICHQ Vanderbilt ADHD assessment scales; and Conners 3 (Conners 3rd Edition). Table 1-3, a sample

---

Box 1-7. Common Factors Mnemonic: HELP Build a Therapeutic Alliance

H = Hope

E = Empathy

L² = Language, Loyalty

P³ = Permission, Partnership, Plan

Adapted from American Academy of Pediatrics. *Addressing Mental Health Concerns in Primary Care: A Clinician's Toolkit.* Elk Grove Village, IL: American Academy of Pediatrics; 2010. For the fully annotated mnemonic, please refer to Chapter 2.

Table 1-3. Sample Office Developmental Surveillance, Screening, and Referral Protocol

Visit	General Screening or Surveillance	Concern	Secondary Screening	Referral or Consultation Source	Intervention
Age: 0–5 y					
1-, 2-, 4-, and 6-mo	Edinburgh Post-natal Depression Scale or PHQ-2	Postpartum depression	ASQ:SE-2 Baby PSC	For mother: MHS, OB, PCC For mother-infant dyad: MHS, DBP	Evidence-based therapy EI Part C
9-mo, 18-mo, 24-mo, or 30-mo	ASQ-3, PEDS, or SWYC ASQ:SE-2, Baby PSC, Preschool PSC, or ECSA	Motor, language Social-emotional	As above Preschool PSC ECSA	DBP MHS	EI Part C Evidence-based therapy
48-mo	ASQ-3, PEDS, or SWYC ASQ:SE-2, Pre-school PSC, or ECSA	Motor, language Social-emotional	ASQ:SE-2, Preschool PSC, ECSA	MHS or DBP	EI Part B Evidence-based therapy
Any age if at-risk psychosocial situation	Family psychosocial questionnaire	Maternal depression, DV, SA, ACE Social determinants	ASQ:SE-2 Baby PSC Preschool PSC ECSA	MHS	Evidence-based therapy
Any age if parent concern	Appropriate general screening as above	Motor, language Social-emotional	As indicated	MHS, DBP as appropriate	EI Evidence-based therapy, EI
18-mo, 24-mo	M-CHAT-R/F	ASD	M-CHAT-R/F follow-up questions	DBP	EI Part C

Age: 6–10 y					
Any age if psychosocial risk identified, or routinely	PSC or SDQ	Depressive symptoms Anxiety Learning, school behavioral problems	CDI, CES-DC SCARED NICHQ Vanderbilt ADHD assessment scales and school records Columbia Impairment Scale	MHS MHS School evaluation	CBT CBT IEP for OHI or LD
Age: 11–21 y					
Every health supervision visit	Bright Futures supplemental questionnaires	Function; risks and strengths	SDQ	MHS; school evaluation	
	HEADSSS	Anxiety Learning, school behavioral problems	SDQ SCARED NICHQ Vanderbilt ADHD assessment scales and school records Columbia Impairment Scale	MHS School evaluation	CBT IEP for OHI or LD
	PHQ-9 Modified for Adolescents	Depression	Ask Suicide-Screening Questions SBQ-R SIQ or SIQ-Jr SAFE-T	MHS	CBT
	S2BI	Substance use, use disorder	CRAFFT	MHS	Evidence-based therapy

Abbreviations: ACE, adverse childhood experience; ADHD, attention-deficit/hyperactivity disorder; ASD, autism spectrum disorder; ASQ, Ages & Stages Questionnaires; ASQ:SE-2, ASQ: Social-Emotional, Second Edition; ASQ-3, ASQ, Third Edition; CBT, cognitive behavioral therapy; CDI, Children's Depression Inventory; CES-DC, Center for Epidemiological Studies Depression Scale for Children; CRAFFT, Car, Relax, Alone, Family/Friends, Forget, Trouble; DBP, developmental-behavioral pediatrician; DV, domestic violence; ECSA, Early Childhood Screening Assessment; EI, early intervention; IEP, Individualized Education Program; LD, learning disability; M-CHAT-R/F, Modified Checklist for Autism in Toddlers, Revised with Follow-Up; MHS, mental health specialist (integrated in practice or in community); OB, obstetrician; OHI, other health impaired; PCC, primary care clinician; PEDS, Parents' Evaluation of Developmental Status; PHQ, Patient Health Questionnaire; PSC, Pediatric Symptom Checklist; S2BI, Screening to Brief Intervention; SA, substance abuse; SBQ-R, Suicide Behaviors Questionnaire Revised; SAFE-T, Suicide Assessment Five-step Evaluation and Triage; SCARED, Screen for Child Anxiety Related Disorders; SDQ, Strengths and Difficulties Questionnaires; SIQ, Suicidal Ideation Questionnaire; SIQ-Jr, SIQ-Junior; SWYC, Survey of Well-being of Young Children.

protocol for surveillance, screening, and referral in primary care, lists sample concerns identified in the course of general screening or surveillance that may call for the use of secondary screening tools and the names of those tools; Appendix 2 provides further descriptions of these and other tools.

Identification of psychosocial concerns in the child or family should trigger assessment of the child's functioning at home, at school, and with peers. Functional assessment is important because as many as 19% of children experience impairment in functioning without meeting the criteria for a mental disorder: their impairment is associated with significant morbidity into adulthood and deserves attention in its own right.[25-27] Functional assessment is also important because knowing the severity of the patient's impairment may assist the PCC in determining whether it is amenable to primary care management or will require the involvement of mental health specialist(s) or a developmental and behavioral pediatrician. The clinician can pose questions about functioning to the child and family or use a standardized tool. The Strengths and Difficulties Questionnaires (SDQ) include a functional assessment scale on their second page, and the NICHQ Vanderbilt ADHD assessment scales incorporate assessment of the child's functioning in the school environment. The Columbia Impairment Scale and Brief Impairment Scale are "stand-alone" functional assessment tools that are amenable to use in primary care. See Appendix 2 for a description of these tools. If functional impairment is severe, the patient will need mental health or developmental specialty care.

If the psychosocial assessment suggests the possibility of harm to self or others, the PCC should assess the patient for suicidality. Tools to assist are described in Appendix 2. If the situation is a psychiatric or social emergency, the practice should be prepared to refer for specialty care, with knowledge of local crisis services and processes.

Problem-solving and Initiation of Care

In some circumstances, the clinician may find (with the help of common factors techniques) that the family is open to practical suggestions. See Table 1-4 for examples of advice appropriate to various developmental concerns.

When the patient manifests certain common symptoms (eg, disruptive behavior and aggression, inattention and impulsivity, anxiety, low mood), the "common elements" approach may be helpful in initiating care. Common elements are psychosocial interventions effective across a variety of related disorders. For example, for a child manifesting symptoms of anxiety, clinicians can coach the family to expose the child gradually to feared objects or activities, reward the child's brave behavior, and teach the child relaxation techniques to cope with anxious feelings. More detail on common elements is available in Appendix 5.

For patients engaged in unhealthy behaviors (eg, substance use, sedentary lifestyle, excessive media use) or for families whose routines, or lack thereof, are contributing to stress in their child or adolescent, motivational interviewing can be effective in overcoming barriers to behavior change. See Chapter 2, Family-Centered Care: Applying Behavior Change Science, for a description of this technique.

Table 1-4. Advice for Parents Regarding Common Developmental Concerns

Concern	Advice for Parents
Infancy (Birth–11 Months)	
Infant-parent attachment	Hold, cuddle, talk to, and sing to your baby often. Respond promptly to your baby's needs. Ask for help from family and friends. Explore and address any sources of stress inside or outside the family that might be affecting your ability to respond to your child.
Difficult temperament (irritable, hard to console, unpredictable needs, difficulty feeding)	Take time for yourself and your partner. Ask for help from family and friends. Explore and address any sources of stress inside or outside the family that might be affecting your own resilience and ability to attend to your child's needs. If you find you are losing patience or control with your child, let your child's primary care clinician know right away.
Delayed development	Read to your child often. Enroll your child in preschool or Head Start. Review developmental screening results with your child's primary care clinician in order to identify strengths, as well as weaknesses. Your child's primary care clinician can help you with referral to Early Intervention services.
Weak attachment	Be alert for your child's spoken and unspoken messages and feelings; respond promptly to needs. Set aside "special time" one-on-one with your child. Play and eat together as a family.
Difficulty forming relationships	Make sure your child has the chance to play with other children. Model kindness to others, taking turns, sharing, and empathy.
Behavioral problem (impulsivity/tantrums/ aggression)	Notice and praise your child's good behavior. Do not hit, spank, or yell at your child. Set age-appropriate limits on your child's behavior, and ensure all caregivers use the same rules. Help your child develop vocabulary to describe his or her feelings. Use positive messages whenever possible (eg, "Please use your inside voice" instead of "Don't yell"). Consider a parenting class. Encourage healthy habits: good diet, sufficient sleep, physical activity, limited screen time, outdoor play.

Table 1-4. Advice for Parents Regarding Common Developmental Concerns (*continued*)

Concern	Advice for Parents
Middle Childhood (5–10 Years)	
Poor success at school, learning difficulties, inattention	Attend parent-teacher meetings and school events. Limit screen time. Show interest in your child's school experiences and homework. If your child is struggling academically, request testing by the school psychologist and convey results to your child's primary care clinician. Avoid battles over homework.
Bullying/violence at school	Talk with your child about bullies and bullying. Discuss bullying concerns with school personnel.
Anxiety, worries	Talk about what worries your child. Show your child techniques for relaxing. Instead of avoiding feared activities or objects, reward small steps toward managing fears/brave behavior. If you learn that your child's worries began after a frightening or painful experience, let your child's primary care clinician know.
Behavioral problems (impulsivity/tantrums/ aggression/oppositionality)	Notice and praise your child's good behavior. Do not hit, spank, or yell at your child. Set age-appropriate limits on your child's behavior and ensure all caregivers use the same rules. Help your child talk about his or her feelings. Consider a parenting class. Encourage healthy habits: good diet, sufficient sleep, physical activity, limited screen time, and outdoor play. Discuss your concerns with your child's teacher.
Depression	Help your child talk about his or her feelings. Encourage activities that make your child feel happy, confident, and generous. Encourage healthy habits: good diet, sufficient sleep, physical activity, limited screen time, and outdoor play.
Late Childhood and Adolescence (11–18 Years)	
School problems	Attend parent-teacher conferences and school events. Monitor and limit screen time and use of social media. Show interest in your child's school experiences and homework. Praise your child's positive accomplishments in school and involvement in extracurricular activities. Check in with your child's teacher about academic progress and relationships with peers. If your child is struggling academically, request testing by the school psychologist and convey results to your child's primary care clinician. Avoid battles over homework.
Depression/suicide	Listen to your adolescent's hopes and concerns. Encourage activities that make your adolescent feel happy, confident, and generous and those that promote his or her sense of belonging (eg, sports team, extracurricular program, group music or arts activities, volunteer project, youth group, boys' or girls' club). Encourage healthy habits: good diet, sleep, physical activity, and limited screen time. Be sure your child does not have access to weapons or medications. With your child's primary care clinician create a plan for emergency care in case your adolescent experiences thoughts of harming self or others.

Table 1-4. Advice for Parents Regarding Common Developmental Concerns (*continued*)

Concern	Advice for Parents
Late Childhood and Adolescence (11–18 Years) (*continued*)	
Anxiety	Set aside time to listen to your teen's hopes and concerns. Encourage healthy habits: good diet, sleep, physical activity, and limited screen time. Support your adolescent as he or she figures out healthy ways other than avoidance to relax and deal with the stress of participating in activities important to his or her development. Monitor and limit screen time and use of social media.
Substance use or abuse	Make sure your son or daughter knows how you feel about alcohol and drugs. Know his or her friends and whereabouts. Be a positive role model. Have a safety plan in case your son or daughter finds himself or herself in a car driven by someone who is high.
Sexual abuse/dating violence	Know your son or daughter's friends and whereabouts. Model and talk with him or her about healthy, respectful relationships.

Adapted from Foy JM. Pediatric care of children and adolescents with mental health problems. In: Foy JM, ed. *Mental Health Care of Children and Adolescents: A Guide for Primary Care Clinicians.* Itasca, IL: American Academy of Pediatrics; 2018:47–49.

Certain natural strategies are applicable to promoting mental health in virtually all children, regardless of whether they are experiencing symptoms of distress. See Box 1-8 for examples of these universal interventions.

In addition, the patient and family may be amenable to using Web resources for gaining a better understanding of their problems and available treatments. See Box 1-9.

Referral and Linkages to Resources

Some children, adolescents, and parents may require services outside the medical home. (See Table 1-4 for examples, see Appendix 3 for an overview of sources of key services, and see Appendix 4 for a synopsis of the evidence supporting various psychosocial interventions.) Since families often encounter delays in connecting with services, it is important to put tracking mechanisms in place when referrals are made and to initiate primary care interventions in parallel with referrals. The clinician's use of common factors techniques can increase the likelihood that families accept referrals. Referral to community resources assumes previous networking by the practice with community partners and a working knowledge of and connection to community providers such as counselors, infant mental health specialists, agencies, EI programs, child care, Head Start, and schools. For newborns, infants, and children aged 0 to 5 years with at-risk scores on

Box 1-8. Universal Strategies for Promoting Mental Health

- Outdoor time (with appropriate skin protection)
- Special one-on-one time for child with caregiver
- Sufficient sleep
- Social connections (child and parent)
- Good nutrition
- Expressions of appreciation and kindness
- Physical activity
- Limited screen time
- Stress management through self-regulation techniques

Adapted from Foy JM. Pediatric care of children and adolescents with mental health problems. In: Foy JM, ed. *Mental Health Care of Children and Adolescents: A Guide for Primary Care Clinicians.* Itasca, IL: American Academy of Pediatrics; 2018:50.

screening tests, referral to EI services should occur. Early intervention for 0- to 3-year-olds is covered under Part C of the federal Individuals with Disabilities Education Act (IDEA); EI for 3- to 5-year-olds is covered by Part B of IDEA and is provided by the school system. A school-aged child or adolescent may need assessment through the school's exceptional children program or through other specialists, as with the young child. For a parent whose child has a medical condition or developmental problem, a connection to a family support network can provide parent-to-parent support.

Box 1-9. Helpful Web Sites for Families of Children With Behavioral Problems

- Healthy Children (www.healthychildren.org)
- Zero to Three (www.zerotothree.org)
- National Alliance on Mental Illness (www.nami.org)
- American Psychological Association (www.apa.org)
- Children and Adults with Attention-Deficit/Hyperactivity Disorder (www.chadd.org)
- National Federation of Families for Children's Mental Health (www.ffcmh.org)
- Substance Abuse and Mental Health Services Administration (www.samhsa.gov)
- American Academy of Child and Adolescent Psychiatry (www.aacap.org)

From Foy JM. Pediatric care of children and adolescents with mental health problems. In: Foy JM, ed. *Mental Health Care of Children and Adolescents: A Guide for Primary Care Clinicians.* Itasca, IL: American Academy of Pediatrics; 2018:51.

Parents with adverse social determinants of health may need a referral to community resources for the parent, other supports for the family, more-frequent follow-ups, or a combination of these. Early empowerment of parents through training in an evidence-based parenting program has positive effects on the child's long-term outcomes, including readiness to learn, school success, and social success. In a family-centered medical home, financial issues need to be considered to assure that the plan of care is realistic and practical (eg, for cost of medication or transportation to a referral).

As long as the patient is progressing, the PCC may continue to schedule brief visits for problem-solving or make periodic contact with the patient or family by phone or text. If concerning findings were originally discovered during a preventive visit, the findings may have distracted from completing other elements of routine care, such as immunizations or nutritional counseling; in this case, it is important to reschedule the patient to complete preventive activities. If the child's condition does not improve or if it worsens, next steps include a full diagnostic assessment and treatment, by the PCC or mental health specialist(s).

Office Process

Integrating psychosocial assessment, screening, and brief mental health interventions, such as those described earlier in this chapter, into the primary care office process and flow is crucial. Appendix 1, A Process for Integrating Mental Health Care Into Pediatric Practice, developed by the AAP Task Force on Mental Health and updated in 2017 by the AAP Mental Health Leadership Work Group, algorithmically depicts the steps in that process.

Once integrated, the process is routine and occurs reliably. Prompts at appropriate ages can be made part of an electronic health record. With the advent of electronic health records and their associated secure patient portals, parents and patients may be able to complete questionnaires and checklists from home before the visit. Use of a portal eliminates the need to scan forms into the record. For those who do not have access to the Internet at home, a kiosk may be made available at the practice for screening and questionnaire completion just before the visit.

Implementation of new screening activities requires that clinicians

1. Assess protocols for screening already in use in the practice.
2. Map the work flow. This process needs to include the PCCs, nursing staff, and office manager and should be tailored to the practice. For

example, the nurse can give the screening tool to the parent at intake to be completed in the examination room so as to be ready for the physician to review and score after coming into the room.

3. Select tool or tools. See the following section for further discussion of this step and Appendix 2 for a comprehensive listing of tools.

4. Identify system supports for parent education, referral, and community services.

    ▶ Meet with key partners. Inviting community partners to a lunch meeting at the practice to share screening plans and align goals is a good idea.

    ▶ Establish a process for referral and communication.

5. Orient all staff members to new procedures.

Billing issues are an important aspect of preventive mental health care. The AAP has coding resources available at www.aap.org/en-us/professional-resources/practice-transformation/getting-paid/Coding-at-the-AAP/Pages/default.aspx and https://shop.aap.org/products/Coding.

In a family-centered medical home, financial issues need to be considered to assure that the plan of care is realistic and practical (eg, transportation to a referral, cost of specialty care, cost of medication). The PCC can enhance the likelihood of the child's completing a referral by using common factors techniques to identify and address barriers to completion of the referral and by offering assistance of a staff member or peer navigator.

Even after the child has connected with other sources of care, the PCC's ongoing involvement is critical to provide primary care, monitor response to specialty mental health care and social services, and convey support and optimism.

Tools to Screen for Social Determinants of Health and Developmental, Behavioral, and Social-Emotional Problems

Family Psychosocial Assessment and Maternal Depression Screening

To assist with family psychosocial and behavioral assessment, a variety of tools are available, ranging from brief and specific to general and incorporating questions on a range of topics, such as maternal depression, domestic violence, and substance use. These can identify both parental adverse childhood experiences (ACEs) and risk for ACEs and toxic stress in the child, that is, psychosocial factors that have significant impact on healthy development. Appendix 2 includes a comprehensive listing of these tools. Examples include

- ▶ Kemper-Kelleher (Pediatric Intake Form in the *Bright Futures Tool and Resource Kit*): includes questions about parent's childhood experiences (eg, substance use and use disorder, discipline, abuse and neglect, foster care) and about child's experiences (eg, depression, substance use, support)
- ▶ Survey of Well-being of Young Children (SWYC): includes questions about smoking, substance use, food availability, depression, and domestic violence
- ▶ SEEK (A Safe Environment for Every Kid): includes questions about smoking, guns, food availability, depression, substance use, discipline, and domestic violence
- ▶ Parents' Assessment of Protective Factors: self-assessment of parents' resilience, parenting skills, and social supports
- ▶ Edinburgh Postnatal Depression Scale: assesses for symptoms of postpartum depression
- ▶ The Hunger Vital Sign: includes 2 validated questions to identify food insecurity and its associated social determinants
- ▶ Health Leads Screening Toolkit (https://healthleadsusa.org): includes 10 questions to assess food insecurity, housing instability, utility needs, strained financial resources, transportation difficulty, exposure to violence, and sociodemographic information

Bright Futures highlights the importance of addressing these risk areas and identifying family protective factors to promote the healthy development of the child.

Use of Child Developmental and Social-Emotional Screening Tools

Parents generally give accurate and high-quality information, and they are good reporters of what their child can do. Parents' concerns are accurate indicators of true problems, particularly for speech and language, fine motor, hearing, and general function. When parents are asked how old their child acts compared with other children, their estimations correlate well with developmental quotients for cognitive, motor, self-help, and academic skills. Recall (eg, milestones) is unreliable, however.[26] For tools completed by a parent, an inclusive reading level must also be considered, although the best tools have been developed with an eye to readability. If parental reading skills are a concern, parents can be asked if they would like to complete the screen independently or have someone go through it with them. Availability of tools in languages other than English is an important consideration in some practices. Several advantages exist to using a parent questionnaire, not the least of which is that it is a family-centered process, recognizing the parent as the expert on the child. The parent is engaged as a partner in the care of the child. A parent-completed tool can address concerns about time and efficiency. A parent tool does not require administration by staff and can be completed while the parent is in the waiting room or examination room so that it does not impinge on visit time or office flow. In the case of young children, it also removes the problem of trying to elicit skills from a toddler or preschooler by a virtual stranger and in a setting that is not the child's natural environment.

Developmental and behavioral and social-emotional screening tools are of different types and include direct elicitation, interview, and questionnaires completed by parents (and the adolescent when there is an adolescent version of the tool). Effective screenings have sensitivity and specificity of at least 70% to 80%. The tools referred to next do not reflect an exhaustive list but are conducive to use, and commonly used, in primary care practice.

Age-Appropriate General Surveillance and Screening

General screenings for young children cover several areas of development, including gross and fine motor, language, learning and problem-solving, social-emotional, and behavioral development. Commonly used (practical in a busy primary care practice) general screenings include the ASQ-3 (ASQ, Third Edition); PEDS (Parents' Evaluation of Developmental Status); PEDS:DM (PEDS:Developmental Milestones); SWYC; and IDI (Infant Developmental Inventory). Any of these can be used for universal screening at ages 9 months, 18 months, and 30 months, per *Bright Futures,* 4th Edition, recommendations. For children born preterm, screenings should be used according to adjusted age until 2 years of age.

The M-CHAT-R/F (Modified Checklist for Autism in Toddlers, Revised with Follow-up) screens specifically for risk for ASD and is recommended universally by the AAP at the 18-month and 24-month visits.[27] The follow-up questions for the M-CHAT-R/F are used to clarify parental responses on the M-CHAT tool and increase the tool's positive predictive value.

For older children and adolescents, the domains of development are reflected in learning skills (reading, written language, organization, attention, and academics) and social skills. General screening tools include the PSC (Pediatric Symptom Checklist) and SDQ, which have versions for the child and adolescent as well as for the parent to complete. The *Bright*

Futures, 4th Edition, periodicity schedule does not include a universal recommendation for general developmental or psychosocial screening of school-aged children. To identify risks and strengths of children and youths, as recommended by *Bright Futures,* 4th Edition, for routine visits, surveillance tools such as *Bright Futures* adolescent supplemental question-naires (or comparable tools) or the interview, using a guide such as the HEADSSS mnemonic, are approaches that elicit both strengths and risks.

Social-Emotional Screening

Although there is not a specific schedule, assessment of social-emotional development is recommended as part of routine care.[28] Specific social-emotional screenings are available for both general screening and secondary screening (which helps the PCC make decisions about referrals and types of interventions when history or a general screening result is positive). In addition, social-emotional screenings can be used by an integrated mental health provider in the practice or by a care manager. Practical tools for the very young child include the ASQ:SE-2 (for 0–5 years) and the ECSA (Early Childhood Screening Assessment) (for 18 months–5 years). The SWYC (for 0- to 5-year-olds) actually incorporates the Baby PSC and the Preschool PSC; therefore, for practices using the SWYC as a general screening tool, a social-emotional screening is also included. For older children, tools include the CES-DC, SCARED, and PHQ-9 Modified for Adolescents. Bright Futures recommends screening for depression at every health supervision visit from ages 11 through 21 years. The US Preventive Services Task Force recommends routine screening for depression in adolescents. Routine screening for depression at age 12 years and older is a Meaningful Use measure (National Quality Forum, Measure No. 0418).

For an overview of how these various tools may be integrated into the health supervision schedule, see Table 1-3. For more information about the tools, see Appendix 2.

Substance Use Screening

American Academy of Pediatrics policy recommends universal screening of adolescents for substance use with a tool such as the S2BI (Screening to Brief Intervention); BSTAD (Brief Screener for Tobacco, Alcohol, and Other Drugs); or National Institute on Alcohol Abuse and Alcoholism youth alcohol screening beginning at age 11 years. For brief evaluation (secondary screening) of youths who screen positive, to determine the extent of their respective uses, several tools are available: CRAFFT (Car, Relax, Alone, Family/Friends, Forget, Trouble), GAIN (Global Appraisal of Individual Needs), or AUDIT (Alcohol Use Disorders Identification Test).

Summary

Promotion of healthy development begins as early as the prenatal visit and continues through the longitudinal relationship of the PCC with the patient and family. Routine discussion of assets and risks is an essential health promotion and preventive strategy. Opportunities for promoting healthy development and identifying developmental and psychosocial problems include psychosocial assessment of both patient and family. The use of routine standardized screening tools at recommended intervals enhances surveillance and the ability to identify risk early.

The roles of the medical home include

▶ Develop a reliable system for systematically integrating into office work flow routine psychosocial assessments, screenings, primary care interventions, and, when needed, referral and follow-up.
▶ Develop relationships with specialists and community agencies to include standardized referral and feedback processes.
▶ Follow criteria for follow-up and referral after a positive screening or identification of developmental concerns, even if planning primary care interventions. There is *no rationale* for a "wait and see" approach because it delays EI.

When developmental and psychosocial problems are identified, the PCC can use the primary care advantage to engage the child or adolescent and the family in developing a plan for further assessment and care in the medical home and, when indicated, through referral to developmental or mental health specialists. If specialty care is necessary, the PCC communicates and collaborates with specialists, schools, and other providers in the monitoring and ongoing care of the child or adolescent.

AAP Policy

American Academy of Pediatrics Committee on Psychosocial Aspects of Child and Family Health and Task Force on Mental Health. The future of pediatrics: mental health competencies for pediatric primary care. *Pediatrics.* 2009;124(1):410–421. Reaffirmed August 2013 (pediatrics.aappublications.org/content/124/1/410)

Cohen GJ; American Academy of Pediatrics Committee on Psychosocial Aspects of Child and Family Health. The prenatal visit. *Pediatrics.* 2009;124(4):1227–1232. Reaffirmed May 2014 (pediatrics.aappublications.org/content/124/4/1227)

Earls MF; American Academy of Pediatrics Committee on Psychosocial Aspects of Child and Family Health. Incorporating perinatal and postpartum depression recognition and management into pediatric practice. *Pediatrics.* 2010;126(5):1032–1039. Reaffirmed December 2014 (pediatrics.aappublications.org/content/126/5/1032)

Foy JM, Kelleher KJ, Laraque D; American Academy of Pediatrics Task Force on Mental Health. Enhancing pediatric mental health care: strategies for preparing a primary care practice. *Pediatrics.* 2010;125(suppl 3):S87–S108 (pediatrics. aappublications.org/content/125/Supplement_3/S87)

Lipkin P, Macias M. Promoting optimal development: identifying infants and young children with developmental disorders through developmental and behavioral screening. *Pediatrics.* In press

Myers SM, Johnson CP; American Academy of Pediatrics Council on Children With Disabilities. Management of children with autism spectrum disorders. *Pediatrics.* 2007;120(5):1162–1182. Reaffirmed August 2014 (pediatrics.aappublications.org/content/120/5/1162)

Johnson CP, Myers SM; American Academy of Pediatrics Council on Children With Disabilities. Identification and evaluation of children with autism spectrum disorders. *Pediatrics.* 2007;120(5):1183–1215. Reaffirmed August 2014 (pediatrics. aappublications.org/content/120/5/1183)

Weitzman C, Wegner L; American Academy of Pediatrics Section on Developmental and Behavioral Pediatrics, Committee on Psychosocial Aspects of Child and Family Health, and Council on Early Childhood; Society for Developmental and Behavioral Pediatrics. Promoting optimal development: screening for behavioral and emotional problems. *Pediatrics.* 2015;135(2):384–395 (pediatrics.aappublications.org/content/135/2/384)

References

1. Garner AS, Shonkoff JP; American Academy of Pediatrics Committee on Psychosocial Aspects of Child and Family Health; Committee on Early Childhood, Adoption, and Dependent Care; and Section on Developmental and Behavioral Pediatrics. Early childhood adversity, toxic stress, and the role of the pediatrician: translating developmental science into lifelong health. *Pediatrics.* 2012;129(1):e224–e231
2. The Adverse Childhood Experiences Study: A Springboard to Hope Web site. http://www. acestudy.org. Accessed May 7, 2018
3. Kemper KJ. *Mental Health, Naturally: The Family Guide to Holistic Care for a Healthy Mind and Body.* Elk Grove Village, IL: American Academy of Pediatrics; 2010
4. Boyle CA, Boulet S, Schieve LA, et al. Trends in the prevalence of developmental disabilities in US children, 1997–2008. *Pediatrics.* 2011;127(6):1034–1042
5. National Center for Health Statistics. QuickStats from the National Center for Health Statistics: percentage of children aged 4–17 years with emotional or behavioral difficulties who used mental health services, by type of service — United States, 2003. In: Centers for Disease Control and Prevention. The role of public health in mental health promotion. *MMWR Morb Mortal Wkly Rep.* 2005;54(34):852
6. Riley AW, Broitman M. *The Effects of Maternal Depression on the School Readiness of Low-Income Children.* Baltimore, MD: Annie E. Casey Foundation, Johns Hopkins Bloomberg School of Public Health; 2003
7. Trapolini T, McMahon CA, Ungerer JA. The effect of maternal depression and marital adjustment on young children's internalizing and externalizing behaviour problems. *Child Care Health Dev.* 2007;33(6):794–803
8. Chronicity of maternal depressive symptoms, maternal sensitivity, and child functioning at 36 months. NICHD Early Child Care Research Network. *Dev Psychol.* 1999;35(5):1297–1310

9. Essex MJ, Klein MH, Cho E, Kalin NH. Maternal stress beginning in infancy may sensitize children to later stress exposure: effects on cortisol and behavior. *Biol Psychiatry.* 2002; 52(8):776–784

10. Glascoe FP. Early detection of developmental and behavioral problems. *Pediatr Rev.* 2000; 21(8):272–279

11. Centers for Disease Control and Prevention. Developmental monitoring and screening. CDC Web site. https://www.cdc.gov/ncbddd/childdevelopment/screening.html. Updated February 20, 2018. Accessed May 7, 2018

12. Rosenberg SA, Zhang D, Robinson CC. Prevalence of developmental delays and participation in early intervention services for young children. *Pediatrics.* 2008;121(6):e1503–e1509

13. Sices L. *Developmental Screening in Primary Care: The Effectiveness of Current Practice and Recommendations for Improvement.* Washington, DC: The Commonwealth Fund; 2007

14. Squires J, Nickel RE, Eisert D. Early detection of developmental problems: strategies for monitoring young children in the practice setting. *J Dev Behav Pediatr.* 1996;17(6):420–427

15. Sand N, Silverstein M, Glascoe FP, Gupta VB, Tonniges TP, O'Connor KG. Pediatricians' reported practices regarding developmental screening: do guidelines work? Do they help? *Pediatrics.* 2005;116(1):174–179

16. ABCD: 12 years of promoting healthy child development. National Academy for State Health Policy Web site. http://www.nashp.org/ABCD. Published October 9, 2012. Accessed May 7, 2018

17. The National Survey of Children's Health. Data Resource Center for Child and Adolescent Health Web site. http://www.childhealthdata.org/learn/NSCH. Accessed May 7, 2018

18. Radecki L, Sand-Loud N, O'Connor KG, Sharp S, Olson LM. Trends in the use of standardized tools for developmental screening in early childhood: 2002–2009. *Pediatrics.* 2011;128(1):14–19

19. Lipkin PH, Macias MM, Hyman SL, Coury DL, O'Connor KG. Identification of children <36 months at risk for developmental delay/autism: results of national survey of pediatricians. Poster presented at: 2016 Society for Developmental and Behavioral Pediatrics Annual Meeting; September 16–19, 2016; Savannah, GA. Abstract 15

20. Hagan JF Jr, Shaw JS, Duncan PM, eds. *Bright Futures: Guidelines for Health Supervision of Infants, Children, and Adolescents.* 4th ed. Elk Grove Village, IL: American Academy of Pediatrics; 2017

21. American Academy of Pediatrics Committee on Psychosocial Aspects of Child and Family Health and Task Force on Mental Health. The future of pediatrics: mental health competencies for pediatric primary care. *Pediatrics.* 2009;124(1):410–421

22. Cohen GJ; American Academy of Pediatrics Committee on Psychosocial Aspects of Child and Family Health. The prenatal visit. *Pediatrics.* 2009;124(4):1227–1232

23. Brendtro LK, Brokenleg M, Van Bockern S. *Reclaiming Youth at Risk: Our Hope for the Future.* Bloomington, IN: National Education Service; 1990

24. Search Institute. Developmental assets. Search Institute Web site. http://www.search-institute. org/research/developmental-assets. Accessed May 7, 2018

25. American Academy of Pediatrics Task Force on Mental Health. *Addressing Mental Health Concerns in Primary Care: A Clinician's Toolkit.* Elk Grove Village, IL: American Academy of Pediatrics; 2010

26. Glascoe FP, Dworkin PH. The role of parents in the detection of developmental and behavioral problems. *Pediatrics.* 1995;95(6):829–836

27. Robins DL. Official M-CHAT Web Site. http://www.mchatscreen.com. Accessed May 7, 2018

28. Weitzman C, Wegner L; American Academy of Pediatrics Section on Developmental and Behavioral Pediatrics, Committee on the Psychosocial Aspects of Child and Family Health, and Council on Early Childhood; Society for Developmental and Behavioral Pediatrics. Promoting optimal development: screening for behavioral and emotional problems. *Pediatrics.* 2015;135(2):384–395

2

Family-Centered Care: Applying Behavior Change Science

Sebastian G. Kaplan, PhD, and Linda Nicolotti, PhD

"From a relational foundation that is empathetic, supportive of autonomy, and nonconfrontational, motivational interviewing seeks to enhance a patient's intrinsic motivation to adopt health behavior changes."

Effective communication is a crucial skill for any clinician. Whether responding to a health risk (eg, inadequate sleep, insufficient physical activity, excessive media use), addressing an identified symptom (eg, avoidant behavior, substance use, family conflict), or recommending involvement of a developmental-behavioral or mental health specialist, the pediatric primary care clinician (eg, pediatrician, family physician, internist, nurse practitioner, physician assistant) or subspecialist engages in communication about patient and caregiver behavior. This chapter addresses the following question: How can a pediatric clinician most effectively engage patients and caregivers in making the behavioral changes that will protect and nurture mental health?

Relationship Between Patient-Centered Care and Health Promotion

In 2001, the Institute of Medicine (IOM) published a report titled *Crossing the Quality Chasm: A New Health System for the 21st Century*.[1] To address growing concerns with the US health care system, the IOM proposed 6 aims for improvement, one of which was patient-centered care. The IOM defines *patient-centered care* as "respectful of and responsive to individual patient preferences, needs, and values, and ensuring that patient values guide all clinical decisions."[1] A similar term used by researchers[2] is *relationship-centered care,* which advocates similar principles as the patient-centered approach but with more emphasis on the collaboration between the patient and clinician. The American Academy of Pediatrics (AAP) has also recommended the use of patient-centered communication strategies (eg, motivational interviewing [MI], described in more detail later in this chapter) for challenging conditions such as pediatric obesity.[3]

Implementing a patient-centered model of health care is easier said than done, in part because of the stark contrast between patient centeredness and the authoritarian role traditionally found in physician-centered doctor-patient relationships. However, the empirical evidence supporting physician adherence to a patient-centered approach is expanding.

Safran and colleagues[4] found that the variables most predictive of patient adherence to physician advice were the physician's comprehensive or whole-person knowledge of the patient as well as the patient's trust in his or her physician. Stewart and collegues[5] examined the effect of patient centeredness during office visits using a cohort of 39 family physicians and 315 of their patients. Patient-centered communication was correlated with improved patient outcomes (eg, improvements with discomfort, pain, and emotional health) as well as reduced need for diagnostic tests and referrals. Finally, Stewart[6] conducted a review of 21 studies on the effect of physician-patient communication on health outcomes and concluded that most published findings support a direct relationship between effective communication and a number of positive patient health outcomes, including emotional health, symptom resolution, function, physiologic measures, and pain control.

Self-determination Theory

Why might patient-centered care lead to such robust patient health outcomes? A number of possible theories and models exist.[7,8] One theory of human motivation, called *self-determination theory* (SDT),[9] differentiates among several types of human motivation rather than focusing on how much motivation a person may have. Self-determination theory also considers how each type of motivation predicts certain outcomes, including those pertaining to health and well-being.

A central tenet in SDT is the distinction between autonomous motivation and controlled motivation.[10] Autonomous motivation includes a range of motivation types, from intrinsic, whereby a person experiences a natural inclination toward a particular behavior purely for its inherent satisfactions, to some forms of extrinsic motivation, whereby the person has largely internalized the value of a particular choice as a result of external forces. Controlled motivation, on the other hand, consists of 2 types of extrinsic motivation whereby the primary forces governing a person's actions are either completely external (ie, contingent rewards or punishments) or partially internalized (ie, internal gratification associated with approval from others or avoidance of shame).

The distinction between autonomous and controlled motivation is important: each type predicts different outcomes. Research has demonstrated that the more an individual is intrinsically motivated, the more likely he or she is to experience improved performance, creativity, self-esteem, and general well-being.[11] Regarding health outcomes, the application of SDT in health care settings has grown as the research supporting the link between autonomously motivated health behavior and positive health outcomes has strengthened.

Williams et al emphasized the importance of physicians being "autonomy supportive" rather than "controlling" in their interactions with patients and patients' families. They reviewed research on the relationship between intrinsic patient motivation, autonomy-supportive physician interaction, and a host of health-related benefits, including engagement in alcoholism treatment,[12] adherence to long-term medication regimens,[13] successful participation in a weight management program,[14] improved glucose control,[15] and smoking cessation.[16] A relevant caveat to these studies is that they all involved adult populations. Can SDT be applied to the practice of pediatrics, and if so, what strategies can be useful in pediatric settings?

Developmental Perspectives on Health Promotion

The practice of pediatrics poses unique challenges that are often absent in other areas of medicine. The clinician must use vastly different approaches when working with newborns, infants, children, and adolescents. Furthermore, engaging the patient's caregivers is frequently a crucial element in implementing preventive health strategies, responding to identified health risks or emerging symptoms, and initiating treatment or referral. How can clinicians apply behavior change science to the range of pediatric clinical situations?

Most research on health behavior change has been conducted with adult populations. As is often the case, a theory first gains empirical support using adult samples, followed by attempts to test the theory with pediatric cohorts. Much of the initial evidence supporting the application of SDT to children and adolescents comes from research in educational settings, in which studies have demonstrated positive relationships between autonomous academic motivation and enhancements in behavioral, cognitive, and affective domains.[17] Furthermore, research has shown that both parents and teachers can effectively support autonomous academic motivation in children and adolescents, which often results in positive educational outcomes.[18,19] Support for SDT as a model for pediatric health promotion has emerged, primarily in the area of increasing physical activity—an example of a health behavior change that is beneficial to both physical health and mental health. (See Chapter 10, Healthy Active Living.)

A school-based intervention using SDT principles was more effective than the control condition in increasing high school students' intention to exercise and self-reported leisure-time physical activity.[20] The authors designed the SDT-based intervention to include 4 important components of autonomy-supportive relationships: (1) providing a rationale for exercise, (2) feedback, (3) choice, and (4) acknowledging barriers to becoming more physically active. The control condition included only components 1 (providing a rationale) and 2 (feedback). Another study that tested a model grounded in SDT found that adolescents whose motivation to exercise was primarily intrinsic (eg, fitness, enjoyment) positively predicted improved quality of life and exercise behavior compared with adolescents whose motivation was primarily extrinsic (eg, pressure from others, weight control).[21] Other studies explicitly testing SDT-based models with younger patient cohorts have found similarly positive outcomes, such as reduced drop-out rates from an eating disorder inpatient program[22] and increased engagement in substance use treatment.[23]

Motivational Interviewing

Given the call to adopt patient-centered care and the science supporting its efficacy, how might a clinician engage with patients and caregivers to promote health behavior change? Motivational interviewing,[24] a counseling method that originated as an intervention for alcohol misuse, has gained empirical support for its effectiveness with adults and children.[25,26] From a relational foundation that is empathetic, supportive of autonomy, and nonconfrontational, MI seeks to enhance a patient's intrinsic motivation to adopt health behavior changes.

An MI practitioner uses a variety of engagement strategies with patients and caregivers, such as reflective listening, open-ended questions, and affirmations, which establish a collaborative relationship that honors a patient's autonomy. In addition to demonstrating the patient-centered style, often referred to as the "MI spirit," MI practitioners strategically elicit and reinforce patient "change talk."[27] For instance, if a patient expresses ambivalence about change ("sustain talk"), citing barriers to implementing a specific plan while also mentioning the desire or need to make lifestyle changes, an MI practitioner intentionally chooses to reflect on the desire and need for change expressed in the patient's statements rather than confronting the patient for a lack of progress. The MI practitioner would engage with the patient in such a way that increases the likelihood that the patient makes the necessary argument for and commitment to health behavior change (Table 2-1).

Rollnick and colleagues[28] described 3 communication styles evident in health care settings: directing, guiding, and following. The authors distinguish the 3 styles on the basis of how much a clinician makes use of 3 communication skills: listening, asking, and informing. A *directing* style

Table 2-1. Features of Motivational Interviewing

Motivational Interviewing Concept	Definition	Application or Examples for Primary Care Practice
"Motivational interviewing spirit"	• A set of professional values that pediatric clinicians can strive for • Critical to establishing a patient-centered climate shown to produce positive health outcomes	Collaboration (Partnership) • Emphasis on the collaborative nature of health care relationships • Thought of as *2 experts:* the patient and the clinician Autonomy (Acceptance) • Acknowledging that patients have freedom to make health choices whether clinicians approve of the choices or not • Highlights the importance of a *nonjudgmental* stance toward the patient as a person, even if the clinician has concerns about the patient's health or health choices or both Compassion • Health care delivered in a way that prioritizes the patient's interests and uses the patient's goals and values as a guide Evocation • Ongoing effort to evoke the patient's story, including the patient's perspective on his or her illness and the patient's thoughts about treatment options, as opposed to relying solely on clinician questions and directives

Table 2-1. Features of Motivational Interviewing (*continued*)

Motivational Interviewing Concept	Definition	Application or Examples for Primary Care Practice
Asking permission	• Patient-centered way to initiate discussion of sensitive subjects • Patient-centered way to initiate advice giving • Maintains collaboration between patient and clinician	• Discussing topics such as depression, substance use, or suicidality • Providing information about treatment options for topics such as depression and substance use • "I have some information about options that have worked for other patients dealing with this issue. Would it be alright if I shared that with you?"
Open-ended questions Affirmations Reflections Summaries	• Core communication skills (OARS) useful throughout conversations with patients and families • Affirmations: reflective statements about patient strengths (not just praise), helps empower and highlights qualities about patients that will be important as they consider and commit to health behavior change • Reflections *critical* for expressing empathy and as a way to elicit information in lieu of questioning	• Open-ended question: "What benefits would you get from getting more sleep?" • Affirmation: "You have already taken an important step in getting enough sleep by setting a consistent bedtime and wake-up time." • Reflection: "It has been challenging at times to get enough sleep because of homework and extracurricular activities, and having more energy is important to you."
4 fundamental processes	• Important processes that occur throughout ≥1 MI encounter • Not a rigid, linear stage model	Engaging • More than brief rapport building, means establishing a sense of trust and nonjudgmental understanding in the clinician-patient relationship Focusing • Collaboratively identifying behavioral health goals with parent or young person or both, particularly if several potential goals exist – Primary care intervention vs referral to a developmental-behavioral pediatrician. "It sounds as if we can start by developing a plan together to help with your daughter's behavior. If we are not satisfied with her progress, we can enlist the help of a developmental specialist. How does that sound to you?"

Table 2-1. Features of Motivational Interviewing (*continued*)

Motivational Interviewing Concept	Definition	Application or Examples for Primary Care Practice
4 fundamental processes (*continued*)		– Plan for increasing physical activity as part of a plan to address depressive symptoms: "You are starting to feel better and perhaps ready to take on a bit more. We could talk about your returning to your soccer team practices or about your spending more time outdoors at home. Which of those topics would be more helpful for you to discuss right now?" Evoking • Evoking "change talk" or language in favor of healthy decision-making – "What are the 3 best reasons for you to improve your sleep routine?" Planning • Developing a change plan with the family or young person or both • Collaborative process through which ideas are shared and a commitment about change takes place
Elicit-Provide-Elicit model	• Sequence to use when providing feedback or advice, similar to the Ask-Tell-Ask sequence. • Clinician first elicits patient's ideas about topic, then provides feedback/advice, and then elicits thoughts or reactions from the patient about what clinician shared.	• Useful for a variety of topics, such as getting more sleep, changing to a safer weight-loss regimen, reducing marijuana use, or seeking help from a mental health specialist. • See Box 2-1.
Ambivalence	• Simultaneous and contradictory attitudes or feelings (as attraction and repulsion) toward an object, a person, or an action (www.merriam-webster.com/dictionary/ambivalence) • Viewed as common human experience when considering and attempting health behavior change	• "Feeling better rested and having more energy is important to you, *and* you are not sure that you can commit yet to getting to sleep earlier." • "Past counseling was not very helpful with this issue, *and* you want your child to get help with his anxiety."

Table 2-1. Features of Motivational Interviewing (*continued*)

Motivational Interviewing Concept	Definition	Application or Examples for Primary Care Practice
"Change talk"	• Patient statements in favor of health behavior change. • Predictive of positive health outcomes.[a] • Clinician can listen for and reflect instances of change talk, as well as ask certain sorts of questions that can evoke change talk.	• "I hear you saying that you would like to feel rested and have more energy throughout the day." • "What are the 3 best reasons for you to start eating breakfast?"
"Sustain talk"	• Patient statements in favor of the status quo (ie, to not change). • Seen as a commonly experienced part of patient ambivalence. • Can be useful to listen to and understand; however, clinicians should be aware not to evoke too much "sustain talk," as this talk might stifle health behavior change.	For example, a patient or caregiver might say, • "Smoking marijuana helps me feel less stressed." – Possible response: "Your stress level is a concern for you." • "We are too busy to make healthy meals at home." – Possible response: "So any changes in your routine will have to account for your busy lives."

Abbreviations: ADHD, attention-deficit/hyperactivity disorder; MI, motivational interviewing.
[a] Amrhein PC, Miller WR, Yahne CE, Palmer M, Fulcher L. Client commitment language during motivational interviewing predicts drug use outcomes. *J Consult Clin Psychol.* 2003;71(5):862–878.

would rely heavily on informing, with less asking and even less listening. The *following* style is an opposite approach whereby the physician primarily listens to the patient's questions, concerns, or ideas about a particular issue, with some asking and very little informing. Although the authors acknowledge that directing and following styles are important in certain clinical situations, they describe MI as most consistent with the *guiding* style, which uses a balance of listening, asking, and informing and which they argue is most effective for health behavior change interventions.

Much of the emphasis in MI is on the listening and asking skills that Rollnick described. The dual processes of the interpersonal MI spirit and the focus on eliciting change talk have been described as the main components of the proposed theory of MI.[26] Maintaining a patient-centered, MI-adherent approach when informing patients and caregivers about an illness or its resulting treatment options can be quite a challenge for clinicians.

The provision of information from clinician to patient or caregiver may seem at odds with a patient-centered model designed to make the patient's goals and values central to the decision-making process. Rollnick and colleagues[28] outlined a simple and useful strategy, the Elicit-Provide-Elicit (E-P-E) model, to help guide clinicians in providing information that maintains the autonomy and collaborative emphasis in MI. The first *Elicit* step is an effort by the clinician to evoke ideas from the patient or caregiver about a condition or its treatment.

The *Provide* step in the sequence is the point at which the clinician shares information or recommendations about the clinical issue at hand. Often the information provided follows a specific request for ideas or recommendations from the patient or caregiver. An MI-adherent strategy often used in the Provide step, if the patient or caregiver does not make such a request, is to ask for permission before giving advice. Although patients or caregivers rarely will turn down this request, the action of asking permission reinforces the collaboration between clinician and patient or caregiver.

The final *Elicit* step occurs when the clinician offers the patient or caregiver an opportunity to comment on the information provided. This step is crucial in helping ensure that the patient or caregiver understands the information or recommendation being shared. It also allows the patient or caregiver a chance to respond, share concerns, or modify the recommendations in a manner that fits better with the patient and caregiver lifestyle. Box 2-1 contains an example of the E-P-E sequence in the context of smoking cessation.

Box 2-1. Example of the Elicit-Provide-Elicit Sequence in the Context of Smoking Cessation

Elicit

Clinician: We've been talking a lot today about your smoking. What thoughts do you have at this point regarding your smoking?

Patient: It's not that I think it's good for me. I know about the risks. It's just that I've tried to quit before, and I never stick with it. It's so hard!

Provide

Clinician: It has been tough to quit on your own, and you are still concerned about the risks to your health. Could I share some information with you about quitting strategies that might help?

Patient: Sure.

Clinician: Some strategies that have been very effective for other people who are trying to quit smoking are nicotine replacements, such as the patch, as well as a support group.

Elicit

Clinician: What are your thoughts about those options?

The E-P-E sequence, asking permission to give advice, and other MI-consistent strategies are quite different from a traditional authoritarian or prescriptive clinical approach. When a clinician encounters patient or caregiver ambivalence about adopting health behavior strategies, confrontation will likely lead to increased resistance. Consistent with patient-centered strategies such as MI, clinicians will be more effective if they avoid statements such as "you must," "you should," and "you need to," which are more controlling and minimize a patient or caregiver's autonomy and responsibility for change. Motivational interviewing is a shared process of decision-making, and the reasons for change should come from the patient's own goals and values. See Table 2-2 for a brief transcript of an MI session in the

Table 2-2. Transcript of a Motivational Interviewing Session With an Adolescent Patient (James), His Mother (Mother), and Their Pediatrician (MD)

Discussion	Motivational Interviewing Principles
MD: Well, James and I have had a chance to discuss how things have been for him over the past few months. Sounds like he's been having a tough time.	NA
Mother: Yes, absolutely. I'm glad he opened up with you. It's frustrating trying to talk with him at home. We can tell he's struggling, but he just wants to be in his room all day.	NA
MD: It can be hard to talk about difficult things. James, would it be OK if I asked you some questions?	Reflection; Asking permission, which supports James' autonomy
James: Sure.	NA
MD: Could you share with your mother some of what you described for me? That way, we are all on the same page as we discuss possible options to help you.	Evoking James' perspective
James: I don't really know what's happening. I just feel tired all the time and don't really want to do anything. My parents then get on my case and constantly ask me what's wrong or why this is happening, and then they get frustrated when I don't give them a simple explanation.	NA
MD: You've noticed that you've felt differently, and it's been confusing for you. Your parents are concerned and are trying to help, but maybe it's led to everyone being more frustrated.	Reflections both of how he feels and his parents' efforts, reframing their questions as concern
James: Yeah, and school is not going well either. My grades are pretty low right now. It's not like I want to do badly; I am trying. It's just that I feel like I'm too behind to catch up.	"Change talk": "It's not like I want to do badly."
MD: Doing well in school is important to you.	Affirmation

Table 2-2. Transcript of a Motivational Interviewing Session With an Adolescent Patient (James), His Mother (Mother), and Their Pediatrician (MD) (*continued*)

Discussion	Motivational Interviewing Principles
James: Right, I mean I still plan to go to college; at least that was my plan.	NA
Mother: James has always been a good student. That's why it worried us so much.	NA
MD: You've noticed these changes in James and want to help. I have some ideas that, according to what you've shared with me, James, might be helpful. But first could you all tell me what you've tried so far to help the situation?	Reflection; Eliciting information about their efforts
James: Not much really. Like I said, they just get on my case, and I just stay in my room to avoid them.	NA
Mother: Well, that's not exactly true. I mean we've tried to encourage him, lecture him, take away his phone.... Nothing really seems to be getting through. He doesn't really care about anything right now.	NA
MD: So, James, your parents have tried a few strategies and so far things haven't changed. And from what I'm hearing, besides talking with me today, all of you haven't sought help from anyone at school or any other resource.	Reflections about efforts so far and that attempts to help have remained only within the family
Mother: That's right. We just weren't sure where to turn next.	NA
MD: OK, I have a couple of ideas, and I'd like to hear your thoughts on them. I'm concerned that James is experiencing symptoms of depression, which is likely affecting his ability to concentrate and perform in school. Many families I've worked with have had success reaching out to their schools to discuss the situation with a school counselor or principal. They might be able to help you, James, create a plan that doesn't feel so over-whelming. Second, given that James has been feeling this way for several weeks and things at home seem to be getting tenser for everyone, I would like to refer James to a therapist who works well with teenagers. What do you think of those options?	Providing information/ suggestions while also eliciting their feedback
Mother: Both of those sound reasonable to me. What do you think James?	NA
James: I don't know about a therapist. I don't see how talking about my feelings would be helpful.	NA
MD: If you were to see a therapist, you would want to make sure it was useful for you.	Reflection focusing on James' apparent desire for any strategy they pursue being helpful
James: I guess. I don't want to waste my time or anything.	Subtle change talk
MD: You really want things to get better.	Reflection change talk

Abbreviation: NA, not applicable.

context of a visit with a teenaged boy, his mother, and their pediatrician, discussing symptoms of depression and academic difficulties.

Motivational Interviewing in Pediatrics: Empirical Support

Suarez and Mullins[26] reviewed the research on MI and pediatric health behavioral interventions. The authors described findings from 15 published studies (9 of which were randomized clinical trials) on the feasibility and efficacy of MI for a range of pediatric conditions and caregiver interventions: diabetes, obesity and diet, dental care, reproductive health, reducing secondhand smoke, and child behavior management interventions. The authors concluded that the emerging evidence is promising and worthy of further study.

For example, Channon and colleagues[29,30] conducted a pilot study and follow-up randomized controlled trial examining the feasibility and efficacy of MI for type 1 diabetes in adolescents. Results from pilot and randomized controlled trial phases demonstrated the utility of MI in reducing A_{1C} levels through a 2-year follow-up period as well as positive outcomes on a number of psychosocial measures, such as well-being, quality of life, anxiety, and perceived impact of diabetes on the adolescents' lives. Another example was an MI intervention for caregivers designed to reduce children's (≤3 years of age) exposure to secondhand smoke.[31] Results at 6-month follow-up showed reduced mean nicotine levels in homes of MI participants relative to controls.

Motivational Interviewing in Combination With Other Evidence-Based Approaches

Can MI be combined with more directive treatment approaches such as cognitive behavioral therapy (CBT) to enhance patient outcome in pediatric practice? Cognitive behavioral therapy has been shown to be efficacious for a number of behavioral health issues (eg, anxiety, depression)[32,33] for which initial presentation is most often to the primary care clinician. However, efficacy of CBT depends on patient and family cooperation and adherence to treatment,[34] which can be limited by the more structured and directive approach of CBT. See Appendix 4, PracticeWise: Evidence-Based Child and Adolescent Psychosocial Interventions, for an overview of evidence-based therapies, including CBT. A growing body of literature indicates that the integration of MI and CBT is complementary, and the combination of these therapeutic techniques can improve treatment initiation, increase treatment response, shorten the treatment process, and maintain treatment gains.[35,36] Common core elements between MI and CBT include problem-oriented focus, case formulation and treatment planning, skills training and cognitive restructuring, and behavioral activation.[37]

Using MI with CBT has been shown to have the following benefits: assisting with patient readiness and motivation to participate in a CBT approach, maintaining motivation and resolving ambivalence throughout CBT to engage in more challenging therapeutic interventions, enhancing relatedness between the clinician and patient or parent, engendering a greater sense of autonomy for change, and increasing motivation to complete between-session therapeutic activities.[35,38–40] The integration of MI and CBT has been useful with a variety of behavioral health issues,[41] including controlling type 1 diabetes,[42] anxiety,[36,38,43] depression,[38,40] eating disorders,[44] substance use,[45] and suicide prevention.[39] A small yet expanding body of research is demonstrating the effectiveness of MI and CBT used jointly to treat pediatric patients specifically,[46–48] and this area is ripe for future research. In a busy practice, the clinician can use a combination of MI and cognitive strategies or behavioral strategies or both to address common pediatric issues such as improving sleep, addressing obesity,[49] and reducing risky adolescent behavior. The clinician can also use MI to enhance CBT by motivating parents or adolescents to follow through with a treatment referral for behavioral health issues beyond the scope of the pediatric practice.[50]

More broadly, MI is central to mental health care in pediatrics. When the pediatric clinician combines MI with communication skills drawn from CBT, family therapy, family-focused pediatrics, family engagement, and solution-focused therapy, collectively known as "common factors" in effective psychosocial interventions, the clinician can target symptoms that occur commonly across multiple mental health problems—feelings of anger, ambivalence, and hopelessness—and the family conflicts frequently associated with these problems. Components of the common factors approach can be represented by the HELP mnemonic in Box 2-2. For more details about this approach, which the AAP has identified as a foundational competency for pediatric practice,[51] see Appendix 2.

Box 2-2. Mnemonic for Common Factors Communication Methods: *HELP*

H = Hope

Hope facilitates coping. Increase the family's hopefulness by describing your realistic expectations for improvement and reinforcing the strengths and assets you see in the child and family. Encourage concrete steps toward whatever is achievable.

E = Empathy

Communicate **empathy** by listening attentively, acknowledging struggles and distress, and sharing happiness experienced by the child and family.

L^2 = Language, Loyalty

Use the child and family's own **language** (not a clinical label) to reflect your understanding of the problem as they see it and to give the child and family an opportunity to correct any misperceptions.

Communicate **loyalty** to the family by expressing your support and your commitment to help now and in the future.

P^3 = Permission, Partnership, Plan

Ask the family's **permission** for you to ask more in-depth and potentially sensitive questions or to make suggestions for further evaluation or management.

Partner with the child and family to identify any barriers or resistance to addressing the problem, find strategies to bypass or overcome barriers, and find agreement on achievable steps (or simply an achievable first step) that are aligned with the family's motivation. The more difficult the problem, the more important is the promise of partnership.

On the basis of the child and family's preferences and sense of urgency, establish a **plan** to expand the assessment, change a behavior or family routine, try out a psychosocial intervention, seek help from others, work toward greater readiness to take one or more of these actions, or monitor the problem and follow up with you. The plan might include, for example, completing additional checklists or questionnaires, keeping a diary of symptoms and triggers, gathering information from other sources such as the child's school or child care center, making lifestyle changes, applying new parenting strategies or self-management techniques, reviewing educational resources about the problem or condition, seeking mental health specialty care or social services, or simply returning to the medical home for further discussion.

Use of the HELP mnemonic builds a therapeutic alliance between the clinician and the patient and family and improves the likelihood of follow-through on a plan of care. This approach is well suited to the care of patients who would benefit from a behavior change, patients whose symptoms are undifferentiated and patients whose symptoms do not reach a diagnostic threshold, patients who are resistant or otherwise not yet ready to pursue further diagnostic assessment or treatment, and patients who are awaiting further diagnostic assessment and treatment. Use of the HELP mnemonic should not delay a full diagnostic evaluation or definitive therapy if the patient's symptoms suggest a psychiatric emergency, severe impairment, or marked distress.

Adapted from American Academy of Pediatrics. *Addressing Mental Health Concerns in Primary Care: A Clinician's Toolkit.* Elk Grove Village, IL: American Academy of Pediatrics; 2010. Updated May 2017.

Conclusion

The complexities of pediatric care require pediatric clinicians to engage with patients and caregivers across a broad developmental spectrum. A major challenge in producing positive clinical outcomes is health promotion for patients and their caregivers. Early evidence supports the application in pediatric settings of models such as SDT, motivational strategies such as MI, and the combination of MI with CBT and other common factors communication skills. Although more research is needed to better understand causal pathways of patient-centered strategies, the IOM and AAP have both placed an increased focus on the use of patient-centered medicine in the promotion of health behavior changes in pediatrics.

References

1. Committee on Quality of Health Care in America. *Crossing the Quality Chasm: A New Health System for the 21st Century.* Washington, DC: National Academy of Sciences; 2001
2. Williams GC, Frankel RM, Campbell TL, Deci EL. Research on relationship-centered care and healthcare outcomes from the Rochester biopsychosocial program: a self-determination theory integration. *Fam Syst Health.* 2000;18(1):79–90
3. Barlow SE; American Academy of Pediatrics Expert Committee. Expert committee recommendations regarding the prevention, assessment, and treatment of child and adolescent overweight and obesity: summary report. *Pediatrics.* 2007;120(suppl 4):S164–S192
4. Safran DG, Taira DA, Rogers WH, Kosinski M, Ware JE, Tarlov AR. Linking primary care performance to outcomes of care. *J Fam Pract.* 1998;47(3):213–220
5. Stewart M, Brown JB, Donner A, et al. The impact of patient-centered care on outcomes. *J Fam Pract.* 2000;49(9):796–804
6. Stewart MA. Effective physician-patient communication and health outcomes: a review. *CMAJ.* 1995;152(9):1423–1433
7. Goldstein MG, DePue J, Kazura AN. Models of provider-patient interaction and shared decision making. In: Shumaker SA, Ockene JK, Riekert KA, eds. *The Handbook of Health Behavior Change.* 3rd ed. New York, NY: Springer Publishing Co LLC; 2009;107–125
8. National Cancer Institute. *Theory at a Glance: A Guide to Health Promotion Practice.* 2nd ed. Washington, DC: US Dept of Health and Human Services; 2005
9. Deci EL, Ryan RM. *Intrinsic Motivation and Self-determination in Human Behavior.* New York, NY: Plenum Press; 1985
10. Deci EL, Ryan RM. Self-determination theory: a macrotheory of human motivation, development, and health. *Can Psychol.* 2008;49(3):182–185
11. Ryan RM, Deci EL. Self-determination theory and the facilitation of intrinsic motivation, social development, and well-being. *Am Psychol.* 2000;55(1):68–78
12. Ryan RM, Plant RW, O'Malley S. Initial motivations for alcohol treatment: relations with patient characteristics, treatment involvement, and dropout. *Addict Behav.* 1995;20(3):279–297
13. Williams GC, Rodin GC, Ryan RM, et al. Autonomous regulation and long-term medication adherence in adult outpatients. *Health Psychol.* 1998;17(3):269–276
14. Williams GC, Grow VM, Freedman ZR, et al. Motivational predictors of weight loss and weight-loss maintenance. *J Pers Soc Psychol.* 1996;70(1):115–126
15. Williams GC, Freedman ZR, Deci EL. Supporting autonomy to motivate patients with diabetes for glucose control. *Diabetes Care.* 1998;21(10):1644–1651

16. Williams GC, Deci EL. Activating patients for smoking cessation through physician autonomy support. *Med Care*. 2001;39(8):813–823

17. Guay F, Ratelle CF, Chanal J. Optimal learning in optimal contexts: the role of self-determination in education. *Can Psychol*. 2008;49(3):233–240

18. Vallerand RJ, Fortier MS, Guay F. Self-determination and persistence in a real-life setting: toward a motivational model of high school dropout. *J Pers Soc Psychol*. 1997;72(5):1161–1176

19. Reeve J, Jang H, Carrell D, Jeon S, Barch J. Enhancing students' engagement by increasing teachers' autonomy support. *Motiv Emot*. 2004;28(2):147–169

20. Chatzisarantis NL, Hagger MS. Effects of an intervention based on self-determination theory on self-reported leisure-time physical activity participation. *Psychol Health*. 2009;24(1):29–48

21. Gillison FB, Standage M, Skevington SM. Relationships among adolescents' weight perceptions, exercise goals, exercise motivation, quality of life and leisure-time exercise behaviour: a self-determination theory approach. *Health Educ Res*. 2006;21(6):836–847

22. Vandereycken W, Vansteenkiste M. Let eating disorder patients decide: providing choice may reduce early drop-out from inpatient treatment. *Eur Eat Disord Rev*. 2009;17(3):177–183

23. Klag SM, Creed P, O'Callaghan F. Early motivation, well-being, and treatment engagement of chronic substance users undergoing treatment in a therapeutic community setting. *Subst Use Misuse*. 2010;45(7–8):1112–1130

24. Miller WR, Rollnick S. *Motivational Interviewing: Preparing People for Change*. 2nd ed. New York, NY: Guilford Press; 2002

25. Hettema J, Steele J, Miller WR. Motivational interviewing. *Annu Rev Clin Psychol*. 2005;1: 91–111

26. Suarez M, Mullins S. Motivational interviewing and pediatric health behavior interventions. *J Dev Behav Pediatr*. 2008;29(5):417–428

27. Miller WR, Rose GS. Toward a theory of motivational interviewing. *Am Psychol*. 2009;64(6):527–537

28. Rollnick S, Miller WR, Butler CC. *Motivational Interviewing in Health Care: Helping Patients Change Behavior*. New York, NY: Guilford Press; 2008

29. Channon S, Smith VJ, Gregory JW. A pilot study of motivational interviewing in adolescents with diabetes. *Arch Dis Child*. 2003;88(8):680–683

30. Channon SJ, Huws-Thomas MV, Rollnick S, et al. A multicenter randomized controlled trial of motivational interviewing in teenagers with diabetes. *Diabetes Care*. 2007;30(6):1390–1395

31. Emmons KM, Hammond SK, Fava JL, et al. A randomized trial to reduce passive smoke exposure in low-income households with young children. *Pediatrics*. 2001;108(1):18–24

32. Butler AC, Chapman JE, Forman EM, Beck AT. The empirical status of cognitive-behavioral therapy: a review of meta-analyses. *Clin Psychol Rev*. 2006;26(1):17–31

33. Hofmann SG, Asnaani A, Vonk IJ, Sawyer AT, Fang A. The efficacy of cognitive behavioral therapy: a review of meta-analyses. *Cognit Ther Res*. 2012;36(5):427–440

34. Burns DD, Nolen-Hoeksema S. Coping style, homework assignments, and the effectiveness of cognitive-behavioral therapy. *J Consult Clin Psychol*. 1991;59(2):305–311

35. Naar-King S, Earnshaw P, Breckon J. Toward a universal maintenance intervention: integrating cognitive-behavioral treatment with motivational interviewing for maintenance of behavior change. *J Cogn Psycho*. 2013;27(2):126–137

36. Randall CL, McNeil DW. Motivational interviewing as an adjunct to cognitive behavior therapy for anxiety disorders: a critical review of the literature. *Cogn Behav Pract*. 2017;24(3):296–311

37. Naar S, Flynn H. Motivational interviewing and the treatment of depression. In: Arkowitz H, Miller WR, Rollnick S, eds. *Motivational Interviewing in the Treatment of Psychological Problems*. 2nd ed. New York, NY: Guilford Press; 2015:170–192

38. Arkowitz H, Westra HA. Integrating motivational interviewing and cognitive behavioral therapy in the treatment of depression and anxiety. *J Cogn Psycho*. 2004;18(4):337–350

39. Britton PC, Patrick H, Wenzel A, Williams GC. Integrating motivational interviewing and self-determination theory with cognitive behavioral therapy to prevent suicide. *Cogn Behav Pract.* 2011;18(1):16–27

40. Flynn H. Setting the stage for the integration of motivational interviewing with cognitive behavioral therapy in the treatment of depression. *Cogn Behav Pract.* 2011;18(1):46–54

41. Westra HA, Arkowitz H. Integrating motivational interviewing with cognitive behavioral therapy for a range of mental health problems. *Cogn Behav Pract.* 2011;18(1):1–4

42. Brennan L. In people with poorly controlled type 1 diabetes, cognitive behavior therapy combined with motivational enhancement therapy reduces HbA_{1c} after 12 months. *Evid Based Nurs.* 2011;14(3):72–73

43. Westra HA, Dozois DJA. Preparing clients for cognitive behavioral therapy: a randomized pilot study of motivational interviewing for anxiety. *Cogn Ther Res.* 2006;30(4):481–498

44. Geller J, Dunn EC. Integrating motivational interviewing and cognitive behavioral therapy in the treatment of eating disorders: tailoring interventions to patient readiness for change. *Cogn Behav Pract.* 2011;18(1):5–15

45. Moyers TB, Houck J. Combining motivational interviewing with cognitive behavioral treatments for substance abuse: lessons from the COMBINE research project. *Cogn Behav Pract.* 2011;18(1):38–45

46. Belur V, Dennis ML, Ives ML, Vincent R, Muck R. Feasibility and impact of implementing motivational enhancement therapy–cognitive behavioral therapy as a substance use treatment intervention in school-based settings. *Adv Sch Ment Health Promot.* 2014;7(2):88–104

47. Merlo LJ, Storch EA, Lehmkuhl HD, et al. Cognitive behavioral therapy plus motivational interviewing improves outcomes for pediatric obsessive-compulsive disorder: a preliminary study. *Cogn Behav Ther.* 2010;39(1):24–27

48. Riley KJ, Rieckmann R, McCarty D. Implementation of MET/CBT 5 for adolescents. *J Behav Health Serv Res.* 2008;35(3):304–314

49. Limbers CA, Turner EA, Varni JW. Promoting healthy lifestyles: behavior modification and motivational interviewing in the treatment of childhood obesity. *J Clin Lipidol.* 2008;2(3):169–178

50. Dean S, Britt E, Bell E, Stanley J, Collings S. Motivational interviewing to enhance adolescent mental health treatment engagement: a randomized clinical trial. *Psychol Med.* 2016;46(9):1961–1969

51. American Academy of Pediatrics Committee on Psychosocial Aspects of Child and Family Health and Task Force on Mental Health. The future of pediatrics: mental health competencies for pediatric primary care. *Pediatrics.* 2009;124(1):410–421

Culturally Effective Care

Kristine Torjesen, MD, MPH, and Karen Olness, MD

"The goal of cultural competency in pediatrics
is to help clinicians set aside their own cultural
lenses for a moment and understand
how high-quality patient care might be
accomplished in the context of the patient
and family's cultural community."

Cultural competency is recognized as an important component of high-quality pediatric practice and is essential to provide safe, effective, and equitable care to the increasingly diverse patient population found in the United States.[1-4] Providing culturally and linguistically appropriate health care services has emerged as a critical intervention in efforts to address racial, ethnic, and socioeconomic disparities in health care, including recommendations for improving cultural diversity of the health care team, clinician training, interpreter services for patients with limited English proficiency (LEP), and other strategies.[5,6] As pediatric clinicians (defined in this chapter as primary care pediatricians; pediatric subspecialists; and family physicians, internists, nurse practitioners, and physician assistants who provide pediatric health care) take on greater responsibility for managing or comanaging the mental health needs of children and adolescents, understanding cultural beliefs and practices is integral to providing effective mental health care.

Pediatric clinicians encounter different types of cross-cultural situations in everyday practice. Whether it is overtly demonstrated or not, children and families carry a cultural framework with them into each patient-clinician encounter. Similarly, pediatric clinicians bring and apply their own cultural frames of reference into patient care, which may be further influenced by the culture of the medical, social, political, and economic communities in which they practice. Generational cultural differences (eg, around communication, social media, and ethnic identity) add further complexity as pediatric clinicians seek to meet diverse patient needs.

Cultures vary for children growing up in different states, in urban or rural settings, in immigrant or nonimmigrant families, in single or married or same-sex parent households, in resource-poor or resource-rich settings, and in many other variations. There are often unique cultural issues around mental health care, including different understanding of what causes emotional, behavioral, or mental health difficulties; greater mistrust and fear of diagnosis or treatment; and complementary and integrative traditional healer or faith-based approaches to mental health. Language barriers, inadequate insurance, and lack of provider diversity are well-recognized access barriers to primary health care; these can be even greater access barriers for families dealing with mental health issues.

Strengthening the awareness, understanding, and ability of pediatric clinicians to communicate and solve problems effectively across cultural perspectives has gained increasing attention within pediatric education. In medical and mental health communities, cultural competency training modules and approaches abound.[7-11] The American Academy of Pediatrics (AAP) provides a Web-based resource, the *Culturally Effective Care Toolkit* (www.aap.org/en-us/professional-resources/practice-transformation/managing-patients/Pages/effective-care.aspx), as a practice management tool to help clinicians learn more about providing culturally effective care to their patients and families. The AAP Task Force on Mental Health has developed a mental health toolkit (www.aap.org/en-us/advocacy-and-policy/aap-health-initiatives/Mental-Health/Pages/Addressing-Mental-Health-Concerns-in-Primary-Care-A-Clinicians-Toolkit.aspx), and the *Bright Futures in Practice: Mental Health Tool Kit* (www.brightfutures.org/mentalhealth/pdf/tools.html) includes a cultural competence assessment tool. Community-based organizations such as the National Alliance on Mental Illness (commonly known as NAMI) have a variety of materials that address cultural competence from the provider and patient perspectives.[12] Additional resources for effective communication, cultural competence, and patient- and family-centered care are available through the Joint Commission Web site as well as the Web site for the National Standards for Culturally and Linguistically Appropriate Services (commonly known as CLAS) in Health and Health Care.[2,3]

In keeping with the nature of medical education, cultural competency requires a lifelong process of self-learning, that is, using each patient-clinician encounter to broaden one's perspective and understanding of the cultural regularity and variation observed. Rogoff writes eloquently in her book *The Cultural Nature of Human Development* about reframing the traditional ethnocentric view of culture to one in which children and families are understood to develop within cultural communities and about how this is a dynamic process that shapes perspective and shifts over time.[13] A large component of primary care practice focuses on behavior and development; primary care clinicians may be dogmatic in asserting the timing of developmental milestones or in giving advice on co-sleeping, eating, and parental discipline. Rogoff provides a lens for viewing how children develop in a myriad of cultural communities that invites the following questions: How much of North American pediatric anticipatory guidance is a reflection of cultural perspective rather than scientific fact? How much of our approach to pain, or childhood disability, or palliative care, or mental health, or gender identity, is influenced by the dominant North American culture?

The goal of cultural competency in pediatrics is to help pediatric clinicians set aside their own cultural lenses for a moment and understand how high-quality patient care might be accomplished in the context of the patient and family's cultural community. Ignoring cultural context can result in poor adherence, misinterpretation of diagnosis and treatment, adverse events, health care disparities, and frustration for the patient and clinician. The goal of this chapter is to sensitize pediatric clinicians to some of the cultural beliefs that may affect families' views of physical and mental health and their treatments, as well as families' expectations of the clinician's role.

Definitions

Americans encounter cultural differences every day. The individual's perceptions of social self and of culture and cultural norms play a part in the way reality is defined. *Social self* refers to the way individuals perceive or present themselves to others. It includes the degree of acceptance of the cultural community in which the individual lives and how individuals project this acceptance or rejection to those around them. *Culture* is defined as a way of life for a group of people, that is, how they work; how they relax; their values, prejudices, and biases; and the way they interact with one another. *Cultural norms* are the ethical, moral, or traditional principles of a given society and include unwritten definitions of health, sickness, and abnormality. Social self, culture, and cultural norms change over generations of families. Persons of the same ethnic group may have very different cultures or cultural norms. Consider, for example, the different cultures of a Chinese farmer living in a rural area of the Shanxi province and a fourth-generation American who is ethnically Chinese, has a doctorate in economics, and lives in a wealthy suburb of Minneapolis, MN. Focusing on individual families as unique cultural units rather than on the cultural origins or ethnic background of the family is preferable because what is typical of a group does not necessarily predict the beliefs of an individual.[14,15] Although medical training traditionally defines competency as mastery of a body of knowledge, *cultural competency* requires a more qualitative definition that emphasizes commitment to a lifelong process of self-reflection that demonstrates a clinician's willingness to listen, learn, and value the cultures of his or her patients and families. To this end, cultural competency may be better described as *cultural humility* as clinicians move beyond factual knowledge to a change in self-awareness, attitudes, and behavior toward diverse populations.[16] The essence of cultural humility is to acknowledge one's own inability to fully understand another culture and be open to new ideas or approaches that fit the specific context of a patient's life.

Explanations of Disease: Cultural Variations

Explanations of disease for both physical health and mental health vary across cultures. It is helpful to learn about how different cultural groups in a practice community think about disease and to, at the same time, take care to avoid stereotyping on the basis of groups or make assumptions about an individual patient's beliefs. Some cultures have more difficulty talking about mental health issues or may use different terms to describe them, resulting in misinterpretation by providers. For example, Latinos may describe symptoms of depression as *nervios* ("nervousness"), tiredness, or a physical ailment.[12] Blacks may perceive mental disorders as a sign of weakness or punishment from God.[12] Asian Americans may not acknowledge mental health needs because of cultural beliefs around social status and family harmony.[17] Namboze[18] notes that cultural beliefs about disease causation in Ugandan society fall under the categories of magical, supernatural, infectious, and hereditary. She notes that some of these beliefs are beneficial and can be included in health teaching; other beliefs are harmless and best left alone by pediatric clinicians. Some cultural practices, however, are harmful. In general, these types of cultural beliefs and practices are common to all societies, and culturally effective care requires understanding the social-ecological model in which a given family or child functions.

Cultural Assessment

Appraising a family's cultural beliefs, values, and customs is as important as a physical or psychological assessment and can help explain behavior that might otherwise be interpreted as negative or nonadherent. Cultural assessments are multilayered. They may involve linkages with local community groups or a narrative approach through which clinicians read and reflect on literature and stories from the communities they serve. At an individual level, a cultural assessment involves creating a safe environment for the patient and family to share their experiences, asking open-ended questions about the family's cultural background and beliefs and listening to the responses in a nonjudgmental way (eg, Does the family consult any traditional healers or use any traditional medicines or herbs? What does the family believe caused the illness?).

The ability to be interculturally sensitive is desirable but can be difficult to achieve. Teufel[19] notes that ethnocentricity counteracts the ability to be interculturally sensitive and describes 6 stages of development toward the ideal change in mind-set. Initially, the other culture is denied, and cultural differences go unrecognized. The second stage is defensive, and a person may either denigrate the other culture or claim the person's own to be superior. In the third stage, differences between cultures are trivialized; such a perspective does not recognize the different social, physical, and spiritual environments in which worldviews are constructed. In the fourth stage, the individual moves toward accepting that a cultural difference exists and that another culture is worthy of understanding. In the fifth stage, the person adapts to the difference and shifts from an ethnocentric worldview to one that is ethnorelative. Finally, the ideal change in mind-set is that the difference is integrated. The individual attains the ability to analyze and evaluate situations from one or more cultural perspectives and is neither totally a part of nor totally apart from the person's own culture but rather lives within comfortable boundaries.

It is essential to avoid stereotypical assumptions and remain sensitive to individual differences within cultural groups while gathering information concerning a particular family. For example, although many Native American adolescents enjoy traditional dancing and powwows, assuming that any Native American adolescent enjoys these activities would be erroneous. A tendency exists to assume that all members of a similar cultural background share commonalities, such as language, religion, and viewpoints. Developing a false sense of cultural knowledge can impede the clinician from learning specific aspects about a particular family.

An accurate understanding of several cultures would take an anthropologist years of study. For pediatric clinicians, a starting point can be to review available literature and interview colleagues who are members of a specific cultural group. Training in narrative medicine and active listening skills can enrich this process.[20] Observation and interviews are useful tools when assessing cultural background. When possible, home visiting can provide a wealth of insight into a patient's cultural community. Adding a few questions to the medical and mental health history can provide insight into cultural context. Although gathering information about a patient's ethnic group affiliation, preferred language, and dietary practices may take a relatively short time, knowing about the values and beliefs, including mental health beliefs, of a given family in the context of the family's unique community may take a long time.[21] The AAP *Culturally Effective Care Toolkit* provides additional online resources for strengthening cultural competency in practice. The American Medical Association also developed several manuals on providing culturally competent care to adolescents, which include open-ended questions to facilitate understanding of how an adolescent from another culture perceives personal health problems (eg, "Apart from me, who do you think can help you get better?").[22,23]

Racial and Ethnic Identities

The racial and ethnic diversity of the United States is increasing, with minority (not single-race white and not Hispanic) births now constituting most births.[24] Although race has historically been viewed as a biological construct based on physical characteristics, it is now better understood to have both a biological dimension and a social dimension that change over time and vary across societies and cultures. Ethnicity is typically understood as a social construct reflecting a shared nationality, ancestry, religion, or language, or other shared cultural and folk traditions. Although there is much discussion about race in the United States, other societies may place more emphasis on class, tribal affiliation, or other characteristics. Within the boundaries of one country, such as Uganda or Laos, may live scores of different tribes varying with respect to physical characteristics, genetically transmitted diseases, and health beliefs. The categorization of race and ethnicity has developed and changed as geographic, social, and cultural forces have shifted. While overall prevalence rates of mental disorders are similar across groups, racial and ethnic minorities have less access to mental health services in the United States than whites, are less likely to receive or seek needed care, and receive care that is of lower quality.[25] The AAP acknowledges that race and ethnicity influence health through social, physical, behavioral, and biological mechanisms as fundamental causes, mediators, and moderators of child health and predictors of adult health status. Their influences are evident in the extensive and persistent racial and ethnic disparities in children's health documented in the literature.[26]

Within the United States, racial and ethnic identities vary in importance and use by different individuals and communities. The effects of racial and ethnic identification may be perceived as positive, negative, or neutral. For example, immersion in a cultural tradition or value system linked to racial or ethnic identity may be perceived as a positive source of strength and confidence for an individual or a community, or, in turn, may result in stigmatization of those perceived to be different. Alternatively, racial or ethnic identity may seem unconscious or invisible to some, particularly those whose culture matches that of mainstream society, but may nevertheless manifest in an individual's attitudes and behavior. As demographics shift, younger people increasingly embrace and express multiracial or multiethnic identities. Although racial or ethnic background is an important variable to assess for clinical and mental health risk factors, it is also important to assess the patient's and family's individual perceptions around race and ethnicity, as well as how these constructs may facilitate or impede effective communication and access to care or contribute to health disparities.

Health Beliefs and Practices

Viewpoints on health, mental health, and healing vary from group to group. Western health beliefs tend to emphasize scientific inquiry and are accompanied by the belief that allopathic treatment is necessary. Other cultures may give more emphasis to social, spiritual, family, or individual causal factors and treatments. For mental health in particular, it is important to understand how patients from a given culture express or manifest symptoms, their own beliefs about underlying causes, their individual coping styles, and how the family or community perceives their symptoms. Similarly, individual providers should assess how their own social and cultural health beliefs influence their responses to a given patient.[27] It takes substantial effort to see illness and healing from a different perspective.

In addition to assessing for varying beliefs, it is important to assess for varying practices. Many ethnic groups within the United States bring their children to both pediatric clinicians and traditional healers within the community.[28-31] Special ceremonies, herbal remedies, chanting, and prayer are often prescribed by the latter. Sharing this information with a clinician is unusual for the family unless the clinician is of the same ethnic group, speaks the same language, or has a long-standing, trusting relationship with the family. Notably, families from many different cultural backgrounds may purchase vitamins, minerals, and food supplements or consult chiropractors for their children and may not inform their pediatric clinicians about all treatments being used.[32] A recent survey of American adults found that 34% reported using at least 1 unconventional therapy in the past year. One-third of these adults saw practitioners of unconventional therapy, making an average of 19 visits in 1 year. The types of therapy included relaxation and imagery techniques, chiropractic and spiritual healing, commercial weight-loss programs, megavitamin therapy, homeopathy, acupuncture, and massage.[33]

Religious Influences or Special Rituals

The dominant North American culture has separated church and state for so many years that separating these specific entities in health care is common as well. However, for many cultures, religion strongly influences beliefs concerning health and illness, death, and treatment. Assessing these beliefs and the role of significant religious leaders is important, especially during times of life-threatening illness. Special religious ceremonies may be comforting to the ill child and family members. These beliefs can be integrated into the treatment plan.

Language Barriers and Communication Styles

Determining which language is spoken at home and assessing a family's ability to read and write in English are parts of a cultural assessment. Although the family and child may speak English, their words and understanding, especially related to abstract concepts, may be limited. Communicating about mental health concepts may be particularly challenging when a language barrier is present. For example, the Latino phrase *me duele el Corazon* ("my heart hurts") is an expression of emotional pain, but it may be interpreted by a clinician as chest pain.[12] Providing linguistically appropriate services is essential for patient safety and effective care. Relying on informal translators, such as family members, friends, or multilingual colleagues, can result in inaccurate or incomplete information being conveyed and can significantly compromise patient safety.

Common translation pitfalls include underestimating the language barriers when patients speak some English, having difficulty translating certain concepts from one language to another, inadequate training or supervision of translators, use of the wrong language or dialect for some ethnic minority groups (eg, speaking Lao to a Hmong patient), and unrecognized sociocultural, political, or hierarchical differences between the interpreter and the patient or family that limit open communication. In addition to needing translation services during a medical visit, LEP patients may also need help filling out forms and navigating the health system to access specialty care or community services. Significant problems may also occur when translations are made of standard research consent forms.[34]

In addition to being attentive to verbal language, pediatric clinicians should be attentive to cultural variation in nonverbal communication, which may have different meanings in different cultures. Many Americans of East Asian descent nod out of respect, not necessarily out of understanding. Some nonverbal behaviors can lead to alienation and eventually withdrawal; thus, their meanings are essential in keeping communication open. For example, crossing the legs in such a way as to point the sole of the foot toward a person from Southeast Asia is interpreted as an insult. In Bulgaria, a person nods the head to mean no and moves the head back and forth to denote yes. It is important to identify communication needs for each patient and family and to provide interpreters or translation services that are culturally, as well as linguistically, competent to address questions and misunderstandings.[35] Many clinics and hospitals have translation services available on-site; others use telephone-based medical translation services. Many resources for physician and care team training on how to provide linguistically appropriate care are now available online.[2,3,36]

Parenting Styles and Role of Family

Understanding that parenting is neither good nor bad in any culture, simply different, is the basis of acknowledging differing cultural attitudes toward the family. Assuming that the dominant American culture has all the answers is inaccurate when parenting is considered.[13] It is important to assess how parenting styles and family roles might influence understanding and willingness to address a child's mental health needs. Although the dominant American culture may value independence in children, another culture may value submissiveness. Attitudes toward family members vary with each culture. Culture will address how different members' advice is regarded and whether these members are involved in decisions. Culture will also affect the values held about children, family structure, and gender.[37] Parental attitudes regarding newborn and infant development and sleeping arrangements often reflect cultural values.[38]

Dietary Practices

Diet is an integral part of a person's culture and may be tied to religious beliefs. Dietary practices can include not only preferences and dislikes of particular foods but also food preparation, consumption, frequency, time of eating, and utensils used. When a prescribed diet is part of a patient's treatment, assessing the cultural influences involved is essential. Consulting a nutritionist, a cultural informant, or colleagues of various ethnic backgrounds can be helpful. In the United States, children from underserved, ethnically diverse population groups are at increased risk for obesity, increased serum lipid levels, and dietary consumption patterns that do not meet the standards in the *Dietary Guidelines for Americans*.[39,40] However, the overall diet and eating styles in the United States represent a unique culture in the world, generally different from that of the countries of origin, and result in more than 80% of US children consuming more than recommended amounts of total fat and saturated fat. This circumstance is a good example of how facets of culture can change dramatically over a few generations.

How People Interact: Expectations for Appropriate Behavior

Perhaps in a century, all people of the world will share a common culture with respect to appropriate interactions. The US population has scores of views regarding appropriate interpersonal interactions.[41] More than a common language is required to develop consensus regarding, for example, eye contact, touching, personal space or territory, appearance, gestures, use of the voice, greetings, partings, and facial expressions. Most humans tend to use the rules regarding these interactions developed from childhood cultural experiences. Complicating this tendency within the United States is that chaotic living situations for children may not provide models for appropriate interpersonal interactions. Young children (aged 2–6 years) who watch television a great deal may be unable to distinguish what is real from what is acting and may imitate unusual or inappropriate interpersonal interactions. An explosion in the use of technology and social media has dramatically changed social norms around communication, particularly for young people and often with a resulting generational gap in expectations around appropriate behavior.

In diplomatic circles, norms can be found, some of them written, with respect to communication. Diplomats are encouraged to learn about cultural norms within their host country (eg, who can shake hands, how close to another one stands at a reception, and how much eye contact is allowed). Nonetheless, diplomats make mistakes and are therefore misinterpreted. Pediatric clinicians who interact with peers from other cultures should study cultural norms when working with foreign colleagues, whether in this country or their own. Visitors from East Africa and Southeast Asia often report that they find American friendliness superficial. In their cultures, the immediate pleasant friendliness of Americans represents a more advanced stage of personal intimacy and friendship, and they are offended when they discover that it does not necessarily reflect depth. They also find difficulty in accepting gifts from Americans because, in many cultures, gifts are given only in exchange for something or to acquire an advantage. Direct expression of feelings is inappropriate and considered bizarre in many cultures. In Thailand, for example, a person turns anger toward another object, either animate or inanimate, called *prachot*. This practice is performed consciously to alert the person (who is the object of the person's displeasure and annoyance) as to how the injured party feels. In Southeast Asia, avoiding confrontation is considered positive, and expressing anger, hatred, and annoyance overtly is considered negative.

In terms of generational cultural gaps around appropriate behavior, clinicians must be aware of their own assumptions as well as those of the family and patient. Generation gaps may be compounded by other cultural influences within a given family, such that talking back to authority figures, strong expressions of emotion, texting at the dinner table, or exploration of gender identity are perceived as much more challenging or stigmatizing within a given family's cultural environment. The AAP provides resources on how to assess and respond to changing norms around the use of social media, including how to talk with children and adolescents about social media use and sexting.[42,43]

Several training programs are available to increase sensitivity among people toward varying cultural norms and values. Clinicians who plan to work in other cultures may benefit from a game (*BaFá BaFá*) in which participants are divided into 2 groups and provided with values, expectations, and customs of a new culture.[44] Training programs that raise awareness of varying cultural norms should be incorporated into standard training of pediatric residents in the United States.[45]

Perceptual Differences Among Cultures

Perceptual differences among various groups of humans relate not only to group beliefs, customs, and experiences but also to differences in sensory systems that may have evolved in response to the need for individual survival or in response to that society's needs. These differences in auditory, visual, musical, and tactile skills are well-documented and may relate to differences in eye-hand coordination, information processing, and language and spatial perceptions.

Some of the differences may be genetic, but others reflect the emphasis, focus, and practice of a skill within a culture. For example, an infant's perceptual abilities are modified by listening to a particular language. Syllables, words, and sentences used in all human languages are formed from a set of speech sounds called *phones.* Only a portion of the phones are used in any particular language. Young infants (aged 5–10 months) can discriminate nearly every phonetic contrast, but this broad-based sensitivity declines by 1 year of age.[46] In contrast to phones, which occur across multiple languages, *phonemes* are speech sounds that are specific to a given language and must be perfectly pronounced for the meaning of a word to be understood. Adults have difficulty discriminating phonemes that do not connote meaning in their own native language and thus have a handicap when learning a new language. For example, English-speaking natives have difficulty in perceiving the difference between 2 *k* phonemes used in Thai. Japanese-speaking adults have difficulty distinguishing between the English /ra/ and /la/. Adults who learn another language early but who do not practice the language as they mature may lose the ability to differentiate among its sounds.

Learning the language of another culture helps in understanding that culture. Dependency on translators is fraught with the likelihood of misunderstanding, especially around mental health issues. In some cultures, the status of the translator affects what information is provided by the patient and how it is prepared for the ears of the foreign clinician. If the patient is of higher social status than the translator, an awkward situation can result: personal questions may be answered to preserve social standing and result in changed meaning. Furthermore, abstract or mental health concepts may not translate well from English to other languages. For example, expressing abstract concepts in Norwegian or in Russian is much more difficult than in English. Many words from Western languages do not exist in Asian languages; therefore, certain concepts may be difficult to convey, even with a translator. Similarly, some Asian concepts are difficult to express in English. The Lao language, for example, is richer in words related to family relationships than is the English language.

Ethical Issues in Cross-cultural Medicine

Many ethical issues operate in making transcultural diagnostic and treatment decisions. These issues relate to communication barriers, varying explanations for disease, and different expectations regarding what is honest or valuable. Mental illness is defined very differently among cultures.[47] Is using psychotherapy considered ethical when therapist and patient are unmatched culturally? Can an American clinician truly explain a surgical consent form to newly arrived parents of a Southeast Asian baby? When newly arrived refugees fear that they will be returned and, therefore, sign anything or do anything to gain favor, is asking them to sign a consent form to have blood drawn for clinical research ethical? Oppenheim and Sprung[48] have reviewed cross-cultural differences in ethical decisions related to critical care. They compare Chinese and Israeli cultures with respect to informed consent in intensive care units. For Chinese, giving all information regarding grave decisions directly and openly to the patient or to the parent of the patient is considered callous and inconsiderate. Therefore, informed consent, as a Western clinician understands it, may not be achieved. Recognizing that clinicians' attitudes may differ from those of the patient is important in considering the ethics of treatment care decisions, even when the clinician and patient are from the same ethnic group.

Education for Health Care Professionals

Megatrends, such as increasing flow of refugees and immigrants, will make all pediatric practices more multicultural and multiethnic.[49] The AAP has issued policy statements defining culturally effective health care and its importance for pediatrics.[10] *Culturally effective pediatric health care* is defined as the delivery of care within the context of appropriate clinician knowledge, understanding, and appreciation of cultural distinctions leading to optimal health outcomes. Such understanding takes into account the beliefs, values, actions, customs, and unique health care needs of distinct population groups. The AAP affirms that such knowledge and skills can be taught and acquired through educational courses. It recommends that the pediatric community develop and evaluate curricular programs in medical schools and residency programs to enhance the provision of culturally effective health care and to develop continuing medical education materials for pediatricians and other clinicians, with the goal of increasing culturally effective health care. Examples of such curricula include the Society for Developmental and Behavioral Pediatrics guidelines for residency training, which emphasize the need for pediatric residents to develop skills in working with diversity in cultural beliefs.[50] Similarly, Ohio State University; University of California, San Francisco; and Maimonides Medical Center have all published examples of programs to help pediatric residents communicate in culturally diverse environments.[51–53]

Summary

Cross-cultural issues in pediatrics affect communication, expectations, medical and mental health explanations, patient safety, quality, and access to care. Pediatric clinicians, although enculturated by their training, also have individual cultural experiences that affect their beliefs and values. A commitment to lifelong learning about the varying beliefs and cultural frames of reference that exist among colleagues and patients will strengthen the ability of clinicians to provide culturally competent and effective care, which is particularly critical for the provision of mental health prevention, early intervention, and treatment services. Wherever a strong belief exists in a folk explanation for the cause of an illness, clinicians are most likely to succeed if they acknowledge the belief and attempt to work with it. When simultaneous use of a traditional and allopathic regimen is possible and will do no harm, it is likely to enhance long-term, trusting relationships. Awareness of cultural evolution, perceptual differences related to cultural background, and implications for decision-making with respect to children's emotional and mental health is essential.

AAP Policy

American Academy of Pediatrics Committee on Pediatric Workforce. Culturally effective pediatric care: education and training issues. *Pediatrics*. 1999;103(1):167–170 (pediatrics.aappublications.org/content/103/1/167)

American Academy of Pediatrics Committee on Pediatric Workforce. Enhancing pediatric workforce diversity and providing culturally effective pediatric care: implications for practice, education, and policy making. *Pediatrics*. 2013;132(4):e1105–e1116. Reaffirmed October 2015 (pediatrics.aappublications.org/content/132/4/e1105)

American Academy of Pediatrics Council on Communications and Media. Children, adolescents, and the media. *Pediatrics*. 2013;132(5):958–961 (pediatrics.aappublications.org/content/132/5/958)

Britton CV; American Academy of Pediatrics Committee on Pediatric Workforce. Ensuring culturally effective pediatric care: implications for education and health policy. *Pediatrics*. 2004;114(6):1677–1685. Reaffirmed February 2008 (pediatrics.aappublications.org/content/114/6/1677)

References

1. Brotanek JM, Seeley CE, Flores G. The importance of cultural competency in general pediatrics. *Curr Opin Pediatr.* 2008;20(6):711–718

2. Joint Commission. *Advancing Effective Communication, Cultural Competence, and Patient- and Family-Centered Care: A Roadmap for Hospitals.* Oakbrook Terrace, IL: Joint Commission; 2010. https://www.jointcommission.org/topics/health_equity.aspx. Accessed January 16, 2018

3. Office of Minority Health, US Department of Health and Human Services. Think Cultural Health: Advancing Health Equity at Every Point of Contact Web site. https://www.ThinkCulturalHealth.hhs.gov. Accessed January 16, 2018

4. Institute of Medicine Forum on the Science of Health Care Quality Improvement and Implementation, Roundtable on Health Disparities, and Roundtable on Health Literacy. *Toward Health Equity and Patient-Centeredness: Integrating Health Literacy, Disparities Reduction, and Quality Improvement; Workshop Summary.* Washington, DC: National Academies Press; 2009

5. Anderson LM, Scrimshaw SC, Fullilove MT, Fielding JE, Normand J; Task Force on Community Preventive Services. Culturally competent healthcare systems. A systematic review. *Am J Prev Med.* 2003;24(3)(suppl):68–79

6. Betancourt JR, Green AR, Carrillo JE, Ananeh-Firempong O. Defining cultural competence: a practical framework for addressing racial/ethnic disparities in health and health care. *Public Health Rep.* 2003;118(4):293–302

7. Paul CR, Devries J, Fliegel J, Van Cleave J, Kish J. Evaluation of a culturally effective health care curriculum integrated into a core pediatric clerkship. *Ambul Pediatr.* 2008;8(3):195–199

8. Macdonald ME, Carnevale FA, Razack S. Understanding what residents want and what residents need: the challenge of cultural training in pediatrics. *Med Teach.* 2007;29(5):444–451

9. Aeder L, Altshuler L, Kachur E, et al. The "Culture OSCE"—introducing a formative assessment into a postgraduate program. *Educ Health (Abingdon).* 2007;20(1):11

10. Britton CV; American Academy of Pediatrics Committee on Pediatric Workforce. Ensuring culturally effective pediatric care: implications for education and health policy. *Pediatrics.* 2004;114(6):1677–1685

11. *Cultural Competence in Mental Health.* Philadelphia, PA: UPenn Collaborative on Community Integration; 2017. http://tucollaborative.org/sdm_downloads/cultural-competence-in-mental-health. Accessed January 16, 2018

12. Diverse communities. National Alliance on Mental Illness Web site. http://www.nami.org/Find-Support/Diverse-Communities. Accessed January 16, 2018

13. Rogoff B. *The Cultural Nature of Human Development.* New York, NY: Oxford University Press; 2003

14. McEvoy M, Lee C, O'Neill A, et al. Are there universal parenting concepts among culturally diverse families in an inner-city pediatric clinic? *J Pediatr Health Care.* 2005;19(3):142–150

15. Kinsman SB, Sally M, Fox K. Multicultural issues in pediatric practice. *Pediatr Rev.* 1996;17(10):349–354

16. Tervalon M, Murray-García J. Cultural humility versus cultural competence: a critical distinction in defining physician training outcomes in multicultural education. *J Health Care Poor Underserved.* 1998;9(2):117–125

17. Meyers L. Asian-American mental health. *Monitor on Psychology.* 2006;37(2):44. http://www.apa.org/monitor/feb06/health.aspx. Published February 2006. Accessed January 16, 2018

18. Namboze JM. Health and culture in an African society. *Soc Sci Med.* 1983;17(24):2041–2043

19. Teufel KW. *A Call for Dialogue: Health Communication Interventions in the Context of Culture* [thesis]. Yellow Springs, OH: Antioch College; 1999

20. DasGupta S, Meyer D, Calero-Breckheimer A, Costley AW, Guillen S. Teaching cultural competency through narrative medicine: intersections of classroom and community. *Teach Learn Med.* 2006;18(1):14–17

21. Rosales NB. Commentary: cultural effectiveness—ask and listen. *Pediatrics*. 2005;115(4) (suppl):1165–1166

22. Davis BJ, Voegtle KH. *Culturally Competent Health Care for Adolescents: A Guide for Primary Care Providers*. Chicago, IL: Dept of Adolescent Health, American Medical Association; 1994

23. Fleming M, Towey K. *Delivering Culturally Effective Health Care to Adolescents*. Chicago, IL; American Medical Association; 2003

24. Most children younger than age 1 are minorities [press release]. Washington, DC: US Census Bureau; May 17, 2012. https://www.census.gov/newsroom/releases/archives/population/cb12-90.html. Accessed January 16, 2018

25. McGuire TG, Miranda J. New evidence regarding racial and ethnic disparities in mental health: policy implications. *Health Aff (Millwood)*. 2008;27(2):393–403

26. Cheng TL, Goodman E; American Academy of Pediatrics Committee on Pediatric Research. Race, ethnicity, and socioeconomic status in research on child health. *Pediatrics*. 2015;135(1): e225–e237

27. Office of the Surgeon General, Center for Mental Health Services, National Institute of Mental Health. Culture counts: the influence of culture and society on mental health. In: *Mental Health: Culture, Race, and Ethnicity; A Supplement to Mental Health: A Report of the Surgeon General*. Rockville, MD: Substance Abuse and Mental Health Services Administration; 2001:chap 2. https://www.ncbi.nlm.nih.gov/books/NBK44249. Accessed January 16, 2018

28. Hufford DJ. Folk medicine and health culture in contemporary society. *Prim Care*. 1997;24(4): 723–741

29. Krajewski-Jaime ER. Folk-healing among Mexican-American families as a consideration in the delivery of child welfare and child health care services. *Child Welfare*. 1991;70(2):157–167

30. Olness K. Cultural aspects in working with Lao refugees. *Minn Med*. 1979;62(12):871–874

31. Barnes LL, Plotnikoff GA, Fox K, Pendleton S. Spirituality, religion, and pediatrics: intersecting worlds of healing. *Pediatrics*. 2000;106(4)(suppl):899–908

32. Carrillo JE, Green AR, Betancourt JR. Cross-cultural primary care: a patient-based approach. *Ann Intern Med*. 1999;130(10):829–834

33. Wolsko PM, Eisenberg DM, Davis RB, Phillips RS. Use of mind-body medical therapies. *J Gen Intern Med*. 2004;19(1):43–50

34. McCabe M, Morgan F, Curley H, Begay R, Gohdes DM. The informed consent process in a cross-cultural setting: is the process achieving the intended result? *Ethn Dis*. 2005;15(2): 300–304

35. Flores G. Culture, ethnicity, and linguistic issues in pediatric care: urgent priorities and unanswered questions. *Ambul Pediatr*. 2004;4(4):276–282

36. *TeamSTEPPS Enhancing Safety for Patients With Limited English Proficiency Module*. Rockville, MD: Agency for Healthcare Research and Quality; 2013. https://www.ahrq.gov/professionals/education/curriculum-tools/teamstepps/lep. Accessed January 16, 2018

37. Harwood RL. The influence of culturally derived values on Anglo and Puerto Rican mothers' perceptions of attachment behavior. *Child Dev*. 1992;63(4):822–839

38. Morelli GA, Rogoff B, Oppenheim D, Goldsmith D. Cultural variation in infants' sleeping arrangements: questions of independence. *Dev Psychol*. 1992;28(4):604–613

39. Bronner YL. Nutritional status outcomes for children: ethnic, cultural, and environmental contexts. *J Am Diet Assoc*. 1996;96(9):891–903

40. Davis SP, Northington L, Kolar K. Cultural considerations for treatment of childhood obesity. *J Cult Divers*. 2000;7(4):128–132

41. Marsh P. *Eye to Eye: How People Interact*. Topsfield, MA: Salem House; 1988

42. Talking to kids and teens about social media and sexting. American Academy of Pediatrics Web site. http://www.aap.org/en-us/about-the-aap/aap-press-room/news-features-and-safety-tips/Pages/Talking-to-Kids-and-Teens-About-Social-Media-and-Sexting.aspx. Published June 2009. Updated May 31, 2013. Accessed January 16, 2018

43. American Academy of Pediatrics Council on Communications and Media. Children, adolescents, and the media. *Pediatrics*. 2013;132(5):958–961

44. Shirts RG. *BaFá BaFá: A Cross-cultural Simulation.* Del Mar, CA: Simile; 1977
45. Sidelinger DE, Meyer D, Blaschke GS, et al. Communities as teachers: learning to deliver culturally effective care in pediatrics. *Pediatrics.* 2005;115(4)(suppl):1160–1164
46. Werker JF. Becoming a native listener. *Am Scientist.* 1989;77(1):54–59
47. Krener PG, Sabin C. Indochinese immigrant children: problems in psychiatric diagnosis. *J Am Acad Child Psychiatry.* 1985;24(4):453–458
48. Oppenheim A, Sprung CL. Cross-cultural ethical decision-making in critical care. *Crit Care Med.* 1998;26(3):423–424
49. Haggerty RJ. Child health 2000: new pediatrics in the changing environment of children's needs in the 21st century. *Pediatrics.* 1995;96(4, pt 2):804–812
50. Coury DL, Berger SP, Stancin T, Tanner JL. Curricular guidelines for residency training in developmental-behavioral pediatrics. *J Dev Behav Pediatr.* 1999;20(2)(suppl):S1–S38
51. Goleman MJ. Teaching pediatrics residents to communicate with patients across differences. *Acad Med.* 2001;76(5):515–516
52. Altshuler L, Kachur E. A culture OSCE: teaching residents to bridge different worlds. *Acad Med.* 2001;76(5):514
53. Takayama JI, Chandran C, Pearl DB. A one-month cultural competency rotation for pediatrics residents. *Acad Med.* 2001;76(5):514–515

Interviewing Adolescents

Melanie A. Gold, DO, DMQ, and Angelica Terepka, PsyD

> "Clinicians can often become involved in their own agenda of asking questions and obtaining answers to specific medical questions, thus missing important clues about their patients' feelings and perspectives."

The skill of interviewing is tested in the practice of adolescent medicine because the relationship between the adolescent patient and the adult in a position of authority changes rapidly and is often fragile. Good interviewing requires establishing a relationship that enhances communication between the interacting parties. The information most relevant and useful to both people emerges when the relationship promotes communication and respect. Conversely, even skillfully formulated questions do not yield useful information if the interaction between the conversing parties is tense, rushed, hostile, or judgmental.

Building rapport is vital for pediatricians, family physicians, internists, nurse practitioners, physician assistants, and other health care professionals who work with adolescents. Establishing a positive provider-patient relationship facilitates communication, and it can improve honest patient disclosure during interviews and on self-report measures. This rapport is particularly important when asking for disclosure of sensitive or stigmatizing topics related to risk-taking behaviors such as sexual behaviors, alcohol and drug use, and emotional problems. Establishing positive rapport can take time; several techniques to increase provider-patient interaction are discussed throughout this chapter.

Whom to Interview

During adolescence, a transition from dependence to independence should be made by the teenager and facilitated by the parents. In early adolescence, the parents are still largely responsible for their teen's health care, although by late adolescence, these patients are often managing their own medical needs completely. These changes occur over a relatively brief period; therefore, the *pediatric clinician* (a term used in this chapter to include all adolescent-serving health care providers), is faced with assessing the stage of transition toward independence each time the adolescent patient is seen. Whom to interview should be decided in the context of this transition, and the following factors need to be considered.

Adolescent's Developmental Level

For many adolescents, feeling that they are being treated as children can be upsetting. This perception is a particular problem in early adolescence, when a teen's lack of sexual maturation can cause insensitive adults to underestimate the youth's psychological age and cognitive abilities. Adolescent patients are often sensitive to the atmosphere of the pediatric clinician's office that emphasizes the interests of the child. Therefore, the clinician should arrange the office waiting area with a section that contains reading material and decor appropriate for adolescent patients. At least 1 examining room should be equipped and decorated with the adolescent patient in mind. The hospital ward and patient lounge areas should also have a section furnished and decorated specifically for adolescent patients, and an interviewing room to be used exclusively for teens should be available.

The need for privacy during the interview is perhaps never more important than in the practice of adolescent medicine. If the adolescent thinks that the conversation will be interrupted or overheard, then important information may not be disclosed. Privacy may be particularly difficult to find on the hospital ward or in the emergency department, but every effort should be made to achieve it.

The interview room should be arranged with the clinician, the patient, and the parents seated at the same level, at comfortable conversational distances, and without desks between the clinician and the other person or people to whom the clinician is speaking. The few moments needed to rearrange the furniture to meet these requirements are well spent.

Establishing Rapport

Establishing rapport with an adolescent can be challenging; therefore, the clinician should take a genuine interest in the adolescent from the beginning of the interview. Establishing a collaborative partnership with the adolescent patient is important to building trust and setting the stage for developing an effective therapeutic relationship. Greeting the adolescent patient before greeting the parent or guardian is best. Asking the patient to introduce the others in the room can be helpful. The adolescent is then given the message that the primary focus is on the adolescent and that he or she is the expert about the other people in the room. Also helpful is to chat informally with the adolescent patient briefly before the interview begins, being careful to gear the conversation to the appropriate developmental level for that patient. To accomplish this task, the clinician should know enough about normal adolescent development to judge the appropriateness of this preinterview conversation. This initial conversation with the adolescent patient can help establish rapport and possibly relieve anxiety the patient may have about the visit.

Parents' Role

Although creating an environment in which the adolescent feels comfortable is essential, the clinician should not ignore the importance of the parents' role. In early and middle adolescence, the parents' input is critical for a thorough evaluation because adolescents may have limited insight about themselves or inadequate perspective on the timing and importance of symptoms. Adolescents may not be familiar with their own perinatal and birth histories, developmental histories, previous illnesses, hospitalizations, surgeries, allergies, medications, immunizations, and family histories. A portion of the interview conducted with the parent present may help elicit important health history information while giving the adolescent the opportunity to hear and learn about these important aspects of his or her own medical history. Interviewing the patient and parent together initially also gives insight into family dynamics and interaction.

Confidentiality

Confidentiality issues should be addressed with both the adolescent patient and the parents before sensitive topics are discussed. The clinician should also explain that the adolescent will be interviewed alone for part of the medical history and that the adolescent may have the physical examination conducted without the parents to ensure confidentiality. Confidentiality and the limits of confidentiality based on state laws as well as clinician comfort should be made clear to the adolescent and the family early in the interview process. The clinician should be aware of the particular state's laws regarding the adolescent's rights to confidential evaluation, and these rights must be respected. State-specific guidelines are available from the American Medical Association and the Center for Adolescent Health & the Law. For more information on confidentiality laws by state, see *State Minor Consent Laws: A Summary,* available from the Center for Adolescent Health & the Law, or visit their Web site at www.cahl.org. To educate adolescents about confidentiality, see "Information for Teens: What You Need to Know About Privacy" at www.healthychildren.org/English/ages-stages/teen/Pages/Information-for-Teens-What-You-Need-to-Know-About-Privacy.aspx.

Although adolescents' independence should be encouraged, and time should always be set aside for the adolescent to see the clinician alone, the appropriate role of the parents should not be ignored. Because of adolescents' possible limited perspective and their need for emotional and financial support, the clinician would be wise in most cases to encourage early adolescents to involve their parents in their medical decision-making. When parents are involved, allowing them time to discuss their concerns *without* their early adolescent present may also be helpful because they may be reluctant to discuss some concerns in front of their child, such as parental conflict or mental health issues.

Clinician Neutrality

If significant disagreements exist between an adolescent and his or her parents, the clinician must avoid the appearance of taking sides on these issues. This task can best be accomplished by interviewing the adolescent and parents together and concentrating on understanding and clarifying their disagreements, thus conveying an appropriately neutral attitude about the conflict. The following vignette illustrates this technique. The evaluation was initiated by the parents, who were concerned that their 15-year-old son had behavioral problems.

> Mr Jones: We think his choice of friends leaves a lot to be desired.
> Jim: What's the matter with my friends?
> Mr Jones: Most of them have no ambition. They don't care about school and spend their time just hanging around.
> Jim: It's just that we're not like you. You don't care about anything except work. At least my friends know how to have fun.
> Clinician: Jim, you think your father devotes too much time to work.
> Jim: Yeah.
> Clinician: And, Mr Jones, you wish Jim were more ambitious and that he would pick friends who are ambitious too.
> Mr Jones: Yes, I worry that Jim isn't going to succeed.
> Jim (to his father): I'll succeed in my own way.
> Clinician: What are your ideas about success, Jim?

In this interaction, the clinician has facilitated communication between the father and son by using reflections and open-ended questions without stating an opinion that would seem to commit to either person's point of view. A review of these issues before the interview helps the clinician make a reasonable decision about whom to interview first; no rigid rules apply. The choice depends on the age of the adolescent patient, the person who initiates the contact, and whether conflict exists between the adolescent and parents regarding the problem.

Interviewing Technique

The key to good interviewing is building a trusting relationship among the clinician, patient, and parents. This relationship can be accomplished if the clinician makes an effort to understand how the adolescent patient perceives the problem and relationships with important people in his or her life. Most clinicians would say that they attempt to understand their patients. However, clinicians can often become involved in their own agenda of asking questions and obtaining answers to specific medical questions, thus missing important clues about their patients' feelings and perspectives. The following vignette illustrates the insensitivity that results when medical issues are pursued vigorously and when the clinician becomes more interested in the answers than in establishing a therapeutic relationship. The patient is a 16-year-old girl who has diabetes.

> Clinician: How much insulin do you take?
> Sarah: 16 units of NPH and 4 units of regular each morning.
> Clinician: Do you test your urine?
> Sarah: Yeah.
> Clinician: How often?
> Sarah: Every morning and in the late afternoon, when my mother doesn't bug me.
> Clinician: Does your urine ever test positive for glucose?
> Sarah: Sometimes, but not too often.
> Clinician: How much? 1 plus, 2 plus?
> Sarah: Just 1 plus a couple of times a week. Mom's always asking me that, but I tell her to leave me alone.
> Clinician: Do you ever have insulin reactions?
> Sarah: Not for a long time.
> Clinician: How's school?

The casual observer can sense the clinician's urgency to fill in the blanks of the medical history and that a rushed demanding of information is taking place, illustrated by the series of closed-ended questions asked of the patient without eliciting more elaboration. In the process, this clinician has failed to pick up the clues of the mother-daughter conflict. The clinician completed the agenda and then turned to a question about the adolescent's life that will probably be perceived by the patient as a mechanical question because the clinician did not *hear* the previous comments and explore them.

Rapport can be better established by using techniques to further open communication based on motivational interviewing. These strategies include using open-ended questions, affirmations, reflections, and summaries (the mnemonic is *OARS*). Open-ended questions encourage adolescents to voice their thoughts or concerns and avoid the feeling of being interrogated by numerous closed-ended questions asked in a row. Affirmations are statements of appreciation of patient strengths or past efforts. Some affirmations show support for patients' sharing information, such as "I really appreciate that you are able to share that information with me" and "That sounds like a really difficult time for you. I'm impressed that you have taken care of yourself so well." Reflections indicate to adolescents that their perspective is being understood. They can be a simple restatement of what the adolescent has said, or they can be made more complex by extending the meaning of the words or emotions that the adolescent has used. Summaries are often helpful to clarify the problem and pull together the discussion, and they can often help encourage the adolescent to make additional comments.

One strategy to identify salient sources of affirmations is to ask every adolescent to tell the clinician about a special attribute or strength by saying, "Tell me something about yourself that is special or unique or a particular strength." Explore this attribute or strength fully with open-ended questions and reflections and document this attribute or strength in the chart. The "special attribute or strength" may be as simple as being on the honor roll, excelling at track, helping a parent care for younger siblings, volunteering in the community, or, for an adolescent patient with special health care needs, having academic success in some area. Giving back this information in the form of an affirmation both establishes rapport by helping adolescents feel they are appreciated by the clinician and helps adolescents feel good about themselves.

Several problems can arise during the adolescent interview. Adolescents may disclose sensitive issues that they do not feel comfortable sharing with their parents. When this disclosure occurs, the clinician should help the adolescent identify, when possible, other trusted adults in the adolescent's life (eg, family member, coach, teacher) who can support the adolescent and be a sounding board for the adolescent to discuss these issues. Rarely, parents may ask for confidential information about their son or daughter, such as whether he or she is using drugs or having sex, or they may request a drug test without their adolescent's knowledge. Additionally, clinicians may hold their own biases or experience discomfort about engaging in discussion of certain topics; these biases or discomforts may prevent clinicians from completing a thorough adolescent interview. Therefore, clinicians are encouraged to be aware of their own biases regarding adolescent engagement in sexual behaviors, drug use, and other risk-taking behaviors. Awareness of biases can also prevent clinicians from making assumptions about their patients' sexual behaviors or drug use instead of directly asking questions regarding these domains. These issues can be addressed by first having discussions with parents and adolescents about confidentiality early, at the first adolescent visit, and, when the request for confidential information arises later, reiterating the limits of confidentiality and when it can and cannot be breached. Often the sharing of confidential information or performing of a drug test can be negotiated with the adolescent, who will agree to limited sharing of some information or will agree to a drug test to "get the parents off my back," without needing to breach confidentiality and injure the therapeutic relationship between the clinician and the adolescent.

Techniques that promote the acquisition of useful information fall into 2 main categories: listening skills and facilitative responses. Component aspects of these techniques, discussed briefly in the next 2 sections, are outlined in Box 4-1.

Listening Skills

Unless clinicians pay attention to the meaning of words, they often think that they understand the patient's perspective when they really do not. Every time a patient uses words that are abstract or unclear, clinicians should ask

Box 4-1. Interview Techniques

- Listening skills
- Clarification of meaning
- Verbal asides
- Nonverbal communication
- Facilitative responses
- Repetition and review
- Acknowledgment of feelings
- Periods of silence

for clarification by using open-ended questions or reflections. Skilled interviewers continually ask themselves if they understand what has just been said. In the following vignette, the importance of this technique is illustrated. The patient is a 15-year-old boy who has problems with school.

> Clinician: Your parents seem concerned about how you are doing in school. What do you think?
>
> Dave: Sometimes I think I'm a wreck.
>
> Clinician: A wreck?
>
> Dave: Yeah, you know, like I'm a mess.
>
> Clinician: I don't know, Dave. What does that feel like?
>
> Dave: Like I get these funny feelings, and I think I'm falling apart.
>
> Clinician: Tell me about one of these funny feelings.
>
> Dave: Well…sometimes it's like my fingers are growing really big, or small. It's weird.
>
> Clinician: You mean like parts of your body are changing size?
>
> Dave: Yeah.
>
> Clinician: What else?
>
> Dave: Sometimes I feel like I'm walking just a little off the ground, like I am floating.

If the clinician did not pursue the meaning of Dave's words, she might have been left with the vague statement that Dave thinks he is a *wreck*, which many people would assume means that he thinks he is a failure. Instead, the clinician now has evidence that Dave is experiencing somatic symptoms of anxiety or psychotic thinking and can pursue the source of these feelings. If the patient is describing symptoms commonly associated with mental health concerns, it is important to explore these symptoms and the patient's perception of the described symptoms using the patient's own words. In the aforementioned example, the clinician reflects Dave's statements using Dave's (the patient's) specific words (ie, "Tell me about one of these *funny feelings*"). Some patients may hold social or cultural stigmas associated with mental health. Therefore, psychoeducation about the connection between mental and physical symptoms, before engaging in open discussion about mental health concerns, may help reduce stigmatization of mental health concerns.

Verbal asides are parenthetical statements that often reveal the patient's true feelings but that are stated as though they are unimportant. They usually reflect the adolescent's ambivalence about exposing real feelings. The patient with diabetes described earlier, who said that she tested her urine twice a day "when my mother doesn't bug me," is giving a verbal aside.

Statements about her mother constitute unsolicited and important information. Clinicians often focus only on the solicited information and therefore fail to hear such asides. All that is usually required to facilitate further communication is to echo the phrase back to the patient in a simple or complex reflection followed by an open-ended question, such as "It sounds like you are annoyed at your mom. What do you mean when you said she bugs you? Tell me more about that."

Nonverbal communication consists of body movements and facial expressions that reveal a person's feelings. A clinician who is preoccupied with asking the right questions, accumulating the answers, and documenting them in the electronic health record will miss these important clues. The skilled interviewer learns to divide attention between the words that are being said and the body language of the person being interviewed. Because body language is usually outside the patient's awareness, commenting immediately on such observations may be premature, which may impart discomfort or anxiety on the patient. Part of the art of interviewing is to sense when such comments may be useful. A good rule to remember is that when body language reveals something that the person seems to be trying to hide, it should be left alone. For example, a patient's clenched fists may indicate tension when the patient's words suggest calm. However, when a facial expression suggests an inner thought or feeling, then commenting is often useful by using a reflection of emotion. The patient may say something funny, for example, and then seem sad. In this instance, saying something such as "It looks as if that thought suddenly made you feel sad" is often helpful.

Facilitative Responses

The person who is talking (the speaker) usually feels good when the listener can synthesize what the speaker has just said into a summary that reflects the speaker's thoughts accurately. If, for example, the patient has had difficulty finding the right words to describe symptoms and the clinician then restates these symptoms briefly and accurately, the patient realizes that the clinician heard and understood what the patient has been experiencing. People like to be understood, and this type of repetition and review using summaries greatly facilitates further communication as well as enhances rapport.

An important component of repetition and review is the acknowledgment of feelings, as well as the recognition of facts and meaning. In many instances, patients make a series of statements that are really meant to build a case for the underlying feelings they are experiencing. If the clinician can hear and then acknowledge these feelings with a reflection of emotion or meaning, the relationship may be significantly enhanced. The following segment of an interview illustrates this interaction. The patient is a 13-year-old girl brought in by her parents because of acting-out behavior.

> Clinician: Your parents are upset over some of the things you have done. What do you think?
>
> Jen: They really bug me. Last week, Mom wouldn't let me go to the mall with my friends. She said that we were too young to go by ourselves, but all my friends' parents let them go. Then, a couple of nights ago, I wanted to stay at Katie's house for dinner, and Dad made me come home. He said that it's getting too dark at night. You'd think I was a baby!
>
> Clinician: You don't feel that your parents trust you.
>
> Jen: I know they don't trust me. It makes me feel like doing whatever I want, since they don't trust me anyway.
>
> Clinician: It makes you angry that they don't give you more freedom.

Another important facilitative response is the carefully timed use of silences, or pauses. This tactic is particularly important when the patient has difficulty with self-expression. Pediatric clinicians are usually highly verbal people and respond to such patients by asking more and more questions. When a question has been asked and the response is not immediate, the interviewer should look closely for cues that the patient is processing the question. If the patient seems to be thinking about the answer, the clinician should pause to allow a response. Further statements might include facilitative responses, such as "What thoughts are you having?" or "It's hard, sometimes, to find the right words." Such replies tend to encourage the response. Similarly, the periods of silence should not be so long that the patient is made to feel uncomfortable. In psychiatric interviews, long silences are sometimes used purposefully; however, this approach would be too threatening for most medical interviews, especially with early adolescents. Instead, the suggested approach is to allow time for the person whose verbal responses are slow.

Approaching the Sensitive Issues of Drugs, Sex, and Emotional Problems

Vital issues in adolescent medicine include a healthy response to emerging sexuality, avoidance of addiction to drugs or alcohol, and emotional state. Pediatric clinicians should address these issues from the perspective of prevention. This approach requires inquiring about these topics throughout the period of adolescent development. However, adolescents and clinicians often feel uncomfortable with these issues. Questions about sexual attraction, sexual orientation, gender identity, sexual activity, the use of drugs and alcohol, and the possibility of emotional problems often seem intrusive and embarrassing. Reassuring the adolescent again about confidentiality is important at this stage of the medical interview. Normalizing questions about sexual behavior, drugs and alcohol, mood, school performance, relationships, and other sensitive topics may also be helpful. Statements such as "People your age may be curious about sexual behavior" can help patients feel more comfortable about engaging in discussion with the clinician. In addition, a useful way to begin the discussion is to explain to the adolescent why these questions are being asked, for example, "I am asking you these questions to help me find out if there is anything that may be putting your health at risk and to tell me what kind of examination and tests I should do."

A tool for assessing the psychosocial history in adolescents is known by the acronym HEEADSSS, used to address issues of *h*ome, *e*ducation, *e*mployment, *e*ating, *a*ctivities, *d*rugs, *d*epression, *s*uicidality, *s*exuality, *s*afety, and *s*pirituality. The HEEADSSS assessment was developed in 1972, refined in 1988, updated in 2004, and updated again in 2014. Examples of HEEADSSS questions are summarized in Table 4-1.

Providing a confidential questionnaire for the adolescent to fill out is another method to help facilitate questioning on more sensitive issues, especially when the questions are administered electronically. For example, the Bright Futures previsit questionnaire (see Appendix 2, Mental Health Tools for Pediatrics) is one such tool that gathers information on physical health, drug and substance use, social and family functioning, sexual activity, and mental health; clinicians can review responses to these questionnaires to guide the interviewing process. Such questionnaires usually begin with questions that are medical, such as questions about the adolescent's perception of his or her own weight, skin condition, and development of secondary sexual characteristics. Such questionnaires should include a review of systems, with questions about the major organ systems; psychiatric issues; sleep; and general concerns such as fatigue and change in appetite. They should ask about prescribed and over-the-counter medications, dietary supplements, and complementary or integrative therapies the adolescent is using. Questions should also include strengths such as trusted adults, connection to school, coping strategies for stress, and regular physical activity. Questions may then move to more sensitive areas such

Table 4-1. The HEEADSSS Interview

Topic	Sample Questions
Home	• Who lives with you at home? • Where do you live? Do you live in a house or an apartment? Tell me about your living situation. • Do you share a room or have your own? • Do any new people live in your home? • How are your relationships with parents, siblings, and other important relatives? • What are the rules like at home? ☐ Have you ever been homeless or in shelter care? ☐ Have you ever been in foster care or a residential group home?
Education	• What school do you go to? What is your grade level? • Are you in gifted, regular, or special education classes? • How do you do in school in terms of grades? ☐ What would you say is contributing to your academic performance? • What are your best and worst subjects? • In the past year, how many days of school have you missed? Why? ☐ Have you ever had to repeat a year of school? Why? ☐ Have you ever been suspended? Why? ▲ What are your educational goals? ▲ How connected do you feel to your school? Do you feel as if you belong? ▲ Which adults at school do you feel you could talk with about something important?
Employment	• Do you work after school? • What type of work do you do? • How many hours a week do you work? • What are your future career goals? What do you want to do as a job when you grow up? ☐ Do you have any home chores? Do you get an allowance?
Eating	• How do you feel about your weight? Do you want to weigh more or less or stay the same? • What do you think your ideal or perfect weight should be? • How many meals and snacks do you eat per day? • Tell me what you would eat in a typical day. ☐ Do you ever skip meals? Why? How often? ☐ How do you control your weight? Do you control it with exercise, vomiting, diuretics, or laxatives? ☐ How often do you have a bowel movement? Do you have any problems with your bowel movements? ▲ What would it be like if you gained (lost) 10 lb?
Activities	• How do you like to spend your free time? What do you like to do for fun? What do you particularly excel at? ☐ What hobbies, clubs, or church or school activities do you have? • What sports do you play, and how many hours a week? ☐ How many hours of TV per week do you watch? How many hours a week are you on the computer (sedentary)? • How much time do you spend with social media such as Facebook and text messaging?

Table 4-1. The HEEADSSS Interview (*continued*)

Topic	Sample Questions
Drugs	• How many of the people with whom you hang out smoke cigarettes, drink alcohol, or use drugs? • How do drinking, smoking, and drugs fit in with your life? • Do you smoke or chew tobacco? • Do you drink alcohol? What kind? Beer, wine, wine coolers, or hard liquor? • How often do you use tobacco, alcohol, or drugs? How much and how often? ☐ Have you ever blacked out or passed out? ☐ Have you ever done anything you regretted while drunk or high? ☐ When do you most often use alcohol or drugs? Socially? Alone? Time of day? Day of week? ☐ How do you feel about cutting back or quitting? • What other drugs have you used or tried? Marijuana, inhalants, cocaine or crack, heroin, pills, LSD, ecstasy, crystal meth, or other drugs? • Do you use anabolic steroids? ▲ Have you ever received drug treatment or counseling? ▲ How do you support your alcohol or drug use? Have you ever had any arrests?
Depression and suicidality	• How do you usually feel: happy, sad, or a bit of both? ☐ How would you describe your mood on most days? • What makes you feel stressed? • What do you do to relieve stress? How do you cope? • Have you ever thought about trying to hurt or kill yourself? ☐ Have you ever tried to hurt or kill yourself? What did you do? Whom did you tell? ☐ Have you ever gotten counseling or therapy? ▲ Have you ever been in a psychiatric hospital? Why? How long did you stay?
Sexuality	For female adolescents • How old were you when you started your menstrual periods? • How often do you have a period? • How long are your periods, and how heavy is your flow? • Do you have menstrual cramps? • How often do you miss school because of cramps? For all adolescents ☐ Do you find yourself sexually attracted to others? ☐ When you think of people to whom you are attracted, are they guys, girls, both, or neither, or are you not sure? How comfortable are you with your feelings? ☐ When you think of yourself as a person, do you think of yourself as male, female, neither, or both? How comfortable are you with your feelings of who you are, in terms of gender, on the inside? • Have you ever had the kind of sex in which [add specific type of contact: penis in vagina, mouth on penis, mouth on vagina, penis in rectum, or other type of contact]? • How old were you when you first [describe sexual contact]? • How often do you have pain during sexual intercourse or other sexual activities?

Table 4-1. The HEEADSSS Interview (*continued*)

Topic	Sample Questions
Sexuality (*continued*)	• How satisfied are you with how often you have sexual relations and with what you do with your sexual partner? □ Do you have any problems becoming aroused, getting an erection, getting lubricated (wet), or having an orgasm? □ Have you ever been pregnant or gotten someone pregnant? What concerns do you have about being able to get pregnant or get someone else pregnant? □ What have you used in the past to prevent pregnancy? What are you using now? For methods that you stopped, why did you stop them? □ How many people have you had sexual relationships with in your lifetime? What about the past 3 mo? □ Have you ever had an STI, such as gonorrhea, chlamydial infection, trichomonal infection, herpes, or warts? What concerns do you have about STIs? □ Has anyone ever asked you to exchange sex for something such as drugs, money, clothing, jewelry, food, or a place to stay? □ Have you ever exchanged sex for drugs, money, clothing, jewelry, food, or a place to stay? □ Have you ever sent nude or partially nude pictures of yourself or someone else via cell phone or over the Internet?
Safety	• Have you ever been forced to have sex or been touched in a sexual way against your will? By whom, and is this still going on? • In what ways does that experience affect your day-to-day life? • In what ways does that experience affect your sexual relationships now? • How often do you wear protective sports gear when you play sports? • Have you ever been seriously injured in your home, neighborhood, or school? (How?) How about anyone else you know? • Have you ever been bullied in your neighborhood, in your school, or anywhere else in your life? • Do you have access to weapons? Is there a gun in your home? □ Do you ever ride in a stolen car, in a car with a drunk driver, or in a car late at night? □ Do you use a cell phone or text while you are driving? If so, how often? □ Do you use sunscreen when in the sun?
Spirituality	• What do you consider to be your religion? ▲ How often do you participate in religious activities? ▲ How important are your spiritual beliefs in your day-to-day life? • How do your beliefs affect your daily eating habits? Are there times of the year that you engage in fasting? • How do your beliefs influence your health and attitudes about drug and alcohol use, sex, and contraception?

• = *essential questions*   □ = *as time permits*   ▲ = *when situation requires*

Abbreviations: STI, sexually transmitted infection; TV, television.
For updates, please see Klein DA, Goldenring JM, Adelman WP. HEEADSSS 3.0: the psychosocial interview for adolescents updated for a new century fueled by media. *Contemp Pediatr*. 2014:16–28. Reprinted with permission from *Contemporary Pediatrics*, Vol. 21, January 1, 2004, pp. 64–90. *Contemporary Pediatrics* is a copyrighted publication of UBM, LLC. All rights reserved. (Some questions added or adapted.)

as gender identity, sexual attraction and sexual activity, use of alcohol and drugs, and exposure to violence and abuse. Questions should also address mental health problems such as feelings of depression, suicidal thoughts, and symptoms of anxiety. The questionnaire should ask about school performance, including possible problems with teachers or peers. The clinician can then use the questionnaire to address issues that are pertinent to the adolescent at the visit. For example, if the adolescent indicates sexual activity is occurring, the clinician can address issues of preventing pregnancy and sexually transmitted infections. If the patient is not sexually active, the clinician can emphasize making informed choices about abstinence and sexual activity in the future. However, a questionnaire should not be a substitute for addressing these issues in person and conducting a thorough history. The questionnaire can be a helpful tool to open up conversation, but questions unanswered or answered as "no problem" should be readdressed during the interview, because problems may be revealed that the adolescent was uncomfortable writing down, especially related to sexuality, substance use, sexual or physical abuse, emotional or relationship problems, and mental illness.

When addressing the issue of sexuality with adolescents, care must be taken to avoid making assumptions regarding gender identity and sexual orientation. Such assumptions may dissuade adolescents from discussing important medical problems related to their respective gender identities, sexual orientations, and overall sexual health. Asking patients about their preferred names and gender pronouns is helpful to ascertain the patient's gender identity early on in the interview. The use of gender-neutral terms such as *partner* can keep communication open for discussion of same-gendered attractions. One way of opening a conversation about sexual orientation is to ask, "Many people have sexual experiences with members of the same sex at some point in their lives. Have you had any experiences with other boys [girls]?" This question can be followed up with questioning regarding whether adolescents consider themselves attracted to boys, girls, or both, or if they are unsure or asexual. The health care professional should recognize that people who have sex with those of the same gender may not consider themselves to be homosexual. In addition, the clinician should be aware that a person's sexual orientation may change throughout the person's life and that adolescents can go through periods of confusion in which they may be unsure or questioning of their respective sexual orientations. For further information on this subject, refer to Chapter 20, Lesbian, Gay, and Bisexual Youths.

Another helpful approach, especially in addressing issues of drug and alcohol use, is to precede any direct questions about such use with indirect normative statements about the possible use of such substances by others. The following vignette illustrates this approach. The patient is a 15-year-old boy.

> Clinician: Sometimes kids your age try alcohol, such as beer, wine, or mixed drinks, when they're at parties or hanging out together. Have you ever had anything with alcohol?
>
> Justin: Yeah, like, a couple of times.
>
> Clinician: What was it like?
>
> Justin: Once I was with a friend who was driving and I thought he was, like, kind of crazy. I was really afraid he might get us in an accident.
>
> Clinician: Was there anything you felt you could do to protect yourself?
>
> Justin: Well, no, but I sure wish there was.
>
> Clinician: How about yourself? Did you ever feel you drank too much?
>
> Justin: Well, yeah, once I woke up the next day and I couldn't remember anything that happened.

These responses would probably not have been forthcoming had the clinician asked directly, "Do you drink alcohol or take drugs?" The indirect approach is face-saving and is therefore likely to yield more truthful information. The clinician can now offer more targeted advice. The importance of drug or alcohol use and of possible drug or alcohol use disorder has also led to screening questionnaires that may be helpful when used with a population of adolescents at particularly high risk for drug or alcohol use disorder. Such questionnaires usually assume some alcohol or drug use and are designed to measure the severity of that use and indicate when a referral might be needed. One such method of assessing the severity of drug and alcohol use is the CRAFFT (Car, Relax, Alone, Forget, Family/Friends, Trouble) interview in Box 4-2.

Similarly, patients may not be forthcoming when clinicians ask direct questions related to other areas of health such as mental health. Assessments such as the Patient Health Questionnaire-9 (PHQ-9) Modified for Teens can be useful in assessing for symptoms of depression that may be indicative of mental health distress. The PHQ-9 is a self-report measure that offers clinicians a guide to the patient's specific symptoms (ie, changes in eating habits, changes in sleep, changes in ability to concentrate, feelings of worthlessness or failure) and the impact of these symptoms on daily

Box 4-2. The CRAFFT Interview

Begin: *"I'm going to ask you a few questions that I ask all my patients. Please be honest. I will keep your answers confidential."*

Part A

During the past 12 months, on how many days did you:

❶ Drink more than a few sips of beer, wine, or any drink containing **alcohol**? Put "0" if none.

☐ # of days

❷ Use any **marijuana** (weed, oil, or hash by smoking, vaping, or in food) or "**synthetic marijuana**" (like "K2," "Spice")? Put "0" if none.

☐ # of days

❸ Use **anything else to get high** (like other illegal drugs, prescription or over-the-counter medications, and things that you sniff, huff, or vape)? Put "0" if none.

☐ # of days

Did the patient answer "0" for all questions in Part A?

Yes ☐   No ☐
↓   ↓

Ask CAR question only, then stop   **Ask all six CRAFFT[a] questions below**

Part B   **No**   **Yes**

C Have you ever ridden in a **CAR** driven by someone (including yourself) who was "high" or had been using alcohol or drugs?   ☐ ☐

R Do you ever use alcohol or drugs to **RELAX,** feel better about yourself, or fit in?   ☐ ☐

A Do you ever use alcohol or drugs while you are by yourself, or **ALONE**?   ☐ ☐

F Do you ever **FORGET** things you did while using alcohol or drugs?   ☐ ☐

F Do your **FAMILY** or **FRIENDS** ever tell you that you should cut down on your drinking or drug use?   ☐ ☐

T Have you gotten into **TROUBLE** while you were using alcohol or drugs?   ☐ ☐

[a] **Two or more YES answers suggest a serious problem and need for further assessment.**

functioning. Other assessments such as the Pediatric Symptom Checklist (commonly known as PSC) and the Strengths and Difficulties Questionnaires (SDQ) can be similarly helpful in serving as a catalyst to further conversation about mental health. See Appendix 2, Mental Health Tools for Pediatrics, for more information about these tools.

Summary

The interviewing techniques described provide some suggestions for the clinician who provides care to adolescents. Effective interviewing requires practice. However, the skill is well worth learning because it leads to the completion of better medical and psychosocial histories and improved patient adherence. The result is improved health care for adolescents and their families.

Acknowledgments: The authors acknowledge the substantive contributions of Esther Wender, Susan Coupey, and Aimee Seningen in authoring the previous versions of this chapter.

Counseling Parents of Adolescents

Jonathan D. Klein, MD, MPH

"By enhancing parents' knowledge and increasing their coping abilities, primary care clinicians can help parents provide a safe harbor for their adolescent patients; they can also help promote appropriate development of responsibility and autonomy, as teenagers mature into adults."

Adolescence is characterized by dramatic and at times uneven integration of developmental changes into the daily lives of young people. Teenagers simultaneously experience changing body image, mood swings, burgeoning sexuality, intense need for peer acceptance, increasing independence from family, expectations to achieve, pressure to "act maturely," and fragile egos. At the conclusion of adolescent development, the emerging young adult needs to understand complex issues, arrive at decisions, have developed an ethical and moral value system, prepare for entry to the workforce, and be capable of intimacy. These tasks occur, for the most part, within families. Parents often view their pediatric primary care clinician (PCC; ie, the pediatrician, family physician, internist, nurse practitioner, or physician assistant who provides their son's or daughter's frontline health care) as a person from whom to seek advice about both physiologic and behavioral issues. The PCC's ongoing relationship with families allows opportunities to provide anticipatory guidance and support parents as their children enter and move through adolescence.

Autonomy and independence evolve over the adolescent years, usually progressing from young people's connectedness to their parents or adult guardians and to their families. This process rarely leads to adolescents achieving independence through a sudden break; rather, the process is a gradual redefinition of relationships, eventually leading to adult interdependence.[1] The adolescent years are one phase of this developmental continuum, as young people continually renegotiate their respective places within their families. Experimentation and risk-taking behaviors are often perceived negatively, as something to be avoided. Nonetheless, assuming some risks, such as those faced by athletes, performers, or peer leaders, has positive development effects, enhancing self-esteem and leading to competence and mastery. Most adolescents need to experience the tension created by experimenting with ideas and lifestyles that contrast with those of their families. However, during this time of *trying on* diverse personalities, the adolescent also needs to know that his or her return to the safety of the family is assured.

A parent's or guardian's greatest challenge is to maintain a balance between fostering adolescents' independent behavior and supporting the adolescent's need for trust and security. The tension created by adolescents' experimentation with ideas and behaviors can be a source of conflict and emotional distress to both parents and adolescents. Parents may feel a loss of control provoked by the young person's independent behavior, and adolescents may struggle with feelings of loss of childhood security and support as they struggle to cope with greater freedom and responsibility. This emotional conflict is often unrecognized and unarticulated, yet these issues underlie many common confrontations between parents and adolescents. Helping parents understand the developmental basis for this conflict may reduce their frustration, as does acknowledging and empathizing with parents about the emotional separation, which may be more painful for them than it is for their adolescent. Development of adolescents during the teen years has been described as fostering the 7 Cs of resilience, that is, competence, confidence, connection, character, contribution, coping, and control, all of which are necessary to equip young people with the skills to manage challenges and excel in life.

Parenting Goals

Primary care clinicians can help parents and their adolescents navigate adolescence, beginning with providing parents information about the physical, cognitive, and psychosocial developmental tasks of adolescence and with helping parents realize that adolescent development is a variable process. Parenting styles may be described as authoritarian, authoritative, permissive, or uninvolved.[2] *Authoritarian* parents are demanding and directive, expecting orders to be obeyed without explanation. *Authoritative* parents are both demanding and responsive, monitoring and communicating standards for children's or adolescents' conduct and expecting their children or adolescents to learn self-regulation of behavior. *Permissive* parents do not require or expect mature behavior and generally avoid confrontation. *Uninvolved* parents are neither responsive nor demanding, and they may be neglectful. Although both authoritarian and authoritative parenting styles have been shown to lead to good social and vocational outcomes,[3] the former style is often associated with much greater conflict and turmoil for all family members.[4] Parents should be encouraged to set clear expectations for their adolescents; however, parents should also be encouraged to communicate with their adolescents with 2 major goals. The first goal is to promote communication and resolution of conflict through mutual respect. Parents should maintain the adolescent's trust in the family by speaking respectfully to their adolescent and ensuring that their adolescent speaks respectfully to them. The second goal for parents is to be able to tolerate the adolescent's expression of differences. When parents can demonstrate this ability, and are able to avoid being provoked, the teenager's perception of parental support is heightened, and the adolescent's ego is nurtured. In this way, parents become leaders in a process in which collaboration and mutuality are affirmed, and interdependent adult partnerships can eventually be achieved.

Parent-Adolescent Communication

Open communication is probably the most important skill for parents to develop and maintain with their maturing adolescent (Box 5-1). Adolescents need a trusted sounding board, and, as facilitators, parents should listen more than speak. When parents lecture, adolescents shut down. The axiom *actions speak louder than words* often makes a more useful parenting motto than *do as I say, not as I do.* This latter philosophy is perceived as hypocritical, often diminishing the adolescent's respect for the parent. Such a situation often results in confrontation, and it weakens the parent-teen relationship.

Box 5-1. Dos and Don'ts of Parent-Adolescent Communication

- Listen more, speak less.
- Respond empathetically rather than intellectually.
- Resist saying, "I told you so!"
- Clarify expectations.
- Discuss consequences.
- Allow adolescents to participate in decision-making.

Adolescents' need for parental affection and acceptance, plus their not yet fully developed sense of self, makes them vulnerable to perceived injustices, put-downs, and negative innuendos. Parents gain immeasurably when they respond to their adolescents' feelings with empathetic rather than intellectual responses. For example, during the teen years, peer relationships are characterized by intense emotions consistent with adolescents' egocentricity. Should a break occur in a heretofore close friendship, the empathetic parent demonstrates support by empathizing with their adolescent's hurt feelings. Statements such as "I'm sorry that you are in such pain," "I can imagine how bad you might be feeling," or "It seems that your friend has really hurt you; do you want to talk about it?" express empathy and allow for continued discussion. Sometimes in an attempt to *make it better,* parents tend to minimize the adolescent's pain, perceiving it as "only" a short-lived adolescent drama. Statements such as "You'll find other friends" or "Don't worry; you're young and have your whole life ahead of you" are rarely received positively. Rather than finding this approach helpful, the adolescent may feel misunderstood and may cut off communication.

If the parent did not approve of the friend, the end of the relationship may be a source of relief for the parent. Telling a teenager to "forget about it" may represent the parent's wish, rather than the teen's. The ultimate negative scenario is a parent who adds, "I told you so!" Thoughtful parents refrain from statements that belittle the adolescent. In fact, adolescents often feel devastated when berated by a parent, despite attempts to defend themselves against the hurt by false bravado or an "I don't care!" response. When parents empathize with their teenagers' emotional intensity and allow their teenagers to express emotions without restraint or embarrassment, adolescents are comforted and feel supported. This approach reinforces open communication with parents and minimizes the need for adolescents to act out angry or hurt feelings.

Parents also have an obligation to clarify expectations, responsibilities, and privileges. However, these decisions are not made in a vacuum, and parents of adolescents should allow teens to participate in decision-making. The success of a contract between 2 parties requires that each person express *without dissent* what the other person wants. Also important is that both sides *gain something* from the outcome. Win-lose outcomes breed discontent and nonadherence by the person who perceives no gain. These guidelines can be useful when thinking about interactions between parents and adolescents. Open communication and decision-making founded on mutual respect are skills that are best learned within a family, and they help ensure win-win outcomes.[5]

The consequences of breaking a contract should be discussed by all involved family members. Few parents have difficulty grounding or otherwise punishing their adolescent for nonadherence, but many have difficulty acknowledging that they, too, have failed to abide by an agreement. As an example of this situation, consider a family in which the parents conceded that they nagged their daughter about not spending enough time on schoolwork, fearing her academic failure. The parents agreed with their PCC's advice that they respect the adolescent's privacy and give her responsibility for her schoolwork. A contract was signed by the PCC (as mediator), parents, and adolescent, with terms including the adolescent's decision about time to set aside for study and the parents' agreement to permit her to experience her decision and avoid questioning her. If the adolescent's grades declined, she would be grounded; if the parents continued to nag, they agreed to consequences too.

Assessing the Parent-Adolescent Relationship

Primary care clinicians can assess how families are coping with their adolescents' development by asking parents how parent-teen decision-making is handled. Curfews and rules are good issues to discuss with parents because they are a frequent source of conflict and because, when parents set rules and expectations for safe and responsible behavior, their guidance helps adolescents maintain healthy behaviors and avoid risky behaviors. Curfew decisions include safety issues (which are and should be subject to parental authority) and the issues of adolescent choice of friends and social functions (decisions which are within the adolescent's jurisdiction); thus, they are ideal for learning about shared decision-making and negotiating. Primary care clinicians should explore whether parents are able to have open discussions with their adolescent about their plans. Do the parents routinely ask about the location of social functions and travel plans? Do they easily agree on curfews with which everyone is reasonably satisfied? In the event of a disagreement, how are compromises negotiated? (See Box 5-2.) Parents should try to avoid arbitrarily rigid limits. An example of the type of statement best avoided is "I have decided that you are to be home no later than midnight." Such unilateral decisions usually end in unresolvable confrontation. Sometimes the rigidity of the curfew time is confounded by the parents' feelings about the adolescent's choice of friends or activities.

Not infrequently, parental disapproval of an adolescent's friends or activities may be the *expressed* reason for parental inflexibility about the teen's curfew. However, the *underlying* cause for concern may have more

Box 5-2. Anticipatory Guidance Mnemonic for Parents of Adolescents

- **Participate as partners with the adolescent.**
- **Acknowledge your parental authority.**
- **Respect each other's differences.**
- **Encourage open communication.**
- **Negotiate win-win agreements.**
- **Tolerate the adolescent's separateness.**

to do with the parents' fear that their adolescent might engage in unsafe sexual activity or substance use. The PCC might ask the parents whether they and their adolescent have been able to share their views about alcohol and drug use or about sexual activity and relationships and, if so, whether the discussion resulted in mutual understanding. The PCC can suggest to both parents and teen that such discussions should take place to make sure that parents have made their values and expectations clear and to encourage communication about responsible behavior and safe decision-making.

Parents may also feel anxious because they fear adverse outcomes from their adolescent's behavioral choices. In particular, parents may be afraid that such behavior will become permanent or will threaten the teen's opportunity to mature into a responsible, productive adult. Knowing that extremes of adolescent behavior are generally transient and that most adolescents mature into adults whose lifestyles, values, and mores are similar to those of their families may reassure parents.[6] However, more rigid parental control often leads to greater adolescent rebellion. The adolescent's perception of parental acceptance, interest, warmth, and respect is associated positively with the adolescent's self-esteem. Nevertheless, parents should be supported in their efforts to protect adolescents from injuries and dangerous behavioral choices.

Parents should also be advised to avoid abdicating their authority. Parental limit-setting is strongly associated with less risky behavior by adolescents. Thus, parents should be encouraged to maintain their authority and clearly negotiate limits, particularly when true issues of safety are involved. Rather than confrontation over who is in control, parents and their teens should both be encouraged to frame these issues to focus on and highlight the safety issues, on which both parents and adolescents can agree.

Management of Parent-Adolescent Conflict

Some families are intuitively or purposefully flexible and reasonable, and others are able to achieve this with their PCCs' counsel. However, some families require the intervention of a mental health specialist. For example, some parents resist understanding adolescent development and choose not to acknowledge the mutuality of parent-adolescent interactions. Instead, they chronically respond to the adolescent's point of view with "Yes…but," followed by a litany of the adolescent's misdeeds. Other parents are themselves immature and needy and may rely inappropriately on the adolescent for nurturing or support. The unmet needs of such adolescents may result in chronic acting-out behaviors, which may include poor school performance, loss of friends, somatic concerns, and, in some situations, depression or suicide attempts. For serious adjustment issues and depressive symptoms, referral to and support by mental health professionals is essential. For less serious adjustment issues, some PCCs may choose to treat these patients by meeting with the parents to assess their willingness and capacity to understand the developmental and family communication issues and to manage change within the family. (See Chapter 2, Family-Centered Care: Applying Behavior Change Science.) If parents are refractory to counseling after 1 or 2 meetings, the PCC will be in a better position to make an appropriate mental health referral than he or she would have been at the initial visit.

Primary care clinicians who counsel parents and adolescents about developing mutually satisfying working relationships can make a significant difference in these families' lives. By enhancing parents' knowledge and increasing their coping abilities, PCCs can help parents provide a safe harbor for their adolescent patients; they can also help promote appropriate development of responsibility and autonomy, as teenagers mature into adults.

References

1. Ginsburg KR. *Building Resilience in Children and Teens: Giving Kids Roots and Wings.* 3rd ed. Elk Grove Village, IL: American Academy of Pediatrics; 2015
2. Baumrind D. Patterns of parental authority and adolescent autonomy. *New Dir Child Adolesc Dev.* 2005;(108):61–69
3. Steinberg L, Lamborn SD, Dornbusch SM, Darling N. Impact of parenting practices on adolescent achievement: authoritative parenting, school involvement, and encouragement to succeed. *Child Dev.* 1992;63(5):1266–1281
4. DeVore ER, Ginsburg KR. The protective effects of good parenting on adolescents. *Curr Opin Pediatr.* 2005;17(4):460–465
5. Fish LS. Hierarchical relationship development: parents and children. *J Marital Fam Ther.* 2000;26(4):501–510
6. Gecas V, Seff MA. Families and adolescent: a review of the 1980s. *J Marriage Fam.* 1990;52(4):941–958

Family Support

James M. Perrin, MD, and Amy Pirretti, MS

"Any clinical encounter offers opportunities for reinforcing the family's strengths and enhancing the family's capacity to support the child or adolescent with challenges that lie ahead."

Background

The definition of family can be complex. Here is a definition shared by the late family advocate Polly Arango in the Bright Futures guidelines.[1]

We all come from families. Families are big, small, extended, nuclear, multigenerational, with 1 parent, 2 parents, and grandparents. We live under one roof or many. A family can be as temporary as a few weeks, as permanent as forever. We become part of a family by birth, adoption, marriage, or from a desire for mutual support. As family members, we nurture, protect, and influence each other. Families are dynamic and are cultures unto themselves, with different values and unique ways of realizing dreams. Together, our families become the source of our rich cultural heritage and spiritual diversity. Each family has strengths and qualities that flow from individual members and from the family as a unit. Our families create neighborhoods, communities, states, and nations.

Developed and adopted by the New Mexico Legislative Young Children's Continuum and New Mexico Coalition for Children, June 1990

The American Academy of Family Physicians defines the family as "a group of individuals with a continuing legal, genetic, or emotional relationship,"[2] indicating the varied nature of families, the complexities of assessing each family constellation, and the importance of recognizing diversity. Every family is an individual system with beliefs and attitudes of its own. Families play an essential role in all aspects of mental health care, that is, in prevention, early identification, help seeking, treatment, and management.

Family Trends

The number of children living with 2 married parents has decreased during the past 40 years (Figure 6-1). In 1970, 85% of children were living with married parents, whereas 67% of children in 2010 did so. During this same period, the number of children being raised by single mothers grew from 11% to 23%. The proportion of children being raised by single fathers has fluctuated from 1% to 5% and was 3% as of 2010. The number of children living without either parent has remained constant at about 4% across the past 4 decades. Other notable family structure trends include nearly 7% of children living with a grandparent, with a parent also present in more than half of these families (data from 2010). Families have become much more diverse in the past few decades. More and more same-sex couples have children. Children and young families have increasing racial and ethnic diversity, with larger numbers of mixed-race families. Family structure also differs significantly when stratified by race (Figure 6-2). Almost 85% of Asian children live in families with 2 married parents, compared with

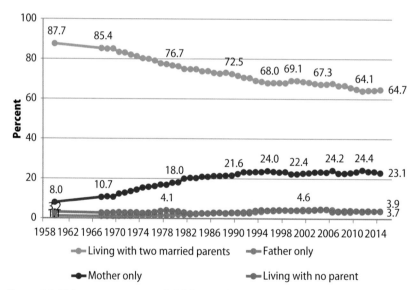

Figure 6-1. Living arrangements of children under 18: 1970–2015.

Note: Children living with two married parents may be living with biological, adoptive, or non-biological parents. Children living with mother only or father only may also be living with the parent's unmarried partner.

Source: Data for 2008-2015: Child Trends calculations of U.S. Census Bureau, Current Population Survey, Annual Social and Economic Supplement. "America's Families and Living Arrangements."

From Child Trends Databank. Family structure. Child Trends Web site. http://www.childtrends.org/?indicators=family-structure. Updated December 2015. Accessed January 18, 2018. Reproduced with permission.

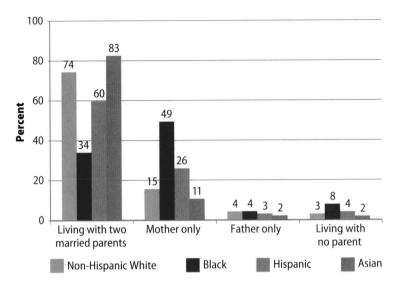

Figure 6-2. Living arrangements of children, by race and Hispanic origin: 2015.
From Child Trends Databank. Family structure. Child Trends Web site. http://www.childtrends.org/
?indicators=family-structure. Updated December 2015. Accessed January 18, 2018. Reproduced
with permission.

71% of whites, 61% of Hispanics, and 35% of blacks,[3] again indicating the
diversity among families and the need to inquire about household structure
with all families.

Family Culture and Behaviors

The growing racial, ethnic, cultural, and gender diversity among US children and their families reflects diverse beliefs about family roles and activities, including child-rearing, discipline, and mental well-being and illness.
Cultural variations may include rituals and activities that help ground a
developing child in his or her community and its stories and beliefs, including those regarding health and living healthy lives. Cultural differences can
influence eating behaviors and foods offered, definitions of appropriate and
inappropriate behaviors, parental efforts at control, time together and activities, and views of medications and other treatments. The family's culture is
an intrinsic part of the child's social environment, and pediatric primary
care clinicians (PCCs) (ie, pediatricians, family physicians, internists, nurse
practitioners, and physician assistants who provide pediatric care) should
develop cultural awareness while learning individual family preferences.

Understanding the cultural context of the family in concert with the
internal family dynamics helps the PCC in forming a therapeutic alliance
with the family that can enhance discussion of mental health issues and

early identification of problems. Clinicians can become familiar with the major cultural groups in their community, develop ways to elicit cultural beliefs that may affect a patient's health and behavior, and implement the culturally competent tools to enhance effective understanding and communication. Guidance for providing culturally effective care can be found in Chapter 3, Culturally Effective Care.

Family and Community Environments

The communities in which children and adolescents live influence their health, mental health, and development. Communities provide different levels of cohesiveness, safety, support, and beliefs, all of which have effects on children and adolescents (collectively called *children* in the remainder of this chapter) and their families. Families with children interact with many community agencies and services, especially schools, which play a major role in prevention and identification of mental health issues and family support. Communities provide variation in opportunities for children, such as areas to play and exercise, access to nutritious foods, and exposure to potential toxins (including poor housing with mold or other antigens).

For an in-depth discussion of promoting the health of children at the community level, see Chapter 29, Promoting the Mental Health of Young Children; Chapter 30, Promoting the Health of Adolescents; and Chapter 31, Promoting Mental Health in Schools. The section, Care of Special Populations, discusses promoting the health of specific populations of high-risk children. The discussion that follows focuses broadly on the role that a child's medical home can play in enhancing families' capacity to support their children.

Enhancing Family Support in the Primary Care Setting

Change, stress, and happiness that affect one family member will have reciprocal effects on all family members. The role of PCCs in promoting families' support of their children may include surveillance of family members' health, mental health, strengths, and challenges; formal screening of caregivers for health and social problems and signs of family dysfunction; evaluation of families' social and financial resources; and anticipatory guidance to enhance the family's resilience and address the challenges parents face in nurturing their child. Medical home principles emphasize partnership with families and providing them with the tools and education to participate actively in health care.

Surveillance

To identify strengths and needs of a child's family, the PCC might explore
the following topic areas in the context of children's routine health supervision care. See Chapter 1, Healthy Child Development, for description of a
process to integrate these topics into the iterative assessment of the family.

Parental Strengths and Challenges

It is important for PCCs to identify and reinforce each parent's strengths.
These may include the parent's commitment to the child's health care, relationship with the other parent, extended family connections, patience,
understanding of the child's developmental needs, use of helping services,
or other ways in which the parent demonstrates his or her capacities as a
caregiver. By recognizing and nurturing these strengths, the PCC can benefit the child and build trust with the family.

It is also important to recognize the parents' health needs and socioeconomic challenges, which may affect the child's well-being. Among
people aged 20 to 40 years, the main use of health care is for mental health
issues and obstetric care, and large numbers of people in this age-group do
not seek medical care regularly. Thus, key issues that parents may face in
their families may go unidentified and untreated. Among the most important are parental depression, substance use, domestic violence, poverty, and
separation and divorce, all of which can affect the mental well-being of their
children. The pediatric encounter may play a role in identifying important
parental health and social issues, especially as they pertain to the family's
ability to care for the child. The following sections provide further guidance
on addressing these issues when they are identified.

Family Configuration

In working with children, PCCs should inquire about the whole family, that
is, who is in it, how they are doing, and how well their activities fit the needs
of the developing child.

In general, having 2 parents, whether in heterosexual or same-sex households, involved in a child's care is associated with a number of improved
outcomes.[4] Ideally, parents share care and care decisions and recognize the
value of collaborating with other adult caregivers in a child's environment.
Both parents should be encouraged to share actively in child care and development; their involvement in the clinical encounter can also be encouraged.

Although many children do well in single-parent households, children
in these circumstances have higher rates of school failure and mental health
and developmental problems, partly reflecting much higher likelihood of

poverty than in 2-parent households, as well as the additional parenting stress that accompanies parenting alone. Close connection with extended family members or other sources of support can significantly enhance the well-being of children in single-parent households.

Children whose parents divorce may have experienced much family discord and conflict and will need to adjust to the intermittent absence of 1 or both parents. Persistent conflict may also affect the child's health and behavior. Divorce may lead to new economic hardship for the child.

Parents involved in adoption or foster care face the relatively sudden inclusion of new children in a household and may know relatively little about the child's previous health, mental health, or development. The children may have difficulties in new settings because of previous losses or inconsistent parenting, attachment, or bonding. Primary care clinicians can help parents gather more information, gain helpful skills, learn about resources, access support, and learn strategies to parent and care for a new child who may have had very different parenting experiences in the past. Identifying support and resources in the extended family may help grandparents (or others) play supportive roles. Adolescent parents may need support in developing their parenting skills, and referrals to parenting education programs that focus on young parents can help in this regard.

Caregiver Roles and Interactions

In modern families, parent roles and responsibilities vary widely, with many ways of distributing tasks, including child care, discipline, and daily activities such as supervision of homework, entertainment, eating, or sleep.[5] Primary care clinicians should seek information about the role of a noncustodial parent in the household and encourage the parent's participation in various care and health areas.[6]

A parent who is out of the home or working may feel too busy or otherwise excluded from interactions with a child's health care providers; encouraging the parent's interaction either in person or through other means of communication can help support these roles and provide broader understanding about the family.

Children With Special Health Care Needs

Children and adolescents with special health care needs substantially increase the time (and often physical work) of parenting. Children with diabetes need attention to diet, blood testing, and insulin treatment. Families should understand how various daily life issues (eg, illness, stress) may influence blood glucose levels. Children with mental health and emotional problems require behavior management and educational guidance. Children with developmental conditions also require family support and accommodation. Asthma, arthritis, epilepsy, leukemia, and other childhood chronic health conditions create demands specific to those conditions. The child's symptoms, absences from school or child care, health care appointments, hospitalizations, and medication management may require that caregivers interface with schools and agencies, miss work, and deplete their emotional and financial resources, compounding the stress on the child and caregivers, individually, and on the family as a unit, including siblings. Primary care clinicians can support the family by identifying and attending to these stressors, making appropriate referrals for both the child and caregivers, and connecting them to sources of peer support and respite care.

Change and Family Stress

Families face many changes that are stressful, and their responses and adjustment to them may affect children's health and mental health. Obvious stresses include transitions, for example, a new (parent) job, a new house, illness or death of a parent, and separation and divorce. Other transitions that the child may experience include discharge from hospital to home as a newborn or after care for a serious chronic or acute condition, entering school, or entering adolescence. Economic stresses, such as a parent's job loss or long-term unemployment, may have a powerful effect on the family's capacity to attend, physically and emotionally, to the child's needs. Indeed, family stressors, large and small, are very common. Chronic toxic stress may have immediate and long-term negative health and especially mental health consequences for the child. (See Chapter 13, Children Exposed to Adverse Childhood Experiences.)

Primary care clinicians can help by querying about recent changes in the household or new stresses that the family may be experiencing. A brief mental health update can be adapted for this purpose.[7]

When the PCC finds stresses that may affect family well-being, she or he can use "common factors" techniques (Chapter 2, Family-Centered Care: Applying Behavior Change Science) to strengthen the therapeutic alliance with the family and develop a family-centered plan of action. The plan may include general steps to improve the family's health and resilience (eg, physical activity, sleep, help from friends or extended family, connection with spiritual resources) and specific referrals for mental health care, marital or financial counseling, social services, or peer support. The PCC's demonstrated empathy, hopefulness, and commitment will likely have their own therapeutic value.

Screening

Parents may hesitate to bring up their stresses or personal health problems during pediatric visits, despite their importance in affecting child care and health. Brief screening tools exist to help pediatricians identify these concerns in a family. Chapter 1, Healthy Child Development, and Appendix 2, Mental Health Tools for Pediatrics, list screening tools that can be readily incorporated into primary care work flow.

Anticipatory Guidance

To nurture a family's capacity to support its children, the PCC will need a relationship of trust with the family. The first 5 chapters of this book provide guidance on making a primary care practice a friendly environment for the discussion of family issues that may affect the child's health and well-being.[8,9] Understanding and supporting the family in a family-centered medical home will, in turn, enhance the child's health and development.[10]

Any clinical encounter offers opportunities for reinforcing the family's strengths and enhancing the family's capacity to support the child with challenges that lie ahead. This guidance may take many forms, depending on the family's readiness to accept help and the needs of the child.[11] For example, the clinician may have an opportunity to advise new parents on the importance of their communication with the PCC and to emphasize that child care providers should not use television screens as babysitters, to encourage the parent of an adolescent to stay involved in the adolescent's daily activities, to recommend a counselor for parents undergoing separation or divorce, or to involve extended family in supporting a parent facing military deployment.

Families needing additional support can be referred to helping agencies or peer support programs. Evidence-based programs such as the Nurse-Family Partnership and early literacy promotion can assist caregivers in strengthening bonds with their children. For children and adolescents with special health care needs, legislative efforts have led to development of Family-to-Family Health Information Centers (F2F HICs) in each state.[12] Staffed by parents of children with special health care needs, the F2F HICs assist families and clinicians in locating community resources. See Appendix 3, Sources of Key Mental Health Services, for a listing of community services and the professionals who provide them.

Summary and Recommendations

In many ways, pediatric PCCs are clinicians for the whole family. Thus, much clinical interaction relates to learning about family strengths and capabilities, understanding circumstances in which family health issues and stressors may affect a child's health, and determining with the family best strategies to identify and address a child's health needs in the family context. Knowledge of community resources will help clinicians make appropriate referrals, when indicated.

Developing therapeutic relationships with children and families involves taking into consideration the diversity of families and family structures, the involvement of various adults in the relationship, variations in household and community culture and language, parental health and socioeconomic status, and the effect of the child's health condition on the family. Providing effective preventive care and anticipatory guidance builds on an understanding of the family and its characteristics, strengths, and challenges.

AAP Policy

American Academy of Pediatrics Committee on Early Childhood, Adoption, and Dependent Care. The pediatrician's role in family support and family support programs. *Pediatrics*. 2011;128(6):e1680–e1684. Reaffirmed December 2016 (pediatrics.aappublications.org/content/128/6/e1680)

American Academy of Pediatrics Committee on Hospital Care, Institute for Patient and Family Centered Care. Patient- and family-centered care and the pediatrician's role. *Pediatrics*. 2012;129(2):394–404 (pediatrics.aappublications.org/content/129/2/394)

Perrin EC, Siegel BS; American Academy of Pediatrics Committee on Psychosocial Aspects of Child and Family Health. Promoting the well-being of children whose parents are gay or lesbian. *Pediatrics*. 2013;131(4):e1374–e1383 (pediatrics. aappublications.org/content/131/4/e1374)

Yogman M, Garfield CF; American Academy of Pediatrics Committee on Psychosocial Aspects of Child and Family Health. Fathers' roles in the care and development of their children: the role of pediatricians. *Pediatrics*. 2016;138(1):e20161128 (pediatrics.aappublications.org/content/138/1/e20161128)

References

1. Hagan JF Jr, Shaw JS, Duncan PM, eds. *Bright Futures: Guidelines for Health Supervision of Infants, Children, and Adolescents.* 4th ed. Elk Grove Village, IL: American Academy of Pediatrics; 2017

2. American Academy of Family Physicians. Family, definition of. AAFP Web site. http://www.aafp.org/about/policies/all/family-definition.html. Accessed January 18, 2018

3. Child Trends. DataBank: family structure. Child Trends Web site. http://www.childtrends.org/?indicators=family-structure. Updated December 2015. Accessed January 18, 2018

4. American Academy of Pediatrics Committee on Psychosocial Aspects of Child and Family Health. Coparent or second-parent adoption by same-sex parents. *Pediatrics.* 2002;109(2):339–340

5. Yogman M, Garfield CF; American Academy of Pediatrics Committee on Psychosocial Aspects of Child and Family Health. Fathers' roles in the care and development of their children: the role of pediatricians. *Pediatrics.* 2016;138(1):e20161128

6. Cabrera NJ, Tamis-LeMonda CS, Bradley RH, Hofferth S, Lamb ME. Fatherhood in the twenty-first century. *Child Dev.* 2000;71(1):127–136

7. Appendix S8: brief mental health update. *Pediatrics.* 2010;125(suppl 3):S159–S160. http://pediatrics.aappublications.org/content/125/Supplement_3/S159. Accessed March 6, 2018

8. American Academy of Pediatrics Committee on Psychosocial Aspects of Child and Family Health and Task Force on Mental Health. The future of pediatrics: mental health competencies for pediatric primary care. *Pediatrics.* 2009;124(1):410–421

9. Radecki L, Olson LM, Frintner MP, Tanner JL, Stein MT. What do families want from well-child care? Including parents in the rethinking discussion. *Pediatrics.* 2009;124(3):858–865

10. Stille C, Turchi RM, Antonelli R, et al; Academic Pediatric Association Task Force on Family-Centered Medical Home. The family-centered medical home: specific considerations for child health research and policy. *Acad Pediatr.* 2010;10(4):211–217

11. Kuhlthau KA, Bloom S, Van Cleave J, et al. Evidence for family-centered care for children with special health care needs: a systematic review. *Acad Pediatr.* 2011;11(2):136–143

12. All about Family-to-Family Health Information Centers. National Center for Family/Professional Partnerships Web site. http://www.fv-ncfpp.org/f2fhic/about_f2fhic. Accessed January 18, 2018

Healthy Sleep

Anne May, MD, and Mark L. Splaingard, MD

> "Guiding parents about ways to foster healthy
> sleep in their children, surveillance of
> children's sleep patterns, and recognizing
> signs and symptoms that may signal a sleep
> disturbance are important components of
> routine health supervision."

Sleep is crucial to the mental and physical health of both children and their parents. When children achieve the recommended amount of sleep for their ages, they have overall better health outcomes.[1] Poor sleep in a child or an adolescent may have a 2-generational effect. Sleep deprivation can cause a young child to be irritable, inattentive, or hyperactive and may make the child less resilient to life's stressors; in the older child or adolescent, sleep deprivation can cause similar symptoms, mimicking common mental health conditions and contributing to poor school performance and risky behaviors. Inability to sleep can also signal the onset of a mood disorder or other serious psychiatric condition. Whatever the cause, poor sleep of a child or an adolescent can, in turn, cause sleep deprivation in the parents, compromising their capacity to respond to their children's needs and to function in their roles inside and outside the home.

Guiding parents about ways to foster healthy sleep in their children, surveillance of children's sleep patterns, and recognizing signs and symptoms that may signal a sleep disturbance are important components of routine health supervision and are the subject of this chapter.

Development of Sleep

The development of physiologic sleep patterns is predictable (Table 7-1). It begins in utero; by 28 weeks' gestational age, rapid eye movement (REM), or active sleep, can be discerned via fetal ultrasound. Non–rapid eye

Table 7-1. Sleep Developmental Milestones

Age (mo)	Sleep Patterns
Birth	Newborn sleeps 16–17 of 24 h. Active sleep occupies 50% of TST by term newborn. Periodic breathing is noted, particularly during active sleep.
4	Sleep shifts to nighttime settling by 12–16 wk. Slow-wave sleep recognized at 3–4 mo. By 16 wk, sustained wake periods are as long as 3–4 h.
6	By 6 mo, 90% of infants have more NREM sleep than REM sleep.
8	REM sleep occupies 30% of TST. Total sleep duration is 13–14 hours a day by 6–8 months of age.

Abbreviations: NREM, non–rapid eye movement; REM, rapid eye movement; TST, total sleep time.

movement (NREM), or quiet sleep, appears at 32 weeks' gestational age. At term, newborns have discrete sleep cycles, lasting 50 to 60 minutes, with awakenings every 2 to 6 hours. These sleep cycles are composed of alternating periods of equal amounts of quiet and active sleep. The total daily amount of reported sleep at 1 month of age ranges widely, from 9 to 19 hours, with an average of 14 hours.[2] As children age through the first decade after birth, the recommended amount of sleep gradually decreases from 12 to 16 hours of sleep per day in the first year to 9 to 12 hours of sleep per day between 6 and 10 years of age.[1] For other recommended sleep durations by age, see Table 7-2.

Humans have internal clocks that operate on a cycle of approximately 24 hours. These 24-hour cycles, known as *circadian rhythms,* are controlled by the hypothalamic suprachiasmatic nucleus. Most people have cycles that are not exactly 24 hours in length, and external time cues help reinforce the 24-hour schedule. The time cues are known as *zeitgebers* (German for "time givers"). The most powerful cue is exposure to bright light; other cues include social interaction, food, and exercise. Circadian rhythms are usually synchronized or *entrained* with light-dark cycles. Newborns and infants develop these circadian rhythms over the first few months after birth, with rhythmic secretion of melatonin by 12 weeks in term infants.

By the time an infant is 4 months of age, mature sleep stages begin to emerge, and day-night sleep patterns are well consolidated. Infants have their longest sleep periods at night and have 3- to 4-hour periods of wakefulness during the day. By the time an infant is 6 months, circadian rhythms begin to display activity similar to rhythms in adults; these

Table 7-2. Recommended Sleep Duration by Age

Age	Recommended Sleep in 24 Hours (h)
4–12 mo	12–16
1–2 y	11–14
3–5 y	10–13
6–12 y	9–12
13–18 y	8–10

Derived from Paruthi S, Brooks LJ, D'Ambrosio C, et al. Recommended amount of sleep for pediatric populations: a consensus statement of the American Academy of Sleep Medicine. *J Clin Sleep Med.* 2016;12(6):785–786.

rhythms are well established by 1 year of age. By 3 years of age, the child reaches an adult pattern of sleep, with each discrete cycle of NREM and REM sleep lasting 70 to 100 minutes.[3]

At the beginning of the night, a child progresses rapidly through the lighter stages of NREM sleep and enters slow-wave sleep (stage N3) for much of the first third of the night. During slow-wave sleep, the child is difficult to awaken. Subsequent sleep cycles have decreased amounts of slow-wave sleep and increased amounts of stage N2 sleep and REM sleep. Dreaming takes place mainly during REM sleep. Rapid eye movement episodes become longer and more intense later in the sleep period; thus, children are more likely to report bad dreams during the last portion of the night. In addition, sleep-disordered breathing (commonly known as SDB) is likely to be most prominent during REM sleep. This tendency is important to recognize, given that this time of night is when parents are least likely to be awake and watching the sleep patterns of their children.

The amount of sleep that children need varies by age. (See Table 7-2.)

Fostering Healthy Sleep: Anticipatory Guidance

Safe Sleep Guidelines

Sudden unexplained infant death (commonly known as SUID) is a term that describes unexpected death during the first year after birth. This category of death includes sudden infant death syndrome (SIDS), for which an etiologic origin is often undefined. In an effort to decrease the frequency of these events, the American Academy of Pediatrics (AAP) recently revised its safe infant sleeping environment guidelines.[4] The following summary of sleep-related "A-level recommendations" from the AAP Task Force on Sudden Infant Death Syndrome applies to all newborns and infants younger than 1 year:

1. Infants should be placed in a supine position for every sleep. This population includes term and preterm infants.
2. Infants should be placed on a firm sleep surface. Room sharing with parents is recommended for the first year, but the infant should be placed on a separate sleep surface. If a full year of room sharing is not a possibility, it is recommended for at least the first 6 months after birth.
3. All soft objects and loose blankets should be kept away from the infant sleep area. This recommendation also includes tiny stuffed animals and blankets ("lovey") in addition to pillows, soft mattresses, crib bumper pads, and blankets.
4. Breastfeeding is recommended.
5. Families should consider offering a pacifier at bedtime and nap times. This pacifier does not need to be replaced if it falls out of the infant's mouth, nor should it be forced if the infant is not interested in taking the pacifier.
6. Avoid overheating.
7. Home cardiorespiratory monitors ("apnea monitors") should not be used as a way to prevent the occurrence of SIDS.
8. Smoke exposure, alcohol, and illicit drugs should be avoided during pregnancy and after birth.
9. Pregnant women should seek routine prenatal care.
10. Infants should be immunized according to recommendations from the AAP and the Centers for Disease Control and Prevention.

Sleep Hygiene Principles

General principles of sleep hygiene apply at any age, but specifics may vary with the child's age. The goal of developing good sleep hygiene is to create and maintain an environment that is conducive to good sleep. Chapter 10, Healthy Active Living, suggests incorporating sleep-related guidance into a broader effort to modify patient and family lifestyles, using a 24-hour movement model that includes physical activity.

1. Establish a good sleep environment that is dark, quiet, and comfortable and has a steady, slightly cool temperature. Sleep should be in the same place for night and naps as much as possible. The bed or crib should be used as a place for sleep and not as a play area or playpen while awake.

2. After bedtime feedings, infants should be placed in bed without a bottle. Parents can teach infants the skill of falling asleep on their own after about 4 months of age by avoiding body contact with the parent as they drift to sleep (self-soothing). This method enables infants to go back to sleep on their own after waking during the night.

3. Establish a soothing bedtime routine that involves friendly interaction between the parent and the child. This routine should involve interactions that decrease the stimulation around the child, and it should last no more than 20 to 30 minutes. Use of electronics as part of this routine is discouraged, as it can increase stimulation. The parent should leave the room while the child is still awake. The child should be put to bed when moderately tired to reduce bedtime resistance.

4. Avoid changing the routine because of demands or tantrums at bedtime, which can quickly develop into a pattern.

5. No television (TV), computer, or any electronic screens should be in the child's room. Research shows that video screens will prolong sleep onset and delay bedtime. It is advisable to enforce an electronic curfew for older children and adolescents to facilitate preparation for sleep and to prevent further use during the night.

6. Try to keep a consistent schedule for bedtime, naps, and morning wake up, which will help the child maintain regular circadian rhythms. Naps should not be taken too close to bedtime.

7. Try to keep the household atmosphere calm in the evening. Remember that TV programs and movies may be frightening or stimulating. Arguments between parents or other family members may also be distressing.

8. Keep track of activities that seem to lead to sleeping problems. If active play or video games lead to problems, stop them 1 or 2 hours before bedtime. Caffeine and nicotine can disrupt sleep. Avoid caffeine at least 6 hours before bedtime.

Surveillance of Children's Sleep Patterns

Monitoring pediatric sleep is an important part of any health supervision visit. It can be overwhelming for a primary care clinician to start getting to the underlying issues when sleep is the topic. A good suggestion is to follow the BEARS Sleep Screening Algorithm (Box 7-1). This algorithm divides sleep into 5 domains. These include bedtime problems, excessive daytime sleepiness, awakenings during the night, regularity and duration of sleep,

Box 7-1. BEARS Sleep Screening Algorithm

The "BEARS" instrument is divided into five major sleep domains, providing a comprehensive screen for the major sleep disorders affecting children in the 2- to 18-year-old range. Each sleep domain has a set of age-appropriate "trigger questions" for use in the clinical interview.

B = bedtime problems

E = excessive daytime sleepiness

A = awakenings during the night

R = regularity and duration of sleep

S = snoring

Examples of developmentally appropriate trigger questions:

(P) Parent-directed question

(C) Child-directed question

	Toddler/ preschool (2-5 years)	School-aged (6-12 years)	Adolescent (13-18 years)	Suggestions
1. Bedtime problems	Does your child have any problems going to bed? Falling asleep?	Does your child have any problems at bedtime? (P) Do you have any problems going to bed? (C)	Do you have any problems falling asleep at bedtime? (C)	Recommend bedtime routine to allow for winding down before bedtime. Consider asking about anxiety in patients unable to fall asleep. Evaluate for stimulating bedtime behaviors such as electronics use, use of video games, and completing homework immediately before bed.
2. Excessive daytime sleepiness	Does your child seem overtired or sleepy a lot during the day? Does she still take naps?	Does your child have difficulty waking in the morning, seem sleepy during the day or take naps? (P) Do you feel tired a lot? (C)	Do you feel sleepy a lot during the day? In school? While driving? (C)	Question whether nighttime sleep is sufficient for age. Consider narcolepsy or hypersomnia if adequate nighttime sleep.

Box 7-1. BEARS Sleep Screening Algorithm (*continued*)

	Toddler/preschool (2-5 years)	School-aged (6-12 years)	Adolescent (13-18 years)	Suggestions
3. Awakenings during the night	Does your child wake up a lot at night?	Does your child seem to wake up a lot at night? Any sleepwalking or nightmares? (P) Do you wake up a lot at night? Have trouble getting back to sleep? (C)	Do you wake up a lot at night? Have trouble getting back to sleep? (C)	Consider sleep environment leading to awakenings. Consider sleep disruption caused by sleep apnea and periodic limb movements. Obtain history about stimulating substances (eg, caffeine, medications) or activities (eg, video games) before bedtime.
4. Regularity and duration of sleep	Does your child have a regular bedtime and wake time? What are they?	What time does your child go to bed and get up on school days? Weekends? Do you think he/she is getting enough sleep? (P)	What time do you usually go to bed on school nights? Weekends? How much sleep do you usually get? (C)	Consider insufficient sleep time. Recommend routine sleep and wake time on both weekends and weekdays. Adjust evening activities if possible to allow for routine bedtime.
5. Snoring	Does your child snore a lot or have difficulty breathing at night?	Does your child have loud or nightly snoring or any breathing difficulties at night? (P)	Does your teenager snore loudly or nightly? (P)	Consider evaluation for sleep-disordered breathing.

From Mindell JA, Owens JA. *A Clinical Guide to Pediatric Sleep: Diagnosis and Management of Sleep Problems.* 3rd ed. Philadelphia, PA: Wolters Kluwer; 2015. Reproduced with permission.

and snoring. For each section, age-appropriate questions for parents and children are provided to initiate conversations on sleep. The idea is to trigger a discussion of sleep issues.

Helpful resources for parents include "Fostering Comfortable Sleep Patterns in Infancy" (www.brightfutures.org/mentalhealth/pdf/families/in/sleep_patterns.pdf) and *Sleep: What Every Parent Needs to Know,* 2nd Edition (book), American Academy of Pediatrics (https://shop.aap.org).

Identification of Concerns

If surveillance suggests any of the following sleep disturbances, the clinician should proceed with further assessment.

- ▶ Day-night reversal
- ▶ Delayed settling
- ▶ Difficulties with night waking
- ▶ Bedtime struggles
- ▶ Inability to sleep when desired
- ▶ Comorbid mental health symptoms
- ▶ Signs or symptoms of sleep deprivation in the child (eg, excessive daytime sleepiness, irritability, hyperactivity)

AAP Policy

American Academy of Pediatrics Task Force on Sudden Infant Death Syndrome. SIDS and other sleep-related infant deaths: updated 2016 recommendations for a safe infant sleeping environment. *Pediatrics.* 2016;138(5):e20162938 (pediatrics.aappublications. org/content/138/5/e20162938)

References

1. Paruthi S, Brooks LJ, D'Ambrosio C, et al. Recommended amount of sleep for pediatric populations: a consensus statement of the American Academy of Sleep Medicine. *J Clin Sleep Med.* 2016;12(6):785–786

2. Iglowstein I, Jenni OG, Molinari L, Largo RH. Sleep duration from infancy to adolescence: reference values and generational trends. *Pediatrics.* 2003;111(2):302–307

3. Sheldon SH. *Evaluating Sleep in Infants and Children.* Philadelphia, PA: Lippincott-Raven Publishers; 1996

4. American Academy of Pediatrics Task Force on Sudden Infant Death Syndrome. SIDS and other sleep-related infant deaths: updated 2016 recommendations for a safe infant sleeping environment. *Pediatrics.* 2016;138(5):e20162938

Chapter

Healthy Weight

Sandra G. Hassink, MD, MS

"Caregivers' distress may affect their ability to establish healthy eating patterns in their children. If primary caregivers are experiencing mental health problems, they may have unhealthy eating patterns themselves and less resilience when faced with the challenges of providing healthy meals for their families."

Introduction

Achieving good nutrition and maintaining a healthy weight are core components of lifelong health and depend on a multiplicity of factors, including individual child, family, and community characteristics. At the systems level, this complex process involves the production and distribution of food, access to health-supporting nutrition, and a marketing environment that promotes healthy eating. If all these factors were in place, making healthy food choices would become easier for families and children.[1,2] That said, negotiating the current toxic obesity-promoting environment means that families, children, and adolescents have to exert tremendous control over day-to-day decisions to achieve a healthy lifestyle. This need places an additional burden on families struggling with other chronic stressors.

Dietary Effects of Family Stress

Caregivers' distress may affect their ability to establish healthy eating patterns in their children. If primary caregivers are experiencing mental health problems, they may have unhealthy eating patterns themselves and less resilience when faced with the challenges of providing healthy meals for their families. In a population of mothers of young infants enrolled in a

Special Supplemental Nutrition Program for Women, Infants, and Children (WIC) clinic, mental health problems (depression, anxiety, stress, and cumulative high mental health symptoms) were associated with high likelihood of emotional eating (a behavior pattern of eating in response to a range of negative emotions),[3] and depression was associated with a high likelihood of restrained eating.[4]

Maternal emotional distress (depression, anxiety, and stress) has also been linked to restrictive feeding,[5] pressure to eat, and an authoritarian, indulgent, and uninvolved feeding style.[6] In a study of parents with low incomes and from ethnic or racial minorities, an uninvolved parental feeding style has been correlated with parental psychological distress and higher child body mass index (BMI).[7] In one study of a low-income minority population, emotional eating was linked to obesity and to a history of childhood emotional abuse, with findings of reduced emotional regulation as a possible mechanism.[8]

Several studies have found a relationship between parental work or life stress and a less healthy family food environment,[9,10] lower level of physical activity,[11] and less time to prepare meals and eat together.[12] Some evidence supports that greater parental stress is correlated with a child's higher level of fast-food consumption and television viewing.[13,14] Perceived stress is the belief that environmental stressors exceed one's adaptive capacity and has been associated with obesity-promoting behaviors in families.[15] Other family stressors found to be associated with child overweight include lack of cognitive stimulation and emotional support in the young child and parental mental and physical health problems and financial strain in the older child.[16]

Social stressors resulting from disadvantages in income, home ownership, education, and race have been associated with obesity.[17] Children from persistently food insecure households had significantly greater increases in BMI from kindergarten to third grade than children in food secure homes did.[18] This finding had led researchers to suggest that incorporating stress reduction techniques and strategies into obesity-prevention programs should be considered.[19] In one study, children with higher dietary restraint and higher reactivity increased their total energy intakes in response to a stressful task, shifting their intakes toward comfort foods, as did children with higher BMI and lower dietary restraint. This shifting indicates that high stress reactivity and high BMI may mediate greater calorie consumption of comfort food.[20]

Dietary Effects of Childhood Mental Health Problems

A study of more than 11,000 children aged 5 to 11 years in California found that poor child mental health, as reported by parents, was associated with increased consumption of french fries and fast food and decreased consumption of vegetables.[21] In a study of adolescents, higher scores on internalizing (withdrawal, somatic concerns, and anxious or depressed behavior), externalizing (delinquency and aggression), and total behavior scores on the Child Behavior Checklist were associated with consumption of a diet of fast food, sweets, red meat, and processed food compared with a diet of fresh fruits and vegetables.[22]

Obesity

This chapter highlights obesity, which has reached epidemic proportions throughout the developed world and is a threat to both child health and adult health.[23,24]

Epidemiology of Obesity

The prevalence of obesity among children, adolescents, and young adults aged 2 to 19 years was 17.0% in 2011–2014 (Figure 8-1). Prevalence increased with age, from 8.9% among preschool children aged 2 to 5 years; to 17.5% among school-aged children 6 to 11 years; to 20.5% among preadolescents, adolescents, and young adults 12 to 19 years; and up to 32.3% among 20- to 39-year-olds.[25,26] The increase in rates since 2000 has slowed among 12- to 19-year-olds and has begun to decline among 6- to 11-year-olds and 2- to 5-year-olds[27]; however, racial and ethnic and socioeconomic disparities in prevalence are still on the upswing, and these populations remain at increased risk for obesity.[28]

Obesity and Chronic Stress

Some emerging literature correlates chronic stress with initiation and maintenance of obesity.[29–31] In cross-sectional studies, children with obesity have shown greater cortisol responses to stress than their peers without obesity have shown.[32] Elevated cortisol level may shift food choices toward energy-dense, high-fat, and sweet foods, further exacerbating weight gain.[33]

Toxic stress in childhood may play a role in the development of unhealthy eating patterns in adults. In fact, these unhealthy patterns have been found to be more likely in adults who had unhappy, violent childhoods, independent of demographic factors, and the likelihood increased when the adults were

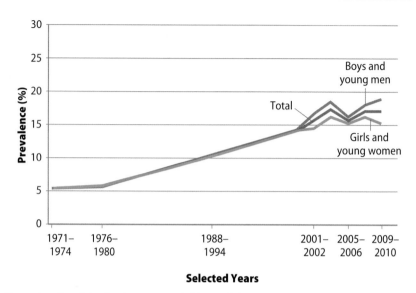

Figure 8-1. Trends in obesity[a] among children, adolescents, and young adults aged 2–19 years by sex: United States, 1971–1974 through 2009–2010.

Abbreviations: BMI, body mass index; CDC, Centers for Disease Control and Prevention.

[a] Obesity is BMI ≥95th percentile of the sex- and age-specific 2000 CDC growth charts.

Adapted from Fryar CD, Carroll MD, Ogden CL. Prevalence of obesity among children and adolescents: United States, trends 1963-1965 through 2009-2010. Centers for Disease Control and Prevention Web site. https://www.cdc.gov/nchs/data/hestat/obesity_child_09_10/obesity_child_09_10.htm. Updated September 13, 2012. Accessed January 18, 2018.

currently experiencing low adult well-being.[34] In the Adverse Childhood Experiences Study, adults who experienced 4 or more adverse childhood experiences had an increased risk of having a greater than 30 BMI.[35]

Risk of Obesity in People With Mental Health Problems

Serious mental illness has been associated with an increased prevalence of obesity in adults: more than 50% of adults with a diagnosis of mental illness have an associated diagnosis of obesity. Factors such as poor nutrition, lack of physical exercise, and weight gain side effects of psychiatric medications, as well as lack of access to preventive and obesity treatment services, may contribute to these elevated rates.[36] In a small group of adolescents with severe mental illness, rates of obesity were 30%; obesity in this population was associated with lack of private insurance, smoking, and antidepressant and antipsychotic treatments.[37]

The relationship between obesity and child mental health has been studied in the context of specific mental health diagnoses. A study of more than 5,000 children and adolescents in the Autism Treatment Network compared with children and adolescents from the National Health and Nutrition Examination Survey demonstrated significantly higher prevalence of obesity among children and adolescents with autism spectrum disorder aged 2 to 5 years and 12 to 17 years but no difference in the prevalence of obesity among children of both groups aged 6 to 11 years.[38]

Children and adolescents with the diagnosis of attention-deficit disorder (ADD) or attention-deficit/hyperactivity disorder (ADHD) who were not taking medication had 1.5 increased odds of having obesity compared with the general population. By contrast, individuals taking medication for ADD or ADHD had 1.6 increased odds of being classified as underweight.[39] Childhood ADHD and conduct problems may predict obesity in adulthood. In a longitudinal study, children with behavioral and conduct problems at age 5 and ADHD and conduct problems at age 10 years had an increased risk of obesity at age 30 years.[40]

In a meta-analysis of longitudinal studies of obesity and depression, a bidirectional relationship was found between depression and obesity in adults. Obesity at baseline increased the risk of onset of depression at follow-up, and baseline depression increased the odds for developing later obesity.[41] Depression in childhood and adolescence has been shown in longitudinal studies to predict obesity into adulthood.[42-44] In a 3-year longitudinal study of children, adolescents, and young adults 8 to 18 years of age, depression and anxiety were associated with higher initial BMI and persistently elevated BMI over 3 years, compared with children, adolescents, and young adults without a mental health diagnosis. In this study, anxiety was associated with elevated BMI in both boys and girls, but elevated BMI with depression was seen only in girls.[45]

Certain psychotropic drugs can cause accelerated weight gain,[46] and children and adolescents on antipsychotics are particularly susceptible to developing type 2 diabetes (Table 8-1).[47]

Risk of Mental Health Problems in Children With Obesity

Children with obesity are more likely than children who do not have obesity to have mental health problems. In a cross-sectional analysis of more than 43,000 children and adolescents (10–17 years) from the 2007 National Survey of Children's Health, children and adolescents with obesity were more likely to have reported internalizing problems, externalizing problems, and school problems. Attention-deficit/hyperactivity disorder, conduct disorder, and depression were also reported more commonly among children and adolescents with obesity as compared with children and adolescents who did not have overweight.[48] In a review of population-based studies, obesity was found

Table 8-1. Classification of Psychotropic Medications

Obesogenic Psychotropic Medications	Non-obesogenic Psychotropic Medications
Antidepressants • Sertraline • Amitriptyline • Nortriptyline • Paroxetine	**Antidepressants** • Bupropion • Venlafaxine • Trazadone • Buspirone • Citalopram • Doxepin • Fluoxetine • Escitalopram • Imipramine HCL • Doxapram HCL • Desipramine HCL • Trimipramine Maleate • Fluvoxamine • Protriptyline HCL
Mood stabilizers/Antimania • Lithium • Valproate • Carbamazepine • Gabapentin	**Mood stabilizers/Antimania** • Topiramate • Lamotrigine • Zonisamide
Antipsychotics • Mirtazapine • Haloperidol • Perphenazine • Clozapine • Olanzapine • Risperidone • Quetiapine • Ziprasidone • Aripiprazole • Thioridazine	**Antipsychotics** • Molindone • Pimozide
Anxiolytics • None applicable	**Anxiolytics** • Alprazolam • Lorazepam
Psychostimulants • None applicable	**Psychostimulants** • Methylphenidate • Amphetamine • Dextroamphetamine Sulfate

From Eneli IU, Wang W, Kelleher K. Identification and counseling for obesity among children on psychotropic medications in ambulatory settings. *Obesity (Silver Spring)*. 2013;21(8):1656–1661. Reproduced with permission.

to be prospectively associated with increased rates of depression, but there was less consistent evidence that depression leads to obesity.[49] Higher rates of anxiety and mood disorders have been identified among children with obesity in clinical populations[50,51] than among children with obesity in the general population.[50]

Obesity, Teasing, and Bullying

One of the most disturbing aspects of having obesity is being bullied. Studies have shown that children with overweight and obesity are more likely to be bullied than their peers with normal weight are.[52] Weight-based teasing has been found to increase the risk of suicidal ideation among girls and has been shown to increase the risk of developing disordered eating behaviors. In addition, lower self-esteem, poorer body image, and higher depressive symptoms have been associated with weight-based teasing in adolescents.[53] In one study, adolescents who experienced social ostracism ate not only more food than adolescents without obesity who experienced ostracism did but also more food than adolescents with obesity who were not ostracized did.[54] Mental health and behavioral problems may be predictive of bullying.[55] Bullying may be more common in subpopulations of children with obesity. In a study of more than 41,000 children and adolescents from 10 to 17 years of age, overweight and obesity were positively associated with bullying; however, this association was no longer significant when controlling for individual, family, and neighborhood factors. For example, current depression, but not ADHD or anxiety, was associated with bullying, as was decreased ability to stay calm when faced with a new challenge. Children with or without obesity who had witnessed domestic violence, or neighborhood violence, or been harmed by violence were more likely to have engaged in bullying other children. Among children with overweight and obesity, ADHD was associated with bullying.[55]

Another study showed that both bullies and those being bullied have been shown to be at greater risk of obesity and eating disorders, as well as injuries, smoking, alcohol abuse, and suicidal ideation or suicidal attempt (or both).[56]

Obesity and School Performance

Children with obesity encounter more behavioral problems in school than children without obesity do. Internalizing problems (eg, low self-esteem, sadness, acting withdrawn) and externalizing problems (eg, arguing, fighting, disobedience) are more common among school-aged children with obesity. School discipline problems (eg, detentions, suspensions) increase significantly with increased weight status.[48,57–59] Problems such as repeating a grade, low school engagement, and increased school absence have been reported to increase with a child's BMI.[60]

Obesity and Unhealthy Weight Control Behaviors

Unhealthy weight control behaviors, involving binge and restrictive eating, are not uncommon in the population of children and adolescents with overweight and obesity. In a study of more than 4,000 middle and high school students, 60% of girls who had overweight and 76% who had obesity reported engaging in unhealthy weight control behaviors (16% and 18% respectively practiced extreme weight control behaviors). Students who had overweight and those who had obesity used weight control strategies that ranged from moderate (dieting and exercising) to unhealthy (skipping meals, using food substrates, fasting, and smoking more cigarettes) to extreme (abuse of laxatives and diuretics, intake of diet pills, and vomiting).[61,62] In another study of more than 30,000 students from seventh to 12th grade, adolescents who had overweight were significantly more likely to engage in weight control and binge-eating behaviors than were their counterparts who did not have overweight.[63] Studies have correlated activation of the reward pathway in the brain with response to high-calorie food cures and compulsive overeating.[64] Studies have also shown neurophysiological overlap between eating palatable (refined) foods and reward pathways activated in drug and alcohol use.[65–67] There is also some evidence that binge eating in childhood and adolescence increases the risk for obesity in adulthood.[68]

Obesity and Self-esteem

In a community-based study, children with overweight or obesity had poorer self-esteem at baseline (ages 5–10 years) than children without obesity did, and higher baseline BMI predicted poorer self-esteem at follow-up, while poorer self-esteem at baseline did not predict higher BMI at follow-up.[69]

Children with obesity are more likely to have low self-esteem than are children with normal weight. Bullying and disturbed eating are highly correlated with low self-esteem in children with overweight and obesity.[8]

Obesity and Quality of Life

In a clinical sample of children with severe obesity, health-related quality of life was comparable to that of children with cancer.[70] Smaller but similar effects in health-related quality of life were seen in a community-based sample of children: children with obesity or overweight scored lower on physical and social functioning compared with children who did not have overweight or obesity.[71]

Promoting Healthy Weight: Implications for Practice

Family Meals

Taking a history of how and when families eat together is an important first step. Encouraging positive, healthy family meals, along with building knowledge and skills for healthy eating, may help support families in establishing healthy eating patterns in their children. Young children who participate in more than 5 family meals per week were less likely to consume sugar-sweetened beverages; adolescents had greater odds of consuming more than 3 fruits and vegetables per day and no sugar-sweetened beverages.[72] Families who ate together were more likely to increase fruit and vegetable consumption, drink water instead of soda, eat whole-grain bread instead of white bread, eat breakfast every morning, and drink low-fat, skimmed, or nonfat milk.[73]

Family meals may also support children's mental health. Frequent family meals (>5 meals per week) in adolescents have been associated with higher well-being scores and lower depression scores, as well as less likelihood of suicidal ideation and attempts. Risk-taking behavior (smoking, binge drinking, unsafe sex, and marijuana use) were also less likely.[74]

Social Support for the Family

Families under stress may benefit from healthy lifestyle counseling and support. Many children with obesity live in poverty and experience food insecurity. Screening for food insecurity and connecting families to federal food programs such as WIC, Supplemental Nutrition Assistance Program (commonly known as SNAP), summer feeding, and local food pantries should be part of the practice routine. Parenting skills targeting healthy routines can be particularly valuable for families coping with mental health issues. Encouraging families to participate in community parenting classes and identifying each family's social networks and strengths are ways to help strengthen family supports.

Universal Care: Anticipatory Guidance, Surveillance, Screening, and Early Identification

Body mass index or weight for length need to be calculated and classified for all children as a first step to assess their obesity risk. This step allows for a targeted approach to prevention, early intervention, or treatment. Unhealthy nutrition and activity behaviors are prevalent and should be assessed and addressed with a counseling technique, such as brief, focused negotiation or motivational interviewing. Physicians should consider referral to a dietician for children and adolescents with persistent unhealthy eating patterns. Because inadequate sleep has been associated with weight gain, attention to sleep hygiene is important to address in all children as part of promoting healthy weight. (See Chapter 7, Healthy Sleep.)

Care of Children With Mental Health Problems

Heightened attention to nutrition is necessary in children with mental health problems. They should have a nutrition and physical activity assessment and counseling aimed at ensuring a healthy lifestyle, no matter what their weights. It is particularly important to help parents create a healthy nutrition and healthy physical activity and screen time environment at home. Counseling should also be aimed at helping parents deal with their child's reactions and behaviors that may arise when they institute changes in food and in physical activity and screen time. Counseling on the risk of weight gain and close monitoring of BMI and metabolic status should be routine for children beginning obesogenic antipsychotic medications.

Care of Children With Obesity

Children with obesity should be routinely screened for mental health symptoms and functional impairment, as well as medical comorbidities, and, as in cases of other chronic diseases, routine medical follow-up is essential. Resources for obesity screening and evaluation can be found at https://ihcw. aap.org. Children with obesity should also be monitored for binge eating and other eating abnormalities. School performance and absences should also be monitored and counseling provided if any problems emerge. Children and adolescents should be asked directly about bullying and teasing; counseling should be offered to children and adolescents being bullied or engaging in bullying behavior.

The basis for obesity treatment is family-based lifestyle behavior change. This change can be challenging for families and children who have experienced the psychological comorbidities of obesity, such as low self-esteem, diminished quality of life, stress, bullying, and teasing. Elements of the family lifestyle plan can include creating a healthy home nutritional and activity environment, including eliminating sugared beverage consumption, having fruits and vegetables at meals and snacks, and reducing or eliminating high energy–dense snack foods. Additional family-based steps such as maintaining a regular schedule of meals and snacks, making sure as many meals as possible are eaten together as a family, no screen time during meals, regular family-based physical activities, limiting eating out, and serving age-appropriate portions of food are also important strategies. Maintaining a positive, supportive relational environment is also important, and eliminating parent or sibling weight-related teasing or bullying is essential.

Children with overweight or obesity should also have an individualized plan of care, taking into consideration presence of mental health problems or risk for mental health problems (or both) and medical comorbidities. Evidence suggests that including stress-reduction techniques may be helpful to some children. "Weight loss and methods used to lose weight should be carefully monitored by the pediatrician to ensure that the child or adolescent does not develop the medical complications of semi starvation."[74]

AAP Policy

American Academy of Pediatrics Council on Communications and Media. Children, adolescents, obesity, and the media. *Pediatrics.* 2011;128(1):201–208 (pediatrics. aappublications.org/content/128/1/201)

Golden NH, Schneider M, Wood C; American Academy of Pediatrics Committee on Nutrition, Committee on Adolescence, and Section on Obesity. Preventing obesity and eating disorders in adolescents. *Pediatrics.* 2016;138(3):e20161649 (pediatrics. aappublications.org/content/138/3/e20161649)

References

1. Rutten LF, Yaroch AL, Patrick H, Story M. Obesity prevention and national food security: a food systems approach. *ISRN Public Health.* 2012;2012:539764
2. Koelen MA, Lindström B. Making healthy choices easy choices: the role of empowerment. *Eur J Clin Nutr.* 2005;59(suppl 1):S10–S15
3. Faith MS, Allison DB, Geliebter A. Emotional eating and obesity: theoretical considerations and practical recommendations. In: Dalton S, ed. *Obesity and Weight Control: The Health Professional's Guide to Understanding and Treatment.* Gaithersburg, MD: Aspen; 1997:439–465
4. Emerson JA, Hurley KM, Caulfield LE, Black MM. Maternal mental health symptoms are positively related to emotional and restrained eating attitudes in a statewide sample of mothers participating in a supplemental nutrition program for women, infants and young children. *Matern Child Nutr.* 2017;13(1)
5. Mitchell S, Brennan L, Hayes L, Miles CL. Maternal psychosocial predictors of controlling parental feeding styles and practices. *Appetite.* 2009;53(3):384–389
6. Hurley KM, Black MM, Papas MA, Caulfield LE. Maternal symptoms of stress, depression, and anxiety are related to nonresponsive feeding styles in a statewide sample of WIC participants. *J Nutr.* 2008;138(4):799–805
7. Hughes SO, Power TG, Liu Y, Sharp C, Nicklas TA. Parent emotional distress and feeding styles in low-income families. The role of parent depression and parenting stress. *Appetite.* 2015;92:337–342
8. Renzaho AM, Kumanyika S, Tucker KL. Family functioning, parental psychological distress, child behavioural problems, socio-economic disadvantage and fruit and vegetable consumption among 4-12 year-old Victorians, Australia. *Health Promot Int.* 2011;26(3):263–275
9. Bauer KW, Hearst MO, Escoto K, Berge JM, Neumark-Sztainer D. Parental employment and work-family stress: associations with family food environments. *Soc Sci Med.* 2012;75(3):496–504

10. Devine CM, Jastran M, Jabs J, Wethington E, Farell TJ, Bisogni CA. "A lot of sacrifices": work-family spillover and the food choice coping strategies of low-wage employed parents. *Soc Sci Med.* 2006;63(10):2591–2603

11. Roost E, Sarlio-Lahteenkorva S, Lallukka T, Lahelma E. Associations of work-family conflicts with food habits and physical activity in children. *Public Health Nutr.* 2007;10(3):222–229

12. Slater J, Sevenhuysen G, Edginton B, O'Neil J. "Trying to make it all come together": structuration and employed mothers' experience of family food provisioning in Canada. *Health Promot Int.* 2012;27(3):405–415

13. Parks EP, Kumanyika S, Moore RH, Settler N, Wrotniak BH, Kazak A. Influences of stress in parents on child obesity and related behaviors. *Pediatrics.* 2012;130(5):1096–1104

14. Stenhammar C, Olsson G, Bahmanyar S, et al. Family stress and BMI in young children. *Acta Paediatr.* 2010;99(8):1205–1212

15. Parks EP, Kumanyika S, Moore RH, Stettler S, Wrotniak BH, Kazak A. Influence of stress in parents on child obesity and related behaviors. *Pediatrics.* 2012;130(5):e1096–e1104

16. Garasky SA, Stewart SD, Gundersen C, Lohman BJ, Eisenmann JC. Family stressors and child obesity. *Soc Sci Res.* 2009;38(4):755–766

17. Grow HM, Cook AJ, Arterburn DE, Saelens BE, Drewnowski A, Lozano P. Child obesity associated with social disadvantage of children's neighborhoods. *Soc Sci Med.* 2010;71(3):584–591

18. Jyoti DF, Frongillo EA, Jones SJ. Food insecurity affects school children's academic performance, weight gain, and social skills. *J Nutr.* 2005;135(12):2831–2839

19. Gundersen C, Mahatmya D, Garasky S, Lohman B. Linking psychosocial stressors and childhood obesity. *Obes Rev.* 2011;12(5):e54–e63

20. Roemmich JN, Lambiase MJ, Lobarinas CL, Balantekin KN. Interactive effects of dietary restraint and adiposity on stress-induced eating and the food choice of children. *Eat Behav.* 2011;12(4):309–312

21. Banta JE, Khoie-Mayer RN, Somaiya CK, McKinney O, Segovia-Siapco G. Mental health and food consumption among California children 5-11 years of age. *Nutr Health.* 2013;22(3–4):237–253

22. Oddy WH, Robinson M, Ambrosini GL, et al. The association between dietary patterns and mental health in early adolescence. *Prev Med.* 2009;49(1):39–44

23. Barlow SE; American Academy of Pediatrics Expert Committee. Expert committee recommendations regarding the prevention, assessment, and treatment of child and adolescent overweight and obesity: summary report. *Pediatrics.* 2007;120(suppl 4):S164–S192

24. Commission on Ending Childhood Obesity. *Report of the Commission on Ending Childhood Obesity.* Geneva, Switzerland: World Health Organization; 2016. http://www.who.int/end-childhood-obesity/info-resources/en. Accessed January 18, 2018

25. Ogden CL, Carroll MD, Fryar CD, Flegal KM. Prevalence of obesity among adults and youth: United States, 2011-2014. *NCHS Data Brief.* 2015;(219):1–8

26. Kamali A, Hameed H, Shih M, Simon P. Turning the curve on obesity prevalence among fifth graders in the Los Angeles unified school district, 2001-2013. *Prev Chronic Dis.* 2017;14:E16

27. Li W, Buszkiewicz JH, Leibowitz RB, Gapinski MA, Nasuti LJ, Land TG. Declining trends and widening disparities in overweight and obesity prevalence among Massachusetts public school districts, 2009-2014. *Am J Public Health.* 2015;105(10):e76–e82

28. Madsen KA, Weedn AE, Crawford PB. Disparities in peaks, plateaus, and declines in prevalence of high BMI among adolescents. *Pediatrics.* 2010;126(3):434–442

29. Roemmich JN, Lambiase MJ, Lobarinas CL, Balantekin KN. Interactive effects of dietary restraint and adiposity on stress-induced eating and the food choice of children. *Eat Behav.* 2011;12(4):309–312

30. Roemmich JN, Smith JR, Epstein LH, Lambiase M. Stress reactivity and adiposity of youth. *Obesity (Silver Spring).* 2007;15(9):2303–2310

31. Lohman BJ, Stewart S, Gundersen C, Garasky S, Eisenmann JC. Adolescent overweight and obesity: links to food insecurity and individual, maternal, and family stressors. *J Adolesc Health.* 2009;45(3):230–237

32. Dockray S, Susman EJ, Dorn LD. Depression, cortisol reactivity, and obesity in childhood and adolescence. *J Adolesc Health.* 2009;45(4):344–350

33. Dallman MF. Stress-induced obesity and the emotional nervous system. *Trends Endocrinol Metab.* 2010;21(3):159–165

34. Russell SJ, Hughes K, Bellis MA. Impact of childhood experience and adult well-being on eating preferences and behaviors. *BMJ Open.* 2016;6(1):e007770

35. Felitti VJ, Anda RF, Nordenberg D, et al. Relationship of childhood abuse and household dysfunction to many of the leading causes of death in adults. The Adverse Childhood Experiences (ACE) Study. *Am J Prev Med.* 1998;14(4):245–258

36. Pratt SI, Jerome GJ, Schneider KL, et al. Increasing US health plan coverage for exercise programming in community mental health settings for people with serious mental illness: a position statement from the Society of Behavior Medicine and the American College of Sports Medicine. *Transl Behav Med.* 2016;6(3):478–481

37. Gracious BL, Cook SR, Meyer AE, et al. Prevalence of overweight and obesity in adolescents with severe mental illness: a cross sectional chart review. *J Clin Psychiatry.* 2010;71(7):949–954

38. Hill AP, Zuckerman KE, Fombonne E. Obesity and autism. *Pediatrics.* 2015;136(6):1051–1061

39. Waring ME, Lapane KL. Overweight in children and adolescents in relation to attention-deficit/hyperactivity disorder: results from a national sample. *Pediatrics.* 2008;122(1):e1–e6

40. White B, Nicholls D, Christie D, Cole TJ, Viner RM. Childhood psychological function and obesity risk across the lifecourse; findings from the 1970 British Cohort Study. *Int J Obes (Lond).* 2012;36(4):511–516

41. Luppino F, de Wit LM, Bouvy PF, et al. Overweight, obesity, and depression: a systematic review and meta-analysis of longitudinal studies. *Arch Gen Psychiatry.* 2010;67(3):220–229

42. Hasler G, Pine DS, Gamma A, et al. The associations between psychopathology and being overweight: a 20-year prospective community study. *Psychol Med.* 2004;34(6):1047–1057

43. Franko DL, Striegel-Moore RH, Thompson D, Schreiber GB, Daniels SR. Does adolescent depression predict obesity in black and white young adult women? *Psychol Med.* 2005;35(10):1505–1513

44. Stice E, Presnell K, Shaw H, Rohde P. Psychological and behavioral risk factors for obesity in adolescent girls: a prospective study. *J Consult Clin Psychol.* 2005;73(2):195–202

45. Rofey DL, Kolko RP, Iosif AM, et al. A longitudinal study of childhood depression and anxiety in relation to weight gain. *Child Psychiatry Hum Dev.* 2009;40(4):517–526

46. Eneli IU, Wang W, Kelleher K. Identification and counseling for obesity among children on psychotropic medications in ambulatory settings. *Obesity (Silver Spring).* 2013;21(8):1656–1661

47. Pramyothin P, Khaodhiar L. Type 2 diabetes in children and adolescents on atypical antipsychotics. *Curr Diab Rep.* 2015;15(8):53

48. Halfon N, Larson K, Slusser W. Associations between obesity and comorbid mental health, developmental, and physical health conditions in a nationally representative sample of US children aged 10 to 17. *Acad Pediatr.* 2013;13(1):6–13

49. Faith MS, Butryn M, Wadden TA, Fabricatore A, Nguyen AM, Heymsfield SB. Evidence for prospective associations among depression and obesity in population-based studies. *Obes Rev.* 2011;12(5):e438–e453

50. Britz B, Siegfried M, Ziegler A, et al. Rates of psychiatric disorders in a clinical study group of adolescents with extreme obesity and in obese adolescents ascertained via a population based study. *Int J Obes Relat Metab Disord.* 2000;24(12):1707–1714

51. Vila G, Zipper E, Dabbas M, et al. Mental disorders in obese children and adolescents. *Psychosom Med.* 2004;66(3):387–394

52. van Geel M, Vedder P, Tanilon J. Are overweight and obese youths more often bullied by their peers? A meta-analysis on the relation between weight status and bullying. *Int J Obesity (Lond).* 2014;38(10):1263–1267

53. Eisenberg ME, Neumark-Sztainer D, Haines J, et al. Weight-teasing and emotional well-being in adolescents: longitudinal findings from Project EAT. *J Adolesc Health.* 2006;38(6):675–683

54. Salvy SJ, Bowker JC, Nitecki LA, Kluczynski MA, Germeroth LJ, Roemmich JN. Impact of simulated ostracism on overweight and normal-weight youths' motivation to eat and food intake. *Appetite.* 2011;56(1):39–45

55. Odar Stough C, Merianos A, Nabors L, Peugh J. Prevalence and predictors of bullying behavior among overweight and obese youth in a nationally representative sample. *Child Obes.* 2016;12(4):263–271

56. Srabstein JC, McCarter RJ, Shao C, Huang ZJ. Morbidities associated with bullying behaviors in adolescents. School based study of American adolescents. *Int J Adolesc Med Health.* 2006; 18(4):587–596

57. Datar A, Sturm R. Childhood overweight and parent- and teacher reported behavior problems: evidence from a prospective study of kindergartners. *Arch Pediatr Adolesc Med.* 2004;158(8):804–810

58. Shore SM, Sachs ML, Lidicker JR, Brett SN, Wright AR, Libonati JR. Decreased scholastic achievement in overweight middle school students. *Obesity (Silver Spring).* 2008;16(7):1535–1538

59. Young-Hyman D, Schlundt DG, Herman-Wenderoth L, Bozylinski K. Obesity, appearance, and psychosocial adaptation in young African American children. *J Pediatr Psychol.* 2003; 28(7):463–472

60. Carey FR, Singh GK, Brown HS III, Wilkinson AV. Educational outcomes associated with childhood obesity in the United States: cross-sectional results from the 2011–2012 National Survey of Children's Health. *Int J Behav Nutr Phys Act.* 2015;12(suppl 1):S3

61. Neumark-Sztainer D, Story M, Hannan PJ, Perry CL, Irving LM. Weight-related concerns and behaviors among overweight and nonoverweight adolescents. *Arch Pediatr Adolesc Med.* 2002;156(2):171–178

62. Boutelle K, Neumark-Sztainer D, Story M, Resnick M. Weight control behaviors among obese, overweight, and nonoverweight adolescents. *J Pediatr Psychol.* 2002;27(6):531–540

63. Neumark-Sztainer D, Story M, French SA, et al. Psychosocial correlates of health compromising behaviors among adolescents. *Health Educ Res.* 1997;12(1):37–52

64. Foley F, Myers U, DeWitt S. Reward circuit function in high BMI individuals with compulsive overeating: similarities with addiction. *Neuroimage.* 2012;63(4):1800–1806

65. Kalra SP, Kalra PS. Overlapping and interactive pathways regulating appetite and craving. *J Addict Dis.* 2004;23(3):5–21

66. Avena NM, Rada P, Hoebel BG. Evidence for sugar addiction: behavioral and neurochemical effects of intermittent, excessive sugar intake. *Neurosci Biobehav Rev.* 2008;32(1):20–39

67. Ifland JR, Preuss HG, Marcus MT, et al. Refined food addiction: a classic substance use disorder. *Med Hypotheses.* 2009;72(5):518–526

68. Stice E, Cameron RP, Killen JD, Hayward C, Taylor CB. Naturalistic weight-reduction efforts prospectively predict growth in relative weight and onset of obesity among female adolescents. *J Consult Clin Psychol.* 1999;67(6):967–974

69. Hesketh K, Wake M, Waters E. Body mass index and parent-reported self-esteem in elementary school children: evidence for a causal relationship. *Int J Obes Relat Metab Disord.* 2004;28(10):1233–1237

70. Schwimmer JB, Burwinkle TM, Varni JW. Health-related quality of life of severely obese children and adolescents. *JAMA.* 2003;289(14):1813–1819

71. Williams J, Wake M, Hesketh K, et al. Health-related quality of life of overweight and obese children. *JAMA.* 2005;293(1):70–76

72. Fink SK, Racine EF, Mueffelmann RE, Dean MN, Herman-Smith R. Family meals and diet quality among children and adolescents in North Carolina. *J Nutr Educ Behav.* 2014;46(5): 418–422

73. Utter J, Denny S, Robinson E, Fleming T, Ameratunga S, Grant S. Family meals and the well-being of adolescents. *J Paediatr Child Health.* 2013;49(11):906–911

74. Golden NH, Schneider M, Wood C; American Academy of Pediatrics Committee on Nutrition, Committee on Adolescence, and Section on Obesity. Preventing obesity and eating disorders in adolescents. *Pediatrics.* 2016;138(3):e20161649

Healthy Use of Media

Yolanda (Linda) Reid Chassiakos, MD

"Pediatric primary care clinicians can not
only help parents coach their children on
media literacy and digital citizenship but also
encourage them to serve as role models for
healthy media choices."

Background

Children and adolescents today are surrounded by and immersed in media, traditional and digital. Television (TV), movies, and video games have been joined by digital media accessed through devices such as tablets, smartphones, and virtual reality headsets; both traditional media and digital media have been integrated into daily life at home and at school. Today's engaging and interactive media bring new risks for health and wellness, such as sexting and cyberbullying, sleep disturbances, problematic Internet use, and Internet gaming disorder; however, evidence-based research also demonstrates benefits to digital media use such as early learning, exposure to new ideas and knowledge, and greater opportunities for social contact and support. Pediatric primary care clinicians (PCCs)—pediatricians, family physicians, internists, nurse practitioners, and physician assistants who provide longitudinal care to children and adolescents—can help families navigate the modern media landscape and develop a family media use plan that can minimize risks and enhance benefits from media use by children, teenagers, and their families.

Traditional vs New Media

Traditional media such as TV, magazines, newspapers, and films were typically created and produced by an external source and passively viewed or read by children and teens. New media, including multiplayer video games, social media, virtual reality, and interactive programs, apps, and Web sites accessed via the Internet, allow users to both consume content and create content. Modern digital media allow users to personalize their media experiences. For children and adolescents today, media options and use have become seamless, blurring the distinctions and boundaries between "types of media." As an example, a "TV show" can now be streamed on a smartphone, which can also facilitate access to a social media site in which "viewers" can actively engage in branded contests or games with other fans or can communicate with the actors and producers of the series. These changes have resulted in new media use patterns among children and adolescents (collectively referred to as *children* in this chapter unless otherwise specified). In 1970, children began watching TV regularly at 4 years of age; today, children begin interacting with digital media at age 4 months.

Media Use Estimates

Data from the National Health and Nutrition Examination Survey (commonly known as NHANES) in 2012 showed that 98.5% of children aged 12 to 15 reported daily TV watching, and 91.1%, daily computer use. Only 27% reported using 2 hours or less of screen time outside of school. However, TV viewing has been significantly displaced by the breadth of digital media available to children and teens. Non-Hispanic white boys showed the greatest decrease in TV viewing from 2001 to 2012, from 2.24 hours of TV per day to 1.59 hours per day.[1] Figure 9-1 shows the percentage of children aged 12 to 15 who report watching TV and using computers daily, correlated with the number of hours of TV and computer use.

According to a Common Sense Media 2011 survey on technology use in 0- to 8-year-olds,[2] 52% could access a mobile device.[2] By 2013, the percentage had risen to 75%. Figure 9-2 identifies screen media time by the platform used.

In 2017, Common Sense Media's Zero to Eight Census showed that digital media use patterns continue to change with the advent of "smart" TVs and expanded internet access.[3] Figure 9-3 compares the evolution of viewing platforms from traditional TV to online/streamed content.

Economic challenges do not seem to preclude digital media use. Kabali et al[4] reported in 2015 that 96.6% of 0- to 4-year-olds in a low-income pediatric clinic had used mobile devices, and three-quarters owned their own devices. However, the Zero-to-Eight study noted that children from higher-income families accessed educational content more often than those from lower-income families did (54% and 28%, respectively).

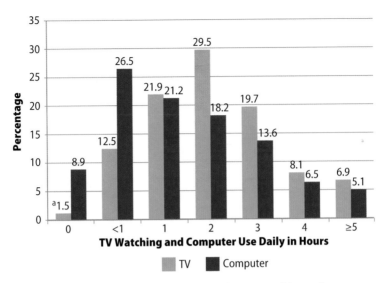

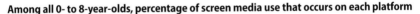

Figure 9-1. Percentage of youth aged 12–15 reporting TV watching and computer use daily, by number of hours: United States, 2012.

[a] Estimate does not meet standards of reliability or precision; relative standard error is greater than 30% but less than 40%.

Note: Access data table for Figure 9-1 at: http://www.cdc.gov/nchs/data/databriefs/db157_table.pdf#1.

Sources: CDC/NCHS, National Health and Nutrition Examination Survey (NHANES) and NHANES National Youth Fitness Survey, 2012.

From Herrick KA, Fakhouri THI, Carlson SA, Fulton JE. TV watching and computer use in U.S. youth aged 12–15, 2012. *NCHS Data Brief*. 2014;(157):1–8.

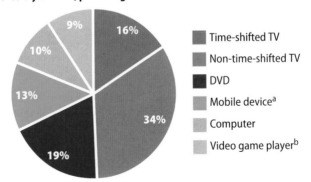

Among all 0- to 8-year-olds, percentage of screen media use that occurs on each platform

Figure 9-2. Screen media time by platform, 2013.

[a] Such as a smartphone or tablet.

[b] Console or handheld.

From Rideout V. *Zero to Eight: Children's Media Use in America*. San Francisco, CA: Common Sense Media; 2013. Reproduced with permission.

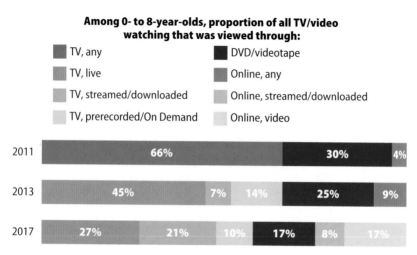

Figure 9-3. TV and video viewing, by delivery, 2011–2017.

Note: Differences between live, streamed/downloaded and prerecorded/OnDemand TV viewing were not measured until 2013, and differences between online viewing of streamed/downloaded content vs. short videos were not measured until 2017.

From Rideout V. *The Common Sense Census: Media Use by Kids Age Zero to Eight.* San Francisco, CA: Common Sense Media; 2017:17.

Social media use rates among children have continued to grow as well. Ninety-nine percent of teens report that they go online daily. More than 95% of teens own a smartphone, 45% report that they are "almost constantly" connected to the Internet, and 44% go online "several times a day."[5] Figure 9-4 shows the frequency of Internet use by adolescents. Fifty percent of teens admit to feeling "addicted" to their phones.[6]

Facebook used to be the most popular social media site for adolescents, but other social media apps, some of which allow temporary posting of photos, videos, or texts, or promise relative anonymity for users, have become more popular (Figure 9-5).

Research shows that girls are drawn to visually oriented social media platforms, whereas boys are attracted by online video games (Figure 9-6). Of teens aged 13 through 17 years, 8 out of 10 have access to a game console (Figure 9-7). Eighty-five percent of teens in households earning less than $30,000 annually now report that they have a game console at home, which has increased from 67% in 2015.[5]

45% of teens say they're online almost constantly
% of U.S. teens who say they use the Internet,
either on a computer or on a cellphone…

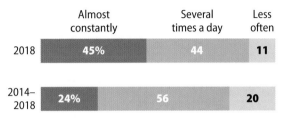

Figure 9-4. Frequency of Internet use by teens.
Note: "Less often" category includes teens who say they use the Internet "about once a day," "several times a week," and "less often."
Source: Pew Research Center survey conducted March 7-April 10, 2018. Trend data from previous Pew Research Center survey conducted 2014-2015.
From Anderson M, Jiang J. Teens, social media and technology 2018. Pew Research Center Web site. http://www.pewinternet.org/2018/05/31/teens-social-media-technology-2018. Published May 31, 2018. Accessed June 4, 2018.

YouTube, Instagram and Snapchat are the most popular online platforms among teens
% of U.S. teens…

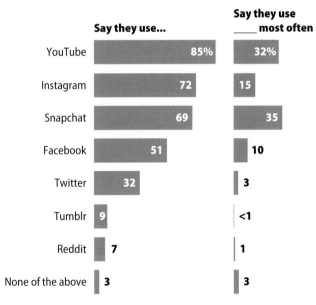

Figure 9-5. Most popular online platforms, by type, among US teens.
Note: Figures in first column add to more than 100% because multiple responses were allowed. Question about most-used site was asked only of respondents who use multiple sites; results have been recalculated to include those who use only one site. Respondents who did not give an answer are not shown.
Source: Pew Research Center survey conducted March 7-April 10, 2018.
From Anderson M, Jiang J. Teens, social media and technology 2018. Pew Research Center Web site. http://www.pewinternet.org/2018/05/31/teens-social-media-technology-2018. Published May 31, 2018. Accessed June 4, 2018.

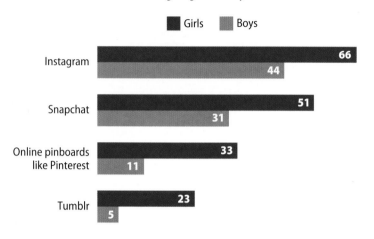

Girls Dominate Visually-Oriented Social Media Platforms
Percentage of girls and boys who use...

■ Girls   ■ Boys

Instagram — Girls 66, Boys 44

Snapchat — Girls 51, Boys 31

Online pinboards like Pinterest — Girls 33, Boys 11

Tumblr — Girls 23, Boys 5

Boys Are More Likely to Play Video Games
Percentage of girls and boys who...

Have or have access to a game console — Girls 70, Boys 91

Play video games online or on their phones — Girls 59, Boys 84

Figure 9-6. Gender variations in digital media use.

Source: Pew Research Center's Teens Relationships Survey, Sept. 25-Oct. 9, 2014 and Feb. 10-Mar. 15, 2015 (n=1,060 teens aged 13 to 17).

From Lenhart A. Teens, social media and technology overview 2015. Pew Research Center Web site. http://www.pewinternet.org/2015/04/09/teens-social-media-technology-2015. Published April 9, 2015. Accessed January 19, 2018.

Benefits of Digital Media

Video chatting can allow families to connect with relatives and friends in distant locations. Co-chatting alongside a parent can help infants and toddlers better communicate and interpret what they are watching on the screen.

Research has shown that, in children aged 3 to 5 years, high-quality TV programs such as *Sesame Street* can improve early social skills as well as

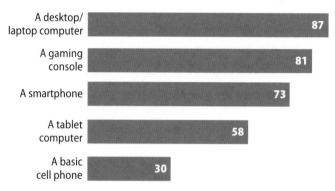

Teens' phone, computer, and console access
% of all teens who have or have access to the following:

Figure 9-7. A majority of US teens report access to a computer, a game console, a smartphone, and a tablet.
Source: Pew Research Center's Teens Relationships Survey, Sept. 25-Oct. 9, 2014 and Feb. 10-Mar. 16, 2015 (n = 1,060 teens aged 13 to 17).

From Lenhart A. Teens, social media and technology overview 2015. Pew Research Center Web site. http://www.pewinternet.org/2015/04/09/teens-social-media-technology-2015. Published April 9, 2015. Accessed January 19, 2018.

promote learning of letters and numbers.[7] These programs also aim to teach families about good health and safety habits. Co-viewing with a parent or caregiver can enhance learning; parents can repeat, discuss, and expand on the media messages face-to-face with their young children.[8]

Digital media can serve as a pathway to new information and ideas for older children and adolescents as well. Children and teens can learn about current events and issues, and they can connect with others online for creative, entertainment, and scholarly activities. Additionally, by developing online networks, facilitated by social media such as Facebook, Twitter, and Instagram, teens can develop empathy. Such networks promote inclusion and a sense of community among adolescents who might otherwise feel excluded or marginalized (eg, adolescents who are lesbian, gay, bisexual, transgender, or questioning).[9]

The Internet's resources can also provide a wealth of information about achieving wellness, as well as about specific, and even rare, medical conditions, to supplement health care visits. Parents and their children with special needs can research medical resources, disabilities services, and assistive technology, and they can participate with other families in online support groups.

Risks of Digital Media to Child Health and Development

Unfortunately, digital media also present potential risks, depending on their type and content, the duration of use, and the age of the child.

Effects on Young Children

Research has shown that excessive TV viewing in childhood is associated with cognitive, language, and social-emotional delays. Viewing of noneducational or non–high-quality content is more likely to result in negative outcomes, such as less impulse control and such as poor self-regulation and poor mental flexibility.[8] Additionally, when the TV is on, fewer parent-child interactions are observed. Screens distract not only children but parents, research has shown. Young children whose parents are focused on their smartphones have been shown to engage in more disruptive behavior as they seek parental attention.[10]

Creators of digital media aimed at young children often seek to make their products distracting, leading to multitasking in children as young as age 4 years. Products, including some e-books with bells and whistles, are often presented as "educational" without supportive research evidence, and they are designed to attract children and keep their attention for extended periods of viewing or engagement.[11]

Violence in the Media

Many programs targeting children contain violent content. Unfortunately, young children, depending on their developmental stages, may be unable to differentiate between virtual violence fantasy and 3-D reality; cartoon characters who are injured or killed on screen arise again unhurt in the next scene, unlike people in "real life." The consequences of risky or dangerous behavior may be misunderstood or underappreciated. Older children can also be negatively affected by virtual violence, although such effects may be subtle and not be recognized or acknowledged.[12] A review and meta-analysis of more than 400 research studies, however, has demonstrated a significant association between exposure to media violence and the development, manifestation, or enhancement (or any combination thereof) of angry feelings, physiologic arousal, and aggressive thoughts and behaviors in children.[13] Another review of 140 studies of video game participation and virtual violence confirmed even greater negative effects.[14] Development and production of high-quality media without violence can provide families with better entertainment options for their children.

Children and Advertising

Young children, as well as older children and adults who have limited media literacy, may be susceptible to targeted marketing and advertising of unhealthy products, including sugary snacks and calorie-laden foods.[15] The Rudd Center for Food Policy and Obesity at UConn reports that children are seeing 57% fewer advertisements for sweet snacks and 37% fewer for cereals and prepared meals; however, exposure to TV advertisements for candy and fast food have risen by 43% and 12%, respectively, in the past decade.[16] Figure 9-8 shows food-related advertising exposure on TV by types of foods and viewer age-groups.

Although advertising of fruits, vegetables, and dairy products has increased in the past few years, Hispanic and black viewers are still exposed to more marketing messages for unhealthy sugar and saturated-fat laden products such as fast foods and sugary drinks that can promote or facilitate health disparities.[17] Figure 9-9 shows the advertisement viewing differences between black and white children and teens.

Older children and teens may also be exposed to advertising[18] for alcohol and e-cigarettes, often in association with other high-risk or unhealthy behaviors. This exposure from TV has been shown to correlate with initiation of such behaviors; TV has been labeled a "super-peer." Researchers are

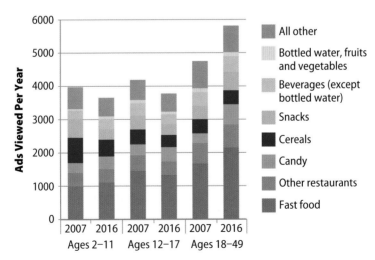

Figure 9-8. Total food-related TV advertising exposure by category.

Source: Nielsen 2017.

From Frazier WC III, Harris JL. *Trends in Television Food Advertising to Young People: 2016 Update.* Hartford, CT: UConn Rudd Center for Food Policy and Obesity; 2017. http://www.uconnruddcenter.org/files/TVAdTrends2017.pdf. Accessed January 19, 2018. Reproduced with permission.

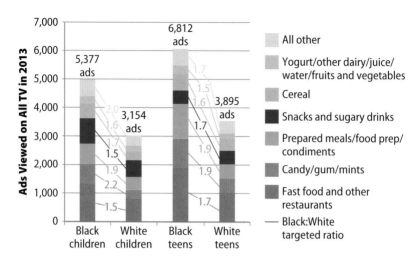

Figure 9-9. Black and white youth exposure to advertising on all TV programming by category.

Source: Nielsen (2015).

From Harris JL, Shehan C, Gross R, et al. *Food Advertising Targeted to Hispanic and Black Youth: Contributing to Health Disparities.* Hartford, CT: UConn Rudd Center for Food Policy and Obesity; 2015. http://www.uconnruddcenter.org/targeted-marketing. Accessed September 27, 2017. Reproduced with permission.

observing similar trends with social media, including alcohol overuse, substance use, self-injury, disordered eating, and high-risk sexual behaviors.

For example, research has identified that major alcohol brands have a strong presence on Facebook, Twitter, and YouTube. Today's technology allows advertisers to use gamification, which applies game elements to attractive sites and apps that integrate advertising and branding with engaging games, information, and activities.[19] The use of cookies that register and store the history of who is participating and returning to a site allows data mining that can be used to target advertising to a specific user, even when the user is surfing on a different Web site. These data can be tied to a specific Internet protocol (commonly known as IP) address, undermining privacy and anonymity. For example, posting content on Facebook about exercise or nutrition can unleash advertisements on diets, exercise equipment, and junk food.

Media and Obesity

One of the most critical risks of digital media use is that this use displaces other activities that are important for healthy growth and development, such as physical activity and exercise. Research has shown that high levels of media use, even in young children, are associated with obesity and long-term cardiovascular risk (Figure 9-10). A recent study in 2-year-olds showed that body mass index (BMI) increased for every hour per week of media consumed.[20] A Dutch study of 4- to 13-year-olds showed that watching TV for more than 1.5 hours per day was a significant risk factor for obesity.[21] A large international study demonstrated that 1 to 3 hours of TV watching resulted in a 10% to 27% increase in obesity risk.[22] Children who have higher BMIs or are more sedentary are at increased risk of remaining overweight or gaining weight. A 1- to 1½-hour cap on TV viewing may help reduce obesity risks.

Media and Sleep

Media use also affects sleep negatively. Research has demonstrated that having a TV, computer, or mobile device in the bedroom is correlated with fewer minutes of sleep, especially among racial/ethnic minority boys when compared with non-Hispanic white boys.[23] Six- to 12-month-olds who were exposed to screen media in the evening had shorter duration of sleep at night.[24] Older children and teens who were greater users of social media or

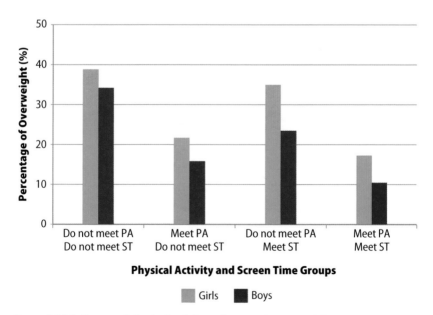

Figure 9-10. Influence of physical activity and screen time on weight.
From Laurson KR, Eisenmann JC, Welk GJ, Wickel EE, Gentile DA, Walsh DA. Combined influence of physical activity and screen time recommendations on childhood overweight. *J Pediatr.* 2008;135(2):209–214. Reproduced with permission.

took their smartphones to bed had more sleep disturbances. Sleep disturbances identified included disrupted sleep, a later sleep time, and fewer total hours of sleep, as well as subsequent daytime dysfunction, which can have a significant negative impact on school performance and mental health.[25]

Media and Mental Health

Excessive media use has also been reported to be associated with mental health concerns in children and teens.[26] There is an opportunity cost when screen time displaces real-life activities that can build self-esteem. Studies have identified an association between Internet and social media use and depression.[27] Depression was more prevalent in teens who passively viewed content, as opposed to teens who posted content and actively communicated with others online.[28]

Children and teens who use media excessively may also develop "problematic Internet use"; those who overuse video games may develop "Internet gaming disorder" (both identified in the fifth edition of the *Diagnostic and Statistical Manual of Mental Disorders* [commonly known as *DSM-5*]). The criteria for these conditions include preoccupation with the Internet or video games, decreased interest in off-line relationships, and difficulty decreasing use with withdrawal symptoms. Four percent to 8% of children and teens may display problematic Internet use,[29] and almost 9%, Internet gaming disorder.[30]

Research on TV viewing in preteens showed that, although white boys exhibited increased self-esteem with greater TV exposure, self-esteem was decreased in white girls and black preteens of both genders.[31] The researchers suggested that the prevalence of positive images for white boys on TV enhanced their self-esteems and promoted perceptions that success was attainable. In contrast, negative stereotypes and representations of girls and minorities were presented as a possible etiology for the negative impacts on self-esteem in the remaining study groups.[31]

Sexting

Traditional media were able to introduce children and teens to inappropriate content, such as high-risk sexual behaviors and violence. Modern digital media offer opportunities for adolescents to themselves initiate dangerous or inappropriate behaviors such as *sexting,* defined as the electronic transmission of nude or seminude images or sexually explicit text messages or both.[32] Twelve percent of 10- to 19-year-olds have admitted sending a sexual photo electronically, often feeling pressured to do so by others. Unfortunately, many teens do not have the experience or skills to resist pressure to send or receive "sexts" or private photos. Surveys of older teens at Children's Hospital Los Angeles reported that half of girls and two-thirds of boys had sent sexts, and 70% of girls and 82% of boys had received a sext.[33] Sexting may precede sexual intercourse, and studies with lesbian, bisexual, and gay teens have found correlations between sexting and the initiation of risky sexual behaviors. Additionally, teens who send or receive sexts may not be aware that photos transmitted of individuals younger than the age of consent may be considered child pornography, and this transmission could lead to prosecution and sex offender status for those convicted.[34] Educating teens about the dangers of sexting and providing them with tools to resist pressure to sext may reduce such risks in today's digital environment.

Privacy and Confidentiality

Children may also not appreciate that content and images posted on the Internet, including social media, can be disseminated widely and remain accessible permanently, despite assurances of "privacy" or the implementation of privacy settings. "Private" photos that have "gone viral" have led to bullying, emotional distress, poor school performance, and, in some cases, suicide. Additionally, an incautious presence on online media can make children vulnerable to contact from sexual predators, who may lie about their ages, genders, and intents to entice their targets.

Cyberbullying

Cyberbullying, using digital media aggressively and repeatedly to bully a vulnerable person, provides new challenges. The attacks are not limited to the school yard; they can reach that person online 24/7, and they can rapidly spread lies, libel, and misinformation to a broad audience in a community and beyond, under cover of anonymity. Sadly, as many as 40% of teens have experienced cyberbullying, and teens orienting or identifying as lesbian, gay, bisexual, transgender, questioning, or intersexual or who have autism spectrum disorder are especially vulnerable. Depression, lower self-esteem, suicidal ideation and suicide are reported consequences of these electronic assaults.[35,36]

Promoting Healthy Use of Media

The Roles of Parents and Caregivers

It is critical for parents and caregivers to familiarize themselves with today's digital media and to understand the benefits and risks of these tools for children and teens. Parents can serve as role models and mentors for their children by using media wisely and in moderation, and they can teach their children age-appropriate digital citizenship. More than a quarter of adults report feeling addicted to their mobile devices; parental screen time pulls parents away from face-to-face communication with their children, results in fewer verbal and nonverbal interactions,[9] and may engender greater parent-child conflicts.[37] Using TV to "calm" misbehaving children is ineffective. Using media to "babysit" reduces adult-child interactions. Adults can incorporate media into their time with children if they co-read e-books, co-view quality programs, or co-use educational apps with their children; they can also use these opportunities to repeat and discuss the presented information and increase their children's media literacy (see the section on Media Literacy). Parents can also set limits on the extent of media use (eg, by pausing an e-book at the end of each chapter and encouraging children to return to real, in-person play). Most important, parents are encouraged by pediatric PCCs, as well as nonprofit organizations promoting children's health and wellness, to "unplug" instead and directly engage with their children, including at family mealtimes, every day. For example, child health advocates Common Sense Media promotes their Device-Free Dinner campaign at www.commonsensemedia.org/device-free-dinner with helpful tips for families to encourage healthy choices regarding media use.

The Role of Health Care Professionals

Pediatric PCCs and other health care professionals can provide helpful guidance and resources to families seeking to use media in healthy and beneficial ways. The American Academy of Pediatrics (AAP) has developed its family media use plan (www.healthychildren.org/English/media/Pages/default.aspx) with which clinicians and parents can work together to develop guidelines for media use that are customized to the needs of each child in the family. The family media use plan allows each family to carve out time for the healthy necessities for every child, ensuring that schoolwork, physical activity, unplugged family mealtimes, and adequate sleep are priorities before entertainment media use. To assist clinicians in these efforts, the AAP has provided a Media and Children Communication Toolkit at www.aap.org/en-us/advocacy-and-policy/aap-health-initiatives/pages/media-and-children.aspx.

Unfortunately, less than 20% of pediatricians ask parents and caregivers about family media use. The AAP Bright Futures materials have provided 2 questions (specific for each child's age-group) that PCCs can ask to assess media use and begin the conversation about healthy media habits. In

November 2016, the AAP presented 2 new policies updating research findings about the risks and benefits of digital media use, along with recommendations for health care professionals, families, researchers, and advocates to promote healthy media use. An updated AAP policy on virtual violence was released in August 2016. The AAP has also provided resources for parents, including "Healthy Digital Media Use Habits for Babies, Toddlers and Preschoolers," available at www.healthychildren.org/English/family-life/Media/Pages/Healthy-Digital-Media-Use-Habits-for-Babies-Toddlers-Preschoolers.aspx, and "How to Connect With Your Teen About Smart and Safe Media Use" at www.healthychildren.org/English/family-life/Media/Pages/Points-to-Make-With-Your-Teen-About-Media.aspx.

Recommendations from the AAP for pediatric PCCs include

For young children
► Educate parents about brain development in the early years and the importance of hands-on, unstructured, and social play to build language, cognitive, and social-emotional skills.
► For newborns, infants, and children younger than 18 months, discourage use of screen media other than video chatting.
► For parents of children 18 to 24 months of age who want to introduce digital media, advise that they choose high-quality programming and apps and use them together with children, because this is how toddlers learn best. Letting children use media by themselves should be avoided.
► Infants and children, especially children younger than 6 years, need to be protected from virtual violence. Parents should understand that young children do not always distinguish fantasy from reality. Cartoon violence can seem very real, and it can have detrimental effects.
► Guide parents to resources for finding quality products (eg, Common Sense Media, PBS Kids, Sesame Workshop).
► For children older than 2 years, limit media to 1 hour or less per day of high-quality programming. Recommend shared use between parent and child to promote enhanced learning, greater interaction, and limit setting.

For school-aged children and teens
► Recommend no screens during meals and for 1 hour before bedtime.
► Problem-solve with parents facing challenges, such as setting limits, finding alternative activities, and calming children. (Serve as role models.)
► Work with families and schools to promote understanding of the benefits and risks of media.

▶ Promote adherence to guidelines for adequate physical activity and sleep via a family media use plan (www.HealthyChildren.org/MediaUsePlan).

▶ Be aware of tools to screen for sexting, cyberbullying, problematic Internet use, and Internet gaming disorder.

▶ First-person shooter games, in which killing others is the central theme, are not appropriate for children. Teens should limit play to games that are rated acceptable for their age-group; however, families are encouraged to avoid violent content and first-person shooter games for all age-groups.

▶ Advocate for and promote information and training in media literacy.

Media Literacy

Media education can reduce harmful media effects by educating children and adults about how to effectively interpret media messages and decipher message goals. By understanding the purpose of a media message, and by accessing, analyzing, and evaluating media products, readers or viewers can make healthier choices and reduce the negative impact of media images and content.

A media-educated individual recognizes that "all media messages are constructed; media messages shape our understanding of the world; individuals interpret media messages uniquely; and mass media has powerful economic implications." He or she can develop critical thinking skills, make positive media choices, and limit the use of media or substitute creative alternatives to minimize negative effects. Evidence-based research has provided confirmation that media education reduces viewer vulnerability for children and teens.[38]

Advocacy

The November 2016 AAP policies recommend that research be continued on the benefits and risks of a breadth of digital media and that legislators and educators be informed about research findings to update guidelines for healthy and effective media use. Researchers and clinicians should also partner with developmental psychologists and educators as well as content creators and producers to design developmentally appropriate interfaces that promote shared parent-child media use and application of learned skills to the "real world." Products should be scientifically evaluated before claims of educational benefit are presented. Products should also be affordable, and they should address and reflect the cultural diversity of our population. Finally, health care professionals can advocate, locally and nationally, for the elimination of advertising and unhealthy messages directed at children on Web sites and apps, because young children cannot differentiate between advertisements and facts and older children may lack media literacy skills to prevent vulnerability to targeted media messages.

Additionally, pediatric advocates can encourage the entertainment industry to develop and produce products that do not contain or promote violence. Verbal or physical assaults should not be presented gratuitously or in ways that trivialize their serious, dangerous, and negative effects.

Summary

The media landscape continues to evolve. More research is needed to fully understand the effects of media use, both positive and negative, on infants, children, and teens, as well as families and communities. We know that excessive media use can displace healthy activities necessary for growth, learning, and wellness, such as adequate sleep, exercise and physical play, and face-to-face communication. We also know that both inappropriate or overuse of media and problematic Internet use can have other adverse health effects, such as depression, weight gain, poor self-esteem, disordered eating, and poor sleep hygiene. In this era of personalized media experiences, pediatric health care professionals can help parents and caregivers prevent or minimize negative media effects and promote positive media benefits by developing a family media use plan that is specific for each child or teen and attends to children's and teens' developmental stages, educational and health needs, and temperaments. Pediatric PCCs can not only help parents coach their children on media literacy and digital citizenship but also encourage them to serve as role models for healthy media choices.

Acknowledgments: Thanks to AAP Fellows Dimitri Christakis, Corinn Cross, David Hill, Megan Moreno, Jenny Radesky, and Vic Strasburger for their valued contributions.

AAP Policy

American Academy of Pediatrics Council on Communications and Media. Media and young minds. *Pediatrics.* 2016;138(5):e20162591 (pediatrics.aappublications.org/content/138/5/e20162591)

American Academy of Pediatrics Council on Communications and Media. Media use in school-aged children and adolescents. *Pediatrics.* 2016;138(5):e20152592 (pediatrics.aappublications.org/content/138/5/e20162592)

American Academy of Pediatrics Council on Communications and Media. Virtual violence. *Pediatrics.* 2016;138(2):e20161298 (pediatrics.aappublications.org/content/early/2016/07/14/peds.2016-1298)

Reid Chassiakos YL, Radesky J, Christakis D, Moreno MA, Cross C; American Academy of Pediatrics Council on Communications and Media. Children and adolescents and digital media. *Pediatrics*. 2016;138(5):e20162593 (pediatrics.aappublications.org/content/138/5/e20162593)

References

1. Loprinzi PD, Davis RE. Secular trends in parent-reported television viewing among children in the United States, 2001-2012. *Child Care Health Dev*. 2016;42(2):288–291
2. Rideout V. *Zero to Eight: Children's Media Use in America*. San Francisco, CA: Common Sense Media; 2011
3. Common Sense Media. *The Common Sense Census: Media Use by Kids Age Zero to Eight*. https://www.commonsensemedia.org/research/the-common-sense-census-media-use-by-kids-age-zero-to-eight-2017. Accessed January 19, 2018
4. Kabali HK, Irigoyen MM, Nunez-Davis R, et al. Exposure and use of mobile media devices by young children. *Pediatrics*. 2015;136(6):1044–1050
5. Anderson M, Jiang J. Teens, social media and technology 2018. Pew Research Center Web site. http://www.pewinternet.org/2018/05/31/teens-social-media-technology-2018. Published May 31, 2018. Accessed June 4, 2018
6. Technology addiction: concern, controversy, and finding a balance. Common Sense Media Web site. https://www.commonsensemedia.org/research/technology-addiction-concern-controversy-and-finding-balance. Accessed January 19, 2018
7. Nathanson AI, Aladé F, Sharp ML, Rasmussen EE, Christy K. The relation between television exposure and executive function among preschoolers. *Dev Psychol*. 2014;50(5):1497–1506
8. Barr R. Memory constraints on infant learning from picture books, television, and touchscreens. *Child Dev Perspect*. 2013;7(4):205–210
9. Moreno MA, Gannon KE. Social media and health. *Adolesc Med State Art Rev*. 2013;24(3):538–552
10. Radesky JS, Kistin CJ, Zuckerman B, et al. Patterns of mobile device use by caregivers and children during meals in fast food restaurants. *Pediatrics*. 2014;133(4):e843–e849
11. Bus AG, Takacs ZK, Kegel CAT. Affordances and limitations of electronic storybooks for young children's emergent literacy. *Dev Rev*. 2015;35:79–97
12. American Academy of Pediatrics Committee on Communications and Media. Virtual violence. *Pediatrics*. 2016;138(2):e20161298
13. Bushman BJ, Huesmann LR. Short-term and long-term effects of violent media on aggression in children and adults. *Arch Pediatr Adolesc Med*. 2006;160(4):348–352
14. Anderson CA, Shibuya A, Ihori N, et al. Violent video game effects on aggression, empathy, and prosocial behavior in eastern and western countries: a meta-analytic review. *Psychol Bull*. 2010;136(2):151–173
15. Fleming-Milici F, Harris JL. Television food advertising viewed by preschoolers, children and adolescents: contributors to differences in exposure for black and white youth in the United States. *Pediatr Obes*. 2016;13(2):103–110
16. Frazier WC III, Harris JL. *Trends in Television Food Advertising to Young People: 2016 Update*. Hartford, CT: UConn Rudd Center for Food Policy and Obesity; 2017. http://www.uconnruddcenter.org/files/TVAdTrends2017.pdf. Accessed January 19, 2018
17. Harris JL, Shehan C, Gross R, et al. *Food Advertising Targeted to Hispanic and Black Youth: Contributing to Health Disparities*. Hartford, CT: UConn Rudd Center for Food Policy and Obesity; 2015. http://www.uconnruddcenter.org/targeted-marketing. Accessed January 19, 2018
18. Elsey JW, Harris JL. Trends in food and beverage television brand appearances viewed by children and adolescents from 2009 to 2014 in the USA. *Public Health Nutr*. 2016:19(11):1928–1933

19. Kim B. The popularity of gamification in the mobile and social era. *Libr Technol Rep.* 2015;51(2):5–9

20. Wen LM, Baur LA, Rissel C, Xu H, Simpson JM. Correlates of body mass index and overweight and obesity of children aged 2 years: findings from the healthy beginnings trial. *Obesity (Silver Spring).* 2014;22(7):1723–1730

21. de Jong E, Visscher TL, HiraSing RA, Heymans MW, Seidell JC, Renders CM. Association between TV viewing, computer use and overweight, determinants and competing activities of screen time in 4- to 13-year-old children. *Int J Obes (Lond).* 2013;37(1):47–53

22. Braithwaite I, Stewart AW, Hancox RJ, Beasley R, Murphy R, Mitchell EA; ISAAC Phase Three Study Group. The worldwide association between television viewing and obesity in children and adolescents: cross sectional study. *PLoS One.* 2013;8(9):e74263

23. Cespedes EM, Gillman MW, Kleinman K, Rifas-Shiman SL, Redline S, Tavares EM. Television viewing, bedroom television, and sleep duration from infancy to mid-childhood. *Pediatrics.* 2014;133(5):e1163–e1171

24. Vijakkhana N, Wilaisakditipakorn T, Ruedeekhajorn K, Pruksananonda C, Chonchaiya W. Evening media exposure reduces night-time sleep. *Acta Pediatr.* 2015;104(3):306–312

25. Bruni O, Sette S, Fontanesi L, Baiocco R, Laghi F, Baumgartner E. Technology use and sleep quality in preadolescence and adolescence. *J Clin Sleep Med.* 2015;11(12):1433–1441

26. Moreno MA, Jelenchick L, Koff R, Eickhoff J. Depression and Internet use among older adolescents: an experience sampling approach. *Psychology.* 2012;3(9A):743–748

27. Lin LY, Sidani JE, Shensa A, et al. Association between social media use and depression among U.S. young adults. *Depress Anxiety.* 2016;33(4):323–331

28. Kross E, Verduyn P, Demiralp E, et al. Facebook use predicts declines in subjective well-being in young adults. *PLoS One.* 2013;8(8):e69841

29. Jelenchick LA, Eickhoff J, Christakis DA. The Problematic and Risky Internet Use Screening Scale (PRIUSS) for adolescents and young adults: scale development and refinement. *Comput Human Behav.* 2014;35

30. Lemmens JS, Valkenburg PM, Gentile DA. The Internet Gaming Disorder Scale. *Psychol Assess.* 2015;27(2):567–582

31. Martins N, Harrison K. Racial and gender differences in the relationship between children's television use and self-esteem: a longitudinal panel study. *Commun Res.* 2012;39(3):338–357

32. McGee JB, Begg M. What medical educators need to know about "Web 2.0." *Med Teach.* 2008;30(2):164–169

33. Moreno MA, Ton A, Selkie E, Evans Y. Secret Society 123: understanding the language of self-harm on Instagram. *J Adolesc Health.* 2016;58(1):78–84

34. Ybarra ML, Mitchell KJ. "Sexting" and its relation to sexual activity and sexual risk behavior in a national survey of adolescents. *J Adolesc Health.* 2014;55(6):757–764

35. Vaillancourt T, Brittain HL, McDougall P, Duku E. Longitudinal links between childhood peer victimization, internalizing and externalizing problems, and academic functioning: developmental cascades. *J Abnorm Child Psychol.* 2013;41(8):1203–1215

36. Selkie E, Kota R, Moreno M. Relationship between cyberbullying experiences and depressive symptoms in female college students. *J Adolesc Health.* 2014;54(2):S28

37. Radesky J, Miller AL, Rosenblum KL, Appugliese D, Kaciroti N, Lumeng JC. Maternal mobile device use during a structured parent-child interaction task. *Acad Pediatr.* 2015;15(2):238–244

38. Five key questions form foundation for media inquiry. Center for Media Literacy Web site. http://www.medialit.org/reading-room/five-key-questions-form-foundation-media-inquiry. Accessed January 19, 2018

Healthy Active Living

Claire M. A. LeBlanc, MD; Gary S. Goldfield, PhD; and
Mark S. Tremblay, PhD, CSEP-CEP

"There is strong evidence to show that sleep,
sedentary behavior, physical activity, and
physical and emotional health outcomes are
interrelated, often bidirectionally."

Background

The World Health Organization defines *health* as a state of complete physical, mental, and social well-being.[1] Thus, primary care clinicians (PCCs) (pediatricians, family physicians, internists, nurse practitioners, and physician assistants who provide frontline care to children and adolescents) should not only address disease but also promote healthy lifestyles. Unfortunately, poor nutrition, inadequate sleep, increasing sedentary behavior, and declining physical activity have resulted in rising pediatric obesity rates and a drop in physical fitness, with adverse physical and emotional health consequences that extend into adulthood. This chapter will help PCCs modify patient and family lifestyles using a 24-hour movement model that integrates promotion of healthy physical activity with themes presented in earlier chapters: healthy sleep (Chapter 7), healthy weight (Chapter 8), and healthy use of media (Chapter 9).

Inadequate Sleep

Sleep has been described as an opportunity for the brain to rest and recover. Research shows that sleep duration in the pediatric age-group has decreased over time by an average of 70 minutes per night throughout the 20th century. An Australian study of more than 4,000 children, adolescents, and young adults aged 9 to 18 years reported that sleep durations decreased with age at a rate of 12 minutes per night per year of age on school nights.[2] American adolescent sleep time is declining, with 15-year-olds (especially girls) sleeping less than 7 hours per night. Although the underlying reasons are unknown, speculation suggests that television (TV) or small screen devices in the bedroom, as well as increased Internet and social media use, may be at play.[3] Insufficient sleep has been associated with a wide range of physical and psychosocial health deficits. Children and adolescents lacking adequate sleep duration or quality have demonstrated impaired academic performance, high-risk behaviors, mental health problems, substance use, and an increased risk of obesity. This relationship is likely bidirectional, as mental disorders, substance use, and obesity may also affect sleep.[4]

Sedentary Behavior

Children and adolescents are increasingly sedentary, with such behaviors promoted by widespread exposure to electronic entertainment technologies, automobile transport, and mechanized living. A recent systematic review of children and adolescents aged 5 to 17 years from 235 studies representing more than 1.6 million participants from 71 different countries showed that, in addition to increasing risk of obesity, higher duration or frequency of screen time, primarily in the form of TV viewing, computer use, or playing video games (or any combination of those activities), was associated with poorer health indicators. These included reduced cardiorespiratory fitness, increased cardiometabolic disease risk, unfavorable behavioral conduct, decreased prosocial behavior, and diminished self-esteem.[5] Screen time behaviors were higher in 13- to 18-year-olds, lower socioeconomic status families, and those with bedroom TV sets, indicating that these populations are more vulnerable to the deleterious effects of excessive screen use. See Chapter 9, Healthy Use of Media, for a robust discussion of media use and its contribution to sedentary behavior. However, higher duration or frequency of reading or doing homework was associated with greater academic achievement, highlighting that the type of sedentary behavior may differentially affect the health and development of children and adolescents.

Inadequate Physical Activity

Most young children accumulate insufficient unstructured free play at home and in family- or center-based child care. Few states have policies and standards to ensure that child care centers contribute to this age-group's achievement of national physical activity guidelines and centers' achievement of national standards for safe outdoor play areas and equipment.[6,7]

School-aged children are also not sufficiently active, and fitness scores have dropped over the past 30 years.[8] According to the 2012 National Health and Nutrition Examination Survey (commonly known as NHANES) report, 16.9% of American children and teens have obesity and an additional 14.9%, overweight.[9] The 2012 National Youth Fitness Survey found that only 25% of 12- to 15-year-olds engaged in moderate-vigorous physical activity for 60 minutes daily. Additionally, the proportion with adequate cardiorespiratory fitness decreased from 52% to 42% from 1999–2000 to 2012, respectively.[10] Physical education recommendations from Healthy People 2010 include 150 minutes per week for elementary students and 225 minutes per week for middle and high school students; however, implementation of these guidelines is inconsistent. Indeed, "No Child Left Behind" elementary schools devote more daily instructional time to reading (47%) and mathematics (37%) and less time to physical education (35%) and recess (28%).[11] School boards often justify such reductions on the grounds that more time at school being physically active will detract from academic achievement, but research suggests otherwise.[12]

In the United States from 1969 to 2001, there was a 68% reduction in the number of children who walked or biked to school.[13] Barriers to active transportation include harsh climate; lack of sidewalks, bike trails, and crosswalks; traffic and safety dangers; and geographic separation of living, working, education, shopping, and leisure activities. Since the 1970s, children have lost about 12 hours per week of free time, which includes a 25% decrease in play and 50% reduction in unstructured outdoor activities.[14] Time spent outdoors increases physical activity levels, yet many children have poor access to parks and open spaces.[15,16] Accessible parks may be underused because they lack playgrounds or sport fields or because they have poor aesthetics, inadequate maintenance, or other safety issues.[12]

Participation in organized sport and recreation programs also increases physical activity. Only 58% of high school students joined at least one school or community-based sports team in 2015 and participation was lower among older students and female students.[17] Cost, sport availability and variety, peer support, peer pressure, and parental time commitments may adversely influence participation. Free recreation facilities are often lacking in low-income communities.[18] Children who are overscheduled and those who are not involved in or dislike sports may be less engaged. Children with a disability often have poor access to affordable quality recreational facilities.[19,20]

Psychosocial Contributors to Unhealthy Living

Stressed or distressed children are more prone to overeating, anxiety, and depression.[21] Chronic stress can also lead to poor sleeping habits, persistent tiredness, and a reluctance to engage in regular physical activity, thereby exacerbating these mental health issues.[21] In turn, stress can stimulate neuroendocrine responses that may promote intra-abdominal adiposity, insulin resistance, and metabolic syndrome through excessive cortisol production.[22,23] Examples of major life stressors include parental separation or divorce, bullying, physical or mental maltreatment or abuse, and living in foster care with frequent placement changes. However, school deadlines, conflict with peers, and other common environmental stressors can accumulate to induce the aforementioned psychobiological responses.

Children and adolescents with obesity represent a population at increased risk of poorer physical and emotional health outcomes.[24] Affected children who also experience bullying, depression, and low self-esteem will have even more difficulty meeting wellness goals. Children and adolescents from economically disadvantaged homes are more likely to fall into unhealthy lifestyle patterns characterized by physical inactivity, poor nutrition, and increased obesity risk.[25]

One source of stress or distress in children and adolescents with obesity is dissatisfaction with body image. This dissatisfaction is defined as the discrepancy between an individual's perceived self-image and the desired image, often internalized by the societal idealized images portrayed in the media.[26,27] More than 50% of children and adolescents report this phenomenon. Most children and adolescents with obesity are dissatisfied with their body weights or shapes, making body dissatisfaction one of the most reliable psychosocial correlates of pediatric obesity.[28] Body-image disturbance is important to identify because it increases the risk of disordered eating practices, which adversely affect weight and healthy active living, which, in turn, exacerbate body-image issues, thereby creating a vicious cycle.

One of the biggest contributors to mental health issues in children and adolescents living with obesity is the prevalence of *weight bias* (defined as the tendency to make unfair judgments based on a person's weight).[29,30] It may lead to bullying, discrimination, and social marginalization, predisposing children and adolescents to stay indoors and further exacerbating anxiety, depression, and other indicators of mental health conditions. It is difficult to facilitate a healthy active lifestyle aimed at improving physical and emotional health outcomes if an unfairly stigmatized child is not identified and well supported. Research has shown that many physicians and health care practitioners hold the same societal weight biases, and this tendency can adversely affect patient care; thus, medical educators, residents, and pediatricians need to bring more sensitivity to treating this population.[31]

Quality of life is another key measure PCCs should address. This measure is low in children and adolescents with obesity and can be associated with poor sleep habits caused by obstructive sleep apnea.[29,32] Children and adolescents with obesity also measure lower than those without obesity on self-esteem scores related to physical self-perception and physical quality of life.[33] Such perceived deficits are often associated with poor physical activity skill development. Both factors can interact and manifest as barriers to participation in games or sports.[34] Low scores on perceived physical competence are consistently associated with reduced physical activity and increased sedentary behavior in children and adolescents.[34]

Health Benefits of Healthy Active Living

Adequate Sleep

Sleep is necessary to provide restoration of molecular, cellular, or network changes that occur in the preceding waking hours. It appears to play an active role in such processes as memory, emotional regulation, metabolic functions and energy balance, and removal of toxic substances and metabolic wastes.[35] Increased sleep duration is associated with lower adiposity indicators, better emotional regulation, and improved quality of life in school-aged children and adolescents. In addition, this age-group demonstrates better academic achievement with longer sleep times.[36]

Limiting Screen Time

It is likely that reducing screen time for newborns, infants, and toddlers will lower obesity rates, improve sleep hygiene, and promote good health and psychosocial development. These outcomes are most likely achieved if parents spend quality time in an interactive format with their young children.[37] In addition, toddlers and preschoolers are more likely to have better attention and language skills with less media exposure and more time being read to by a parent.[38] They also tend to engage in more creative playtime.[38] School-aged children may gain access to valuable support networks through social media, but this possibility should be weighed against the likelihood of experiencing hostile communications, including cyberbullying. Reducing older children and adolescents' screen time has been shown to have a positive impact on sleep quality and duration and also leads to healthier behaviors.[39] Research on school-aged children and adolescents suggests that lower durations or frequencies of screen time and TV viewing are significantly associated with favorable measures of body composition, enhanced fitness, and lower cardiometabolic risk scores. Reduced durations of TV viewing and video game playing are associated with better behavioral conduct and prosocial behaviors. Greater lengths of time spent reading and doing homework outside of school are significantly associated with higher academic achievement, whereas less screen time and computer use are associated with better self-esteem.[5]

Regular Physical Activity

The health benefits of habitual aerobic physical activity include weight reduction or maintenance, improved body composition, lower blood pressure, improved dyslipidemia, reduced biomarkers of inflammation and atherosclerosis, and enhanced self-concept and other indicators of mental wellness.[40] Other benefits include reduction in insulin resistance, risk for type 2 diabetes, nonalcoholic steatohepatitis, and sleep-disordered breathing.[19] Experts suggest that exergaming (playing active computer games) may be a suitable replacement for sedentary activities if the whole body is moved, but evidence is mixed on whether cardiorespiratory fitness improves. Indeed, these indoor screen-based activities should not replace outdoor active play, physical education, or sports.[41]

Strength, anaerobic, high-impact, skill-based, and flexibility exercises provide many other health benefits. Although bone mass is largely determined by genotype, weight-bearing physical activity can enhance bone mass acquisition and structural adaptation during childhood and adolescence.[42,43] Weight training improves neuromuscular learning and muscle and bone strength in both sexes during puberty.[44] Team sports can lead to new skill acquisition, increased self-confidence, and better problem-solving and conflict resolution.[45] Growing children and those with neuromuscular disabilities require stretching programs to improve flexibility and prevent injury.[46] Most children and adolescents with chronic disease can benefit from a variety of exercises and physical activities.[47] At school, all students should have regular access to physical education classes and recess to develop the physical skills necessary to play sports and optimize each child's and adolescent's cognitive, social, physical, and emotional development.[48]

As demonstrated previously, there is strong evidence to show that sleep, sedentary behavior, physical activity, and physical and emotional health outcomes are interrelated, often bidirectionally. In recognition of this complex pattern, Canada and other countries have moved away from individual health behavior guidelines in favor of a more integrated approach, such as the Canadian 24-Hour Movement Guidelines for Children and Youth: An Integration of Physical Activity, Sedentary Behavior, and Sleep.

24-Hour Movement Recommendations

While the importance of a good night's sleep, reducing extended sedentary behavior, and increasing habitual physical activity levels are generally universally accepted and promoted, it is less common to provide counseling for all these movement behaviors in an integrated fashion that respects the inherent interactions among these behaviors. Recently, the Canadian 24-Hour Movement Guidelines were released in an effort to overcome the traditional approach of segregating rather than integrating counseling related to healthy movement behaviors.[49] Such an approach provides greater clinical flexibility in dealing with lifestyle-related issues. For example, when counseling a child with obesity, rather than simply recommending the child get more physical activity, a more nuanced approach may be to understand the child's sleep behaviors and provide guidance on healthy sleep hygiene, leading to a more restful sleep, more energy the next day, and a greater likelihood of receptivity to messages to be more active and to reduce screen time.

Background research from a systematic review and from novel compositional analyses revealed that the health benefits of physical activity, sedentary behavior, and sleep are interdependent, such that "the whole day matters."[50,51] For example, the potential beneficial effects of 60 minutes of exercise will be significantly influenced by how sedentary the child is through the rest of the day and how well the child slept the night before. Efforts should be made to counsel families to understand and appreciate what a healthy day looks like (Figure 10-1). Tools to assist implementing an integrated approach include "Build Your Best Day" at www.buildyourbestday.com, "Caring for Kids" at www.caringforkids.cps.ca, and "ParticipACTION" at www.participaction.com/en-ca/home.

The current American Academy of Pediatrics recommendations discourage media use by children younger than 2 years and advise limiting recreational screen time for 2- to 5-year-olds to less than 1 hour per day.[38] School-aged children and adolescents should also limit recreational screen time to less than 2 hours per day and accumulate (in small increments) at least 60 minutes of moderate to vigorous physical activity per day.[20,52] Healthy sleep parameters vary with age, as outlined in Chapter 7, Healthy Sleep. American national physical activity guidelines are under review, and updated versions will be released in 2018. Ideally, physical activities would include enjoyable group and individual activities through sport, recreation, transportation, chores, and planned exercise. Activities

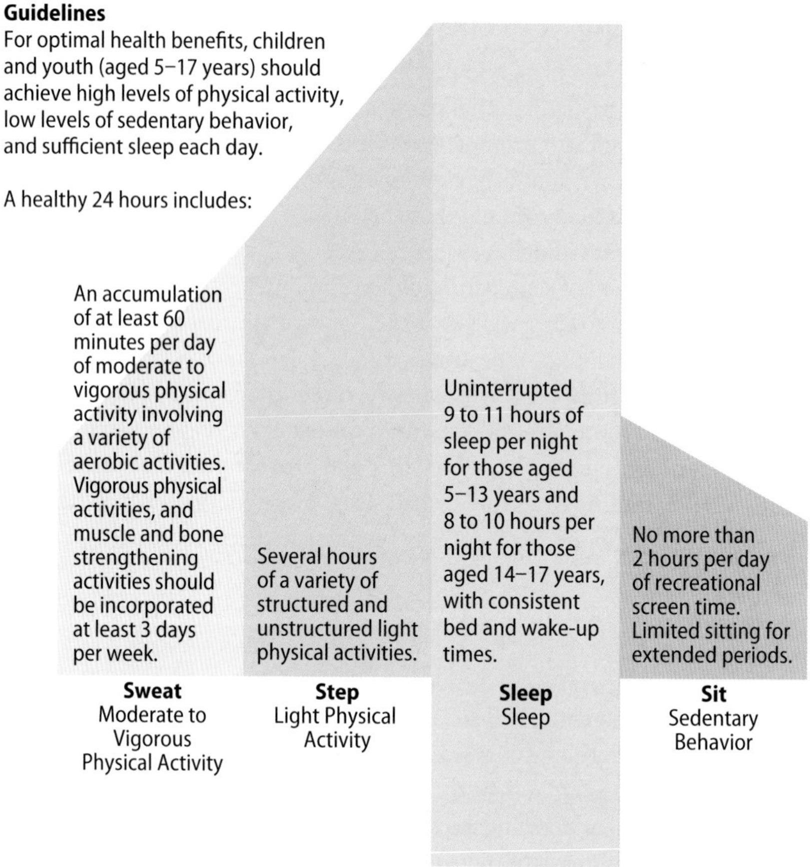

Guidelines

For optimal health benefits, children and youth (aged 5–17 years) should achieve high levels of physical activity, low levels of sedentary behavior, and sufficient sleep each day.

A healthy 24 hours includes:

An accumulation of at least 60 minutes per day of moderate to vigorous physical activity involving a variety of aerobic activities. Vigorous physical activities, and muscle and bone strengthening activities should be incorporated at least 3 days per week.

Several hours of a variety of structured and unstructured light physical activities.

Uninterrupted 9 to 11 hours of sleep per night for those aged 5–13 years and 8 to 10 hours per night for those aged 14–17 years, with consistent bed and wake-up times.

No more than 2 hours per day of recreational screen time. Limited sitting for extended periods.

Sweat
Moderate to Vigorous Physical Activity

Step
Light Physical Activity

Sleep
Sleep

Sit
Sedentary Behavior

Preserving sufficient sleep, trading indoor time for outdoor time, and replacing sedentary behaviors and light physical activity with additional moderate to vigorous physical activity can provide greater health benefits.

Figure 10-1. Canadian 24-Hour Movement Guidelines for Children and Youth: An Integration of Physical Activity, Sedentary Behaviour, and Sleep.
From the Canadian Society for Exercise Physiology. Reproduced with permission.

should be structured (eg, organized sports) and unstructured (free play). Safety should be a priority through the use of appropriate protective equipment, adult supervision, and the promotion of fair play. (For resources to assist parents, see "Let's Move!" at https://letsmove. obamawhitehouse.archives.gov.) Specific recommendations (Table 10-1) should be age and developmentally appropriate.[19]

Table 10-1. Physical Activity for Children and Adolescents

Age-group	Physical Activity	Skills	Activity/Sports
Newborns and infants (0–12 mo)	Be active for short periods several times a day.	Physical activity should promote movement skill development.	• Active play with caregivers, especially through fun floor-based activities • Tummy time, reaching, pushing, pulling, and crawling
Toddlers (1–2 y) Preschoolers (3–5 y)	• At least 60 min, up to several hours, of physical activity through the day. Should include unorganized free play. At least 30 min should be structured. • Young children should accumulate at least 60 min of structured energetic play (moderate to vigorous intensity).	• Limited balance and fundamental skills. Very short attention span. • Learn by trial and error. • Farsighted, difficulty tracking + judging velocity of moving objects.	• Toddlers should develop movement skills, explore their environment, and try new things. • Young children should develop fundamental motor skills for future sports. • Playing tag, tumbling, dancing, throwing, and catching. Start swimming from at least 4 years of age.
Children (6–9 y)	At least 60 min of physical activity with moderate to vigorous intensity every day, including • Vigorous-intensity activities at least 3 days a week • Activities that strengthen muscle and bone at least 3 days a week	• Fundamental skills improving. Posture + balance becoming more automatic. Improved reaction time. • Beginning transitional skills. • Short attention span. Limited memory and rapid decision-making.	• A variety of fun activities. • Sports should have short instruction times, have flexible rules, offer free time in practices, and focus on fun. • Playing tag, soccer, baseball, gymnastics, skating, and skiing.
Children (10–12 y)	At least 60 min of physical activity with moderate to vigorous intensity every day, including • Vigorous-intensity activities at least 3 days a week • Activities that strengthen muscle and bone at least 3 days a week • Regular flexibility exercises	• Fully developed visual tracking, balance, and motor skills • Improved transitional skills • Can understand some sport tactics and strategy	• A variety of fun activities • Fun team sports by maturity, not age • Basketball, football, and martial arts • Weight training using small free weights, high repetitions, proper technique, and appropriate supervision

Table 10-1. Physical Activity for Children and Adolescents (*continued*)

Age-group	Physical Activity	Skills	Activity/Sports
Teens (13–17 y)	At least 60 min of physical activity with moderate to vigorous intensity every day, including • Vigorous-intensity activities at least 3 days a week • Activities that strengthen muscle and bone at least 3 days a week • Regular flexibility exercises	• Fun, preferred variety of activities, including friends • Lifelong physical activity	• A variety of fun activities. • Personal fitness, active transportation, household chores, workplace-related activity, and competitive and noncompetitive sports. • Contact and collision sports based on size and ability, not age. Keep it fun. • Weight training: longer sets using heavier weights; proper technique and appropriate supervision.

Derived from Harris SS, Anderson SJ, eds. *Care of the Young Athlete.* 2nd ed. Elk Grove Village, IL: American Academy of Pediatrics; 2009; and Hagan JF Jr, Shaw JS, Duncan PM, eds. *Bright Futures Guidelines for Health Supervision of Infants, Children, and Adolescents.* 4th ed. Elk Grove Village, IL: American Academy of Pediatrics; 2017.

Active Healthy Living Strategies: Implications for Practice

Primary care clinicians can assess children's and adolescents' lifestyle risks for chronic disease by identifying sleep patterns, unhealthy eating tendencies, sedentary behaviors, and physical activity habits and by calculating and plotting body mass index (commonly known as BMI).[53] Active healthy living promotion begins with a baseline individual and family history, which can be obtained through administering waiting area surveys. Estimating current sleep hygiene, sedentary behavior, and physical activity levels; discovering existing barriers to healthy active living; and assessing the individual's self-efficacy to make change are essential.[54,55] (See Table 10-2.) (See also Chapter 2, Family-Centered Care: Applying Behavior Change Science.)

Working With Families in the Clinical Setting

Parenting plays a pivotal role in the promotion of healthy active living, which includes the formation of psychosocial vitality.[21] Responsibilities include role modeling healthy habits, setting limits, purchasing healthy foods for family consumption, being active together, and managing time

Table 10-2. Office-Based Strategies to Increase Physical Activity

Physical Activities	Strategies to Improve
Ask about existing family physical activity routines and other lifestyle-related activities.	Place active living posters and educational information in waiting areas. Recommend the use of the Build Your Best Day interactive Web site, designed to promote healthy 24-h movement behaviors (www.buildyourbestday.com).
Tabulate amounts of daily physical activity in all settings: home, school, work, transportation, recreation, dance, outside play, and organized and unorganized sports.	Age-specific exercise prescription using a 24-h movement approach and ensuring appropriate sleep and sedentary time. When applicable, include moderate-vigorous and vigorous intensities, bone + muscle strengthening. Promote outdoor play.
Determine whether adequate parental role modeling is occurring.	Post photos or posters in office demonstrating active families. Suggest family-based activities.
Determine access to free play, parks, and green spaces.	Identify and promote nearby open spaces and recreation centers. Increase school physical activity.
Determine access to sport and recreation programs.	Promote affordable recreation centers. Increase physical activity at school.
Determine child/adolescent access to high-quality school physical education.	Advocate for compulsory quality daily physical education (kindergarten through grade 12) taught by qualified trained educators.
Establish family and child/adolescent levels of active transportation.	Promote walking and biking, especially to and from school daily.
Determine whether time barriers exist to physical activity participation.	Encourage increasing incidental movement, taking breaks from inactivity and from sitting for long periods, walking throughout the day, and taking the stairs.
Determine whether safety barriers exist to physical activity participation.	Suggest working out or dancing in the home, a community recreation facility, or school recreation programs before, during, or after school. Recommend neighborhood supervision for outdoor activities.
Determine child/adolescent preferred recreation or sport.	Recommend preferred sport or recreational activity, especially activities that promote energetic play.
Determine whether sport enjoyment and ability are barriers to participation.	Promote enjoyable activities with friend or older buddy (eg, walking, dancing, swimming). Pedometers or exergaming may be motivational.
Determine whether overweight or low fitness is a barrier to participation.	Decrease inactivity. Start slow with 10-min bouts of physical activity with light intensity. Encourage enrolling in an after-school or a community program to learn a new skill. Suggest considering water-based sports or strength training, with less focus on competition.
Assess need for more personalized and ongoing guidance.	Refer to qualified exercise professional (eg, certified exercise physiologist).

Derived from Perrin EM, Finkle JP, Benjamin JT. Obesity prevention and the primary care pediatrician's office. *Curr Opin Pediatr.* 2007;19(3):354–361; and Harris SS, Anderson SJ, eds. *Care of the Young Athlete.* 2nd ed. Elk Grove Village, IL: American Academy of Pediatrics; 2009.

and money effectively. Families may require a concrete medical reason to increase the motivation to change existing behaviors.[21] This reason might be illness in the child (high blood pressure, insulin resistance, fatty liver, musculoskeletal condition such as Blount disease or slipped capital femoral epiphysis, or fracture) or a family history of cardiovascular disease or diabetes.[56] Sometimes children are already participating in sport but are being pushed too hard by parents to excel, which can result in an aversion to sport and exercise.[57] These children and adolescents may become more sedentary because of burnout or disillusionment and may abandon any form of physical activity.[57] Primary care clinicians need to help educate parents to be nonjudgmental in the promotion of wellness for their children.[21]

Social adversities experienced by the family may negatively affect a child's sleep pattern and strain parental resources (eg, time, money, and energy), making healthy eating and regular physical activity more challenging. Identifying family stressors (eg, limited finances, separation or divorce, physical or mental abuse, other adverse social determinants) before embarking on healthy active living counseling allows appropriate primary care intervention or referral to a mental health specialist and a greater likelihood of behavior change.

The focus should be on helping an entire family become healthier. Reinforcing existing family strengths and supports helps families meet their goals. Two key strategies are to determine whether changing family behavior is a priority and to determine how confident the parent is about achieving the necessary changes. Primary care clinicians need to convey their confidence that a family can achieve a healthier lifestyle. Tabulating all family members' current sleep habits, sedentary behaviors, and physical activities through work and play provides a good base from which to start. Sleep quantity can be gathered and compared with age norms provided by the American Academy of Sleep Medicine.[58] Sleep quality can be assessed in children older than 2 years using the BEARS Sleep Screening Algorithm. (See Chapter 7, Healthy Sleep, for the algorithm.) Advising parents how to improve sleep hygiene can follow. Sedentary behaviors might be characterized using the SITT (sedentary behavior frequency, interruptions, time, and type) formula to get a true estimate of total inactivity.[59] Counseling parents on how to set limits on screen time is key.[55] Activity promotion can start by identifying all barriers the family may have to becoming more active and developing strategies to overcome these obstacles. Subsequent action plans might include encouraging parents to become more active themselves and including all members of the family, especially with infants, toddlers, or preschoolers in the home; ensuring children play more outside; and supporting children in developmentally appropriate and age-appropriate sports and recreational activities using standard safety measures (see Table 10-2).

Parents can then be encouraged to select the area of the 24-hour movement guidelines they wish to focus on initially. Visualizing the entire day in activity time portions makes it easier to see that the relationships between sleep, sedentary behavior, and physical activity are interactive, and modifying one has an impact on the others (see Figure 10-1). Should the parents want to begin by improving their child's sleep, they will need to get the child off the couch and away from screens to engage the child in regular, heart-pumping physical activity. Similarly, improving sleep hygiene alone might lead to the child's feeling more energetic and being able to spend a greater portion of time the following day being more physically active.

Behavior Change Strategies and Tools for Primary Care Clinicians

Inactive children and adolescents may not be ready to adopt an active lifestyle and may resist change. Addressing all barriers to change, including emotional factors such as underlying bullying, anxiety, depression, and low self-esteem, is important before developing an action plan. Motivational interviewing is defined as a person-centered, goal-oriented method of communicating that elicits and strengthens intrinsic motivation for positive change. It may elicit and strengthen the patient's intrinsic incentive to identify reasons to change behavior and move toward agreed-on goals.[60,61] (See Chapter 2, Family-Centered Care: Applying Behavior Change Science.) Children and adolescents typically have little concern for any future health benefits of good sleep hygiene, reducing screen time, and adopting regular physical activity; hence, emphasis should be placed on the immediate and short-term rewards. These rewards might include feeling less tired, increasing energy levels, having fun, spending time with friends, improving endurance for sports and hobbies, feeling stronger and getting more muscular, and improving self-image.

After a patient is engaged, the patient should be encouraged to identify a particular goal within the 24-hour movement guidelines (see Figure 10-1) that he or she wishes to target first. Many young people may not realize that they are not sleeping well, often because of screen-based media devices in their bedrooms. The presence of screens has a direct impact on sleep quantity and quality, and it can affect their energy levels the following day. (See Chapter 9 on healthy use of media and Chapter 7 on healthy sleep.) Improving sleep alone can lead to increased physical activity as a result of feeling well rested and having more energy.

Individual sedentary behavior and physical activity prescriptions can be written to reflect agreements reached with the patient on incremental steps. Sedentary behaviors can be reduced using the SITT formula, that is, reducing the most common sedentary activity duration and frequency and increasing the number of interruptions during sedentary time. Physical activity and exercise prescriptions can employ the FITT (frequency, intensity, time, and type) formula. Prescriptions can specify the frequency (daily), intensity (moderate to vigorous), time (accumulate ≥60 minutes), and type (variety of primarily aerobic activities with some strengthening and vigorous-intensity exercise) of activity.[46] Should a PCC require assistance with patient evaluation or prescription, consultation with an exercise specialist or a certified exercise physiologist may be useful. Specific prescriptions ideally promote the child's or adolescent's favorite types of physical activity. These can be integrated into the daily schedule in ways that make them fun, easy, natural, and desirable; can be done with family and friends; involve unstructured and structured play; and can include sports that promote equal participation, enjoyment, safety, and nonviolence.

Primary care clinicians should collaborate with patients and families to find practical interpersonal strategies to approach lifestyle changes. Families should be praised for positive changes, no matter how small, in the achievement of better sleep and physical activity times using the 24-hour movement guidelines. Counseling on the improvement of sleep hygiene and the reduction of recreational screen time may be made easier with the family media use plan teaching tool. (See Chapter 9, Healthy Use of Media.) This tool provides information about the benefits and health risks of both traditional media and new media.[37] A resource used to identify health-related quality of life is the Sizing Them Up score. This resource addresses emotional and physical functioning, teasing, marginalization, positive social attitudes, mealtime challenges, and school functioning.[62]

Motivational interviewing and other evidence-based communication techniques can be incorporated into the office visit. (See Chapter 2, Family-Centered Care: Applying Behavior Change Science.) These techniques are especially useful for individuals who are less confident about their ability to change existing behaviors. Combining supportive and empathetic counseling with more directive methods, PCCs can help these patients move from ambivalence to commitment to adoption of healthier active lifestyles.[60,61] Development of a personal action plan using the Behavior Change Model (assess, advise, agree, assist, and arrange) is a valuable tool for PCCs (Figure 10-2).

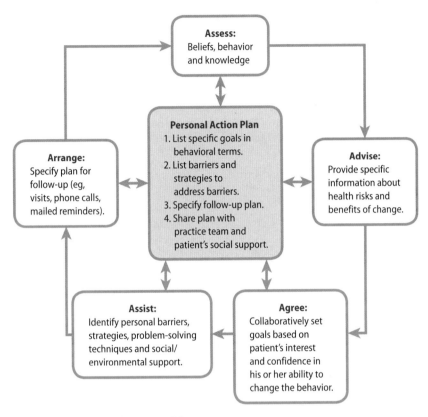

Figure 10-2. Behavior change model.
From US Preventive Services Task Force. 5 A's Behavior Change Model. https://www.uspreventive
servicestaskforce.org/Home/GetFileByID/440. Accessed May 21, 2018. Derived from Glasgow RE, et
al. Self-management aspects of the improving chronic illness care breakthrough series: implementation with diabetes and heart failure teams. *Ann Behav Med.* 2002;24(2):80–87; and Whitlock EP, et al.
Evaluating primary care behavioral counseling interventions: an evidence-based approach. *Am J Prev
Med.* 2002;22(4):267–284.

AAP Policy

American Academy of Pediatrics Adolescent Sleep Working Group, Committee on
Adolescence, and Council on School Health. School start times for adolescents.
Pediatrics. 2014;134(3):642–649 (pediatrics.aappublications.org/content/134/3/642)

American Academy of Pediatrics Committee on Communications. Children, adolescents, and advertising. *Pediatrics.* 2006;118(6):2563–2569. Reaffirmed March 2010
(pediatrics.aappublications.org/content/118/6/2563)

American Academy of Pediatrics Committee on Environmental Health. The
built environment: designing communities to promote physical activity in
children. *Pediatrics.* 2009;123(6):1591–1598. Reaffirmed January 2013 (pediatrics.
aappublications.org/content/123/6/1591)

American Academy of Pediatrics Council on Communications and Media. Children, adolescents, obesity, and the media. *Pediatrics.* 2011;128(1):201–208 (pediatrics. aappublications.org/content/128/1/201)

American Academy of Pediatrics Council on Communications and Media. Media and young minds. *Pediatrics.* 2016;138(5):e20162591 (pediatrics.aappublications.org/content/138/5/e20162591)

American Academy of Pediatrics Council on Communications and Media. Media use in school-aged children and adolescents. *Pediatrics.* 2016;138(5):e20152592 (pediatrics.aappublications.org/content/138/5/e20162592)

American Academy of Pediatrics Council on Communications and Media. Virtual violence. *Pediatrics.* 2016;138(2):e20161298 (pediatrics.aappublications.org/content/138/2/e20161298)

American Academy of Pediatrics Council on Early Childhood. Literacy promotion: an essential component of primary care pediatric practice. *Pediatrics.* 2014;134(2): 404–409 (pediatrics.aappublications.org/content/134/2/404)

American Academy of Pediatrics Council on Early Childhood, Committee on Psychosocial Aspects of Child and Family Health, and Section on Developmental and Behavioral Pediatrics. Addressing early childhood emotional and behavioral problems. *Pediatrics.* 2016;138(6):e20163023 (pediatrics.aappublications.org/content/138/6/e20163023)

American Academy of Pediatrics Council on School Health. The crucial role of recess in school. *Pediatrics.* 2013;131(1):183–188. Reaffirmed August 2016 (pediatrics. aappublications.org/content/131/1/183)

American Academy of Pediatrics Council on Sports Medicine and Fitness. Strength training by children and adolescents. *Pediatrics.* 2008;121(4):835–840. Reaffirmed June 2011 (pediatrics.aappublications.org/content/121/4/835)

Daniels SR, Hassink SG; American Academy of Pediatrics Committee on Nutrition. The role of the pediatrician in primary prevention of obesity. *Pediatrics.* 2015;136(1): e275–e292 (pediatrics.aappublications.org/content/136/1/e275)

Golden NH, Abrams SA; American Academy of Pediatrics Committee on Nutrition. Optimizing bone health in children and adolescents. *Pediatrics.* 2014;134(4):e1229–e1243 (pediatrics.aappublications.org/content/134/4/e1229)

Golden NH, Schneider M, Wood C; American Academy of Pediatrics Committee on Nutrition, Committee on Adolescence, and Section on Obesity. Preventing obesity and eating disorders in adolescents. *Pediatrics.* 2016;138(3):e20161649 (pediatrics. aappublications.org/content/138/3/e20161649)

Owens J; American Academy of Pediatrics Adolescent Sleep Working Group and Committee on Adolescence. Insufficient sleep in adolescents and young adults: an update on causes and consequences. *Pediatrics.* 2014;134(3):e921–e932 (pediatrics. aappublications.org/content/134/3/e921)

Paruthi S, Brooks LJ, D'Ambrosio C, et al. Recommended amount of sleep for pediatric populations: a consensus statement of the American Academy of Sleep Medicine. *J Clin Sleep Med.* 2016;12(6):785–786. AAP endorsed (www.aasmnet.org/Resources/pdf/Pediatricsleepdurationconsensus.pdf)

References

1. Preamble to the constitution of the World Health Organization. *Off Rec World Health Organ.* 1948;(2):100
2. Olds T, Maher C, Blunden S, Matricciani L. Normative data on the sleep habits of Australian children and adolescents. *Sleep.* 2010;33(10):1381–1388
3. Keyes KM, Maslowsky J, Hamilton A, Schulenberg J. The great sleep recession: changes in sleep duration among US adolescents, 1991–2012. *Pediatrics.* 2015;135(3):460–468
4. Owens J; American Academy of Pediatrics Adolescent Sleep Working Group and Committee on Adolescence. Insufficient sleep in adolescents and young adults: an update on causes and consequences. *Pediatrics.* 2014;134(3):e921–e932
5. Carson V, Hunter S, Kuzik N, et al. Systematic review of sedentary behaviour and health indicators in school-aged children and youth: an update. *Appl Physiol Nutr Metab.* 2016; 41(6)(suppl 3):S240–S265
6. McWilliams C, McWilliams C, Ball SC, et al. Best-practice guidelines for physical activity at childcare. *Pediatrics.* 2009;124(6):1650–1659
7. Cradock AL, O'Donnell EM, Benjamin SE, Walker E, Slining M. A review of state regulations to promote physical activity and safety on playgrounds in child care centers and family child care homes. *J Phys Act Health.* 2010;7(suppl 1):S108–S119
8. Tremblay MS, Shields M, Laviolette M, Craig CL, Janssen I, Connor Gorber S. Fitness of Canadian children and youth: results from the 2007-2009 Canadian Health Measures Survey. *Health Rep.* 2010;21(1):7–20
9. Fryar CD, Carroll MD, Ogden CL. Prevalence of overweight and obesity among children and adolescents: United States, 1963–1965 through 2011–2012. Centers for Disease Control and Prevention Web site. https://www.cdc.gov/nchs/data/hestat/obesity_child_11_12/obesity_child_11_12.htm. Updated September 19, 2014. Accessed January 22, 2018
10. Gahche J, Fakhouri T, Carroll DD, Burt VL, Wang CY, Fulton JE. Cardiorespiratory fitness levels among U.S. youth aged 12–15 years: United States, 1999–2004 and 2012. *NCHS Data Brief.* 2014;(153):1–8
11. Steinberger J, Daniels SR, Eckel RH, et al. Progress and challenges in metabolic syndrome in children and adolescents: a scientific statement from the American Heart Association Atherosclerosis, Hypertension, and Obesity in the Young Committee of the Council on Cardiovascular Disease in the Young; Council on Cardiovascular Nursing; and Council on Nutrition, Physical Activity, and Metabolism. *Circulation.* 2009;119(4):628–647
12. Donnelly JE, Hillman CH, Castelli D, et al. Physical activity, fitness, cognitive function and academy achievement in children: a systematic review. *Med Sci Sports Exerc.* 2016;48(6): 1197–1222
13. Rodriguez DA. Active transportation: making the link from transportation to physical activity and obesity. Active Living Research Web site. http://activelivingresearch.org/active-transportation-making-link-transportation-physical-activity-and-obesity. Published June 2009. Accessed January 22, 2018
14. McCurdy LE, Winterbottom KE, Mehta SS, Roberts JR. Using nature and outdoor activity to improve children's health. *Curr Probl Pediatr Adolesc Health Care.* 2010;40(5):102–117
15. Tremblay MS, Gray C, Babcock S, et al. Position statement on active outdoor play. *Int J Environ Res Public Health.* 2015;12(6):6475–6505

16. Gray C, Gibbons R, Larouche R, et al. What is the relationship between outdoor time and physical activity, sedentary behaviour, and physical fitness in children? A systematic review. *Int J Environ Res Public Health.* 2015;12(6):6455–6474

17. Kann L, McManus T, Harris WA, et al. Youth Risk Behavior Surveillance—United States, 2015. *MMWR Surveill Summ.* 2016;65(6):1–174

18. Mowen AJ, Baker BL. Park, recreation, fitness, and sport sector recommendations for a more physically active America: a white paper for the United States national physical activity plan. *J Phys Act Health.* 2009;(6)(suppl 2):S236–S244

19. Lipnowski S, LeBlanc CM; Canadian Paediatric Society Healthy Active Living and Sports Medicine Committee. Healthy active living: physical activity guidelines for children and adolescents. *Paediatr Child Health.* 2012;17(4):209–212

20. American Academy of Pediatrics Council on Sports Medicine and Fitness and Council on School Health. Active healthy living: prevention of childhood obesity through increased physical activity. *Pediatrics.* 2006;117(5):1834–1842

21. Nieman P, LeBlanc CM; Canadian Paediatric Society Healthy Active Living and Sports Medicine Committee. Psychosocial aspects of child and adolescent obesity. *Paediatr Child Health.* 2012;17(4):205–208

22. Goldfield GS, Moore C, Henderson K, Buchholz A, Obeid N, Flament MF. Body dissatisfaction, dietary restraint, depression, and weight status in adolescents. *J Sch Health.* 2010;80(4):186–192

23. Dion J, Hains J, Vachon P, et al. Correlates of body dissatisfaction in children. *J Pediatr.* 2016; 171:202–207

24. Braet C, Van Strien T. Assessment of emotional, externally induced and restrained eating behaviour in nine to twelve-year-old obese and non-obese children. *Behav Res Ther.* 1997; 35(9):863–873

25. Singh GK, Kogan MD, Siahpush M, van Dyck PC. Independent and joint effects of socioeconomic, behavioral, and neighborhood characteristics on physical inactivity and activity levels among US children and adolescents. *J Community Health.* 2008;33(4):206–216

26. Tatangelo G, McCabe M, Mellor D, Mealey A. A systematic review of body dissatisfaction and sociocultural messages related to the body among preschool children. *Body Image.* 2016;18: 86–95

27. Quick V, Eisenberg ME, Bucchianeri MM, Neumark-Sztainer D. Prospective predictors of body dissatisfaction in young adults: 10-year longitudinal findings. *Emerg Adulthood.* 2013; 1(4):271–282

28. Washington RL. Childhood obesity: issues of weight bias. *Prev Chronic Dis.* 2011;8(5):A94

29. Puhl RM, Latner JD. Stigma, obesity, and the health of the nation's children. *Psychol Bull.* 2007;133(4):557–580

30. Schwartz MB, Chambliss HO, Brownell KD, Blair SN, Billington C. Weight bias among health professionals specializing in obesity. *Obes Res.* 2003;11(9):1033–1039

31. Phelan SM, Puhl RM, Burke SE, et al. The mixed impact of medical school on medical students' implicit and explicit weight bias. *Med Educ.* 2015;49(10):983–992

32. Schwimmer JB, Burwinkle TM, Varni JW. Health-related quality of life of severely obese children and adolescents [comment]. *JAMA.* 2003;289(14):1813–1819

33. Morgan PJ, Okely AD, Cliff DP, Jones RA, Baur LA. Correlates of objectively measured physical activity in obese children. *Obesity (Silver Spring).* 2008;16(12):2634–2641

34. Haga M. Physical fitness in children with high motor competence is different from that in children with low motor competence. *Phys Ther.* 2009;89(10):1089–1097

35. Vyazovskiy VV. Sleep, recovery, and metaregulation: explaining the benefits of sleep. *Nat Sci Sleep.* 2015;7:171–184

36. Chaput JP, Gray CE, Poitras VJ, et al. Systematic review of the relationships between sleep duration and health indicators in school-aged children and youth. *Appl Physiol Nutr Metab.* 2016;41(6)(suppl 3):S266–S282

37. American Academy of Pediatrics Council on Communications and Media. Media and young minds. *Pediatrics.* 2016;138(5):e20162591

38. American Academy of Pediatrics Council on Communications and Media. Media use by children younger than 2 years. *Pediatrics.* 2011;128(5);1040–1045

39. Reid Chassiakos Y, Radesky J, Christakis D, Moreno MA, Cross C; American Academy of Pediatrics Council on Communications and Media. Children and adolescents and digital media. *Pediatrics.* 2016;138(5):e1–e18

40. Poitras VJ, Gray CE, Borghese MM, et al. Systematic review of the relationships between objectively measured physical activity and health indicators in school-aged children and youth. *Appl Physiol Nutr Metab.* 2016;41(6)(suppl 3):S197–S239

41. Daley AJ. Can exergaming contribute to improving physical activity levels and health outcomes in children? *Pediatrics.* 2009;124(2):763–771

42. Janz KF, Burns TL, Levy SM, et al. Everyday activity predicts bone geometry in children: the Iowa Bone Development Study. *Med Sci Sports Exerc.* 2004;36(7):1124–1131

43. Golden NH, Abrams SA; American Academy of Pediatrics Committee on Nutrition. Optimizing bone health in children and adolescents. *Pediatrics.* 2014;134(4):e1229–e1243

44. McCambridge TM, Stricker PR; American Academy of Pediatrics Council on Sports Medicine and Fitness. Strength training by children and adolescents. *Pediatrics.* 2008;121(4):835–840

45. Landry GL. Benefits of sports participation. In: Harris SS, Anderson SJ, eds. *Care of the Young Athlete.* 2nd ed. Elk Grove Village, IL: American Academy of Pediatrics; 2009

46. Murphy NA, Carbone PS; American Academy of Pediatrics Council on Children With Disabilities. Promoting the participation of children with disabilities in sports, recreation, and physical activities. *Pediatrics.* 2008;121(5):1057–1061

47. Philpott J, Houghton K, Luke A; Canadian Paediatric Society Healthy Active Living and Sports Medicine Committee, Canadian Academy of Sport Medicine Paediatric Sport and Exercise Medicine Committee. Physical activity recommendations for children with specific chronic health conditions: juvenile idiopathic arthritis, hemophilia, asthma and cystic fibrosis. *Paediatr Child Health.* 2010;15(4):213–225

48. American Academy of Pediatrics Council on School Health. The crucial role of recess in school. *Pediatrics.* 2013;131(1):183–188

49. Tremblay MS, Carson V, Chaput JP, et al. Canadian 24-hour movement guidelines for children and youth: an integration of physical activity, sedentary behaviour, and sleep. *Appl Physiol Nutr Metab.* 2016;41(6)(suppl 3):S311–S327

50. Saunders TJ, Gray CE, Poitras VJ, et al. Combinations of physical activity, sedentary behaviour and sleep: relationships with health indicators in school-aged children and youth. *Appl Physiol Nutr Metab.* 2016;41(6)(suppl 3):S283–S293

51. Carson V, Tremblay MS, Chaput JP, Chastin SF. Associations between sleep duration, sedentary time, physical activity, and health indicators among Canadian children and youth using compositional analyses. *Appl Physiol Nutr Metab.* 2016;41(6)(suppl 3):S294–S302

52. American Academy of Pediatrics Council on Communications and Media. Children, adolescents, and the media. *Pediatrics.* 2013;132(5):958–961

53. Daniels SR, Hassink SG; American Academy of Pediatrics Committee on Nutrition. The role of the pediatrician in primary prevention of obesity. *Pediatrics.* 2015;136(1):e275–e292

54. Perrin EM, Finkle JP, Benjamin JT. Obesity prevention and the primary care pediatrician's office. *Curr Opin Pediatr.* 2007;19(3):354–361

55. Mindell JA, Owens JA. *A Clinical Guide to Pediatric Sleep: Diagnosis and Management of Sleep Problems.* Philadelphia, PA: Lippincott Williams & Wilkins; 2003

56. Carlson SA, Fulton JE, Lee SM, et al. Influence of limit-setting and participation in physical activity on youth screen time. *Pediatrics.* 2010;126(1):e89–e96

57. Brenner JS; American Academy of Pediatrics Council on Sports Medicine and Fitness. Overuse injuries, overtraining, and burnout in child and adolescent athletes. *Pediatrics.* 2007;119(6):1242–1245

58. Paruthi S, Brooks LJ, D'Ambrosio C, et al. Recommended amount of sleep for pediatric populations: a consensus statement of the American Academy of Sleep Medicine. *J Clin Sleep Med.* 2016;12(6):785–786

59. Tremblay MS, Colley RC, Saunders TJ, Healy GN, Owen N. Physiological and health implications of a sedentary lifestyle. *Appl Physiol Nutr Metab.* 2010;35(6):725–740

60. Hettema J, Steele J, Miller WR. Motivational interviewing. *Annu Rev Clin Psychol.* 2005;1: 91–111

61. Miller WR, Rose GS. Toward a theory of motivational interviewing. *Am Psychol.* 2009;64(6): 527–537

62. Modi AC, Zeller MH. Validation of a parent-proxy, obesity-specific quality-of-life measure: sizing them up. *Obesity (Silver Spring).* 2008;16(12):2624–2633

Violence Prevention

Marlene D. Melzer-Lange, MD

"Research has demonstrated the effectiveness
of focused guidance in encouraging parental
use of alternatives to corporal punishment
and awareness of the effects of television
violence during early childhood."

Understanding Violence

Violence is recognized by the World Health Organization (WHO) as a leading worldwide public health problem. The WHO defines violence as the
"intentional use of physical force or power, threatened or actual, against
oneself, [against] another person, or against a group or community that
either results in or has a high likelihood of resulting in injury, death,
psychologic harm, maldevelopment or deprivation."[1] While many parents
worry about strangers hurting their children, most violence occurs when
friends or family members argue or fight. Thus, it is to the child's home,
school, and peer groups that the most attention should be given. Also,
violence or the threat of violence may affect a child's school attendance and
educational success. According to the Centers for Disease Control and
Prevention, 6% of US high school students reported staying home from
school at least 1 day in the past month out of fear of violence.[2]

It is important as a pediatric primary care clinician (PCC) (ie, pediatrician, family physician, internist, nurse practitioner, or physician assistant
providing frontline care to children and adolescents) to guide parents to help
their *children* (a term used in this chapter to encompass both children and
adolescents unless otherwise specified) learn nonviolent problem-solving
skills. By providing parents with ways that they can raise children who do
not use violence to solve their frustrations, PCCs are practicing primary
violence prevention. In addition, parents can help reduce the risk of serious
violence through attention to the child's environment, that is, by decreasing

exposure to media and domestic violence and by decreasing access to firearms. Parents can encourage a nonviolent attitude by resisting toys that promote violence, such as toy guns, violent video games, and toys that encourage racial or ethnic stereotypes. Primary care clinician counseling around violence-related issues has been demonstrated to be effective.[3-5]

Opportunities to Prevent Violence

Aggression naturally increases during early childhood; parents serve to temper and redirect these impulses before school entry.[6,7] It is likely that the foundations of antisocial behavior may begin with coercive or inadequate parenting in early childhood. Children whose parents are unable to set effective limits, particularly in households where corporal punishment is extensively used, develop dysfunctional behavior patterns in interactions with their peers and with adult authorities, including teachers. These children then have behavioral problems even before they enter school. In school, they are rejected by peers and have difficulties academically. In later childhood and adolescence, these ostracized children find each other and form peer groups that reward violence and antisocial behavior.[8,9]

In violent urban settings, children may find themselves in situations during which fighting seems to be customary, and perhaps necessary. Boys, in particular, may feel that they need to fight to be respected and safe. Understanding how to negotiate one's safety in communities where violence is prevalent is an important skill. Primary care clinicians play an important role in developing resiliency in their young patients in these urban settings.[10]

Primary care clinicians have a significant role in promoting peaceful, nonviolent children and adolescents. The 2009 American Academy of Pediatrics (AAP) policy statement on the role of pediatricians in youth violence prevention describes the clinical implications of a far-reaching model that traces the origins of violent behavior to earliest childhood.[11] Use of Connected Kids: Safe, Strong, Secure anticipatory guidance program (https://patiented.solutions.aap.org/DocumentLibrary/Connected%20 Kids%20Clinical%20Guide.pdf) encourages the development of resilience as a means of preventing child abuse and youth violence.[12] Much of this material is incorporated in the fourth edition of *Bright Futures: Guidelines for Health Supervision of Infants, Children, and Adolescents*.[13] Tools for parents are available from the AAP, including such handouts as "Discipline and Your Child" and "Teaching Good Behavior: Tips on How to Discipline" at https://patiented.solutions.aap.org and "How to Handle Anger" at www.brightfutures.org/mentalhealth/pdf/families/mc/handle_ anger.pdf.

Although many social and environmental factors place children at high risk for violence, countervailing resilience factors, many beginning in early childhood, help reduce the risk.

Witnessing Domestic Violence

Witnessing violence in the home may lead to long-term health consequences[14] because of the influence of toxic stress on the growing brain.[15] One of the goals of the PCC in speaking to families with new babies should be to assess family functioning, including the risk for domestic violence. Because the prevalence of domestic violence for women is highest during pregnancy and the first year following birth, PCCs have an opportunity to assist parents at this vulnerable time. Screening all parents for domestic violence in a direct but confidential manner is appropriate. See Appendix 2 for a description of tools useful to PCCs for this purpose. The PCC should have information available in the office concerning domestic violence advocates, shelters, legal aid resources, and safety plans. For resources, see the National Health Resource Center on Domestic Violence Web site (http://ipvhealth. org). Many offices place small cards with relevant telephone numbers in the restroom so this information can be obtained discreetly.[16]

Witnessing Television Violence

Children in the United States spend more time watching television (TV) than in any other activity except sleep. While watching TV, they observe an enormous amount of violence: the average child will see, on TV, more than 10,000 deaths resulting from violence before completing high school.[17] New media, including interactive games and mobile platforms, contribute to the high levels of violence exposure among children.[18] However, many Americans resist the idea that exposure to violence in the media may be associated with subsequent violent behavior.[19] Television violence differs from real-life violence in quality and quantity. On TV, violence is used by both heroes and villains. As a result, young viewers generally view violence as socially acceptable behavior.

Children, because they have more difficulty separating facts from fantasy, are even more likely to be affected by TV violence. The American Psychological Association, in reviewing hundreds of research studies, has concluded that exposure to TV violence is a major risk for children.[20] Children who view violent TV are more likely to experience violence as victims or aggressors and are much less likely to intervene in tense situations, as bystanders, to reduce the likelihood of violence.

The AAP Council on Communications and Media recommends that PCCs counsel families to reduce the amount of TV viewed by young children (aged 0–8 years). Both TV and its influence on children are discussed further in Chapter 9, Healthy Use of Media.

Violence Counseling for Families in High-risk Urban Communities

Neighborhood effects[21] profoundly influence rates of violence, as young people develop strategies for living in violent neighborhoods and adopt behaviors that conform to their perceived social norms.[22] Ethnographic research conducted in poor urban neighborhoods has identified another pattern of violence in which fighting and the willingness to fight are key components of a broader protective strategy for coping with extremely dangerous environments. Young people have observed that individuals who are unable to defend themselves are likely to fall prey to multiple and repeated attacks. Parents also understand this phenomenon and encourage their children to stand up for themselves by becoming able fighters.[8] Other parents adopt protective strategies that keep their children out of harm's way in the first place, often by enrolling them in supervised after-school programs or keeping them safely in the house rather than risking participation in the street culture.

A hopeful sense for the future promotes positive development in children but is challenging in urban environments where violence, racism, and poverty may dash that hope. Adverse childhood experiences (ACEs) with an expanded (community-level) ACE showed that community-level factors such as violence affect youths.[23] In counseling patients in these communities, PCCs need to be aware of community assets and leaders who may benefit young people. Using the strengths of urban neighborhoods to promote hope and resiliency for its young people is an important strategy. Primary care clinicians should be aware of resources such as youth centers, faith-based institutions, and recreation centers that may boost the hope of their young patients.

It is important to remember that these same communities also contain nonviolent problem-solvers who are well-known to their peers. Thus, the reality of the code of the streets need not prevent individual children and adolescents from avoiding violent injuries through avoiding the culture of violence.

Young Children

Primary Prevention: Anticipatory Guidance

During the newborn period, infancy, and early childhood, patterns of behavior and family interactions are established. The proper role of the PCC is to ameliorate risk factors and reinforce factors that protect the child from harm. In this age-group, the following topics should be addressed when providing anticipatory guidance to parents: reduction in exposure to violence, including both domestic violence and TV violence, and teaching appropriate, nonviolent methods of discipline (violence-free parenting). Because patients and families see their PCCs often during this period, opportunities for brief, focused interventions are numerous. Research has demonstrated the effectiveness of focused guidance in encouraging parental use of alternatives to corporal punishment and awareness of the effects of TV violence during early childhood.[3–5,20,24,25]

Violence-Free Parenting: Effective Parenting Without Corporal Punishment

As children enter the second year after birth, patterns of discipline become established in families. Developmentally, this is the age when children are typically separating emotionally and cognitively from their parents, that is, a time of potential stress in the family. Inappropriate discipline, such as the use of corporal punishment, is a risk factor for future aggression and violence in the child. The toxic stress involved may lead to future lifelong consequences in both physical health and mental health.[15] *Bright Futures*, 4th Edition, advises that corporal punishment is unnecessary and destructive.[13]

Providing families with effective, specific alternatives to corporal punishment is the best strategy that PCCs can offer. Here are some specific techniques.

▶ **Praise.** Because toddlers crave parental attention, positive reinforcement for good behavior works best. "I love it when you…" helps children understand what their parents value.

▶ **Act early.** If you notice that a child is getting upset, help him understand his feelings before he may start hitting.

▶ **Closer supervision.** If you find children are fighting, try closer supervision.

▶ **Separate children who are fighting.** Comfort the child who was hit and then address the child who was aggressive.

▶ **Time-outs.** Used judiciously and consistently, time-outs should last 1 minute per year of age during which parents explain clearly why the time-out was deserved.

▶ **Encourage families** to learn more from Play Nicely,[26] an educational program developed to teach discipline in primary care and early education settings.

School-aged Children

As children get older, the external influences of their behaviors become more important. Television, gaming, and social media violence have an enormous effect at this age, and children also begin dealing with playground fights, bullying, and cyberbullying.[27]

Bullying

Bullying, that is, the *repeated infliction* of harm on younger, smaller, or less powerful peers, is a nearly universal problem for school-aged children. Severe and even lethal bullying has been described in the United Kingdom, Japan, and Scandinavia, as well as in the United States. Bullies are usually larger and stronger (among boys) or more socially powerful (among girls) than are their peers whom they bully. Typically, bullies will begin the school year by trying to pick on several children. Children who become singled out as targets are weaker, physically and emotionally, and are unable to strike back, either physically or verbally. Although bullying is a problem of school-aged children, the negative behaviors often happen outside of school supervision: before school, after school, or at recess. Thus, classroom teachers are often unaware of the problem and are almost always unable to solve it without significant support from their administrators.

Bullying has severe adverse consequences for both the bully and the child being bullied. Children being bullied may be hurt physically, often cannot concentrate on their studies, and develop poor self-esteem. Recent news reports suggest that several perpetrators in school shootings in the United States were bullied, and their lethal outbursts may have resulted from the effects of being bullied. Bullying may lead to a variety of behavioral presentations in the primary care office.[28]

Children who are bullies, in contrast, often feel powerful and effective. They typically come from chaotic households, and their parents feel ineffective in controlling their children's behaviors. In many instances, bullies do not experience effective limit setting at home. In the long-term, the outcome for bullies is poor: by age 30, they are more likely to be incarcerated and less likely to be employed, married, or in other stable adult relationships than their peers.[28]

Olweus has developed an effective antibullying program in Scandinavia that has led to a dramatic reduction in bullying.[29] On the basis of this proto-type, current antibullying programs begin with information gathering. Students who are asked to complete anonymous surveys are quite willing to report to school administrators where and when bullying usually occurs. Active efforts to control bullying occur on 3 levels: in the school building and grounds, in the classroom, and with individual students.

Primary care clinicians should screen for bullying in their patients, either as bullied or aggressor, because bullying affects healthy development, may precipitate psychosomatic symptoms, and may interfere with school success. Signs that a child is being bullied include unexplainable injuries, lost or damaged clothing or electronics, difficulty sleeping, and not wanting to go to school. Helping families negotiate bullying situations either through counseling for aggressive children or support for children who have been bullied is an important role of the health care professional. In a bullying situation, parents and teachers should stay calm, separate the children who are involved, make sure everyone is safe, and model respectful behavior when intervening. Young people who are being bullied should be advised to look at the young person bullying them and tell her to stop in a calm, clear voice. If speaking up seems too hard or not safe, the bullied child should be counseled to walk away and stay away and not fight back. Staying near adults and other young people is another tactic, because most bullying happens when adults are not around. Children should also be encouraged to be kind to others who are being bullied and show them that they care. Parents should be advised to work with their child's school if bullying has become an issue for their child. The US government has launched an impor-tant resource, StopBullying.gov, a comprehensive set of resources for parents, schools, and communities (www.stopbullying.gov).

Cyberbullying is the use of electronic communication to bully a person, typically by sending messages of an intimidating or threating nature.[30] With the advent of cell phone use, as many as 60% of children aged 10 and 11 have their own cell phones, capable of receiving and sending text messages. Also, many school-aged children use social media sites, Web sites, text messages, and chat via phones, computers, and tablets. The National Center for Educa-tion Statistics estimates that approximately 21% of students 12 to 18 years of age experienced cyberbullying. While bullying happens in person, cyber-bullying can happen 24 hours a day, 7 days a week; messages can be posted anonymously and distributed quickly to a very wide audience; and messages can be difficult to delete once the message is sent. Parents need to understand the cyberbullying risks that cell phones, computers, and tablets may present to their children so they can monitor their children's use. Primary care clinicians can reinforce the need for parents to know their own children's use and the growing capabilities of the digital world. (See Chapter 9, Healthy Use of Media.)

Adolescents

Violence among adolescents has long been a major concern of teens who live in urban settings and their parents. While rates of firearm violence had been decreasing since the 1990s, there has been a recent upturn in firearm shootings and deaths since 2015. Recent outbreaks of school violence have led to the same concerns among many other groups. Primary care clinicians have several clear roles to play in working with their adolescent patients to reduce the risk of violence: screening all adolescents to identify those at high risk, preventing reinjury to injured adolescents, and referring high-risk or traumatized adolescents for appropriate treatment. Many adolescents begin to form intimate relationships during their teen years. Because these relationships set the tone of an individual's expectations for interactions during intimate relationships for a lifetime, it is important that health care professionals screen and educate their young patients about healthy, respectful intimate relationships.

Recent research strongly supports identifying and reinforcing teen resilience factors in addition to screening for risk. Attachment to school, family, community, and prosocial peer groups all exert strong protective effects, even in the face of risk factors. Programs that provide opportunities for teenagers to belong to prosocial groups and develop mastery of particular activities, ranging from academics to dance, protect them from having health-risk behaviors, including fighting, not only as teenagers but also as young adults. Increasingly, programs for young people are based on the positive youth development model, which has been demonstrated to reduce high-risk behaviors. A focused social history might include questions about engagement in after-school activities, arts programs, athletics, faith-based youth programs, or other activities that engage adolescents and young adults in prosocial activities. Appendix 2 includes a number of screening tools, amenable to use in the primary care setting, for identifying both risks and strengths. Chapter 1, Healthy Child Development, offers guidance in the selection of tools and the timing of screening within the routine health supervision schedule.

Screening

Screening for violence risk can take the form of either a specific violence history or a general screening for related risk factors.

Violence History

Teenagers or young adults can be asked directly about their experiences with violence, using the acronym FISTS and asking the screening questions listed in Box 11-1.

Fighting

Teens and young adults who have been in more than 1 physical fight in the preceding 12 months are at increased risk of violence-related injury.

Injuries

A review of medical records of teens and young adults who were seriously injured or killed through violence usually reveals previous episodes of injuries that required medical attention. Multiple or serious previous injuries may indicate an increased risk of future injury.

Sexual Violence

Teen dating violence is both a serious problem in itself and a harbinger of future domestic violence. Adolescents who use violence against both peers and dates use more of each type of violence compared with those who used only one type of violence.[31] School- and community-based strategies to promote healthy teen relationships include Dating Matters, a program developed by the Centers for Disease Control and Prevention.

Box 11-1. Taking a Violence History: Adolescents and Young Adults (FISTS)

- Fighting: When was your last pushing or shoving fight? How many fights have you been in over the past month? In the past year?

- Injuries: Have you ever been injured in a fight? Has anyone you know been injured in a fight? Has anyone you know been injured or killed?

- Sexual violence: What happens when you and your boyfriend or girlfriend have an argument? Have you ever been forced to have sex against your will?

- Threats: Have you ever been threatened with a knife? With a gun?

- Self-defense: How do you avoid getting into fights? Do you carry a weapon for self-defense?

Threats

Previous threats with a weapon indicate that the patient is at future risk of weapons-related injury, either through the circumstances that led to the original threat or because these young people are far more likely to arm themselves than are those who have never been threatened directly.

Self-defense

Young people who have learned to de-escalate situations of conflict (or to avoid them altogether) deserve praise and encouragement. On the other hand, teens and young adults who arm themselves in self-defense are at extremely high risk.

Violence-Related Risk Factor Screening

A second, broader set of risk factors influences the likelihood of serious violence-related injury (Figure 11-1). Problem teen behaviors tend to cluster as a result of intrapersonal and social factors. Analysis of office-based risk factor screening results has identified 3 classes of risk. Young people in school who report neither drug use nor fighting to their PCC are at low risk of violence-related injuries.[32] Teens who are in school and are passing their courses but who report either fighting or drug use are at medium risk, that is, approximately 3 times that of low-risk students. Adolescents who are failing school, who have already dropped out of school, or who report both fighting and drug use are at approximately 7 times the risk for future violence-related injury as low-risk students. In the clinical setting, most PCCs already inquire about school performance and drug use as part of the adolescent risk behavior screening (eg, HEADSSS mnemonic [home/environment, education and employment, activities, drugs, sexuality, suicide/depression, and safety]); the addition of a single question, "How many fights have you been in over the past 12 months?" completes the screening. Patients who have dropped out of school or who report both drug use and fighting are at high risk and should be referred to appropriate community-based intervention services.

Finally, PCCs should be aware of the strong clustering of health risk behaviors among teens. For example, male teenagers who smoke are at increased risk for carrying weapons. See Appendix 2 for a list and description of tools that can be used for screening teens for this and other health risk behaviors.

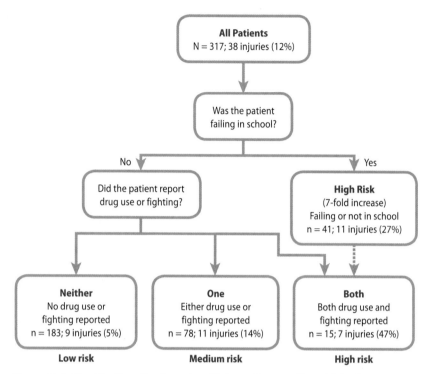

Figure 11-1. Classification of patients into high, medium, and low risk for future violence-related injury.

Modified with permission from Sege RD, Stringham P, Short S, Griffith J. Ten years after: examination of adolescent screening questions that predict future violence-related injury. *J Adolesc Health.* 1999;24(6):395–402.

Counseling and Referral for Adolescents at Increased Risk

Intervention for patients who are identified as being at increased risk for violence-related injuries through either screening approach must be tailored to fit both the degree of risk and the individual circumstances of each teen. Teens at low risk deserve acknowledgment of their respective successes at avoiding this problem, particularly noting that courage is often needed to walk away from a fight. Teens at moderate risk need to hear that the risks are real and individual: "You are strong and healthy. However, I am worried about your telling me that you have been in several fights this year." Basic information concerning techniques for defusing particularly tense situations should be discussed. Teens who carry weapons, have left school, or are otherwise at high risk deserve intense social service or mental health intervention. Primary care clinicians who provide health care to adolescents need to maintain a roster of appropriate trauma-informed referral agencies or individual counselors for these adolescents and emphasize the importance of follow-up to both patient and parents.

After a Fight (Secondary Prevention)

Patients who have been hurt in a fight are at high risk for further violence, either as the injured person of another violence-related injury or by attempting to exact revenge on the assailants. The immediate need after an injury is for crisis intervention. Ask the patient the following questions: "Is the fight over? Do you feel safe leaving here? If the fight is ongoing, is there someone who can mediate?" If the situation is volatile, the patient and family should be referred to social services or, if necessary, the police. Police intervention is warranted whenever the patient is in danger or reveals specific plans to harm another person. At a minimum, parents and patients should be advised of the risk of serious injury and that their safety depends on learning how to de-escalate conflicts. While the immediate concerns of reinjury are significant, PCCs and other health care professionals need to also consider the mental health ramifications, such as acute stress and post-traumatic stress for these young people and their families.[33]

After a fight or violent injury, the following steps are recommended:

▶ Ask the parents to remove any handguns from the home, or, if that is not possible, to store them locked and unloaded with ammunition stored separately. Teen homicide and suicide rates are increased when firearms are available at home,[34] and PCC counseling in this setting seems to be effective.[24]

▶ Have the child or teen tell you about the problem. Allow the narrative to flow freely, avoiding judgments. This approach allows feelings of revenge to be expressed and offers an opportunity to learn the patient's perspective before offering advice.

▶ Evaluate the youth's other risks: Does he or she carry a weapon? Does he or she use alcohol or other drugs? Is he or she involved in a gang?

▶ Discuss with the patient the known risk factors for violence, including the fact that most violent injuries occur between friends or acquaintances and often involve alcohol or drugs.[35] Carrying weapons *increases* the risk of serious injury by encouraging the patient to take unnecessary risks and by encouraging his or her opponent to *draw first*.

► Develop a plan to stay safe after leaving the hospital or clinic. Does the patient have a relative with whom to stay who lives outside of the neighborhood? Do the police need to be involved?

► Discuss conflict avoidance strategies. This discussion can start with the particular incident involved and may need to be continued during subsequent visits. Health care professionals need to understand the patient's need to not be disrespected or belittled by peers.

► Refer to others, including a psychologist or social worker. For many patients, this referral may involve reaching out to mental health providers, church members, recreation departments, or mentoring programs.

► Use referrals to community- or hospital-based violence intervention programs that specialize in after-care of the violently injured youth.[36,37]

Advocacy

Youth violence, although a serious health risk, is a complex social problem that requires broad-based public action. Primary care clinicians, in addition to caring for their own patients, are often able to influence public debate in areas that affect child health. The AAP and other organizations advocate for social policies that benefit children. Pediatricians and other PCCs who serve as school consultants have a critical role. School boards and principals should be advised of the importance of age-appropriate violence prevention programs such as Dating Matters and StopBullying.gov. School districts have antibullying programs as required by state laws. Primary care clinicians may review these policies and their implementations. Also, PCCs may assist in locating high-quality mental health and parenting resources for affected children, either in the community or in schools.

Primary care clinicians have a significant impact on their communities and hospital systems. One opportunity to address violence is to develop systems within community-based organizations, clinics, emergency departments, or hospitals to address the needs of young people who have been injured through violence. The National Network of Hospital-based Violence Intervention Programs has resources on how to start programs within one's community.[37]

Primary care clinicians and child psychologists continue to call attention to the dangers of excess exposure to media violence. In addition to counseling individual families, many PCCs provide testimony at public hearings or endorse community TV "tune-out" weeks.

Despite a general reduction in trauma and death, child and adolescent deaths caused by firearms continue. Individual families can be counseled that the safest home for children is a home without handguns and that any guns present in the home should be locked and unloaded. Primary care clinician testimony and endorsement by medical professional organizations may help support stronger legislation and regulation to reduce minors' access to firearms.

Summary

Violence is a major cause of death and disability for children in the United States. Although the problem has complex social roots and requires multi-faceted solutions, pediatric PCCs have important roles to play. Primary prevention of violence begins with anticipatory guidance for parents of newborns, infants, and toddlers. Secondary prevention involves the identification, counseling, and referral of high-risk patients and should be a part of standard care for older children and adolescents. Finally, PCCs can advocate for school policies, community support of children being bullied, and state and federal legislation to reduce the risk of violence for children.

Acknowledgments: Thank you to Robert Sege, MD, PhD, for authoring the original version of this chapter.

AAP Policy

American Academy of Pediatrics Committee on Injury, Violence, and Poison Prevention. Role of the pediatrician in youth violence prevention. *Pediatrics.* 2009;124(1): 393–402 (pediatrics.aappublications.org/content/124/1/393)

Dowd MD, Sege RD; American Academy of Pediatrics Council on Injury, Violence, and Poison Prevention Executive Committee. Firearm-related injuries affecting the pediatric population. *Pediatrics.* 2012;130(5):e1416–e1423. Reaffirmed December 2016 (pediatrics.aappublications.org/content/130/5/e1416)

Garner AS, Shonkoff JP; American Academy of Pediatrics Committee on Psychosocial Aspects of Child and Family Health; Committee on Early Childhood, Adoption, and Dependent Care; and Section on Developmental and Behavioral Pediatrics. Early childhood adversity, toxic stress, and the role of the pediatrician: translating developmental science into lifelong health. *Pediatrics.* 2012;129(1):e224–e231. Reaffirmed July 2016 (pediatrics.aappublications.org/content/129/1/e224)

Thackeray JD, Hibbard R, Dowd MD; American Academy of Pediatrics Committee on Child Abuse and Neglect and Committee on Injury, Violence, and Poison Prevention. Intimate partner violence: the role of the pediatrician. *Pediatrics.* 2010; 125(5):1094–1100. Reaffirmed January 2014 (pediatrics.aappublications.org/content/125/5/1094)

References

1. World Health Organization. *Preventing Youth Violence: An Overview of the Evidence.* Geneva, Switzerland: WHO Press; 2015
2. Centers for Disease Control and Prevention. Youth Risk Behavior Surveillance System (YRBSS). CDC Web site. http://www.cdc.gov/healthyyouth/data/yrbs/index.htm. Updated August 11, 2016. Accessed January 22, 2018
3. Barkin SL, Finch SA, Ip EH, et al. Is office-based counseling about media use, timeouts, and firearm storage effective? Results from a cluster-randomized, controlled trial. *Pediatrics.* 2008;122(1):e15–e25
4. Scholer SJ, Hudnut-Beumler J, Dietrich MS. A brief primary care intervention helps parents develop plans to discipline. *Pediatrics.* 2010;125(2):e242–e249
5. Chavis A, Hudnut-Beumler J, Webb MW, et al. A brief intervention affects parents' attitudes toward using less physical punishment. *Child Abuse Negl.* 2013;37(12):1192–1201
6. Zahrt DM, Melzer-Lange MD. Aggressive behavior in children and adolescents. *Pediatr Rev.* 2011;32(8):325–332
7. Tremblay RE, Nagin DS, Séguin JR, et al. Physical aggression during early childhood: trajectories and predictors. *Pediatrics.* 2004;114(1):e43–e50
8. Canada G. *Fist, Stick, Knife, Gun: A Personal History of Violence in America.* Boston, MA: Beacon Press; 1995
9. Stoddard SA, Henly SJ, Sieving RE, Bolland J. Social connections, trajectories of hopelessness, and serious violence in impoverished urban youth. *J Youth Adolesc.* 2011;40(3):278–295
10. Kochanska G, Kim S. Toward a new understanding of legacy of early attachments for future antisocial trajectories: evidence from two longitudinal studies. *Dev Psychopathol.* 2012;24(3):783–806
11. American Academy of Pediatrics Committee on Injury, Violence, and Poison Prevention. Role of the pediatrician in youth violence prevention. *Pediatrics.* 2009;124(1):393–402
12. Sege RD, Flanigan E, Levin-Goodman R, Licenziato VG, De Vos E, Spivak H. American Academy of Pediatrics' Connected Kids program: case study. *Am J Prev Med.* 2005;29(5) (suppl 2):215–219
13. Hagan JF Jr, Shaw JS, Duncan PM, eds. *Bright Futures: Guidelines for Health Supervision of Infants, Children, and Adolescents.* 4th ed. Elk Grove Village, IL: American Academy of Pediatrics; 2017
14. Anda RF, Brown DW, Felitti VJ, Dube SR, Giles WH. Adverse childhood experiences and prescription drug use in a cohort study of adult HMO patients. *BMC Public Health.* 2008; 8:198
15. Shonkoff JP, Garner AS; American Academy of Pediatrics Committee on Psychosocial Aspects of Child and Family Health; Committee on Early Childhood, Adoption, and Dependent Care; and Section on Developmental and Behavioral Pediatrics. The lifelong effects of early childhood adversity and toxic stress. *Pediatrics.* 2012;129(1):e232–e246
16. Ambuel B, Hamberger LK, Guse CE, Melzer-Lange M, Phelan MB, Kistner A. Healthcare can change from within: sustained response to the healthcare response to intimate partner violence. *J Fam Violence.* 2013;28(8):833–847
17. American Academy of Pediatrics Council on Communications and Media. Children, adolescents, and the media. *Pediatrics.* 2013;132(5):958–961
18. Strasburger VC, Jordan AB, Donnerstein E. Health effects of media on children and adolescents. *Pediatrics.* 2010;125(4):756–767
19. Strasburger VC, Donnerstein E, Bushman BJ. Why is it so hard to believe that media influence children and adolescents? *Pediatrics.* 2014;133(4):571–573
20. Donnerstein E, Slaby R, Eron LD. The mass media and youth aggression. In: Eron LD, Gentry JH, Schlegel P, eds. *Reason to Hope: A Psychosocial Perspective on Violence and Youth.* Washington, DC: American Psychological Association; 1996:219–250

21. Tolan PH, Gorman-Smith D, Henry DB. The developmental ecology of urban males' youth violence. *Dev Psychol.* 2003;39(2):274–291

22. Robinson WL, Paxton KC, Jonen LP. Pathways to aggression and violence among African American adolescent males: the influence of normative beliefs, neighborhood, and depressive symptomatology. *J Prev Interv Community.* 2011;39(2):132–148

23. Cronholm PF, Forke CM, Wade R, et al. Adverse childhood experiences: expanding the concept of adversity. *Am J Prev Med.* 2015;49(3):354–361

24. Sege RD, Perry C, Stigol L, et al. Short-term effectiveness of anticipatory guidance to reduce early childhood risks for subsequent violence. *Arch Pediatr Adolesc Med.* 1997;151(4):392–397

25. Sege RD, Hatmaker-Flanigan E, De Vos E, Levin-Goodman R, Spivak H. Anticipatory guidance and violence prevention: results from family and pediatrician focus groups. *Pediatrics.* 2006;117(2):455–463

26. Play Nicely: The Healthy Discipline Program. Monroe Carrell Jr. Children's Hospital at Vanderbilt Web site. http://www.playnicely.org. Updated August 23, 2017. Accessed January 22, 2018

27. O'Keeffe GS, Clarke-Pearson K; American Academy of Pediatrics Council on Communications and Media. The impact of social media on children, adolescents, and families. *Pediatrics.* 2011;217(4):800–804

28. Keder R, Sege R, Raffalli PC, Augustyn M. Bullying and ADHD: which came first and does it matter? *J Dev Behav Pediatr.* 2013;34(8):623–635

29. Olweus D. *Bullying at School.* Oxford, UK: Blackwell Publishing Ltd; 1993

30. Brewer G, Kerslake J. Cyberbullying, self-esteem, empathy and loneliness. *Comput Human Behav.* 2015;48:255–260

31. Foshee VA, Reyes HLM, Ennett ST, et al. Risk and protective factors distinguishing profiles of adolescent peer and dating violence perpetration. *J Adolesc Health.* 2011;48(4):344–350

32. Sege R, Stringham P, Short S, Griffith J. Ten years after: examination of adolescent screening questions that predict future violence-related injury. *J Adolesc Health.* 1999;24(6):395–402

33. Ranney ML, Patena JV, Nugent N, et al. PTSD, cyberbullying and peer violence: prevalence and correlates among adolescent emergency department patients. *Gen Hosp Psychiatry.* 2016;39:32–38

34. Dowd MD, Sege RD; American Academy of Pediatrics Council on Injury, Violence, and Poison Prevention Executive Committee. Firearm-related injuries affecting the pediatric population. *Pediatrics.* 2012;130(5):e1416–e1423

35. Zatzick D, Russo J, Lord SP, et al. Collaborative care intervention targeting violence risk behaviors, substance use, and posttraumatic stress and depressive symptoms in injured adolescents: a randomized clinical trial. *JAMA Pediatr.* 2014;168(6):532–539

36. Purtle J, Dicker R, Cooper C, et al. Hospital-based violence intervention programs save lives and money. *J Trauma Acute Care Surg.* 2013;75(2):331–333

37. Youth ALIVE! National Network of Hospital-based Violence Intervention Programs Web site. http://nnhvip.org. Accessed January 22, 2018

Healthy Sexual Development and Sexuality

Sarah Garwood, MD, and Tamera Coyne-Beasley, MD, MPH

"In addition to their role in performing a
sensitive, age-appropriate genital
examination..., primary care clinicians play
an important role in discussing sexual health,
sexuality, and safety with both typical
children and special needs children in a
developmentally appropriate manner,
beginning in the child's infancy and
continuing through adolescence."

Discussion of sexual development and healthy sexuality is important in understanding psychosocial development in children and adolescents. This chapter focuses on the role of primary care clinicians (PCCs) (pediatricians, family physicians, internists, nurse practitioners, and physician assistants providing frontline care to children and adolescents) in partnership with parents in promoting healthy sexual development and addressing sexual health issues and concerns during child and adolescent health supervision visits. Throughout this chapter are examples of various questions that may come up during a pediatric visit. Some of these issues are addressed in this chapter, whereas others are discussed in more detail in other chapters in this book. Issues specific to youths who are lesbian, gay, bisexual, or transgender are addressed elsewhere (see Chapter 20, Lesbian, Gay, and Bisexual Youths, and Chapter 21, Children With Gender Expression and Identity Issues).

The concepts of sexuality and sexual health refer not only to the sexual organs and their functions but also to a child's or an adolescent's gender identity, gender roles, sexual orientation, sexual behavior, emotional health, and physical safety (see Box 12-1 for a glossary of terms associated with gender identity and sexual orientation). Children and adolescents ideally learn about themselves and their respective sexualities and sexual health

Box 12-1. Glossary of Terms

- **Gender identity:** Personal sense of one's integral maleness or femaleness, a blend of both, or neither.
- **Gender roles:** Behaviors within a culture commonly thought to be associated with masculinity or femininity.
- **Sexual orientation:** Persistent pattern of emotional attraction, romantic attraction, or sexual attraction, or any combination of those attractions, to other people. Included are homosexuality (same-sex attractions), bisexuality (attractions to members of both sexes), heterosexuality (opposite-sex attractions), and asexuality (persistent lack of attraction toward any gender).
- **Sexual behavior:** The sexual acts in which an individual engages.[a]

[a] During adolescence, sexual orientation and sexual behavior are not necessarily congruent.

from infancy through adolescence, at the appropriate developmental level. It is the role of the PCC to assist them in achieving this understanding. Table 12-1 describes developmental theories and their applications to child and adolescent sexuality.

Sexuality and sexual health are generally perceived as sensitive and private issues. It is essential for the PCC to create a sense of trust with the family and patient.[1] Communication about this topic can be effective only after families have developed confidence in their PCC. Primary care clinicians should be honest with the family and themselves about their comfort level and expertise in the realm of sexual health. Furthermore, the PCC needs to be capable of discussing sexuality and sexual health without bias. This discussion can include, but is not limited to, homosexuality, masturbation, gender identity, and adolescent sexual behavior. Primary care clinicians who are managing a sexuality or sexual health issue that is beyond their comfort level or expertise can seek assistance from a colleague or make referrals to an appropriate clinician or agency.[1]

In addition to the discussion of sexual health and sexuality, the genital examination is essential during routine child health supervision examinations and the adolescent physical examination. The genital examination not only is essential for a proper complete physical examination but also demystifies the genital area and possibly offers opportunities to discuss concerns the parent, child, or adolescent may have regarding the genital organs, sexual health, sexuality, or reproduction.

Children and adolescents observe other people's attitudes toward sexuality and affection. These can include their parents' or caregivers' reactions

Table 12-1. Developmental Theories and Their Applications to Sexuality

Erickson	Piaget	Application
Trust vs mistrust (newborn/infancy) Basic trust learned by having needs met	**Sensorimotor (birth–2 y)** Coordinating sensations and perceptions with own actions	Learning to trust people because basic needs are satisfied Learning to trust oneself and own body as control over body movements is developed
Autonomy vs shame (toddlerhood) Gaining independent control over own body	Coordinating sensations and perceptions with own actions	Beginning understanding of relationship between actions and consequences (eg, pleasure sensations elicited when genitalia are touched) Intense curiosity about own body
Initiative vs guilt (preschool) Initiating actions to overcome feelings of powerlessness Oedipal conflict	**Preoperational (2–7 y)** Symbolic system enlarges. Here-and-now reasoning only. Egocentric (ie, see only own perspective).	Knowing and interested in genital differences between boys and girls. Developing love-hate feelings for parent of opposite sex with fear of fulfilling sexual fantasies. Imitating behavior strengthens sense of male or female.
Industry vs inferiority (middle childhood) Developing feelings of competency in intellectual and physical skills	**Concrete operations (7–11 y)** Increasing intellectual capacity Able to think from different perspectives and about ≥2 aspects of a problem, but relies on concrete events to think in this way	Curious, with some ideas and questions about where babies come from Period of expanding factual knowledge about oneself, including physical aspects, and the world around oneself Compares accomplishment to peers
Identity vs role confusion (puberty and adolescence) Establishing one's personal identity through socially accepted vocational decisions	**Formal operations (11–14 y)** Develops abstract thinking Able to conceptualize Able to use symbols and logic	Discovering one's identity through experimentation with ideas, behavior, and relationships, including the same and opposite sex, without having to commit oneself. Moving toward acceptance of consequences for behavior and fitting into society. Peer groups and youthful romances serve as mechanism for identity development.

Table 12-1. Developmental Theories and Their Applications to Sexuality (*continued*)

Erickson	Piaget	Application
Intimacy vs isolation (young adulthood) Ability to establish close, intimate relationships with the same or opposite sex that include openness, sharing, trust, self-abandon, and commitment	No theory	Being able to identify sexual needs and establish healthy intimate relationships

Adapted, with permission, from Smith M. Pediatric sexuality: promoting normal sexual development in children. *Nurse Pract.* 1993;18(8):37–38, 41–44.

to each other, to their children, and to others in their children's environ-ment. Children and adolescents also observe actions, including gender roles, nudity, and displays of affection toward a spouse, children, and adult friends. These observations, from infancy through adolescence, affect a child and adolescent's own perception of his or her sexuality and his or her body. Behaviors that involve touch, such as hugging, kissing, and cuddling, are ways of expressing affection that may or may not be sexual in nature, and children process this information from an early age.

Newborns and Infants

Newborns and infants (babies) learn and derive a sense of security from their respective environments, from physical and emotional stimulation, and from having their basic needs met. Caregivers, in the process of caring for a baby, teach the baby about his or her own body. In the process of being cared for during feeding, changing, playing, cuddling, and receiving positive reinforcement, the baby learns about security in a comforting way. Caregivers also teach the baby that caring, love, and affection should not be intrusive or cause discomfort in any way. Nonsex-ual contact with the baby such as kissing and cuddling gives the baby a feeling of security, enhances the baby's emotional health, and teaches the baby empirically about physical boundaries.

During the newborn period and infancy, babies begin to form patterns of trust in their caregivers. Parents should realize that hugging, kissing, loving, and caring for their babies contribute to a trusting relationship. When parents make appropriate arrangements for child care, this contrib-utes to the creation of trust between parent and child, including monitoring the care the babysitter or child care provider gives the baby.

Infants begin to explore their bodies and occasionally elicit the pleasurable sensation that can come from touching their own genitalia. It is not uncommon for infants to reach for their genitalia when their diapers come off during diaper changes. Parents can be counseled that this exploratory behavior is normal at this age and not a cause for concern.[2] Box 12-2 contains questions that parents of babies may have pertaining, directly or indirectly, to their baby's sexual organs, sexual health, or establishment of appropriate boundaries. Primary care clinicians can prepare themselves to answer them with patience and understanding.

Toddlers

Toddlers, by nature, are curious about everything around them, including their bodies and the bodies of others. It is also during toddlerhood that voluntary sphincter control and toilet training begin. At this stage, toddlers are also curious about differentiating between males and females, and gender identity begins to emerge (see Table 12-1).

At child health supervision visits, parents of toddlers may need advice on a variety of topics regarding sexuality and sexual health. First and foremost, they will need guidance in addressing children's questions about the body parts of females vs males. Primary care clinicians can urge parents to use correct terms for the male and female anatomy because this practice promotes open communication with the child and allows the child to accurately describe any pain or problems he or she may have with his or her genitalia.

Gender identity becomes more established at this age, and a toddler will typically identify with his or her same-gender caregivers and other children. Some toddlers may be interested in traditionally opposite or other-gender

Box 12-2. Questions and Concerns Parents of Babies May Have

- Why does my newborn look as if she is having a period?
- How do I clean my newborn's genital area? How far in do I need to go to clean my daughter's genital area?
- How do I care for my son's circumcision?
- How do I care for my son's uncircumcised penis?
- Why does my son/daughter put his/her hands into his/her diaper or touch his/her genitalia during diaper changes?
- Why does it seem that my baby boy has an erection when he is urinating or when I am changing his diaper?

activities or roles, such as boys wanting to wear dresses or makeup or girls wanting to wear boys' clothes or underwear. These behaviors manifest the natural curiosity of the toddler. A separate chapter discusses in further detail issues surrounding gender identity and offers guidance in addressing issues that pose a concern for the family (Chapter 21, Children With Gender Expression and Identity Issues). Parents need to be advised that there are many behaviors that may be alarming or perceived as improper yet are within the range of normal behavior for a toddler. Examples include masturbation, curiosity about their own genitalia or those of their peers, and curiosity about the nude adult body.[2] Table 12-2 provides examples of common, less common, uncommon, and rarely seen behaviors in children aged 2 to 6 years.[3] This information may be valuable in discussing parents' concerns and in deciding which behaviors are normal and which behaviors are concerning, requiring further assessment. Box 12-3 lists several questions common among parents of toddlers.

Parents of a toddler who masturbates can be reassured that this is a normal behavior. They can be guided as to when the behavior is concerning, such as chronic, repetitive masturbation that the child is not able to control or behavior that causes injury to the genitalia. Parents can instruct their toddlers that masturbation, although not wrong, should be done in private and not in public places. Often the toddler learns that masturbating is a way to self-soothe during stressful situations, relieve boredom, or relax at nap time or bedtime.

Trust that is established during the newborn and infant period continues developing into the toddler years. These years are a good time to bring up ideas of body safety, private parts of the body, and modesty. Children should know that only certain caregivers are allowed to assist them with their bodily needs and that no one should make them feel uncomfortable when it comes to touching their bodies. Such behaviors include actions that come in the form of play, such as games that result in discomfort (including excessive tickling), or showing or touching private parts of the body.

The PCC and parents can tell toddlers that no one should ask children to keep any secrets from a parent. Primary care clinicians may want to guide parents into discussing with their older toddler that any games or interactions that result in a secret should be revealed to the parent to make sure the child is safe. Toddlers can begin learning that they should always tell someone they trust (eg, parent, grandparent, teacher, police officer, clinician) if someone has touched them or made them feel uncomfortable in any manner. Other topics the PCC may want to discuss during the child health

Table 12-2. Examples of Sexual Behaviors in Children 2 to 6 Years of Age

Normal, Common Behaviors	Less Common, Normal Behaviors	Uncommon Behaviors in Normal Children	Rarely Normal Behaviors
Touching/masturbating genitalia in public/private	Rubbing body against others	Asking peer/adult to engage in ≥1 specific sexual act	Any sexual behaviors that involve children who are ≥4 y apart
Viewing/touching peer or new sibling genitalia	Trying to insert tongue into mouth while kissing	Inserting objects into genitalia	A variety of sexual behaviors displayed daily
Showing genitalia to peers	Touching peer/adult genitalia	Explicitly imitating intercourse	Sexual behavior that results in emotional distress or physical pain
Standing/sitting too close	Crude mimicking of movements associated with sexual acts	Touching animal genitalia	Sexual behaviors associated with other physically aggressive behaviors
Trying to view peer/adult nudity	Sexual behaviors that are occasionally, but persistently, disruptive to others	Sexual behaviors that are often disruptive to others	Sexual behaviors that involve coercion
Behaviors are transient, few, and responsive to distraction.	Behaviors are transient and moderately responsive to distraction.	Behaviors are persistent and resistant to parental distraction.	Behaviors are persistent and child becomes angry if distracted.

Adapted from Kellogg ND; American Academy of Pediatrics Committee on Child Abuse and Neglect. The evaluation of sexual behaviors in children. *Pediatrics*. 2009;124(3):992–998.

Box 12-3. Questions and Concerns Parents of Toddlers May Have

- How do I potty-train my son? How do I potty-train my daughter?
- My toddler wants to know about boy and girl parts.... What do I tell him/her?
- I am having a baby, and my toddler is curious. What do I tell him/her?
- My daughter is playing with her clitoris with her fingers. What do I do?
- My son lies on his tummy and puts his hands into his diaper and humps in the bed. Is that normal?
- My toddler is curious about the new baby's genitalia. What should I tell him/her?
- How much should I say to my child about good touch/bad touch? I do not want to scare him/her.

supervision visits include developmentally appropriate parental privacy, as well as prevention of children's access to sexually explicit materials and witness of adult's sexual behaviors.[3]

Toddlers may become curious about reproduction and where babies come from. This curiosity may arise from a mother who is pregnant, a friend who is about to become a big brother or sister, or a family pet that has given birth. Such occurrences create the opportunity for parents to discuss the topics of birth and the birthing process. The PCC can advise parents to answer the child's question in a clear and concise manner that is appropriate to the child's age and level of understanding. In addition, there are many child-oriented books relating to new babies in the family that may help parents discuss the topic with their child.

Finally, the PCC can raise the issue of the effect of media on the toddler's perception of sexuality and sexual behaviors.[4] This topic will be further discussed in the next sections.

Preschool-aged Children

As the curious toddler grows into the more inquisitive and assertive preschool-aged child, parents and PCCs may revisit sexuality topics from the past, as well as begin new conversations. Toilet training and sphincter control are maturing at this stage. Masturbation continues at this age, and this topic is an important lead-in to discussion of parental values regarding normal sexual exploration in the preschool-aged child. The PCC can assess the parents' perceptions and responses to this behavior, reassuring them that in most cases masturbation is a normal act. Parents can reinforce to the child who masturbates that masturbation is to be done in private. This assessment is also an important time to discuss with the parent and child issues of personal safety, including (if this is an issue for the child) the discovery of body orifices and refraining from inserting foreign objects into the body, including vaginal, urethral, rectal, nasal, oral, and aural orifices. Preschool-aged children should also be told that their bodies are their own property and should be kept private. The concept of body safety, that is, safe touch vs unsafe touch and not keeping secrets, can be reinforced.

Preschool-aged children have a desire to know how things work, including the human body. Thus, they may want to see how other people are made and what is under their clothes. It is also during this stage that children may be interested in playing "doctor" with others. As long as this type of play is with peers, parents can be reassured that this play is not sexual in nature but rather a natural extension of the child's curiosity and need to explore.

Preschool-aged children are also becoming more aware of gender identity and gender roles. In fact, some preschool-aged children may go through a period in which they express the desire to marry one of their parents and seem to be in competition with the other. In families where this period occurs and seems to be a concern, parents can be advised that this is a normal part of the preschool-aged child's development. Parents can explain in a nonjudgmental manner that the parent already has a partner or that the child needs to be much older to marry someone. Gender role play is also common at this stage, as is cross-gender role play. Most children who engage in cross-gender role play or identify as a different gender than their natal sex will eventually accept their natal sex. Some children will persist in cross-gender or non-binary gender identification and develop an adult transgender or non-binary gender identity.[5]

As mentioned in the previous section, the toddler and preschool-aged child may become curious about where babies come from. It is important for the parent to address this in terms the child understands, using appropriate terminology about parts of the body, but to remember that the child may just want basic facts rather than an entire discussion about sex education. The parent can be guided to give simple answers appropriate to the child's level of understanding (eg, when parents love each other, they can make a baby) and allow the child to maintain control of the conversation, initiating his or her own questions. Parents should be clear that they understand the child's questions and give the child the sense that they are available for future questions. Box 12-4 is a guide for parents whose children ask about sex, and Box 12-5 lists questions that parents of preschool-aged children may ask the clinician. Many age-appropriate books and Web

Box 12-4. Guide for Parents When Children Ask About Sex

- Do not make your child feel ashamed for being curious.
- Be honest and use appropriate terms for all body parts.
- Determine whether your child's question has been answered or if he/she has more questions.
- Listen to your child's responses and reactions.
- Be prepared to repeat yourself.

Adapted from American Academy of Pediatrics. Talking to your young child about sex. HealthyChildren.org Web site. https://www.healthychildren.org/English/ages-stages/preschool/Pages/Talking-to-Your-Young-Child-About-Sex.aspx. Updated November 21, 2015. Accessed January 24, 2018.

resources are available to help parents talk with young children about sex, reproduction, and anatomy.

As during all other stages of development, the PCC will find it helpful to inquire about the child's exposure to media. In the preschool years, children begin to access television (TV), video games, electronic devices, and computers more independently. Child health supervision visits provide an opportunity to address exposure to media and limitations parents should place on screen time for their child. Exposure to sexually explicit and violent media may influence some children's behaviors and decrease their sensitivity to sexual violence and behaviors such as premarital sex and infidelity.[4] Parents should monitor their child's viewing and never allow young children to access electronic devices without adult supervision.

Box 12-5. Questions and Concerns Parents of a Preschool-aged Child May Have

- My child is asking questions about body parts when taking a bath with a sibling. What should I tell him/her?
- My child masturbates at preschool at nap time, and the teachers are worried. What should I tell my child? What should I tell the teachers?
- My daughter tries to put the beak of her bathtub duck in her genital area. What should I do?
- How do I get my son/daughter who used to breastfeed to stop grabbing my breasts?
- We have a babysitter coming to watch the kids. What should I tell my children about safe touch?
- I turned on the TV with my child present. There was a nude scene, and now he/she is asking questions. What should I tell him/her?

Abbreviation: TV, television.

School-aged Children and Preadolescents

The early school-age years are a time when children are less interested in their bodies and those of others and are more focused on school, friends, and activities.[6] Sexual behaviors generally peak at 5 years of age and then begin to diminish.[2] During this time, parents will often find that their child has fewer questions that are sexual in nature. However, it is important for parents to continue to communicate with their child about sexuality and sexual health.

In assessing sexual behaviors of school-aged children, the PCC should pay attention to both child variables and family variables, including the developmental level of the child, presence of family violence in the home, and nonfamily influences such as child care.[3] More than two-thirds of children with sexual behavioral problems have witnessed intimate partner violence.[7] If behavior falls out of the typical range, or a parent is concerned about the child's behavior, a referral to a therapist may be necessary. The Child Sexual Behavior Inventory (commonly known as CSBI), a 38-item scale that assesses a broad range of sexual behaviors as a means to clarify concerning behavior, may be administered.[2,8] Other referral options include a pediatrician or other clinician specializing in child abuse or maltreatment. Of course, if at any time there is a suspicion of child abuse or neglect, a referral to child protective services is mandatory.

Because the school-aged child's body is changing and preparing for puberty, the PCC should encourage parents to discuss topics of body cleanliness, body safety, and changes the body will go through. Physiologic changes such as erections and ejaculations in boys, development of pubic hair, and development of breast buds and physiologic vaginal discharge in girls should all be discussed. It is important to speak in clear, concise, and concrete terms because school-aged children and early adolescents may not understand abstract terms at this stage in development. Parents need to be skilled in maintaining open communication with their child during the school-age and preteen years. Parents who are prepared to handle questions and situations that may arise with their school-aged child or preteen are better equipped to communicate confidently regarding matters that are of a sexual nature. That said, many parents feel uncomfortable talking about sexuality. Thus, the PCC should explore how parents feel about talking with their children and, if parents are uncomfortable, should empower them to talk with their children.

Generally speaking, mothers seem to be the primary educator for their school-aged daughters regarding sexual health, whereas fathers were found to be the primary educator for their sons.[9] However, both parents' involvement in their child's sexual health education is important. Cooperation among both parents allows the child to go to either one if questions regarding sexuality arise (Box 12-6). Effective communication about sexual health is best achieved through early and repeated conversations.[10,11]

Parental monitoring of a child's recreational activities before adolescence has been found to create a strong foundation for healthy sexual attitudes of adolescents. When it comes to sexual behaviors and attitudes, children are influenced by a variety of factors, including peer groups, dating partners (as children enter adolescence), media exposure, and their respective communities; however, it is parental monitoring that has been found to be the most influential of societal factors in creating healthy sexual attitudes in adolescents.

Parents are seen as "nonreplaceable significant others" who are responsible for the socialization of children and adolescents.[10] Parental monitoring, control, supervision, closeness, and support all influence sexual attitudes and behaviors; this groundwork is begun in the school-age and preteen years. By adolescence, the groundwork is nearly complete.

In the prepubertal years, patients should be given the opportunity to speak alone with their PCCs to discuss subjects they would rather not address in front of a parent. During the physical examination of a school-aged child and that of a preadolescent, the PCC should be aware of and emphasize the patient's right to privacy and modesty. The examiner should always have a chaperone present, and the entire examination, especially the genital examination, should be explained to the patient in concrete terms. While examining the patient, the PCC may want to continue to inquire about concerns or questions the patient or parent may have, including pubertal changes in the body. It is also a good idea to address the importance of body safety at the onset of the examination, clarifying that it is OK for a

---

Box 12-6. Questions and Concerns Parents of a School-aged Child May Have

- I found my child masturbating in his/her bed the other night. Is this behavior normal?
- What is your opinion about overnight summer camps? Sleepovers? I am worried about what other children know about sex and what they will share with my child.
- My child is beginning to develop pubic hair. Should I tell him/her about puberty now?
- Should both parents sit together to talk with my child about puberty? How much do I tell my child?
- In school, the kids are talking about same-sex relationships. What should I tell my child about these relationships?

clinician to examine the patient's genital area because of the nature of the visit *and* because the parent and patient have both given permission to do so. If during the examination the patient seems uncomfortable, the examiner must stop examining the patient and address the discomfort. The PCC should then discuss with the patient the possibility of another appointment when the patient is more comfortable.

As in all previous sections, the concept of safe and unsafe touch should also be discussed in an age-appropriate and nonthreatening manner. Appropriate boundaries around the need for privacy for family members and the school-aged child or preadolescent should be discussed.

Adolescents

Interest in sexuality peaks during adolescence because of pubertal changes, the need for independence, and the increased role of societal and peer influences. At this stage, sexual curiosity can manifest in several ways, from thoughts and questions about sexuality to masturbation and sexual behaviors with other adolescents.

The cognitive developmental changes in adolescents increase their risk for participation in unsafe sexual practices and are caused by increases in novelty-seeking behavior and a relatively weak prefrontal cortex. Sexual risk-taking can lead to adverse sexual consequences, such as a sexually transmitted infection (STI), an unintended pregnancy, sexual abuse, social stigma, and bullying. These issues can be especially challenging for lesbian, gay, bisexual, transgender, and questioning youths. (See Chapter 20, Lesbian, Gay, and Bisexual Youths, and Chapter 21, Children With Gender Expression and Identity Issues.) Although there are no firm guidelines about how much sexual behavior is appropriate, the general goals of PCCs and adolescent caregivers are to help adolescents delay sexual initiation, minimize unsafe sexual practices, prevent STI acquisition, prevent unintended pregnancy, and develop a personal values system about sexual behavior.

Sexual behaviors are extremely common in adolescence. The average age of sexual initiation is 16 years for boys and 17 years for girls.[12] In 2015, 24% of teenagers had heterosexual vaginal intercourse by ninth grade and 58%, by 12th grade[12] (Table 12-3). By age 13, 5.6% of boys and 2.2% of girls have had intercourse. These numbers are concerning because children who have had vaginal intercourse at an early age are at great risk for coercion. In fact, 60% of girls who had sex before the age of 15 years reported that at least 1 episode was involuntary.[13] Rates of sexual activity vary by gender and race. See Table 12-3.

Table 12-3. Reported Sexual Behaviors Among High School Students in the United States, 2015

Information Surveyed	All (%)	Boys (%)	Girls (%)
Ever Sexually Active			
Students who have ever had sexual intercourse	17.2	43.2	39.2
Race-Ethnicity			
White	39.9	39.5	40.3
Black	48.5	58.8	37.4
Hispanic	42.5	45.1	39.8
Grade			
Ninth grade	24.1	27.3	20.7
12th grade	58.1	59.0	57.2
Students who had first sexual intercourse before age 13 y	3.9	5.6	2.2
Students who have ever been physically forced to have sexual intercourse	6.7	3.1	10.3
Currently Sexually Active			
Students who have had sexual intercourse within the previous 3 mo	30.1	30.3	29.8
High-risk Sexual Behaviors			
Students who have had ≥4 lifetime sexual partners	11.5	14.1	8.8
Currently active students who used drugs or alcohol at last intercourse	20.6	24.6	16.4
Healthy Behaviors			
Currently active students who used a condom at last intercourse	56.9	61.5	52.0
Students who were ever tested for HIV	10.2	9.3	11.1

Data from Kann L, McManus T, Harris WA, et al. Youth risk behavior surveillance - United States, 2015. *MMWR Surveill Summ.* 2016;65(6):1–174.

In one study, nearly 4 in 10 sexually active adolescents did not use a condom with their most recent intercourse, and almost 80% did not use a hormonal contraceptive method.[12] In another, one-third of adolescent girls and young women became pregnant at least once by the age of 20 years, and approximately 90% of these pregnancies were unintended.[14] Rates of STI acquisition increased from 2014 to 2015 for both chlamydia and gonorrhea.[15]

Development of Adolescent Sexual Behaviors

Social factors can either facilitate or inhibit sexual expression. Researchers who propose a biopsychosocial model have identified individual attributes correlated with adolescent sexual behavior, such as testosterone levels,[16] physical maturation,[17] and temperament and personality,[18] as well as social influences such as religiosity[19] and friends' behaviors.[20] Differences by gender are found for some adolescent-reported sexual behaviors. Postponing sexual initiation in girls is also associated with later pubertal development (menarche at 13 years or older), higher parental education, 2-parent families, careful parental supervision, good communication with mother, and high educational aspirations.[21] Sociocultural influences are less well understood for male coital behavior, and few studies have looked at factors that are associated with postponing sexual initiation in boys.[22]

More than half of adolescents want to know more about how to bring up sexual health issues with a physician, particularly questions about the symptoms and diagnoses of STIs and about contraceptive options (Table 12-4). The social and societal pressures to have sex can be difficult for adolescents to manage. Sixty percent had felt pressured to have sex "by a certain age," and most agreed that abstinence is "a nice idea" but not realistic.[23] Adolescents get most of their sexual health information from peers, the media, and their parents. Importantly, the influence of parents on adolescent sexual behavior is strong and seems to be at least equal to that of peers and the media.[23]

Table 12-4. Percentage of Young (13–14 y) and Older (15–17 y) Adolescents Who Want to Know More About Common Sexual Health Issues

Sexual Health Issue	13- to 14-Year-Olds (%)	15- to 17-Year-Olds (%)
How to know if you have an STI	70	67
How to protect yourself from STIs	69	66
Where to get tested for STIs	59	59
What is involved in STI testing	56	62
Birth control options	55	63
How to deal with pressure to have sex	54	46
How to bring up sexual health issues with a physician	52	51
How to talk with a partner about sexual health issues	46	50
How to use condoms	33	29

Abbreviation: STI, sexually transmitted infection.

Adolescents generally think that sexual behaviors should progress incrementally with age from less invasive public displays of affection (such as holding hands, hugging, and kissing) to more private activities (such as touching of the breasts, touching of the genitalia, oral sex, and vaginal intercourse) (Table 12-5).[24]

Oral sex and mutual masturbation are 2 sexual behaviors that often precede vaginal intercourse.[25,26] Nearly half of all adolescents have engaged in oral sex before engaging in vaginal intercourse. In fact, among young adolescents, oral sex is more common than vaginal sex. Teens generally view oral sex as safer and less immoral compared with vaginal intercourse.[27] Similarly, mutual masturbation is a well-accepted behavior among adolescents. By the age of 15 years, most adolescents think that this activity is acceptable (Table 12-6). Self-masturbation is another common sexual behavior of adolescents. By the age of 15 years, nearly 70% of boys had masturbated weekly and 30% of girls had masturbated monthly.[28] No evidence suggests that masturbation has any effect on sexual initiation or the frequency of vaginal intercourse.

Homosexual Behavior

Historically, homosexual behavior was often overlooked in studies of adolescent sexuality, but current research more often documents trends in homosexual and bisexual behaviors among adolescents. Only in the past few decades have any studies of large representative populations tackled the issue of sexual orientation in adolescence. (See Chapter 20, Lesbian, Gay, and Bisexual Youths, and Chapter 21, Children With Gender Expression and Identity Issues.) Data from the 2008 National Survey of Family Growth indicated that 3% of young men and 8% of young women aged 18 to 19 years identify themselves as homosexual or bisexual.[29] The 2001–2002 National Longitudinal Study of Adolescent to Adult Health (commonly known as Add Health) found that 5% to 13% of students in grades 7 through 12 reported some degree of same-sex romantic attraction and 1% to 3% reported same-sex behaviors.[30] In addition, of the students identifying themselves as "mostly heterosexual," almost 6% of boys and 15% of girls reported bisexual behavior. The 2015 Youth Risk Behavior Surveillance System (commonly known as YRBSS) found similar rates of US high school students identifying themselves as gay or lesbian (1%–3%) and bisexual (3%–5%).[12]

In the past, girls were thought to develop a homosexual identity at an older age than boys were, often not until young adulthood or later. In a study of 100 bisexual and lesbian adolescent girls and young women (aged 16–23 years), who were followed for 10 years, Diamond found that

Table 12-5. Percentage of Adolescent Boys and Girls Indicating the Ages at Which It Is OK to Begin Engaging in a Range of Sexual Behaviors

Sexual Behavior	Girls and Young Women (%)			Boys and Young Men (%)		
	12–14 y	15–17 y	18–20 y	12–14 y	15–17 y	18–20 y
At which age is it OK for a girl to engage in the following behaviors with a boy?						
Briefly kiss him on the mouth.	96.5	2.7	0.8	92.6	6.9	0.5
Tongue kiss him.	68.9	30.4	0.8	55.8	41.9	2.3
Have him touch her breast underneath clothes.	22.6	70.0	6.2	16.6	74.7	7.8
Have him touch her between the legs underneath clothes.	12.5	68.5	16.0	10.1	75.6	11.5
Touch his genitalia underneath his clothes.	12.1	70.4	14.0	9.2	74.7	13.8
Have sexual intercourse with him.	1.9	58.8	32.3	3.2	64.5	28.6
Have oral sex with him.	6.6	57.2	27.6	5.1	65.9	23.5
At which age is it OK for a boy to engage in the following behaviors with a girl?						
Briefly kiss her on the mouth.	96.1	3.1	0.8	94.0	5.5	0.5
Tongue kiss her.	69.3	30.0	0.8	59.0	39.2	1.8
Touch her breast underneath her clothes.	22.2	70.8	6.2	25.3	65.9	7.8
Touch her between the legs underneath her clothes.	13.2	67.3	16.7	16.6	69.6	11.5
Have her touch his genitalia underneath his clothes.	12.8	68.9	15.6	15.2	69.1	13.4
Have sexual intercourse with her.	2.3	59.1	32.7	5.5	65.4	25.3
Have oral sex with her.	6.2	57.2	29.2	8.8	63.1	23.0

Adapted, with permission, from Rosenthal D, Smith AMA. Adolescent sexual timetables. *J Youth Adolesc.* 1997;26(5):619–663.

Table 12-6. Mistakes That Parents Commonly Make in Discussing Sexuality and Sexual Health With Their Adolescent

Common Pitfalls by Parents in Discussing Sexuality With Their Teen	How the Pediatrician Should Respond
Not discussing it because of their personal discomfort	Prepare for discussions about sexuality and sexual health by first asking your friends and neighbors, "How did you discuss this with your children?" Next, read books and Web sites about the topic. Several books on this topic exist.
Not wanting to embarrass the child or adolescent	Even if your child is embarrassed by the discussion, this does not mean that he/she does not want your input. Most adolescents want more information from their parents, but they are often too ashamed to ask for it.
Not discussing it because they assume that someone else (eg, school, the other parent) will discuss it with their teen	Discussing sexuality is a great opportunity for parents to give their adolescents accurate information and reinforce their own values and expectations. Nobody else can do that. Fathers, in particular, have experiences and opinions that can be very helpful to their adolescents' emerging sexualities. It's surprising how much teenagers can value their fathers' input.
Talking about it too late (eg, after the child has already formed strong attitudes about sexuality or has already engaged in vaginal intercourse or has already done both)	Sexuality and sexual health conversations should not wait until adolescence. Discuss these issues early and often with your children. In the school-age years, they will be influenced by the media and peers, who often glamorize sex without discussing consequences. Your children need *you* to help provide a counterpoint.
Not setting clear expectations about sexual behavior	Be clear but leave the door open for future conversations. Try, "I want to be clear about this. I don't want you to have sex until you… (eg, are ready, have completed high school, are married). I would not be happy if you had sex before then, but if you are even beginning to think about it, I need you to speak with me first."
Talking about sex in a single "birds and bees" conversation	Sexuality is a complex issue and cannot possibly be covered in a single conversation. Talk about sex with your children early and often. Repeated conversations will reinforce the lessons you taught earlier.
Assuming that abstinence is not an option	Children who choose to abstain from sex often do so because of the influence of their parents. If you assume that abstinence is not an option, so will they. Keep in mind that it is possible to abstain from sex even after losing one's virginity. The most common reason for having sex the first time is curiosity. Once they have explored sex, it is realistic that they may not want to do it again for quite some time.

Table 12-6. Mistakes That Parents Commonly Make in Discussing Sexuality and Sexual Health With Their Adolescent (*continued*)

Common Pitfalls by Parents in Discussing Sexuality With Their Teen	How the Pediatrician Should Respond
Not supporting their children with alternatives to sex	Keep your children busy, especially during after-school hours, with organized adult-supervised activities such as athletics and interest clubs.
Inadvertently promoting sexual behavior by allowing their children to have unlimited and unmonitored exposure to sexual media, particularly the Internet	Limit your children to <2 h of screen time per day and be sure that they are watching age-appropriate media. Become familiar with content labels that come with music, movies, video games, and TV programming.
Discussing sex at a cognitive level beyond the adolescent's understanding	Adolescents are concrete thinkers and often cannot think 2, 3, or 4 steps ahead. For example, making abstract comments such as, "Having sex as a teenager will destroy your life," is incomprehensible for many teenagers. They cannot connect the 2 dots. Try talking about some of the more short-term consequences of unsafe sex.
Making the teenager afraid to ask them questions	Avoid threatening your teen for engaging in sexual behavior, such as, "If you have sex, I'll make you very sorry you did." Clearly this threat will close off any future communication about this topic. Be clear about your expectations but leave the door open for future conversations.
Not practicing what they preach	Discuss your mistakes with your children. This type of reciprocal conversation is vital to effective adolescent communication. If you or another family member has made mistakes regarding sexuality, you should discuss them with your children. For example, let's say you had an unintended pregnancy at a time when you were not ready for it. Discuss with your child how you got into that situation and what you wish you had done differently.

Abbreviation: TV, television.
Adapted from Rosenthal DA, Feldman SS. The importance of importance: adolescents' perceptions of parental communication about sexuality. *J Adolesc*. 1999;22(6):835–851; and Martino SC, Elliott MN, Corona R, Kanouse DE, Schuster MA. Beyond the "big talk": the roles of breadth and repetition in parent-adolescent communication about sexual topics. *Pediatrics*. 2008;121(3):e612–e618.

homosexual female behaviors varied over time in a nonlinear fashion; some of the females experienced what the authors termed "an abrupt emergence of novel erotic feelings and experiences," whereas others reported "periodic episodes of reorganization in sexual identity."[31] The authors found that females were more likely to report bisexual attractions than to report exclusive same-sex attractions.

Adolescent Sexuality and the Media

Adolescents seek and receive a great deal of information about sexual behavior and sexuality from media, whether actively going to Web sites for answers to questions or passively watching sexualized programs on TV.[32] In the United States, 95% of adolescents regularly "go online," and 71% use more than one social networking site (SNS).[33] The Media Practice Model suggests that the "media diet" chosen by adolescents is a reflection of not only who they think they are but also who they want to be.[34] Studies show that social media use may have a significant effect on the social and sexual well-being of adolescents. Multiple studies found a significant relationship between viewing sex in the media and adolescent sexual behavior (including early sexual debut) as well as influence on youths' attitudes and beliefs about sex and sexuality.[35] Online disinhibition may lead to divulging private information more readily than in a face-to-face interaction.[36] In addition, daring and high-risk behaviors may lead to more "likes" by the audience, thus perpetuating such behavior. In a cross-sectional study, 54% of SNS profiles were found to contain one or more references to a high-risk behavior such as sexual activity, substance use, or violence.[37] Self-exploitative behaviors such as creation and distribution of explicit or inappropriate materials, photos, comments, and suggestions may also occur on Internet sites.[38]

Other adolescents may participate in *sexting,* which refers to the sending, receiving, or forwarding of sexually explicit messages, photographs, images, or videos through the Internet, by cell phone, or by another digital device.[36] In a longitudinal study, Temple and colleagues reported that 28% of their research participants had received a "sext" and 57% had been asked to send a sext. In addition, sexting increased the likelihood of high-risk sexual behaviors in female adolescents.[39]

Despite these real concerns, digital media have afforded opportunities for the breakdown of geographic boundaries in health promotion, especially sexuality education. Web-based interventions can be tailored to the cognitive developmental stage of the target audience and can reach underserved youths more easily, especially when it comes to dissemination of sensitive information that adolescents may not feel comfortable discussing in face-to-face interactions. In a review summarizing the effectiveness of digital media–based sexual health interventions in adolescents, Guse and colleagues reported a positive attitude of adolescents toward Web-based interventions.[40] From studies using SNSs to prevent the decline of condom use among adolescents[41] to investigators using SNSs to provide accurate and age-appropriate STI information, educators are working to take advantage of SNS popularity among adolescents.[42] Thus, despite the potential negative consequences of digital media, SNSs can serve as valuable tools for adolescent care providers and educators. Continuing challenges include providing accurate, relevant information and ensuring confidentiality for youths.[43]

Role of Parents and Primary Care Clinician in Guiding Sexuality in Adolescence

Parents must recognize the tremendous effect that they have in guiding adolescent attitudes about sexuality and sexual behavior. Parents who have effective discussions with their adolescents about sexuality can delay sexual initiation, increase the use of condoms and contraceptives during vaginal intercourse, and improve the ability of their teens to discuss sexual health issues with their partners.[44] Primary care clinicians can guide parents who are struggling with how and when to discuss these issues both with their children and with their teens. See Chapter 5, Counseling Parents of Adolescents, for guidance.

Box 12-7 lists common questions from parents of adolescents. In particular, PCCs can steer parents away from some very common mistakes (Table 12-6). Some of these include avoiding or curtailing the discussion because of discomfort or embarrassment, assuming that the teen has already learned about this topic from other sources, and trying to have a single, comprehensive "birds and bees" conversation. One of the major principles of effective parental discussions about sexuality is repetition.[11] Sexuality and sexual health cannot be discussed in a single conversation; rather, the principles should be reiterated and reviewed over and over again. Conversations about this topic should be longitudinal, open, reciprocal, and honest. Such conversations can result in improved connectedness between parent and child, increased adolescent adoption of parental value systems, and decreased risk for unsafe sexual practices.[45]

Parents can apply several other techniques to assist them in curbing the sexual risk-taking behavior of their children. These include monitoring the

---

Box 12-7. Questions and Concerns Parents of an Adolescent May Have

- I found my teen masturbating in his/her bed the other night. Is this behavior normal?
- When should I let my teen have a boyfriend/girlfriend?
- Do I need to talk with my teen about sex? He/she already learns about it in school.
- How can I tell if my daughter/son is still a virgin?
- How can I keep my daughter/son from having sex?

whereabouts of their children (ie, knowing where the child is at all times), relating to their children with an authoritative (firm yet supportive) parenting style, minimizing exposure to sexual content in social media, participating in religious activities (if applicable), and involving their children in adult-supervised after-school activities.[1,46,47] When combined, these activities can modify an adolescent's attitudes about sexual behavior. Parental monitoring is important because it eliminates the perception of privacy required for sexual activity to take place and reminds the adolescent to behave in accordance with parental values. Minimizing exposure to sexual media content is also extremely important. Adolescents spend more than 7 hours daily exposed to music, movies, TV, the Internet, and video games. These forums often glamorize sexual behavior and minimize its potential consequences. In fact, adolescents with unlimited and unmonitored exposure to the media are more likely to participate in unsafe sexual practices and initiate sex at a younger age.[4] Parents should also consider monitoring their adolescent's access to SNSs, as well as reviewing the content of their adolescent's cell phone text messages. Parents should know who their adolescent's friends are and should have a relationship with those friends' parents. Parents must recognize that most adolescents have sex after school in their own home or the home of their partner while parents are away at work.[48] This tendency underscores the importance of organized, adult-supervised after-school activities for adolescents.

The role of the PCC is to support parents in these efforts; to ensure the sexual health of the adolescent by performing routine, opt-out screening of adolescents for STIs and pregnancy[49,50]; and to provide adolescents with confidential counseling about sexual health and sexual abuse prevention.[1,51] State laws on providing these and other reproductive services to minors are often unclear or not well understood. A series of brochures from the Center for Adolescent Health & the Law (www.cahl.org/helping-teens-stay-healthy-and-safe-health-carebirth-control-and-confidential-services-2007) offers guidance to health care professionals, teens, and parents of teens about ways they can deliver, receive, and support adolescents' access to these confidential services.

Sexual Dysfunction

Sexual dysfunction is an area not well studied in adolescence, although the prevalence in both boys and girls is probably quite high. Clinical reports indicate that many sexually active adolescent girls do not enjoy sexual intercourse and have never reached orgasm. Reasons for engaging in the behavior have more to do with intimacy and closeness to the partner than with personal sexual gratification.[52] Occasionally, a girl who is anxious and unsure about sexual activity or who has previously been abused develops vaginismus. Large numbers of adolescent boys are thought to have premature ejaculation, but they rarely report the problem. Erectile dysfunction does occur in adolescence, often as a result of performance anxiety and other psychogenic causes.[53] Heavy alcohol or marijuana use can be responsible for erectile dysfunction and should be explored in the medical history. Prescription medications (eg, antihypertensives, antipsychotics, and antidepressants) are often implicated in erectile dysfunction in men and anorgasmia in women. Other drugs that cause sexual dysfunction and that may be taken by adolescents are cimetidine, ranitidine, meclizine, sulfasalazine, captopril, ketoconazole, atropine, and some anticonvulsants.

Sexual Exploitation

Sexual abuse should always be considered a possibility when an adolescent has very early onset of sexual activity. Both adolescent boys and adolescent girls who have been forced to have sex, either as young children by an adult perpetrator or as adolescents, have higher rates of health risk behaviors and mental health problems. Prevalence rates of child and adolescent sexual abuse vary in the literature depending on the definition of abuse. A study conducted in 2013 using national telephone surveys showed that the lifetime experience of 17-year-olds with sexual abuse and sexual assault was 26.6% for girls and 5.1% for boys.[54] The survey found that a prior history of sexual abuse correlated significantly with young age at onset of voluntary sexual intercourse, unintended pregnancy, suicide attempts, drug and alcohol use, eating disorders, and violence. Girls who have been sexually abused are twice as likely as those not abused to have had intercourse by age 15 years and 3 times more likely to have been pregnant.[55] Thus, it is important to explore the possibility of sexual abuse when an adolescent has very early onset of sexual intercourse or has multiple behavioral problems.

An often-overlooked subset of adolescents who are sexually exploited are those involved in sex trafficking. Sex trafficking is defined as the recruitment, harboring, transportation, provision, or obtaining of a person for the purpose of a commercial sex act.[56] Seventy percent of women involved in prostitution were introduced into the commercial sex industry before age 18 years. The average age at which children and adolescents are being lured into commercial sex exploitation is between 11 and 14 years.[56] In the United States, a total of 5,544 unique cases (incidents) of potential human trafficking were reported to the National Human Trafficking Hotline in 2015. Of these, 74.6% were instances of sex trafficking, 13.0% were instances of labor trafficking, and the remainder of instances were either combinations of sex and labor trafficking or unspecified.[57] Adolescents from any socioeconomic background and any ethnic or racial group can be exploited through sex trafficking. However, poverty, isolation, drug use, violence in the family, school failures, a history of childhood sexual abuse, family dysfunction, or criminal behavior makes adolescents both emotionally vulnerable and economically vulnerable.[58]

Children With Special Health Care Needs

Taking time to discuss sexual health with families of children with special health care needs is important but has often been overlooked while addressing general health concerns. In addition, these children are often erroneously thought to be childlike and asexual. Barriers to discussing sexuality include these factors, as well as the fact that the amount of time allotted for a special health care needs visit may not lend itself to a discussion of a topic that can be both sensitive and extensive. Box 12-8 lists some of the clinician and parental barriers to discussing sexual health in the special needs population.

Box 12-8. Barriers to Discussing Sexual Health of Children With Special Health Care Needs

Clinician Barriers
- Child possibly perceived as asexual
- Paternalistic attitude on the part of the clinician
- Time limitation during the visit
- Parental concerns about other health issues
- Child unable to communicate concerns to clinician

Parental Barriers
- Parental desire to keep child innocent
- Parental desire to discuss sexuality in his/her own way
- Parent possibly too preoccupied with medical concerns to raise issues of sexual health
- Parent perception of child as asexual

Derived from Murphy NA, Elias ER; American Academy of Pediatrics Council on Children With Disabilities. Sexuality of children and adolescents with developmental disabilities. *Pediatrics.* 2006;118(1):398–403.

Primary care clinicians can foster open discussion by calling attention to pubertal changes in the body and mind of the child. These changes may affect the child's self-image, self-esteem, and interaction with peers. The special health care needs population can present some additional challenges; for example, patients with neurodevelopmental disabilities may experience pubertal changes earlier than their peers do. Early maturation requires the parents to begin learning about and accepting these changes sooner than planned.

Children and adolescents with autism spectrum disorder (ASD) may not have experienced social learning opportunities such as school dances or sleepovers. Some girls with ASD or special needs find menstruation distressing, and they may need options to control periods.[59]

Several sexual health topics are appropriate for child and adolescent health supervision visits with patients with special health care needs, including the patient's level of understanding regarding sexuality and sexual health, understanding of his or her body and changes to it, and his or her ability to self-protect. These topics are important to discuss not only with the parent but also with the adolescent while the parent is not present. The PCC can provide education while performing the genital examination and pelvic examination. These can be done in a modified position for patients with orthopedic or neuromuscular disorders.[60] Primary care clinicians can supply the parent and patient information on abstinence. They can also supply information on pregnancy and contraception and how each would interfere with the patient's physical health and medication regimens. Some parents of children or adolescents with special health care needs may bring up the possibility of permanent sterilization as a way to prevent pregnancy. The American Academy of Pediatrics (AAP) Committee on Bioethics recommends that clinicians discuss such an option if the parent expresses concern but also discuss less permanent contraceptive options with the parent and the patient.[61] It is also recommended that the PCC become familiar with the applicable laws regarding sterilization of persons who have developmental disabilities.

The PCC's role includes assessing the expectations of the patient and parents with regard to dating, sexual intercourse, and contraception. The PCC can serve as a source of information and assist in finding information regarding sexuality in patients with similar disabilities. The PCC can recommend that the Individualized Education Program (commonly known as IEP) developed by the child's school include the provision of sexuality education to children with disabilities, including a discussion of body parts, pubertal changes, hygiene, personal care, social skills, sexual expression, the medical examination, contraception, and rights and responsibilities of sexual behavior.[61,62]

When it comes to cautioning parents and their children with special health care needs on sexual abuse, the PCC's role is crucial. Such children are at an especially higher risk for being sexually exploited for several reasons (Box 12-9).

Masturbation in this population should not be seen as a concerning behavior unless it is done in public, is obsessive, or is causing injury to the patient. It is important to note that a patient's developmental age is a critical factor in considering masturbation behaviors; for example, if a patient has a chronological age of 9 years but is developmentally a preschooler, the child's sexual curiosity and masturbation should be seen within the context of a preschooler's development.

In caring for the special needs population, as in caring for any other pediatric population, the PCC's role includes discussion of sexual health and sexuality with the child and parents, especially of the increased vulnerability to abuse in this population. Box 12-10 summarizes important discussion points.

Minimizing Risk of Exploitation and Talking About Safe and Unsafe Touch With Children

Much has been said about talking with children about safe and unsafe touch, yet information on what to discuss with children, at what age to start such discussions, and how much to tell them is a source of much

---

Box 12-9. Why Special Needs Patients May Be at Increased Risk for Sexual Abuse or Exploitation

- May be vulnerable because of disability
- May be more trusting
- May have more care providers
- May have reliance on assistance for toileting
- May not be able to communicate or describe what has happened to them
- May have limited capacity for self-defense

Derived from Murphy NA, Elias ER; American Academy of Pediatrics Council on Children With Disabilities. Sexuality of children and adolescents with developmental disabilities. *Pediatrics.* 2006;118(1):398–403.

Box 12-10. Guide for Discussions With the Special Needs Patient and Parent

- Discuss regularly issues of physical development, maturity, and sexuality, starting early in childhood and continuing through the adolescent years.
- Ensure the privacy of each child and adolescent.
- Assist parents in understanding how the cognitive abilities of their children affect behavior and socialization.
- Encourage children with disabilities and their parents to optimize independence, particularly as related to self-care and social skills.
- Be aware of special medical needs, such as modified gynecologic examinations, latex-free protection from STIs, unplanned pregnancies, and genetic counseling when appropriate.
- Recognize that children with disabilities are at an increased risk for sexual abuse, and monitor for early indications of abuse.
- Advocate for developmentally appropriate sexuality education in home, community, and school settings.
- Encourage parents to be the principal source of developmentally appropriate sexuality education for their children, incorporating family values, cultural traditions, and religious beliefs.
- Provide families with information regarding appropriate community programs that address issues of sexuality for children and adolescents with disabilities.

Abbreviation: STI, sexually transmitted infection.

Derived from Murphy NA, Elias ER; American Academy of Pediatrics Council on Children With Disabilities. Sexuality of children and adolescents with developmental disabilities. *Pediatrics.* 2006;118(1):398–403.

controversy. Current literature supports educational prevention programs on safe and unsafe touch.[63]

There is general agreement on the need for age-appropriate discussions of sexuality and sexual health; use of correct names for body parts; differentiation between appropriate and inappropriate touch, realizing that inappropriate touch may sometimes feel good too; empowering children to say no; and making sure they know to whom they can go for help. Box 12-11 outlines the AAP recommendations to minimize a child's risk for sexual molestation.

Summary

In addition to their role in performing a sensitive, age-appropriate genital examination on children and adolescents during child and adolescent health supervision care, PCCs play an important role in discussing sexual health, sexuality, and safety with both typical children and special needs children in a developmentally appropriate manner, beginning in the child's

Box 12-11. Guidance From the American Academy of Pediatrics to Minimize a Child's Risk for Molestation

❶ Teach your children about privacy of body parts and that no one has the right to touch them.

❷ Teach your children to be able to differentiate between appropriate and inappropriate touching (loving hug vs touching private areas, but be aware that if a loving hug is unwanted or undesired, then this touching is also considered inappropriate).

❸ Teach your children and empower them that they have the right to say no to any unwanted touching.

❹ Teach your children about potentially dangerous situations in which a stranger may lure them into being alone or separated from their parent or group of friends.

❺ Teach your children about the dangers of being offered drugs or mind-altering substances by friends, familiar adults, or strangers.

❻ Teach your children that threats from a molester are against the law and not to keep secrets regardless of what the threat may be.

❼ Teach your children never to go door-to-door without an adult and never to go into someone else's home without parental/adult permission or supervision.

❽ Spend time with your children and give them a sense of love and attention so they do not seek it elsewhere and become an easy target.

❾ Know whom your children spend time with and where your children are when with friends, at parties, or in other social situations.

❿ At the community level, know the abuse prevention programs offered at local libraries, schools, and police or fire departments.

⓫ Monitor activities at your children's child care programs, day care, summer camp, or other places outside the home.

Adapted from American Academy of Pediatrics. Sexual abuse. HealthyChildren.org Web site. https://www.healthychildren.org/English/safety-prevention/at-home/Pages/Sexual-Abuse.aspx. Updated November 21, 2015. Accessed January 24, 2018.

infancy and continuing through adolescence. The PCC's role also includes discussing these topics with parents, encouraging them to discuss these topics with their child regularly, and promoting open communication about sexual issues between the child, or adolescent, and parents. Sexual curiosity and exploration can be normal behavior at each stage of childhood and adolescence. Children and adolescents whose sexual behavior falls outside the range of normal or common sexual behaviors may require the assistance of a specialist.

Acknowledgments: Thank you to Leena Shrivastava Dev, MD, and Mario Cruz, MD, who authored the original version of this chapter.

AAP Policy

American Academy of Pediatrics Committee on Adolescence. Condom use by adolescents. *Pediatrics*. 2013;132(5):973–981 (pediatrics.aappublications.org/content/132/5/973)

American Academy of Pediatrics Committee on Adolescence. Contraception for adolescents. *Pediatrics*. 2014;134(4):e1244–e1256 (pediatrics.aappublications.org/content/134/4/e1244)

American Academy of Pediatrics Committee on Adolescence. Emergency contraception. *Pediatrics*. 2012;130(6):1174–1182. Reaffirmed July 2016 (pediatrics.aappublications.org/content/130/6/1174)

American Academy of Pediatrics Committee on Child Abuse and Committee on Adolescence. Care of the adolescent after acute sexual assault. *Pediatrics*. 2017;139(3):e20164243 (pediatrics.aappublications.org/content/139/3/e20164243)

Breuner CC, Mattson G; American Academy of Pediatrics Committee on Adolescence and Committee on Psychosocial Aspects of Child and Family Health. Sexuality education for children and adolescents. *Pediatrics*. 2016;138(2):e20161348 (pediatrics.aappublications.org/content/138/2/e20161348)

Murphy NA, Elias ER; American Academy of Pediatrics Council on Children With Disabilities. Sexuality of children and adolescents with developmental disabilities. *Pediatrics*. 2006;118(1):398–403. Reaffirmed November 2017 (pediatrics.aappublications.org/content/118/1/398)

Ott MA, Sucato GS; American Academy of Pediatrics Committee on Adolescence. Contraception for adolescents. *Pediatrics*. 2014;134(4):e1257–e1281 (pediatrics.aappublications.org/content/134/4/e1257)

References

1. American Academy of Pediatrics Committee on Psychosocial Aspects of Child and Family Health and Committee on Adolescence. Sexuality education for children and adolescents. *Pediatrics*. 2001;108(2):498–502
2. Friedrich WN, Fisher J, Broughton D, Houston M, Shafran CR. Normative sexual behavior in children: a contemporary sample. *Pediatrics*. 1998;101(4):e9
3. Kellogg ND; American Academy of Pediatrics Committee on Child Abuse and Neglect. The evaluation of sexual behaviors in children. *Pediatrics*. 2009;124(3):992–998
4. American Academy of Pediatrics Council on Communications and Media. Sexuality, contraception, and the media. *Pediatrics*. 2010;126(3):576–582
5. Ruble DN, Martin C. Gender development. In: Damon W, Eisenberg N, eds. *Handbook of Child Psychology*. 5th ed. Hoboken, NJ: Wiley; 1998:933–1016
6. Smith M. Pediatric sexuality: promoting normal sexual development in children. *Nurse Pract*. 1993;18(8):37–38, 41–44
7. Silovsky JF, Niec L. Characteristics of young children with sexual behavior problems: a pilot study. *Child Maltreat*. 2002;7(3):187–197
8. Friedrich WN, Grambsch P, Damon L, et al. Child Sexual Behavior Inventory: normative and clinical comparisons. *Psychol Assess*. 1992;4(3):303–311
9. Wyckoff SC, Miller KS, Forehand R, et al. Patterns of sexuality communication between preadolescents and their mothers and fathers. *J Child Fam Stud*. 2008;17(5):649–662

10. Miller KS, Fasula AM, Dittus P, Wiegand RE, Wyckoff SC, McNair L. Barriers and facilitators to maternal communication with preadolescents about age-relevant sexual topics. *AIDS Behav.* 2009;13(2):365–374

11. Martino SC, Elliott MN, Corona R, Kanouse DE, Schuster MA. Beyond the "big talk": the roles of breadth and repetition in parent-adolescent communication about sexual topics. *Pediatrics.* 2008;121(3):e612–e618

12. Kann L, McManus T, Harris WA, et al. Youth risk behavior surveillance - United States, 2015. *MMWR Surveill Summ.* 2016;65(6):1–174

13. Haffner DW. Facing facts: sexual health for American adolescents. *J Adolesc Health.* 1998;22(6):453–459

14. Martinez G, Copen CE, Abma JC; Centers for Disease Control and Prevention; US Department of Health and Human Services. Teenagers in the United States: sexual activity, contraceptive use, and childbearing, 2006-2010 national survey of family growth. *Vital Health Stat 23.* 2011;(31):1–35

15. Centers for Disease Control and Prevention. *Sexually Transmitted Disease Surveillance 2015.* Atlanta, GA: US Dept of Health and Human Services; 2016

16. Halpern CT, Udry JR, Campbell B, Suchindran C. Testosterone and pubertal development as predictors of sexual activity: a panel analysis of adolescent males. *Psychosom Med.* 1993;55(5):436–447

17. Halpern CT, Udry JR, Suchindran C. Testosterone predicts initiation of coitus in adolescent females. *Psychosom Med.* 1997;59(2):161–171

18. Udry JR, Talbert LM. Sex hormone effects on personality at puberty. *J Pers Soc Psychol.* 1988;54(2):291–295

19. Hipwell AE, Keenan K, Loeber R, Battista D. Early predictors of sexually intimate behaviors in an urban sample of young girls. *Dev Psychol.* 2010;46(2):366–378

20. Smith EA, Udry JR, Morris NM. Pubertal development and friends: a biosocial explanation of adolescent sexual behavior. *J Health Soc Behav.* 1985;26(3):183–192

21. Rosenthal SL, Von Ranson KM, Cotton S, Biro FM, Mills L, Succop PA. Sexual initiation: predictors and developmental trends. *Sex Transm Dis.* 2001;28(9):527–532

22. Lammers C, Ireland M, Resnick M, Blum R. Influences on adolescents' decision to postpone onset of sexual intercourse: a survival analysis of virginity among youths aged 13 to 18 years. *J Adolesc Health.* 2000;26(1):42–48

23. Hoff T, Greene L, Davis J. *National Survey of Adolescents and Young Adults: Sexual Health Knowledge, Attitudes and Experiences.* Menlo Park, CA: Kaiser Family Foundation; 2003

24. Rosenthal DA, Smith AMA. Adolescent sexual timetables. *J Youth Adolesc.* 1997;26(5):619–636

25. Schwartz IM. Sexual activity prior to coital initiation: a comparison between males and females. *Arch Sex Behav.* 1999;28(1):63–69

26. Song AV, Halpern-Felsher BL. Predictive relationship between adolescent oral and vaginal sex: results from a prospective, longitudinal study. *Arch Pediatr Adolesc Med.* 2011;165(3):243–249

27. Halpern-Felsher BL, Cornell JL, Kropp RY, Tschann JM. Oral versus vaginal sex among adolescents: perceptions, attitudes, and behavior. *Pediatrics.* 2005;115(4):845–851

28. Leitenberg H, Detzer MJ, Srebnik D. Gender differences in masturbation and the relation of masturbation experience in preadolescence and/or early adolescence to sexual behavior and sexual adjustment in young adulthood. *Arch Sex Behav.* 1993;22(2):87–98

29. Chandra A, Mosher WD, Copen C, Sionean C. Sexual behavior, sexual attraction, and sexual identity in the United States: data from the 2006-2008 National Survey of Family Growth. *Natl Health Stat Report.* 2011;19(36):1–36

30. Savin-Williams RC, Ream GL. Prevalence and stability of sexual orientation components during adolescence and young adulthood. *Arch Sex Behav.* 2007;36(3):385–394

31. Diamond LM. A dynamical systems approach to the development and expression of female same-sex sexuality. *Perspect Psychol Sci.* 2007;2(2):142–161

32. Strasburger VC, Jordan AB, Donnerstein E. Children, adolescents, and the media: health effects. *Pediatr Clin North Am.* 2012;59(3):533–587

33. Lenhart A. *Teens, Social Media and Technology Overview 2015.* Washington, DC: Pew Research Center; 2015:2–6

34. Brown JD. Adolescents' sexual media diets. *J Adolesc Health.* 2000;27(2)(suppl):35–40

35. Ybarra ML, Strasburger VC, Mitchell KJ. Sexual media exposure, sexual behavior, and sexual violence victimization in adolescence. *Clin Pediatr (Phila).* 2014;53(13):1239–1247

36. Suler J. The online disinhibition effect. *CyberPsychol Behav.* 2004;7(3):321–326

37. Moreno MA, Parks MR, Zimmerman FJ, Brito TE, Christakis DA. Display of health risk behaviors on MySpace by adolescents: prevalence and associations. *Arch Pediatr Adolesc Med.* 2009;163(1):27–34

38. Dowdell EB, Burgess AW, Flores JR. Original research: online social networking patterns among adolescents, young adults, and sexual offenders. *Am J Nurs.* 2011;111(7):28–36

39. Temple JR, Paul JA, van den Berg P, Le VD, McElhany A, Temple BW. Teen sexting and its association with sexual behaviors. *Arch Pediatr Adolesc Med.* 2012;166(9):828–833

40. Guse K, Levine D, Martins S, et al. Interventions using new digital media to improve adolescent sexual health: a systematic review. *J Adolesc Health.* 2012;51(6):535–543

41. Bull SS, Levine D, Black SR, Schmiege S, Santelli J. Social media-delivered sexual health intervention: a cluster randomized controlled trial. *Am J Prev Med.* 2012;43(5):467–474

42. Yager AM, O'Keefe C. Adolescent use of social networking to gain sexual health information. *J Nurse Pract.* 2012;8(4):294–298

43. Selkie EM, Benson M, Moreno M. Adolescents' views regarding uses of social networking websites and text messaging for adolescent sexual health education. *Am J Health Educ.* 2011; 42(4):205–212

44. DiClemente RJ, Wingood GM, Crosby R, Cobb BK, Harrington K, Davies SL. Parent-adolescent communication and sexual risk behaviors among African American adolescent females. *J Pediatr.* 2001;139(3):407–412

45. Markham CM, Lormand D, Gloppen KM, et al. Connectedness as a predictor of sexual and reproductive health outcomes for youth. *J Adolesc Health.* 2010;46(3)(suppl):S23–S41

46. Meier AM. Adolescents' transition to first intercourse, religiosity, and attitudes about sex. *Soc Forces.* 2003;81(3):1031–1052

47. Sieverding JA, Adler N, Witt S, Ellen J. The influence of parental monitoring on adolescent sexual initiation. *Arch Pediatr Adolesc Med.* 2005;159(8):724–729

48. Cohen DA, Farley TA, Taylor SN, Martin DH, Schuster MA. When and where do youths have sex? The potential role of adult supervision. *Pediatrics.* 2002;110(6):e66

49. American Academy of Pediatrics Committee on Practice and Ambulatory Medicine and Bright Futures Periodicity Schedule Workgroup. 2017 recommendations for preventative pediatric health care. *Pediatrics.* 2017;139(4):e20170254

50. Branson BM, Handsfield HH, Lampe MA, et al; Centers for Disease Control and Prevention. Revised recommendations for HIV testing of adults, adolescents, and pregnant women in health-care settings. *MMWR Recomm Rep.* 2006;55(RR-14):1–17

51. Thomas D, Flaherty E, Binns H. Parent expectations and comfort with discussion of normal childhood sexuality and sexual abuse prevention during office visits. *Ambul Pediatr.* 2004;4(3):232–236

52. Ott MA, Millstein SG, Ofner S, Halpern-Felsher BL. Greater expectations: adolescents' positive motivations for sex. *Perspect Sex Reprod Health.* 2006;38(2):84–89

53. Farrow JA. An approach to the management of sexual dysfunction in the adolescent male. *J Adolesc Health Care.* 1985;6(5):397–400

54. Finkelhor D, Shattuck A, Turner HA, Hamby SL. The lifetime prevalence of child sexual abuse and sexual assault assessed in late adolescence. *J Adolesc Health.* 2014;55(3):329–333

55. Stock JL, Bell MA, Boyer DK, Connell FA. Adolescent pregnancy and sexual risk-taking among sexually abused girls. *Fam Plan Perspect.* 1997;29(5):200–203, 227

56. Kotrla K. Domestic minor sex trafficking in the United States. *Soc Work.* 2010;55(2):181–187

57. Comprehensive human trafficking assessment tool. National Human Trafficking Hotline Web site. https://humantraffickinghotline.org/resources/comprehensive-human-trafficking-assessment-tool. Published January 2011. Accessed January 24, 2018

58. McClain NM, Garrity SE. Sex trafficking and the exploitation of adolescents. *J Obstet Gynecol Neonatal Nurs.* 2011;40(2):243–252

59. Chan J, John RM. Sexuality and sexual health in children and adolescents with autism. *J Nurse Pract.* 2012;8(4):306–315

60. Murphy NA, Elias ER; American Academy of Pediatrics Council on Children With Disabilities. Sexuality of children and adolescents with developmental disabilities. *Pediatrics.* 2006;118(1):398–403

61. American Academy of Pediatrics Committee on Bioethics. Sterilization of minors with developmental disabilities. *Pediatrics.* 1999;104(2, pt 1):337–340

62. Holland-Hall C, Quint E. Sexuality and disability in adolescents. *Pediatr Clin North Am.* 2017;64(2):235–449

63. Finkelhor D. Prevention of sexual abuse through educational programs directed toward children. *Pediatrics.* 2007;120(3):640–645

Children Exposed to Adverse Childhood Experiences

Andrew Garner, MD, PhD

"Clinicians in general and pediatric primary care clinicians in particular have an ethical obligation to address childhood adversity and toxic stress because they are important childhood antecedents, perhaps even determinants, of adult disease."

Childhood adversity plays a prominent role in influencing a child's development and eventual life course. A wide array of adverse childhood experiences (ACEs) have been associated with poor developmental outcomes, as diverse as depression, substance use disorder, teenage pregnancy, incarceration, emphysema, obesity, type 2 diabetes, and cardiovascular disease.[1-3] Only recently, however, have advances in the neurosciences, epigenetics, and the physiology of stress begun to reveal the biological mechanisms that might underlie these well-established associations.[4-6] This chapter briefly reviews the epidemiological associations between childhood adversity and less than optimal life course trajectories, including poor mental health outcomes and the adoption of unhealthy behaviors such as smoking, promiscuity, and substance use disorder. This chapter then defines toxic stress and discusses its effect on brain development. Finally, this chapter discusses ways in which pediatric primary care clinicians (PCCs) (pediatricians, family physicians, internists, nurse practitioners, and physician assistants who provide frontline care to children and adolescents) and other child health professionals might intervene to minimize the potentially lifelong effects of childhood adversity on both mental wellness and physical wellness.

Childhood Adversity and Life Course Trajectories

Adversity can take many forms and can be either catastrophic/traumatic (eg, being abused, witnessing violence) or almost routine (eg, experiencing poverty or parental separation). Defining and measuring what makes an event adverse for a particular individual can be problematic. Does adversity depend on characteristics unique to the child (eg, the child's previous experiences, temperament, developmental state, or unusual physical or personal traits), the family situation (eg, childhood experiences of the parents, parental mental illness, intimate partner violence), or broader societal issues (eg, poverty, unemployment, poor housing, neighborhood violence, limited access to medical or mental health care)? Or, more likely, is adversity caused by complex interactions among all 3 ecological levels? The perception of adversity or a threat can be quite variable: some children might have horrific experiences (eg, witnessing interpersonal violence) yet do very well, whereas other children might have long-lasting physiologic and behavior changes resulting from relatively minor trauma (such as seeing a barking and growling dog or falling off a bike).

Despite this ambiguity about what constitutes adversity, numerous epidemiological studies have demonstrated clear associations between various forms of childhood adversity and multiple markers of poor physical and mental health as an adult. The Adverse Childhood Experiences Study looked at more than 17,000 middle-class, middle-aged Americans (average age in the 50s) and found dose-dependent associations between the number of ACEs (Table 13-1) and a wide array of outcomes, including markers for social functioning, sexual health, and mental health; risk factors for common diseases; and prevalent diseases (Box 13-1).[1,3] The retrospective Adverse Childhood Experiences Study and several smaller, prospective studies indicate that ACEs influence behavior, learning, mental wellness, physical health, and economic productivity decades later.[2,7–9]

Because these epidemiological studies are descriptive, no causal mechanisms can be asserted. However, interventional studies such as the Perry Preschool Project[10] and the Abecedarian Project[11–13] have demonstrated that alterations in a child's developmental milieu have profound and enduring effects on behavior and health decades later, suggesting that early childhood experiences alter life course trajectories in a meaningful way. Although econometric analyses of these early childhood interventions suggest a high return on investment, the salient features of these programs (child centered vs family or community centered) and the mechanisms

Table 13-1. Adverse Childhood Experiences[a] Are Not Rare

Type of Experience	Women (n = 9,367) (%)	Men (n = 7,970) (%)	Total (N = 17,337) (%)
Abuse			
Emotional	13.1	7.6	10.6
Physical	27.0	29.9	28.3
Sexual	24.7	16.0	20.7
Household Dysfunction			
Mother treated violently	13.7	11.5	12.7
Household substance use	29.5	23.8	26.9
Household mental illness	23.3	14.8	19.4
Parental separation or divorce	24.5	21.8	23.3
Incarcerated household member	5.2	4.1	4.7
Neglect[b]			
Emotional	16.7	12.4	14.8
Physical	9.2	10.7	9.9

Abbreviation: ACE, adverse childhood experience.
[a] The Adverse Childhood Experiences Study asked >17,000 middle-class adults to recall if they had experienced any of these 10 ACEs prior to the age of 18 y. The prevalence of each ACE is given for both women and men. To determine an individual's ACE score, 1 point was given for each type of ACE recalled (for a maximum score of 10). Only 36% of the participants had an ACE score of 0, and 1 in 8 had an ACE score of ≥4.
[b] Wave 2 data only (N = 8,667).

underlying their success (promoting cognitive vs noncognitive skills) remain a topic of much debate.[14,15]

Measuring Adversity: The Physiologic Stress Response

Among the problems with quantifying childhood adversity are its subjective nature and the variability of individual responses. These problems suggest that the metric of adversity cannot be the precipitants of stress (or the adverse experiences themselves) but rather the individual's physiologic response to those precipitants. The physiologic mediators of stress (eg, cortisol, adrenaline) are quantifiable and can be measured both acutely (as stress reactivity [ie, the magnitude of an acute stress response]) or chronically (as

Box 13-1. Adverse Childhood Experiences Are Associated With Numerous Measures of Poor Health

Social Functioning
❶ High perceived stress
❷ Relationship problems
❸ Married to an alcoholic
❹ Difficulty with job

Mental Health
❶ Anxiety
❷ Depression
❸ Poor anger control
❹ Panic reactions
❺ Sleep disturbances
❻ Memory disturbances
❼ Hallucinations

Sexual Health
❶ Young age of first intercourse
❷ Unintended pregnancy
❸ Teen pregnancy
❹ Teen paternity
❺ Fetal death
❻ Sexual dissatisfaction

Risk Factors for Common Diseases
❶ Obesity
❷ Promiscuity
❸ Alcoholism
❹ Smoking
❺ Illicit drugs
❻ Intravenous drugs
❼ High perceived risk of human immunodeficiency virus (HIV)
❽ Multiple somatic symptoms

Prevalent Diseases
❶ Ischemic heart disease
❷ Chronic lung disease
❸ Liver disease
❹ Cancer
❺ Skeletal fractures
❻ Sexual transmitted infections

All of these adolescent and adult outcomes are associated with Adverse Childhood Experiences (ACE) scores in a dose-dependent and statistically significant manner.

From Garner AS. Home visiting and the biology of toxic stress: opportunities to address early childhood adversity. *Pediatrics*. 2013;132(suppl 2):S65–S73.

elevated basal levels). Obradović and colleagues have looked at stress reactivity in children and have shown a high degree of variability.[16] Traditionally, genetic predispositions were thought to play a major role in determining stress reactivity, but more recent data suggest that previous experiences also play an important role.[17] Stress reactivity, much like brain development itself, results from a complex but cumulative interaction between genes (nature) and the environment (nurture) over time. Neural pathways activated in response to frequent environmental stimuli are strengthened by use. Frequent, strong, or prolonged stress responses early in life are thus able to "set" a relatively lower threshold for future stress responses and to promote a high degree of stress reactivity.[18] Thus, although stress reactivity may be, to an extent, genetically programmed, it is nonetheless shaped by early individual experiences as well. This individual variability in stress reactivity might explain, at least in part, the wide range of long-term responses to adversity. In sum, it may not be the adverse entity itself that matters as much as the nature of the physiologic stress response that it invokes.

Adversity and Stress Are Not Always Negative

High stress reactivity, however, is not always a negative trait or one that invariably leads to maladaptive behavioral responses. In the context of low adversity, children with a high reactivity to stress (the so-called orchids) are actually more social and academically successful than their peers with a low reactivity to stress (the so-called dandelions). However, in the context of high adversity, children with high reactivity to stress fare worse than their peers with low reactivity to stress.[16] Hence, the consequences of high stress reactivity are contextual, with high reactivity promoting adaptive responses in the context of low adversity but maladaptive responses in the context of high adversity. The relationship between adversity and stress is therefore complex. Adversity can promote stress reactivity, but stress reactivity can be beneficial in the context of low adversity.

In an attempt to refine this complex relationship between adversity and stress, the National Scientific Council on the Developing Child has proposed a taxonomy of stress based on the physiologic response to the event (Figure 13-1).[19] Physiologic stress can be positive, tolerable, or toxic. Positive stress is infrequent, mild, or brief and is characterized by strong social-emotional supports. These strong social-emotional supports, that is, engaged, nurturing, and invested caregivers, allow the child's physiology to return to baseline, and they minimize the child's exposure to the

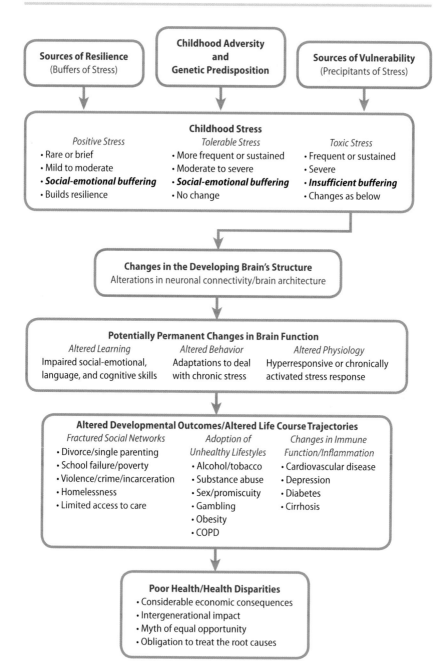

Figure 13-1. Toxic stress in childhood links adversity with poor health and health disparities. ACEs and genetic predispositions regarding stress reactivity interact to determine the type of childhood stress. Sources of resilience (strong social-emotional supports, previous adaptive experiences in which adversity was successfully overcome, and the 7 Cs of Resilience: competence, confidence, connection, character, contribution, coping, and control) buffer this stress, whereas sources of vulnerability (poor social-emotional supports, previous maladaptive experiences in which adversity was not dealt with in a healthy manner, and harsh or abusive parenting) precipitate even more stress. Positive stress is rare or brief, is mild to moderate in intensity, and builds resilience because of appropriate levels of social-emotional buffering by invested, caring adults. Tolerable stress is more frequent or sustained, is moderate to severe in intensity, and has the potential to alter life courses but does not because of adequate levels of social-emotional buffering. Toxic stress is often frequent, sustained, and severe in intensity and is distinguished by the lack of sufficient levels of social-emotional buffering. Consequently, the physiologic mediators of stress (such as cortisol and adrenaline) become "toxic" to the developing brain, resulting in changes in brain architecture and functioning. These changes in brain structure and function are in turn associated with many of the adolescent and adult outcomes seen in the Adverse Childhood Experiences Study (see Box 13-1). Taken together, these altered developmental outcomes and maladaptive life course trajectories contribute to poor adult health and the intergenerational propagation of health disparities.

Abbreviations: ACE, adverse childhood experience; COPD, chronic obstructive pulmonary disease.

Adapted from Garner AS. Home visiting and the biology of toxic stress: opportunities to address early childhood adversity. *Pediatrics.* 2013;132(suppl 2):S65.

physiologic mediators of stress (such as cortisol and adrenaline). Examples of adverse experiences that could trigger a positive stress response (and the social-emotional supports needed to buffer that stress) include a toddler's stumble or fall (under the reassuring eyes of a caregiver), a child's anxiety over beginning kindergarten or child care (and an invested parent's firm but sympathetic response), and the adolescent's fear of failure on a long-term school project (that is overcome by a parent's assistance in organizing time). Social-emotional supports effectively buffer the potentially "toxic" consequences of prolonged exposure to the physiologic mediators of stress (see the following section of this chapter, Brain Development and Toxic Stress). More important, strong social-emotional supports model effective social interactions and promote emotional regulation in the face of adversity, thereby building resilience. It is important to note that positive stress is not the absence of physiologic stress; rather, it reflects an ability to adapt to that stress in a healthy manner.

When compared with positive stress, tolerable stress is more frequent, intense, or sustained. Precipitants of tolerable stress might include the death of a loved one, a natural disaster, or a bully on the bus. Although these experiences have the potential to trigger physiologic responses that are stronger or more sustained, caregivers who are engaged, nurturing, and invested usually allow the child's physiologic stress response to return to baseline. When compared with toxic stress, tolerable stress is distinguished by the presence of sufficient social-emotional supports.

Conversely, toxic stress results from the frequent, strong, or prolonged activation of the body's stress-response system in the absence of sufficient social-emotional supports. Physiologic stress becomes toxic when it overwhelms the available social-emotional supports and the child's physiologic stress response is unable to return to baseline. The 10 childhood adversities studied in the Adverse Childhood Experiences Study (see Table 13-1) are examples of potential precipitants of toxic stress. When a child's social-emotional supports are not engaged (eg, a caregiver who is impaired by mental health or substance use disorders) or nurturing (eg, a caregiver's use of corporal punishment or verbal abuse), the child's physiologic stress response is sustained, and biological adaptations and disruptions begin to occur. Disengaged, non-nurturing caregivers may actually become sources of vulnerability, whereas engaged, nurturing caregivers are important sources of resilience. In sum, the relationship between adversity and stress is both complicated and dynamic. The type of stress response precipitated by adversity is influenced by the nature of the adversity, the individual's stress reactivity, and the level of social-emotional supports. (Are caregivers engaged and nurturing and building resilience, or are they disengaged and non-nurturing and generating additional vulnerabilities?)

Brain Development and Toxic Stress

The process of brain development is driven by a dynamic interaction between the genome (nature) and the environment (nurture).[20] Epigenetic mechanisms such as DNA methylation and histone acetylation are able to transduce experiences with the environment into long-lasting, even intergenerational, changes in gene expression.[21,22] Thus, while the inherited genetic program is thought to provide a general blueprint for brain architecture, the environment is able to influence which genes are expressed, when they are expressed during the course of development, and where they are expressed within the developing brain. Environmental experiences and the neuronal activity that they generate literally sculpt brain architecture and neuronal connectivity.

Understanding the effect of adverse experiences on the developing brain requires a brief review of where the physiologic mediators of toxic stress are acting in the brain. Glucocorticoid receptors are numerous in 3 prominent brain structures: the amygdala, the hippocampus, and the prefrontal cortex. The amygdala is part of the limbic system, is activated during stress, and is thought to play an important role in generating impulsive or aggressive behaviors. That the amygdala is enlarged and more reactive in patients with post-traumatic stress disorder (PTSD) reinforces the notion that the neuronal pathways underlying the stress response (such as those in the amygdala) are built up, reinforced, and strengthened by adverse experiences, leading to a hyperresponsive or chronically active stress response.[23,24]

Another example of how stress might alter brain architecture is seen in the hippocampus. Although neuronal proliferation was once thought to occur only prenatally, new neurons are continuously being generated in the adult hippocampus, and these new neurons play an important role in learning and in the formation of new memories. In animal studies, chronic stress decreases this neuronal proliferation and results in impaired learning.[25] Recent magnetic resonance imaging (commonly known as MRI) data suggest that decreased hippocampal neurogenesis may well play a role in patients with PTSD, as they have selective volume losses in specific hippocampal areas known to be important for learning. While acute deficits in learning and memory might be an evolutionarily advantageous, protective mechanism that allows individuals to get over very traumatic experiences, chronic or ongoing impairments in learning might also delay the development of critical social, emotional, language, and cognitive skills.

The prefrontal cortex is also altered by stress. The prefrontal cortex is thought to play an important role in executive function, including the regulation of behavior by suppressing impulses and emotions arising from the amygdala and other parts of the limbic system. Exposure to chronic stress or glucocorticoids alters the synaptic connectivity within the prefrontal cortex,[26] and this alteration may limit the ability of the prefrontal cortex to suppress the impulsivity and aggression of the limbic system and to execute adaptive responses (rather than maladaptive responses) to future stress.[27,28] Toxic stress–induced changes in brain structure explain, at least in part, the well-described effect of adversity on a variety of brain functions, including dysregulated physiologic responses (a hyperresponsive or chronically active stress response), poor learning (impaired memory), and maladaptive behaviors (difficulty in adopting adaptive responses to adversity).

Toxic Stress, Developmental Outcomes, and Life Course Trajectories

The toxic stress–induced changes in brain structure and function discussed earlier mediate, at least in part, the well-described relationship between adversity and altered life trajectories.[1,3] A hyperresponsive or chronically activated stress response is likely to contribute to the dysregulated immune function and inflammation that are seen with chronic diseases often associated with childhood adversity, such as chronic obstructive pulmonary disease (COPD), cirrhosis, type 2 diabetes, depression, and cardiovascular disease.[29] Toxic stress–induced impairments in critical social-emotional skills and executive functions[30] are likely to contribute to the fractured social networks associated with adults who have experienced childhood adversity. Examples include school failure, divorce, homelessness, poverty, violence, and limited access to health care. Finally, the adoption of maladaptive behaviors to deal or cope with chronic stress explains, at least in part, the association between childhood adversity and unhealthy lifestyle choices, such as alcohol, tobacco, and substance use; promiscuity; gambling; and obesity. Taken together, these 3 general classes of altered developmental outcomes or altered life trajectories (changes in immune function, fractured social networks, and unhealthy lifestyles) encompass many of the morbidities associated epidemiologically with childhood adversity,[1,3] suggesting that these morbidities might be more accurately labeled "adult-manifest" diseases with childhood origins.

Implications of Childhood Adversity and Toxic Stress

Childhood adversity and toxic stress are fundamental concerns for the medical community because unhealthy lifestyles, changes in immune function, and fractured social networks are important markers of higher mortality, morbidity, and medical expenditures. Up to 40% of premature deaths are caused by behavioral patterns.[31] The unhealthy lifestyles associated with childhood adversity are, at least in part, maladaptive coping responses to toxic stress. Another 25% to 30% of premature deaths are thought to be attributable to either social circumstances or shortfalls in medical care.[31] Many of the consequences of fractured social networks associated with childhood adversity are known to contribute to these health care disparities. Toxic stress is also known to alter immune function and increase inflammatory markers, changes that are associated with morbidities as diverse as cardiovascular disease, viral hepatitis, liver cancer, asthma, COPD, autoimmune diseases, and depression.[29] Childhood adversity and toxic stress are inherently medical concerns because they contribute significantly to poor health across the life span by encouraging the adoption of unhealthy lifestyles, widening social inequities and health disparities, and increasing incidence of stress-associated, inflammatory diseases. Clinicians in general and pediatric PCCs in particular have an ethical obligation to address childhood adversity and toxic stress because they are important childhood antecedents, perhaps even determinants, of adult disease.

The consequences of toxic stress are enormous medically, socially, and economically. Advances in epigenetics demonstrate that early adverse experiences can alter gene expression patterns not only in the current generation but in subsequent generations as well. Moreover, the fractured social networks and social inequities that often result from childhood adversity are prominent sources of toxic stress vulnerability for the next generation. These 2 facts, the epigenetic imprinting of the genome and the intergenerational cycle of social inequities, challenge assertions of equal opportunity and underscore the urgent need to address childhood toxic stress as a public health crisis.

Childhood Adversity, Toxic Stress, and Pediatric Care

Primary care clinicians cannot address childhood adversity alone. Many of the systems that generate adversity for children (or serve as sources of vulnerability, such as family structure, income, housing, and violence) lie outside the walls of the pediatric clinic. Productive collaborations between PCCs, other child health professionals, family advocates, educators, judges, business leaders, and other stakeholders are needed to drive fundamental shifts in public policy and to promote more nurturing environments for children to live, grow, and learn.

Childhood toxic stress is a public health crisis, and addressing it will require a public health approach that includes treatment, targeted interventions for those at risk, and universal preventive measures. For children who have already experienced significant adversity, or have had previously supportive connections to family and community interrupted or severed by foster care or adoption, PCCs play several critical roles. These include the recognition of potential signs of toxic stress at various developmental stages, comfort in discussing possible precipitants of toxic stress with families, and familiarity with the available community resources that support the needs of families with children.[32,33]

In addition to treatment, a public health approach to toxic stress would also embrace targeted interventions for those at risk. Routinely screening families for risk factors such as the parent's experiences as a child, substance use disorder, mental illness, intimate partner violence, or food insecurity could identify children at risk for toxic stress. When linked to interventions, as in the SEEK (A Safe Environment for Every Kid) model, these targeted screenings are able to decrease important measures of childhood adversity such as harsh parenting, maltreatment, and referrals to child protective services.[34,35] See Appendix 2 for a list and description of these tools and The Resilience Project: Clinical Assessment Tools at www.aap.org/en-us/advocacy-and-policy/aap-health-initiatives/resilience/Pages/Clinical-Assessment-Tools.aspx.

A public health approach to toxic stress must also include universal primary preventive measures. From a practical standpoint, however, eliminating all childhood adversity is both unfeasible and unadvisable. Some degree of adversity, once overcome, builds resilience, and some degree of stress, if not toxic, motivates behavior change and learning (adaptation). The issue facing PCCs and all other professionals caring for children is how to turn toxic stress into tolerable stress and how to turn tolerable stress into positive stress. Recall that the 3 different types of stress are not defined by the stressors or adverse experiences themselves but rather by the frequency, duration, and intensity of the physiologic stress response to those stressors. As seen in Figure 13-1, a very important determinant of the physiologic stress response is the degree of social-emotional support or buffering.

At the practice level, then, pediatric PCCs can assist parents and caregivers in providing developmentally appropriate forms of social-emotional support. Resources are available to assist the clinician (eg, *Partnering with Parents: Apps for Raising Happy, Healthy Children* from the Institute for Safe Families at www.instituteforsafefamilies.org/materials/partnering-with-parents and *The First 1,000 Days: Bright Futures Examples for Promoting EBCD* from the AAP at www.aap.org/en-us/advocacy-and-policy/aap-health-initiatives/EBCD/Documents/EBCD_Well_Child_Grid.pdf). Beginning as early as the 2-month visit (see *Connected Kids Clinical Guide* at https://patiented.solutions.aap.org/DocumentLibrary/Connected%20Kids%20Clinical%20Guide.pdf and *Bright Futures* at https://brightfutures.aap.org), anticipatory guidance could address the appropriate response to the developing social smile, particularly for parents who might be depressed or overwhelmed. By nurturing the serve-and-return or transactional nature of the social smile, parents are strengthening attachment, promoting rudimentary social skills, and setting the foundation for language. As infants begin to coo and make happy vocalizations, parents need to reinforce those efforts (by cooing and smiling back) as effective alternatives to crying for attention. Attentive, calm, reassuring, and nurturing responses to infant distress model and promote emotional regulation.

In the second year after birth, parents need to acknowledge and encourage the toddler's attempts to be competent and independent while, at the same time, acknowledging that some important and consistent limits need to be maintained for safety. Continued vigilance for and reinforcement of emerging verbal and nonverbal modes of communication will stop or shorten many tantrums. As children reach their third and fourth years, tantrums and conflicts are opportunities to address the behavior ("no biting") and, more important, to demystify the strong emotions that are often underlying the behavior ("I understand that you are angry, but biting doesn't help anger. Next time you are angry, let's try to use our words, or maybe we can take turns, or maybe we can find something else to do"). This sort of emotion coaching models problem-solving, teaches new coping strategies, buffers future stress, and builds resilience, even in the face of severe adversities.[36] These positive parenting techniques (building on strengths while teaching and nurturing emerging new skills) build resilience, in contrast with harsh or physical means of discipline that, while sometimes effective in the short-term, only promote aggression and serve as sources of vulnerability in the future.[37]

For young children, social-emotional supports are primarily external. Parents and invested caregivers provide a predictable, nurturing environment to minimize the child's exposure to the physiologic mediators of stress; model healthy, adaptive responses to stress; and reinforce the child's rudimentary or emerging social-emotional skills (eg, engaging others, language skills, self-soothing). For parents and caregivers who are unable to provide these supports, medical homes must be familiar with evidence-based parenting programs. Table 13-2 gives examples of these programs.

In adolescence, however, the peer group may become a major source of social-emotional support, in some cases eclipsing the support provided by family. This can leave some young people susceptible to peer pressure and to the temptation to act in a certain way to receive additional social-emotional support. Adolescents who are experiencing toxic stress may be more likely to seek this additional social-emotional support from their peer group, even if those peers are less than ideal social-emotional role models.

Table 13-2. Evidence-Based Parenting Programs for Young Children

Cluster Area	Parenting Program
For disruptive behavioral problems	• The Incredible Years (www.incredibleyears.com) • Triple P – Positive Parenting Program (www.triplep.net) • Parent-Child Interaction Therapy (www.pcit.org) • "Helping the Noncompliant Child" parent training program (www.guilford.com/books/ Helping-the-Noncompliant-Child/ McMahon- Forehand/9781593852412)
For first-time pregnant, low-income women prior to 28 weeks' gestation	• Nurse-Family Partnership (www.nursefamilypartnership.org)
For children in foster care	• Attachment and Biobehavioral Catch-up (www.infantcaregiverproject.com) • Multidimensional Treatment Foster Care Program for Preschoolers (www.tfcoregon.com) • Parent-Child Interaction Therapy[a]
For parent-child relationship disturbances and high-risk parenting situations	• Promoting First Relationships (http://pfrprogram.org) • Parents as Teachers (http://parentsasteachers.org) • Child-Parent Psychotherapy (http://nctsn.org/sites/default/files/assets/pdfs/cpp_general.pdf)
For children exposed to trauma, including sexual abuse or domestic violence	• Child-Parent Psychotherapy (www.cebc4cw.org/program/child-parent-psychotherapy/detailed) • CBT[b-d] (www.cebc4cw.org/program/preschool-ptsd-treatment/detailed)

Abbreviation: CBT, cognitive behavioral therapy.
Updates are available at www.aap.org/mentalhealth.
[a] Chaffin M, Funderburk B, Bard D, Valle LA, Gurwitch R. A combined motivation and parent-child interaction therapy package reduces child welfare recidivism in a randomized dismantling field trial. *J Consult Clin Psychol.* 2011;79(1):84–95.
[b] Cohen JA, Mannarino AP. Factors that mediate treatment outcome of sexually abused preschool children: six- and 12-month follow-up. *J Am Acad Child Adolesc Psychiatry.* 1998;37(1):44–51.
[c] Cohen JA, Mannarino AP. A treatment study for sexually abuse preschool children: outcome during a one-year follow-up. *J Am Acad Child Adolesc Psychiatry.* 1997;36(9):1228–1235.
[d] Scheeringa MS, Weems CF, Cohen JA, Amaya-Jackson L, Guthrie D. Trauma-focused cognitive-behavioral therapy for posttraumatic stress disorder in three-through six year-old children: a randomized clinical trial. *J Child Psychol Psychiatry.* 2011;52(8):853–860.

The primary goal for older children, therefore, is to build internal social-emotional supports prior to adolescence. Internal social-emotional skills (such as the 7 Cs of Resilience [ie, a child's internal sense of competence, confidence, connection, character, contribution, coping, and control])[38] need to be the objectives of parents, PCCs, teachers, and all other professionals who care for children. These critical social-emotional skills will not insulate children from all adversity, but they may turn tolerable or even toxic stress responses into positive ones.

Summary

Framing childhood adversity in the context of the physiologic response begins to explain the strong associations between ACEs and a wide array of altered developmental outcomes, including mental illness and substance use disorder. This physiologic framework also suggests a generalizable, proactive approach to mitigating the potentially lifelong consequences of childhood adversity: minimize toxic stress by assisting families of young children and strengthening critical social-emotional supports early in life.

AAP Policy

American Academy of Pediatrics Committee on Early Childhood, Adoption, and Dependent Care. The pediatrician's role in family support and family support programs. *Pediatrics*. 2011;128(6):e1680–e1684. Reaffirmed December 2016 (pediatrics.aappublications.org/content/128/6/e1680)

Earls MF; American Academy of Pediatrics Committee on Psychosocial Aspects of Child and Family Health. Incorporating recognition and management of perinatal and postpartum depression into pediatric practice. *Pediatrics*. 2010;126(5):1032–1039. Reaffirmed December 2014 (pediatrics.aappublications.org/content/126/5/1032)

Flaherty EG, Stirling J Jr; American Academy of Pediatrics Committee on Child Abuse and Neglect. The pediatrician's role in child maltreatment prevention. *Pediatrics*. 2010;126(4):833–841. Reaffirmed January 2014 (pediatrics.aappublications. org/content/126/4/833)

Garner AS, Shonkoff JP; American Academy of Pediatrics Committee on Psychosocial Aspects of Child and Family Health; Committee on Early Childhood, Adoption, and Dependent Care; and Section on Developmental and Behavioral Pediatrics. Early childhood adversity, toxic stress, and the role of the pediatrician: translating developmental science into lifelong health. *Pediatrics*. 2012;129(1):e224–e231. Reaffirmed July 2016 (pediatrics.aappublications.org/content/129/1/e224)

Hibbard R, Barlow J, MacMillan H; American Academy of Pediatrics Committee on Child Abuse and Neglect, American Academy of Child and Adolescent Psychiatry Child Maltreatment and Violence Committee. Psychological maltreatment. *Pediatrics*. 2012;130(2):372–378. Reaffirmed April 2016 (pediatrics.aappublications. org/content/130/2/372)

Jenny C, Crawford-Jakubiak JE; American Academy of Pediatrics Committee on Child Abuse and Neglect. The evaluation of children in the primary care setting when sexual abuse is suspected. *Pediatrics*. 2013;132(2):e558–567 (pediatrics. aappublications.org/content/132/2/e558)

Milteer RM, Ginsburg KR; American Academy of Pediatrics Council on Communications and Media and Committee on Psychosocial Aspects of Child and Family Health. The importance of play in promoting healthy child development and maintaining strong parent-child bond: focus on children in poverty. *Pediatrics*.

2012;129(1):e204–e213. Reaffirmed September 2015 (pediatrics.aappublications.org/content/129/1/e204)

Shonkoff JP, Garner AS; American Academy of Pediatrics Committee on Psychosocial Aspects of Child and Family Health; Committee on Early Childhood, Adoption, and Dependent Care; and Section on Developmental and Behavioral Pediatrics. The lifelong effects of early childhood adversity and toxic stress. *Pediatrics*. 2012;129(1): e232–e246. Reaffirmed July 2016 (pediatrics.aappublications.org/content/129/1/e232)

Stirling J Jr, Amaya-Jackson L; American Academy of Pediatrics Committee on Child Abuse and Neglect and Section on Adoption and Foster Care; American Academy of Child and Adolescent Psychiatry; National Center for Child Traumatic Stress. Understanding the behavioral and emotional consequences of child abuse. *Pediatrics*. 2008;122(3):667–673. Reaffirmed August 2012 (pediatrics.aappublications.org/content/122/3/667)

Thackeray JD, Hibbard R, Dowd MD; American Academy of Pediatrics Committee on Child Abuse and Neglect and Committee on Injury, Violence, and Poison Prevention. Intimate partner violence: the role of the pediatrician. *Pediatrics*. 2010;125(5): 1094–1100. Reaffirmed January 2014 (pediatrics.aappublications.org/content/125/5/1094)

References

1. Anda RF, Felitti VJ, Bremner JD, et al. The enduring effects of abuse and related adverse experiences in childhood. A convergence of evidence from neurobiology and epidemiology. *Eur Arch Psychiatry Clin Neurosci*. 2006;256(3):174–186
2. Danese A, Moffitt TE, Harrington H, et al. Adverse childhood experiences and adult risk factors for age-related disease: depression, inflammation, and clustering of metabolic risk markers. *Arch Pediatr Adolesc Med*. 2009;163(12):1135–1143
3. Felitti VJ, Anda RF, Nordenberg D, et al. Relationship of childhood abuse and household dysfunction to many of the leading causes of death in adults. The Adverse Childhood Experiences (ACE) Study. *Am J Prev Med*. 1998;14(4):245–258
4. Knudsen EI, Heckman JJ, Cameron JL, Shonkoff JP. Economic, neurobiological, and behavioral perspectives on building America's future workforce. *Proc Natl Acad Sci U S A*. 2006;103(27):10155–10162
5. Shonkoff JP. Building a new biodevelopmental framework to guide the future of early childhood policy. *Child Dev*. 2010;81(1):357–367
6. Shonkoff JP, Boyce WT, McEwen BS. Neuroscience, molecular biology, and the childhood roots of health disparities: building a new framework for health promotion and disease prevention. *JAMA*. 2009;301(21):2252–2259
7. Koenen KC, Moffitt TE, Poulton R, Martin J, Caspi A. Early childhood factors associated with the development of post-traumatic stress disorder: results from a longitudinal birth cohort. *Psychol Med*. 2007;37(2):181–192
8. Flaherty EG, Thompson R, Litrownik AJ, et al. Effect of early childhood adversity on child health. *Arch Pediatr Adolesc Med*. 2006;160(12):1232–1238
9. Flaherty EG, Thompson R, Litrownik AJ, et al. Adverse childhood exposures and reported child health at age 12. *Acad Pediatr*. 2009;9(3):150–156
10. Schweinhart LJ. *Lifetime Effects: The High/Scope Perry Preschool Study Through Age 40*. Ypsilanti, MI: High/Scope Press; 2005
11. Campbell FA, Pungello EP, Miller-Johnson S, Burchinal M, Ramey CT. The development of cognitive and academic abilities: growth curves from an early childhood educational experiment. *Dev Psychol*. 2001;37(2):231–242

12. McLaughlin AE, Campbell FA, Pungello EP, Skinner M. Depressive symptoms in young adults: the influences of the early home environment and early educational child care. *Child Dev.* 2007;78(3):746–756

13. Campbell F, Conti G, Heckman JJ, et al. Early childhood investments substantially boost adult health. *Science.* 2014;343(6178):1478–1485

14. Heckman JJ. Skill formation and the economics of investing in disadvantaged children. *Science.* 2006;312(5782):1900–1902

15. Heckman JJ. The economics, technology, and neuroscience of human capability formation. *Proc Natl Acad Sci U S A.* 2007;104(33):13250–13255

16. Obradović J, Bush NR, Stamperdahl J, Adler NE, Boyce WT. Biological sensitivity to context: the interactive effects of stress reactivity and family adversity on socioemotional behavior and school readiness. *Child Dev.* 2010;81(1):270–289

17. Ouellet-Morin I, Boivin M, Dionne G, et al. Variations in heritability of cortisol reactivity to stress as a function of early familial adversity among 19-month-old twins. *Arch Gen Psychiatry.* 2008;65(2):211–218

18. McEwen BS, Gianaros PJ. Central role of the brain in stress and adaptation: links to socioeconomic status, health, and disease. *Ann N Y Acad Sci.* 2010;1186:190–222

19. National Scientific Counsel on the Developing Child. Excessive stress disrupts the architecture of the developing brain. Working paper 3. Published 2005

20. Shonkoff JP, Phillips DA; Committee on Integrating the Science of Early Childhood Development. *From Neurons to Neighborhoods: The Science of Early Child Development.* Washington, DC: National Academies Press; 2000

21. Anacker C, O'Donnell KJ, Meaney MJ. Early life adversity and the epigenetic programming of hypothalamic-pituitary-adrenal function. *Dialogues Clin Neurosci.* 2014;16(3):321–333

22. Kanherkar RR, Bhatia-Dey N, Csoka AB. Epigenetics across the human lifespan. *Front Cell Dev Biol.* 2014;2:49

23. Tottenham N, Hare TA, Quinn BT, et al. Prolonged institutional rearing is associated with atypically large amygdala volume and difficulties in emotion regulation. *Dev Sci.* 2010;13(1):46–61

24. Tottenham N, Sheridan MA. A review of adversity, the amygdala and the hippocampus: a consideration of developmental timing. *Front Hum Neurosci.* 2010;3:68

25. Lagace DC, Donovan MH, DeCarolis NA, et al. Adult hippocampal neurogenesis is functionally important for stress-induced social avoidance. *Proc Natl Acad Sci U S A.* 2010;107(9):4436–4441

26. Hains AB, Vu MA, Maciejewski PK, van Dyck CH, Gottron M, Arnsten AF. Inhibition of protein kinase C signaling protects prefrontal cortex dendritic spines and cognition from the effects of chronic stress. *Proc Natl Acad Sci U S A.* 2009;106(42):17957–17962

27. Holmes A, Wellman CL. Stress-induced prefrontal reorganization and executive dysfunction in rodents. *Neurosci Biobehav Rev.* 2009;33(6):773–783

28. Peters J, Dieppa-Perea LM, Melendez LM, Quirk GJ. Induction of fear extinction with hippocampal-infralimbic BDNF. *Science.* 2010;328(5983):1288–1290

29. Shonkoff JP, Garner AS; American Academy of Pediatrics Committee on Psychosocial Aspects of Child and Family Health; Committee on Early Childhood, Adoption, and Dependent Care; and Section on Developmental and Behavioral Pediatrics. The lifelong effects of early childhood adversity and toxic stress. *Pediatrics.* 2012;129(1):e232–e246

30. Blair C, Granger DA, Willoughby M, et al. Salivary cortisol mediates effects of poverty and parenting on executive functions in early childhood. *Child Dev.* 2011;82(6):1970–1984

31. McGinnis JM, Williams-Russo P, Knickman JR. The case for more active policy attention to health promotion. *Health Aff (Millwood).* 2002;21(2):78–93

32. Dowd MD, ed. *Trauma Toolbox for Primary Care.* Elk Grove Village, IL: American Academy of Pediatrics; 2014. https://www.aap.org/traumaguide. Accessed January 22, 2018

33. American Academy of Pediatrics, Dave Thomas Foundation for Adoption. *Helping Foster and Adoptive Families Cope With Trauma*. Elk Grove Village, IL: American Academy of Pediatrics; 2016. https://www.aap.org/en-us/Documents/hfca_foster_trauma_guide.pdf. Accessed January 22, 2018

34. Dubowitz H, Feigelman S, Lane W, Kim J. Pediatric primary care to help prevent child maltreatment: the Safe Environment for Every Kid (SEEK) Model. *Pediatrics*. 2009;123(3): 858–864

35. Dubowitz H, Lane WG, Semiatin JN, Magder LS. The SEEK model of pediatric primary care: can child maltreatment be prevented in a low-risk population? *Acad Pediatr*. 2012;12(4): 259–268

36. Gottman J, DeClaire J. *The Heart of Parenting: How to Raise an Emotionally Intelligent Child*. New York, NY: Simon & Schuster; 1997

37. Taylor CA, Manganello JA, Lee SJ, Rice JC. Mothers' spanking of 3-year-old children and subsequent risk of children's aggressive behavior. *Pediatrics*. 2010;125(5):e1057–e1065

38. Ginsburg KR, Jablow MM. *Building Resilience in Children and Teens: Giving Kids Roots and Wings*. Elk Grove Village, IL: American Academy of Pediatrics; 2015

Families New to the United States

Rashmi Shetgiri, MD; Paul L. Geltman, MD, MPH; and
Glenn Flores, MD

"Prior violence exposure in the country of origin, ongoing exposure to violence in their neighborhoods in the United States, and migration-related stress increase the risk for post-traumatic stress disorder, adjustment disorder, depression, and other mood disorders in immigrants."

Introduction

The United States is a nation of immigrants. Since 1820, an estimated 81,551,120 people (excluding those who are undocumented) have immigrated to the United States.[1] Currently, almost 19 million immigrant children live in the United States, including approximately 3 million first-generation and 16 million second-generation (with at least one foreign-born parent) immigrants, accounting for a total of 22% of all children.[2] Twenty percent of newborns, infants, and children 0 to 5 years of age are children of immigrants and are the fastest growing population of children in the United States.[3] This chapter provides a comprehensive approach to providing high-quality mental health care to immigrant children. Recent detailed reviews of immigrant health care have focused on screening tests and checklists.[4,5] In addition to reviewing important mental health care, medical, and health-promotion topics for immigrant children, this chapter addresses basic demographics, barriers to health care, and linguistic and cultural issues for immigrant and refugee children in the United States.

Demographics of Immigrants and Refugees

In 2015, 1,051,031 immigrants received legal resident status in the United States, of which 151,995 were refugees or asylees.[1] The 5 largest countries of origin of immigrants to the United States are (in order) Mexico, China, India, the Philippines, and Cuba (Figure 14-1). Most US immigration is through sponsorship by relatives, with 44% being immediate family members of US citizens and 20% receiving family sponsorship (Figure 14-2).

Official immigration figures, however, do not account for the large numbers of undocumented immigrants living and working in the United States. Among the estimated 11.1 million undocumented immigrants in the United States, 10%, or 1.1 million, are children.[6] The annual flow of undocumented immigrants into the United States declined from 2007 and has remained unchanged since 2009.[6]

Access to Health Care in the United States

Pediatric clinicians (ie, primary care pediatricians, pediatric subspecialists, and family physicians, internists, nurse practitioners, and physician assistants

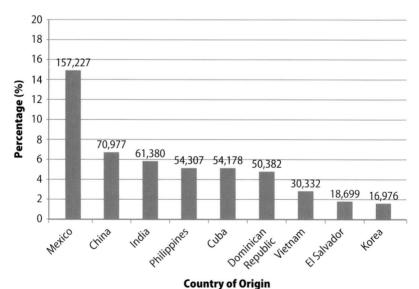

Top 9 Countries of Origin
Of 1,051,031 Total Immigrants to the United States, 2015

Figure 14-1. Top countries of origin of immigrants to the United States, 2015.

Data derived from Office of Immigration Statistics. *Yearbook of Immigration Statistics 2015.* Washington, DC: Office of Immigration Statistics, US Dept of Homeland Security; 2016. https://www.dhs.gov/immigration-statistics/yearbook/2015/table2#. Accessed May 29, 2018.

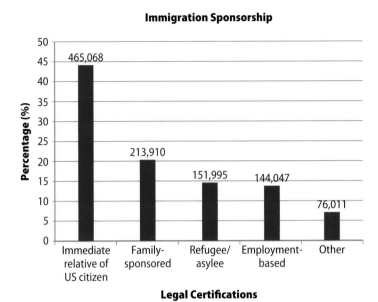

Figure 14-2. Distribution of major classes of admission for immigrants in the United States obtaining "lawful" permanent resident status in 2015.
Data derived from Office of Immigration Statistics. *Yearbook of Immigration Statistics 2015.* Washington, DC: Office of Immigration Statistics, US Dept of Homeland Security; 2016. https://www.dhs.gov/immigration-statistics/yearbook/2015/table6. Accessed May 29, 2018.

who provide health care to children and adolescents) should consider financial issues and insurance coverage when providing care to immigrant families. At present, they pose significant barriers to care for many families. For example, 52% of foreign-born children in noncitizen families are uninsured, compared with 15% of US-born children in citizen families.[7] More than one-fourth (28%) of foreign-born noncitizen children have no usual source of care (other than the emergency department [ED]), compared with approximately 6% of US-born children in citizen families.[7] Foreign-born noncitizen children are also less likely than US-born children to have visited a physician, dentist, or mental health specialist.[7] Noncitizen children from families with low income are approximately 5 times more likely to be uninsured as similar children in citizen families, and only 20% of low-income noncitizen children participate in Medicaid or the Children's Health Insurance Program (CHIP), compared with approximately one-half of low-income citizen children (49% for citizen children in noncitizen families and 41% for citizen children in citizen families).[7] The American Academy of Pediatrics (AAP) advocates for "comprehensive, coordinated, and continuous health services provided within a medical home…" for immigrant children and for awareness of and sensitivity to financial and other barriers that "interfere with achieving optimal health status."[8] An unfortunate start to a clinician's relationship with new patients who are uninsured immigrants would be to perform a large battery of screening laboratory tests that unintentionally cause financial burden to the family.

Studies of Latino children indicate a wide variety of other access barriers to care for immigrant *children* (a term used in this chapter to encompass infants, children, and adolescents unless otherwise specified). For example, a study of a predominantly immigrant Latino population revealed that more than one-quarter of parents (26%) said that language problems were the single greatest barrier to getting health care for their child (specifically, 15% of parents said that the greatest obstacle was physicians and nurses who do not speak Spanish, and 11% cited lack of interpreters).[9] A long wait at the physician's office was reported as the greatest barrier by 15%, 13% mentioned the lack of medical insurance, 7% cited difficulty paying for medical bills, and 6% identified transportation issues. Parents who participated in the study also identified several barriers to care that had caused them not to bring their children in for medical visits in the past; transportation problems were reported most often (21%), followed by not being able to afford health care (18%), excessive waits to see the physician (17%), lack of health insurance (16%), inconvenient clinic hours (14%), difficulty making appointments (13%), and culture and language problems (11%).

Access to primary care and other medical services can be highly variable among immigrant communities. Racial and ethnic minorities and low-income children in the United States have consistently had significantly worse rates of having a usual source of care and other health care indicators.[10] In addition, specific ethnic groups have varying levels of access to and use of health care, even within their own communities.[11] These differences, independent of income and educational levels, underscore the importance of cultural and linguistic barriers to health care access. Accordingly, outreach to ethnic communities and the provision of comprehensive language services to all those who need them are important steps in improving access to health care.

Other research on Latinos, the largest racial and ethnic group among US immigrants, suggests that health insurance coverage is a major determinant of access to and use of care.[12] A large study of Latino people in Los Angeles found that a lack of employment-linked health insurance posed a significant barrier to care for children.[13] Many Latino immigrant children live in 2-parent households, with parents (particularly noncitizens) working in entry-level jobs without benefits or the ability to afford health care insurance premiums. Similarly, children with working parents who were eligible for Medicaid were less likely than others to be continuously enrolled. Children in this category also had less access to care in all measures studied. Indeed, research documents that, after adjustment, parental noncitizenship, having 2 parents work, low family income, and older child age are associated with being an uninsured child, but Latino ethnicity is not.[14] In states where undocumented immigrant children are eligible for at least limited health insurance coverage, *promotoras* (lay Latino community health workers) and other community health workers can be highly effective means of insurance outreach and enrollment. For example, one randomized controlled trial of an insurance intervention for Latino children that included many immigrant families documented that community health workers were substantially more effective than traditional Medicaid and CHIP outreach and enrollment in insuring children (at 96% vs 57%, respectively), and community health workers insured children significantly faster, more continually, and with higher parent satisfaction with the process.[15]

Federal welfare and immigration reform legislation in 1996 further restricted access to Medicaid for noncitizens to reduce expenditures and discourage immigrants from becoming public charges. Nonetheless, research has documented that in the 2 years before enactment of this legislation, immigrants had substantially lower per-capita health care expenditures (55%) than their US-born counterparts.[16] Among children, expenditures were 74% lower among immigrants, yet ED expenditures were 3 times higher. The latter finding suggests that immigrant children are going without basic primary care services and are missing out on the benefits of a medical home. A recent study of immigrant children's use of public health insurance since reform legislation shows that foreign-born children were 1.6 times more likely to be uninsured after 2001 than before 2001, and they are 3 times more likely to be uninsured than to have public insurance.[17] The federal Patient Protection and Affordable Care Act (ACA) of 2010 increased Medicaid coverage to 133% of federal poverty level and restricted access to the health insurance exchange to US citizens and legal residents.[18] It did not alter current restrictions on Medicaid and CHIP eligibility for legal permanent residents within the first 5 years of residency or for undocumented immigrants. Although the ACA contains a provision for the development of guidelines to reduce health disparities through methods such as the use of language services and cultural competency training, the payment mechanism for these services is incentive based. The ACA does not require insurance plans to reimburse for language services or translation of materials into languages other than English, and only 12 states and the District of Columbia currently provide third-party reimbursement for interpreter services.

Of note, there are nearly 4 million children born in the United States to undocumented immigrants who may encounter even further barriers to productive and healthy futures, despite their citizenship status.[19] Recent research found that children of undocumented immigrants may have lower early cognitive and language skills than children of documented immigrants of similar socioeconomic backgrounds.[19] Undocumented parents may share circumstances that adversely affect their children's outcomes, such as avoidance of programs and authorities, social isolation, and poor work conditions. Fearing deportation, undocumented immigrants may be reluctant to access services such as early education programs and food subsidies that could be essential to improving child development. Poor work conditions, including lower rates of benefits and lower wages, may also lead to less access to child care subsidies and center-based care. These factors may contribute to ongoing parental stress and economic hardship, which may result in less of the parent-child interaction that is critical to early skill development in children.[19]

Pediatric clinicians and hospitals that care for children are increasingly facing the dilemma of rationing care to uninsured, undocumented immigrant children, particularly for expensive, lifesaving pediatric care, including transplants, chemotherapy, and dialysis.[20] For example, some hospitals have policies to provide neither dialysis nor kidney transplantation to undocumented, uninsured patients with end-stage renal disease.[20] In such cases, it can be argued that the high costs associated with providing expensive lifesaving care to undocumented children can compromise existing or new clinical programs. On the other hand, denying immediate and long-term care to undocumented immigrant children may result in higher overall expenditures related to preventable hospitalizations and more expensive therapies and have unintended public-health consequences, including significant long-term morbidity and a high risk of early mortality.[20] One potential solution that has been suggested[20] is to have hospitals and clinics establish a structured process with a panel of clinicians and hospital staff who would evaluate these considerations and make a recommendation case by case. This approach could result in formulating a medical individual expense plan for uninsured, undocumented children that could include providing financial aid, discounted treatment, payment plans, and philanthropic support and active fundraising for lifesaving care.

Health Promotion

Primary care clinicians (PCCs) working with families new to the United States must first establish linguistically and culturally effective relationships with the families (see details on cultural competency action steps later in this chapter). By showing interest in the families' backgrounds, cultures, and community issues, the PCC may also gain a reputation as a sympathetic and supportive health care professional whom other members of that ethnic community can trust. The following section describes in more detail the issues associated with this task. An important point to remember is that postponing medical screening is reasonable if it seems inappropriate on the basis of cultural, linguistic, or economic reasons.

The concepts of health promotion and preventive medicine may be new to the family. In introducing these concepts, the clinician will embark on a journey of communication with new Americans. This journey may be relatively straightforward and brief with patients and families who share more Western beliefs, or it may involve multiple levels of complexity that will require a fair amount of time and effort. It can include efforts to understand immigrant families' cultural expectations and previous experiences with the health care system in their native countries; to educate them about basic issues in the American health care system, such as assessing eligibility for and access to health insurance; and to provide practical tips, such as instructions on where to go for urgent care and when to go the ED.

Language Barriers to Care and Providing Adequate Language Access

Approximately 65 million Americans speak a language other than English at home, and 25.9 million have *limited English proficiency* (LEP), defined as a self-rated English-speaking ability of less than "very well."[21] As of 2015, approximately 12 million (21%) US school-aged children and adolescents (5–17 years of age) spoke a language other than English at home, almost triple the number reported in 1979, and 4.5 million (9.3%) had LEP.[22,23] Between 1980 and 2015, the number of people in the United States speaking a language other than English at home increased from 23 million to 65 million.[21] The number of LEP Americans rose from 14 million in 1990 to 25.9 million in 2015.[21]

This marked growth in the number of Americans who speak a language other than English at home or who have LEP can be attributed to the rapid increase in the foreign-born population in the United States, which grew from 9.6 million in 1970 to 43.3 million in 2015.[21] Most LEP Americans speak Spanish (64%, or 16.4 million); Asian and Pacific Island languages (led by Chinese languages) are the next most common among LEP Americans (comprising 19%, or 5 million), followed by other Indo-European languages (14%, or 3.5 million) and all other languages (4%, or 953,484).[21]

Language barriers have many adverse consequences in health care,[24,25] including impaired health status[26,27]; a lower likelihood of having a usual source of medical care[24,25,28]; lower rates of screening and other preventive services[28–30]; nonadherence to medications[31]; a greater likelihood of a diagnosis of more severe psychopathology and leaving the hospital against medical advice among psychiatric patients[32,33]; a lower likelihood of being given a follow-up appointment after an ED visit[34]; an increased risk of intubation in children with asthma[35]; an increased risk of drug complications[36]; higher resource use for diagnostic testing[37]; lower patient satisfaction[24,38,39]; impaired patient understanding of diagnoses, medications, and follow-up[40,41]; fewer telephone calls to physicians' offices[42]; fewer referrals to specialists[42]; and an increased risk of medical errors and injuries.[43–46] Use of ad hoc interpreters (untrained family members, friends, and people pulled from the waiting area or streets) can have particularly deleterious consequences for mental health care. A study of suicides by LEP patients who had been treated by monolingual English-proficient psychiatrists using ad hoc interpreters suggested that utilizing ad hoc interpreters can result in overemphasizing psychotic features and underemphasizing affective components, thus underestimating suicide risk.[47] Another study found that for LEP patients undergoing psychiatric evaluations, relatives who are used as interpreters tend to either minimize or emphasize psychopathology and often answer the clinician's questions without asking the patient.[47] For example, the son of a patient was asked to inquire about his father's possible suicidal ideation; without asking his father, he insisted on a negative answer.[48] Latino parents consider the lack of interpreters and Spanish-speaking staff to be the greatest barrier to health care for their children, and 1 out of every 17 parents in one study reported not bringing his or her child in for needed medical care because of these language issues.[9]

To assess the language needs of patients and caregivers accurately, determining whether a child's caregiver has LEP is essential. Determining English proficiency has been shown to be superior to the primary language spoken at home as a measure of the effect of language barriers on children's health and health care.[49] The following questions, which come from the US Census,[50] are an excellent means of quickly assessing English proficiency and language service needs and should be asked routinely of the primary caregiver during the first visit:

1. Does this person speak a language other than English at home?
   - ▶ Yes
   - ▶ No *[Stop here; person is considered English proficient.]*

2. What is this language?

   (For example: Korean, Italian, Spanish, Vietnamese)

3. How well does this person speak English?
   - ▶ Very well
   - ▶ Well
   - ▶ Not well
   - ▶ Not at all

   [Person has LEP if reply is anything other than "very well" and requires medical interpreter or bilingual provider.]

Although millions of Americans have LEP, many patients who need medical interpreters are not provided with interpreters. Every LEP patient should have access to a trained medical interpreter or bilingual health care professional.[51] Ample scientific evidence documents that optimal communication, patient satisfaction, and outcomes, and minimal interpreter errors, occur when LEP patients have access to trained professional interpreters or bilingual providers.[24] In addition, federal guidance on Title VI of the Civil Rights Act of 1964 has established that denial or delay of medical care for patients who have LEP because of language barriers constitutes a form of discrimination and requires all recipients of federal funds, including Medicaid, CHIP, and Medicare, to provide adequate language assistance to those who need it.[52] Key mechanisms for ensuring adequate language access for patients and families who have LEP are summarized in Box 14-1.

Detailed information on improving language access in health care is available in the Office of Minority Health's *A Patient-Centered Guide to Implementing Language Access Services in Healthcare Organizations.*[53]

Cultural Issues

Cultural issues affect multiple aspects of pediatric care, including outcomes, quality, costs, satisfaction with care, and patient safety.[45,54,55] Failing to appreciate the importance of culture in pediatrics can result in a variety of adverse consequences, including difficulties with informed consent, miscommunication, inadequate understanding of diagnoses and treatment

Box 14-1. Key Mechanisms for Ensuring Adequate Language Access for Patients, Caregivers, and Families With Limited English Proficiency

- **Ensure that a trained medical interpreter or bilingual provider is available for each medical encounter.** Making language available throughout the encounter is especially important, including during registration, the history and physical examination, procedures, visits to the laboratory and radiology department, and scheduling of follow-up appointments.

- **Use telephone or video interpreter services when in-person interpreters or bilingual providers are unavailable.**

- **Ensure adequate language access *door-to-door* (ie, at all points of interaction with the health care system).** This provision includes multilingual operators, telephone trees, or both (for scheduling appointments, leaving messages, and getting phone advice), multilingual signage at all key wayfaring points (parking garages, clinic entrances, registration, paths to the ED, laboratory, radiology facility, and pharmacy), and multilingual registration clerks.

- **Routinely collect and record patient and family data on primary language spoken at home and LEP.** This provision permits efficiently meeting the language needs of the patient population and scheduling interpreters in advance for all future medical visits.

- **Use pharmacies that can print prescription labels, provide medication information packets, and communicate in non-English languages.** Failure to do so can result in medical errors and injuries.[42–45] Printing clinic prescription pads with check boxes such as ☐ *Spanish* or ☐ *Mandarin* is particularly helpful and is a useful reminder.

- **Have patient information and anticipatory guidance pamphlets available in non-English languages common in the physician's practice.** Ideally, certified translators should be available to translate written documents for patients. Useful Web resources with materials already translated include the National Network of Libraries of Medicine Consumer Health Information in Many Languages Resources site (https://nnlm.gov/outreach/consumer/multi.html), US Department of Health and Human Services Español-Healthfinder (www.healthfinder.gov/espanol), CDC en Español (www.cdc.gov/spanish), and Selected Patient Information Resources in Asian Languages (http://spiral.tufts.edu).

- **Translate consent forms into all relevant non-English languages for your patient population.**

- **Help patients and families who have LEP learn English through referrals to free or low-cost English as second language courses.** This excellent resource (www.literacydirectory.org) locates classes according to zip code.

- **Increase the number of bilingual health care providers and staff.** This provision can be achieved through enhanced efforts to recruit bilingual staff, continuing professional education, intensive language courses, and bonuses for demonstrating foreign language fluency.

Abbreviations: CDC, Centers for Disease Control and Prevention; ED, emergency department; LEP, limited English proficiency.

plans by families, dissatisfaction with care, preventable morbidity and mortality, unnecessary child-abuse evaluations, and disparities in prescriptions, analgesia, and diagnostic evaluations.[45,54,55] On the other hand, providing culturally competent health care to children is associated with better health outcomes. For example, pediatric patients with asthma receiving care at practice sites with the highest cultural competence scores are significantly less likely to be underusing preventive asthma medications and have better parental ratings of the quality of care.[56] Similarly, the impact of culturally competent practice in mental health is highlighted in the "Practice Parameter for Cultural Competence in Child and Adolescent Psychiatric Practice," which reviews the interplay between culture and the mental health of children and describes best practices in provision of care.[57]

Because culture can profoundly affect the care of immigrant children, pediatric clinicians should be familiar with the most important cultural issues that affect clinical care, including folk illnesses with symptoms that overlap with biomedical conditions, biomedical conditions that can result from harmful folk illness remedies or parental beliefs and practices, and cultural healing practices that can be confused with child abuse.[45,54,55] Folk illnesses may overlap with several biomedical conditions, including gastroenteritis, parasitic infections, heavy metal poisoning, dehydration, and respiratory illnesses. Certain folk illnesses are of particular relevance to mental health, such as *kitsune-tsuki* (fox possession), a Japanese ethnomedical syndrome consisting of delusions, disordered thinking, auditory hallucinations, and paranoia, thereby overlapping with biomedical conditions that can include psychosis, schizophrenia, and mercury poisoning.[55] Some folk illness remedies or parental beliefs and practices may lead to unintended complications, such as unintentional poisoning caused by herbal treatments of children's symptoms.[54,55] Awareness of these cultural beliefs and practices is helpful in obtaining accurate histories and improving patient satisfaction through the use of culturally acceptable complementary and integrative treatments, generating rapid differential diagnoses and treatment plans, and making informed decisions about child abuse (Table 14-1).

Cultural competency is defined as the recognition of and appropriate response to key cultural features that affect clinical care.[45,54] Providing culturally competent health care should be the goal of every clinician caring for immigrant children. Box 14-2 summarizes a model of cultural competency that can be helpful in clinical encounters with patients from any cultural group.

For further discussion of cultural competency, see Chapter 3, Culturally Effective Care. Helpful Web-based resources for addressing the cultural

Table 14-1. Cultural Healing Practices That Can Be Confused With Child Abuse

Regional Origin	Clinical Presentation	Cultural Practice	Ethnicity or Nationality Associated With Practice	Symptoms or Illnesses Treated
Latin America	Patterned circular erythema, petechiae, occasional burns	*Ventosas* (cupping): vacuum created in cup by burning alcohol over inverted cup, cup placed on affected anatomy	Latino	Pain, fever, poor appetite, congestion
Asia and Pacific Islands	Circular burns (second or third degree) and scars	Moxibustion: moxa herb or yarn rolled into ball or cone, ignited, applied to body part and allowed to burn to point of pain	Laotian Cambodian Chinese Japanese	Fever, abdominal pain, ear infections, enuresis, tantrums
	Linear ecchymoses, hyperpigmentation, transient microscopic hematuria	*Cao gio* ("scratch the wind"), or coin rubbing: symptomatic area covered with mentholated oil or balsam, then rubbed linearly with coin or other object until ecchymoses occurs	Vietnamese	Fever, cough, vomiting, headaches, chills, seizures, myalgias
	Linear ecchymoses	*Quat sha* (spoon scratching): porcelain spoon used to rub skin on back (after water or saline applied) until ecchymoses appear	Chinese	Fever, headache

Adapted from Flores G, Rabke-Verani J, Pine W, Sabharwal A. The importance of cultural and linguistic issues in the emergency care of children. *Pediatr Emerg Care.* 2002;18(4):271–284. Copyright © Lippincott Williams & Wilkins. Reprinted with permission.

issues in pediatric care include DiversityRx (www.diversityrx.org), the Office of Minority Health Web site (https://minorityhealth.hhs.gov), and the University of Michigan Health System Program for Multicultural Health (www.med.umich.edu/multicultural).

Mental Health, Developmental Issues, and Functional Health Screening

Mental health and behavioral problems are common among immigrant and refugee children, in part because many such families experience traumas. Prior violence exposure in the country of origin, ongoing exposure to violence in their neighborhoods in the United States, and migration-related

Box 14-2. Model for Cultural Competency in Health Care

❶ Normative cultural values
  - Identify values that affect care.
  - Accommodate for these values in clinical encounter.

❷ Language issues
  - Use interpreter services unless fluent in patient's primary language.
  - Follow guidelines for effective interpreter use.
  - Encourage efforts to increase foreign language skills of staff and English skills of patients who are LEP.

❸ Folk illnesses
  - Recognize those that may affect clinical care.
  - Suggest alternatives to harmful folk remedies.
  - Accommodate nonjudgmentally into clinical encounter.
  - Integrate into biomedical treatment plan whenever possible.

❹ Parent and patient beliefs
  - Identify beliefs that may affect clinical care.
  - Suggest alternatives to harmful home remedies.
  - Carefully explain etiology and treatment rationale for given biomedical condition.

❺ Provider practices
  - Maintain vigilance for ethnic disparities in screening, prescriptions, procedures, and outcomes.
  - When disparities occur, determine problem's source and address practices that might be responsible.

From Flores G, Abreu M, Schwartz I, Hill M. The importance of language and culture in pediatric care: case studies from the Latino community. *J Pediatrics*. 2000;137(6):842–848, with permission from Elsevier.

stress increase the risk for post-traumatic stress disorder (PTSD), adjustment disorder, depression, and other mood disorders in immigrants.[58] In a large meta-analysis of studies of children who had been internationally adopted, researchers found an elevated prevalence of behavioral problems and use of mental health services compared with nonadopted children.[59] A study of Haitian immigrant students in Boston public schools revealed the prevalence of depression to be 14% and of PTSD to be 12%.[60] Behavioral disorders among traumatized immigrant families may be difficult to diagnose and treat in primary care settings. Even in situations in which parents identify behavioral symptoms in their children, parents may be reluctant to have children treated for behavioral disorders because of cultural beliefs or concerns about immigration status.[58,61] Cultural factors may present similar challenges for diagnosing and treating behavioral disorders among nontraumatized children as well. Many immigrants and refugee families will visit clinicians with symptoms or concerns such as headache or stomachache because of underlying behavioral or emotional problems or somatization.

Somatization is common in many cultures around the world. Studies have documented the high prevalence of somatization and its association with increased clinic visits in immigrant and refugee communities in the United States.[62,63] Caring for patients with somatization may be challenging.[64] The clinician's validation of the impairment from somatic symptoms and focus on functional improvement, however, may facilitate the establishment of trust necessary for uncovering the emotional basis for the symptoms. In the setting of pediatric primary care, the clinician may find simple screening instruments, such as the Pediatric Symptom Checklist (www.massgeneral.org/psychiatry/services/psc_home.aspx), the Strengths and Difficulties Questionnaire (www.sdqinfo.com), or the Child Health Questionnaire (www.healthactchq.com/survey/chq), helpful in identifying social-emotional problems and documenting functional impairment from somatization and behavioral health problems. (See Appendix 2, Mental Health Tools for Pediatrics.) Although all 3 questionnaires are available in multiple languages, literacy barriers can complicate administering these written screening questionnaires with immigrant and refugee patients. Such screening may obviate the need for disease-specific diagnostic questionnaires that either are too lengthy for practical use or may be emotionally upsetting to patients and families. Resources and online training for PCCs wishing to work with traumatized immigrants (or any patients who are survivors of significant violence) are also available from the Harvard Program in Refugee Trauma (www.hprt-cambridge.org). A child-specific resource available to help pediatricians handle mental health issues is the Refugee Services Toolkit (RST), designed by the Refugee Trauma and Resilience Center at Boston Children's Hospital (www.childrenshospital.org/centers-and-services/refugee-trauma-and-resilience-center-program/training-and-resource-development). The RST is a Web-based tool designed to help providers understand the experience of refugee children and families, identify needs associated with their mental health, and ensure that they are connected with the most appropriate available interventions.

Immigrant children are at particularly high risk for impaired access to and knowledge about mental health services. Compared with US-born citizen children, undocumented immigrant children are almost 4 times more likely and second-generation children with undocumented immigrant parents are more than twice as likely to have made no visit to a mental health specialist in the past 12 months.[7] A recent Canadian study revealed that, compared with refugee children, undocumented and new permanent-resident immigrant children significantly more often present to EDs with mental health problems, including approximately 8-fold higher rates of depression or anxiety, 4-fold higher rates of substance abuse, 3-fold higher rates of suicidal ideation, and substantially higher PTSD rates.[65] Indeed, it has been argued that children of undocumented immigrants are at especially high risk for anxiety and PTSD, because their families may be hiding from authorities, may be living in fear of discovery, may include parents who are incarcerated or deported because of their undocumented status, or may experience Immigration and Customs Enforcement raids and deportation sweeps,[66] a particular concern of late because of increased immigration restrictions and deportations under the current federal administration. A survey of immigrant Latino adolescents and adults documented that fewer than 1 in 5 knew of a place in the community that could help an adolescent with a mental health problem or specifically with depression, and fewer than 1 in 4 knew of a place or resource for an adolescent contemplating suicide.[67] Immigrants at particularly high risk of these knowledge deficits included rural residents, males, and those who had lived in the community for less than 1 year.[67]

Immigrant children are also at higher risk of not being screened for behavioral and developmental disorders. Nationally representative data reveal that elicitation of developmental concerns from parents occurs for significantly fewer Latino children in households whose primary language is not English, at 33%, compared with 55% of white children.[68] A survey of California pediatricians showed that only 29% offered Spanish autism spectrum disorder (ASD) screening per AAP guidelines, and only 10% offered both Spanish general developmental and Spanish ASD screening per AAP guidelines.[69] This study also showed that language issues were one of the most important barriers to ASD care for Latino children, with 56% citing these issues as a barrier.[69]

Certain practices and resources have been shown to enhance mental health and developmental outcomes and screening. For Latino children in households whose primary language is not English, having a usual source of care, a personal physician or nurse, and adequate family-centered care are associated with higher adjusted odds of provider elicitation of developmental concerns from parents.[68] Working closely with schools can be particularly useful in identifying immigrant children with mental health issues;

one study in Italy showed that immigrant children were 4 times more likely than nonimmigrant children to be referred by teachers to mental health services.[70] In the United Kingdom, mental health walk-in clinics were found to result in significantly better mental health outcomes than was traditional care for a predominantly immigrant population of children.[71] For children of physically abused immigrant mothers, placement in a domestic violence shelter or issuance of a protective order by the justice system was associated with significant improvements in child functioning and scores for behavioral problems.[72]

Common Medical Issues in Immigrant Children Relevant to Behavioral Health

Growth, Nutrition, and Elevated Blood Lead Level

Growth abnormalities and nutritional disorders are among the most common health problems of immigrant children, particularly refugees,[73] adoptees,[74] and immigrants from similarly deprived backgrounds. Common nutritional disorders, such as iron deficiency, may be seen in a significant portion of some populations of immigrant children, including young refugees. Nutritional deficiencies, such as in iron and calcium, may also increase the susceptibility of immigrant and refugee children to environmental toxins, including lead.[75-79] (See the CDC Web page at www.cdc.gov/lead.) With known neurodevelopmental consequences, many of these disorders, and food insecurity and hunger in general, may have direct behavioral manifestations among affected children.

With hunger and food insecurity well-documented among US immigrant and refugee populations,[80] the PCC should assess growth and the nutritional status of immigrant and refugee children. See Appendix 2 for tools to assist in screening. Eligible families should be referred for nutritional support to available programs, such as the Special Supplemental Nutrition Program for Women, Infants, and Children (commonly known as WIC) and subsidized school meals programs. A multivitamin with iron and minerals is likely to be beneficial for most immigrant children.

Oral Health

A high prevalence of dental caries has been documented among immigrant[81,82] and refugee children.[83] Many immigrants will lack experience with preventive oral health measures, including topical fluoride and water fluoridation, and face significant barriers to care in the United States. Research on the association of acculturation with oral health practices among refugees and immigrants has demonstrated that the many LEP immigrants adopt American lifestyle behaviors that are associated with poor oral health outcomes while giving up protective behaviors from their home countries.[84] Because of LEP and partial acculturation, however, these immigrants do not fully adopt Western preventive oral health practices.[85,86] To the extent that dental pain from untreated caries may cause symptoms of inattention and fidgeting or may cause missed school, the clinician should be cognizant of his or her potential importance in the larger picture of the emotional and behavioral status of immigrant children.

The PCC can play an important role in promoting healthy personal oral hygiene practices and supporting traditional customs and related behaviors (eg, breastfeeding, diets low in refined sugar, use of chewing sticks with antimicrobial properties, incorporation of oral hygiene into existing cultural or religious behaviors) that may provide oral health, nutritional, and other benefits to the child while also promoting proven oral hygiene practices in the United States (eg, consumption of fluoridated water or oral supplementation, use of fluoride-containing toothpaste).[87,88]

A Note on Abdominal Pain and Parasite Infections

As noted previously, clinicians may encounter immigrant children presenting with a variety of somatic concerns, among the most common being abdominal pain. Clinicians should perform a careful assessment of historical and physical findings and include a detailed social history to look for clues suggesting behavioral or emotional etiologies related to trauma, adjustment issues, depression, or anxiety. Mental health problems are well-known to be among the most common etiologies of abdominal pain in children.[89,90]

The situation of the Sudanese refugees who resettled in the United States around 2000–2001 provides an excellent example of this pain. Service providers working with the Sudanese refugees reported extensive concerns of abdominal pain among these adolescents and young adults to the Centers for Disease Control and Prevention (CDC). In response, the CDC conducted a unique assessment of 800 of these refugees at a reunion several years after their resettlement in the United States. This assessment was focused on invasive parasites, such as *Schistosoma* and *Strongyloides* species. Although finding substantial evidence of these infections, the CDC found no associations with abdominal pain.[91] At the same time, other research reported a very high prevalence of likely somatization, including abdominal pain, among the younger members of this group of Sudanese refugees.[92]

Conclusion

Primary care clinicians caring for children new to the United States serve an important role as the gateway to the medical home. Language and cultural divides that separate clinician from patient may be bridged by providing access to language services for LEP patients and ensuring the delivery of culturally competent care. At the same time, pediatric clinicians should be attentive to the acute and chronic health issues specific to immigrant children and their families. Foreign-born children and children of immigrants may continue to encounter significant challenges to their health and well-being caused by the numerous cultural, linguistic, and legal barriers to accessing services discussed in this chapter. Immigrant children and adolescents may experience significant stress, anxiety, and depression related to issues of acculturation and immigration. Immigrant children and adolescents are at particularly high risk for impaired access to and knowledge about mental health services and of not being screened for behavioral and developmental disorders. Children with LEP attending schools whose staff and students have limited experience with this population may have academic difficulties related to English proficiency that may be mistaken for pathology, such as learning disabilities or developmental delay. These children may therefore need continued follow-up in primary care to discuss school progress and related issues.

Primary care clinicians should work to anticipate and integrate potential health and development issues into the health screening and long-term care of immigrant families. By effectively screening for and treating these issues and promoting wellness with cultural sensitivity, the PCC can create strong bonds with immigrant families and communities and ensure that immigrant children receive the highest quality pediatric care with high levels of patient and parent satisfaction.

AAP Policy

American Academy of Pediatrics Council on Community Pediatrics. Providing care for immigrant, migrant, and border children. *Pediatrics*. 2013;131(6):e2028–e2034 (pediatrics.aappublications.org/content/131/6/e2028)

American Academy of Pediatrics Section on Oral Health. Maintaining and improving the oral health of young children. *Pediatrics*. 2014;134(6):1224–1229 (pediatrics.aappublications.org/content/134/6/1224)

References

1. Office of Immigration Statistics. *Yearbook of Immigration Statistics 2015*. Washington, DC: Office of Immigration Statistics, US Dept of Homeland Security; 2016. https://www.dhs.gov/sites/default/files/publications/Yearbook_Immigration_Statistics_2015.pdf. Accessed January 24, 2018

2. Child Trends DataBank. *Immigrant Children: Indicators on Children and Youth*. Bethesda, MD: Child Trends; 2014. http://www.childtrends.org/wp-content/uploads/2012/07/110_Immigrant_Children.pdf. Accessed January 24, 2018

3. Chilton M, Black MM, Berkowitz C, et al. Food insecurity and risk of poor health among US-born children of immigrants. *Am J Public Health*. 2009;99(3):556–562

4. Adams KM, Gardiner LD, Assefi N. Healthcare challenges from the developing world: post-immigration refugee medicine. *BMJ*. 2004;328(7455):1548–1552

5. Jenista JA. The immigrant, refugee, or internationally adopted child. *Pediatr Rev*. 2001;22(12): 419–429

6. Passel JS, Cohn D. *Overall Number of U.S. Unauthorized Immigrants Holds Steady Since 2009*. Washington, DC: Hispanic Trends, Pew Research Center; 2016. http://www.pewhispanic. org/2016/09/20/overall-number-of-u-s-unauthorized-immigrants-holds-steady-since-2009. Accessed January 24, 2018

7. Huang ZJ, Yu SM, Ledsky R. Health status and health service access and use among children in U.S. immigrant families. *Am J Public Health*. 2006;96(4):634–640

8. DuPlessis HM, Cora-Bramble D; American Academy of Pediatrics Committee on Community Health Services. Providing care for immigrant, homeless, and migrant children. *Pediatrics*. 2005;115(4):1095–1100

9. Flores G, Abreu M, Olivar MA, Kastner B. Access barriers to health care for Latino children. *Arch Pediatr Adolesc Med*. 1998;152(11):1119–1125

10. Newacheck PW, Hughes DC, Stoddard JJ. Children's access to primary care: differences by race, income, and insurance status. *Pediatrics*. 1996;97(1):26–32

11. Flores G, Bauchner H, Feinstein AR, Nguyen US. The impact of ethnicity, family income, and parental education on children's health and use of health services. *Am J Public Health*. 1999;89(7):1066–1071

12. Hubbell FA, Waitzkin H, Mishra SI, Dombrink J, Chavez LR. Access to medical care for documented and undocumented Latinos in a southern California county. *West J Med*. 1991; 154(4):414–417

13. Halfon N, Wood DL, Valdez RB, Pereyra M, Duan N. Medicaid enrollment and health services access by Latino children in inner-city Los Angeles. *JAMA*. 1997;277(8):636–641

14. Flores G, Abreu M, Tomany-Korman SC. Why are Latinos the most uninsured racial/ethnic group of US children? A community-based study of risk factors for and consequences of being an uninsured Latino child. *Pediatrics*. 2006;118(3):e730–e740

15. Flores G, Abreu M, Chaisson CE, et al. A randomized, controlled trial of the effectiveness of community-based case management in insuring uninsured Latino children. *Pediatrics*. 2005;116(6):1433–1441

16. Mohanty SA, Woolhandler S, Himmelstein DU, Pati S, Carrasquillo O, Bor DH. Health care expenditures of immigrants in the United States: a nationally representative analysis. *Am J Public Health*. 2005;95(8):1431–1438

17. Pati S, Danagoulian S. Immigrant children's reliance on public health insurance in the wake of immigration reform. *Am J Public Health*. 2008;98(11):2004–2010

18. *Patient Protection and Affordable Care Act Health-Related Portions of the Health Care and Education Reconciliation Act of 2010*. Washington, DC: Office of the Legislative Counsel; 2010. http://docs.house.gov/energycommerce/ppacacon.pdf. Accessed January 24, 2018

19. Yoshikawa H. *Immigrants Raising Citizens: Undocumented Parents and Their Young Children*. New York, NY: Russell Sage Foundation; 2011

20. Young J, Flores G, Berman S. Providing life-saving health care to undocumented children: controversies and ethical issues. *Pediatrics.* 2004;114(5):1316–1320

21. US Census Bureau. Selected social characteristics in the United States: 2015 American Community Survey 1-year estimates. US Census Bureau Web site. https://factfinder. census.gov/faces/tableservices/jsf/pages/productview.xhtml?pid=ACS_15_1YR_ DP02&prodType=table. Accessed January 24, 2018

22. Kids Count Data Center. Children who speak a language other than English at home. Kids Count Data Center Web site. http://datacenter.kidscount.org/data/tables/81-children-who-speak-a-language-other-than-english-at-home#detailed/1/any/false/573,869,36,868,867/ any/396,397. Accessed January 24, 2018

23. National Center for Education Statistics. English language learners. National Center for Education Statistics Web site. https://nces.ed.gov/fastfacts/display.asp?id=96. Accessed January 24, 2018

24. Flores G. The impact of medical interpreter services on the quality of health care: a systematic review. *Med Care Res Rev.* 2005;62(3):255–299

25. Flores G, Laws MB, Mayo SJ, et al. Errors in medical interpretation and their potential clinical consequences in pediatric encounters. *Pediatrics.* 2003;111(1):6–14

26. Kirkman-Liff B, Mondragón D. Language of interview: relevance for research of southwest Hispanics. *Am J Pub Health.* 1991;81(11):1399–1404

27. Hu DJ, Covell RM. Health care usage by Hispanic outpatients as a function of primary language. *West J Med.* 1986;144(4):490–493

28. Weinick RM, Krauss NA. Racial/ethnic differences in children's access to care. *Am J Pub Health.* 2000;90(11):1771–1774

29. Marks G, Solis J, Richardson JL, et al. Health behavior of elderly Hispanic women: does cultural assimilation make a difference? *Am J Pub Health.* 1987;77(10):1315–1319

30. Woloshin S, Schwartz LM, Katz SJ, Welch HG. Is language a barrier to the use of preventive services? *J Gen Intern Med.* 1997;12(8):472–477

31. Manson A. Language concordance as a determinant of patient compliance and emergency room use in patients with asthma. *Med Care.* 1988;26(12):1119–1128

32. Marcos LR, Uruyo L, Kesselman M, Alpert M. The language barrier in evaluating Spanish-American patients. *Arch Gen Psychiatry.* 1973;29(5):655–659

33. Baxter M, Bucci W. Studies in linguistic ambiguity and insecurity. *Urban Health.* 1981;10(5): 36–40

34. Sarver J, Baker DW. Effect of language barriers on follow-up appointments after an emergency department visit. *J Gen Intern Med.* 2000;15(4):256–264

35. LeSon S, Gershwin ME. Risk factors for asthmatic patients requiring intubation. I. Observations in children. *J Asthma.* 1995;32(4):285–294

36. Gandhi TK, Burstin HR, Cook EF, et al. Drug complications in outpatients. *J Gen Intern Med.* 2000;15(3):149–154

37. Hampers LC, Cha S, Gutglass DJ, Binns HJ, Krug SE. Language barriers and resource utilization in a pediatric emergency department. *Pediatrics.* 1999;103(6, pt 1):1253–1256

38. Carrasquillo O, Orav EJ, Brennan TA, Burstin HR. Impact of language barriers on patient satisfaction in an emergency department. *J Gen Intern Med.* 1999;14(2):82–87

39. Morales LS, Cunningham WE, Brown JA, Liu H, Hays RD. Are Latinos less satisfied with communication by health care providers? *J Gen Intern Med.* 1999;14(7):409–417

40. Baker DW, Parker RM, Williams MV, Coates WC, Pitkin K. Use and effectiveness of interpreters in an emergency department. *JAMA.* 1996;275(10):783–738

41. Crane JA. Patient comprehension of doctor-patient communication on discharge from the emergency department. *J Emerg Med.* 1997;15(1):1–7

42. Flores G, Olson L, Tomany-Korman SC. Racial and ethnic disparities in early childhood health and health care. *Pediatrics.* 2005;115(2):e183–e193

43. Harsham P. A misinterpreted word worth $71 million. *Med Econ.* 1984;61:289–292

44. Koren G, Barzilay Z, Greenwald M. Tenfold errors in administration of drug doses: a neglected iatrogenic disease in pediatrics. *Pediatrics.* 1986;77(6):848–849

45. Flores G, Abreu M, Schwartz I, Hill M. The importance of language and culture in pediatric care: case studies from the Latino community. *J Pediatrics.* 2000;137(6):842–848

46. Flores G. Language barrier. WebM&M (Morbidity & Mortality Rounds on the Web) Web site. https://psnet.ahrq.gov/webmm/case/123/language-barrier?q=Flores+G+Language+barrier. Published April 2006. Accessed January 24, 2018

47. Sabin JE. Translating despair. *Am J Psychiatry.* 1975;132(2):197–199

48. Marcos LR. Effects of interpreters on the evaluation of psychopathology in non-English-speaking patients. *Am J Psychiatry.* 1979;136(2):171–174

49. Flores G, Abreu M, Tomany-Korman SC. Limited English proficiency, primary language at home, and disparities in children's health care: how language barriers are measured matters. *Public Health Rep.* 2000;120(4):418–430

50. Shin HB. *Language Use and English-Speaking Ability: 2000.* Washington, DC: US Census Bureau, Economics and Statistics Administration, US Dept of Commerce; 2003. https://www.census.gov/prod/2003pubs/c2kbr-29.pdf. Accessed January 24, 2018

51. Flores G. Language barriers to health care in the United States. *N Engl J Med.* 2006;355(3):229–231

52. Office for Civil Rights. *Title VI Prohibition Against National Origin Discrimination—Persons With Limited-English Proficiency* [guidance memorandum]. Washington, DC: Office for Civil Rights, Dept of Health and Human Services; 1998

53. American Institutes for Research. *A Patient-Centered Guide to Implementing Language Access Services in Healthcare Organizations.* Washington, DC: Office of Minority Health, US Dept of Health and Human Services; 2005. https://minorityhealth.hhs.gov/assets/pdf/checked/hc-lsig.pdf. Accessed January 24, 2018

54. Flores G. Culture and the patient-physician relationship: achieving cultural competency in health care. *J Pediatrics.* 2000;136(1):14–23

55. Flores G, Rabke-Verani J, Pine W, Sabharwal A. The importance of cultural and linguistic issues in the emergency care of children. *Pediatr Emerg Care.* 2002;18(4):271–284

56. Lieu TA, Finkelstein JA, Lozano P, et al. Cultural competence policies and other predictors of asthma care quality for Medicaid-insured children. *Pediatrics.* 2004;114(1):e102–e110

57. Pumariega AJ, Rothe E, Mian A, et al; American Academy of Child and Adolescent Psychiatry Committee on Quality Issues. Practice parameter for cultural competence in child and adolescent psychiatric practice. *J Am Acad Child Adolesc Psychiatry.* 2013;52(10):1101–1115

58. Yearwood EL, Crawford S, Kelly M, Moreno N. Immigrant youth at risk for disorders of mood: recognizing complex dynamics. *Arch Psychiatr Nurs.* 2007;21(3):162–171

59. Juffer F, van Ijzendoorn MH. Behavior problems and mental health referrals of international adoptees: a meta-analysis. *JAMA.* 2005;293(20):2501–2515

60. Fawzi MC, Betancourt TS, Marcelin L, et al. Depression and post-traumatic stress disorder among Haitian immigrant students: implications for access to mental health services and educational programming. *BMC Public Health.* 2009;9:482

61. Geltman PL, Augustyn M, Barnett ED, Klass PE, Groves BM. War trauma experience and behavioral screening of Bosnian refugee children resettled in Massachusetts. *J Dev Behav Pediatr.* 2000;21(4):257–263

62. Lin EH, Carter WB, Kleinman AM. An exploration of somatization among Asian refugees and immigrants in primary care. *Am J Public Health.* 1985;75(9):1080–1084

63. Jamil H, Hakim-Larson J, Farrag M, Kafaji T, Jamil LH, Hammad A. Medical complaints among Iraqi American refugees with mental disorders. *J Immigr Health.* 2005;7(3):145–152

64. Junod Perron N, Hudelson P. How do junior doctors working in a multicultural context make sense of somatisation? *Swiss Med Wkly.* 2005;135(31–32):475–479

65. Rousseau C, Laurin-Lamothe A, Rummens JA, Meloni F, Steinmetz N, Alvaréz F. Uninsured immigrant and refugee children presenting to Canadian paediatric emergency departments: disparities in help-seeking and service delivery. *Paediatr Child Health.* 2013;18(9):465–469

66. Cudara ME. Anxiety and PTSD in Latino children of immigrants: the INS raid connection to the development of these disorders. National Association of Social Workers Web site. http://www.helpstartshere.org/helpstartshere/?p=1780. Published March 2009. Accessed January 24, 2018

67. García CM, Gilchrist L, Vazquez G, Leite A, Raymond N. Urban and rural immigrant Latino youths' and adults' knowledge and beliefs about mental health resources. *J Immigr Minor Health.* 2011;13(3):500–509

68. Guerrero AD, Rodriguez MA, Flores G. Disparities in provider elicitation of parents' developmental concerns for US children. *Pediatrics.* 2011;128(5):901–909

69. Zuckerman KE, Mattox K, Donelan K, Batbayar O, Baghaee A, Bethell C. Pediatrician identification of Latino children at risk for autism spectrum disorder. *Pediatrics.* 2013;132(3): 445–453

70. Pedrini L, Sisti D, Tiberti A, et al. Reasons and pathways of first-time consultations at child and adolescent mental health services in Italy: an observational study. *Child Adolesc Psychiatry Ment Health.* 2015;9:29

71. Barwick M, Urajnik D, Sumner L, et al. Profiles and service utilization for children accessing a mental health walk-in clinic versus usual care. *J Evid Based Soc Work.* 2013;10(4):338–352

72. Cesario SK, Nava A, Bianchi A, McFarlane J, Maddoux J. Functioning outcomes for abused immigrant women and their children 4 months after initiating intervention. *Rev Panam Salud Publica.* 2014;35(1):8–14

73. Geltman PL, Radin M, Zhang Z, Cochran J, Meyers AF. Growth status and related medical conditions among refugee children in Massachusetts, 1995-1998. *Am J Public Health.* 2001; 91(11):1800–1805

74. Albers LH, Johnson DE, Hostetter MK, Iverson S, Miller LC. Health of children adopted from the former Soviet Union and Eastern Europe. Comparison with preadoptive medical records. *JAMA.* 1997;278(11):922–924

75. Centers for Disease Control and Prevention. Elevated blood lead levels among internationally adopted children—United States, 1998. *MMWR Morb Mortal Wkly Rep.* 2000;49(5):97–100

76. Geltman PL, Brown MJ, Cochran J. Lead poisoning among refugee children resettled in Massachusetts, 1995 to 1999. *Pediatrics.* 2001;108(1):158–162

77. Seal AJ, Creeke PI, Mirghani Z, et al. Iron and vitamin A deficiency in long-term African refugees. *J Nutr.* 2005;135(4):808–813

78. Wishart HD, Reeve AM, Grant CC. Vitamin D deficiency in a multinational refugee population. *Intern Med J.* 2007;37(12):792–797

79. Centers for Disease Control and Prevention. Vitamin B_{12} deficiency in resettled Bhutanese refugees—United States, 2008-2011. *MMWR Morb Mortal Wkly Rep.* 2011;60(11):343–346

80. Kasper J, Gupta SK, Tran P, Cook JT, Meyers AF. Hunger in legal immigrants in California, Texas, and Illinois. *Am J Public Health.* 2000;90(10):1629–1633

81. Pollick HF, Rice AJ, Echenberg D. Dental health of recent immigrant children in the Newcomer schools, San Francisco. *Am J Public Health.* 1987;77(6):731–732

82. Sgan-Cohen HD, Steinberg D, Zusman SP, Sela MN. Dental caries and its determinants among recent immigrants from rural Ethiopia. *Community Dent Oral Epidemiol.* 1992;20(6):338–342

83. Cote S, Geltman P, Nunn M, et al. Dental caries of refugee children compared with US children. *Pediatrics.* 2004;114(6):e733–e740

84. Culhane-Pera KA, Naftali ED, Jacobson C, Xiong ZB. Cultural feeding practices and child-raising philosophy contribute to iron-deficiency anemia in refugee Hmong children. *Ethn Dis.* 2002;12(2):199–205

85. Cruz GD, Shore R, Le Geros RZ, Tavares M. Effect of acculturation on objective measures of oral health in Haitian immigrants in New York City. *J Dent Res.* 2004;83(2):180–184

86. Mariño R, Stuart GW, Wright FA, Minas IH, Klimidis S. Acculturation and dental health among Vietnamese living in Melbourne, Australia. *Community Dent Oral Epidemiol.* 2001;29(2):107–119

87. Adams JH, Young S, Laird LD, et al. The cultural basis for oral health practices among Somali refugees pre- and post-resettlement in Massachusetts. *J Health Care Poor Underserved.* 2013;24(4):1474–1485

88. Laird LD, Barnes LL, Hunter-Adams J, et al. Looking Islam in the teeth: the social life of a Somali toothbrush. *Med Anthropol Q.* 2015;29(3):334–356

89. von Gontard A, Moritz AM, Thome-Granz S, Equit M. Abdominal pain symptoms are associated with anxiety and depression in young children. *Acta Paediatr.* 2015;104(11):1156–1163

90. Saps M, Seshadri R, Sztainberg M, Schaffer G, Marshall BM, Di Lorenzo C. A prospective school-based study of abdominal pain and other common somatic complaints in children. *J Pediatr.* 2009;154(3):322–326

91. Posey DL, Blackburn BG, Weinberg M, et al. High prevalence and presumptive treatment of schistosomiasis and strongyloidiasis among African refugees. *Clin Infect Dis.* 2007;45(10):1310–1315

92. Geltman PL, Grant-Knight W, Ellis H, Landgraf JM. The "lost boys" of Sudan: use of health services and functional health outcomes of unaccompanied refugee minors resettled in the U. S. *J Immigr Minor Health.* 2008;109(5):389–396

15

Children in Foster or Kinship Care or Involved With Child Welfare

Moira Szilagyi, MD, PhD, and Sandra H. Jee, MD, MPH

"Entry into foster care and placement in a good home environment may remediate emotional disorders or may exacerbate them because of the trauma of separation from families and the emotional turmoil of living as a child in an uncertain world."

In an ideal world, every child and adolescent would be reared by nurturing and caring birth parents. Many children and adolescents, however, cannot reside with their birth families for reasons of health and safety, and they require care in other settings. In 2014, approximately 3.6 million reports alleging child abuse and neglect and involving 6.6 million children and adolescents were investigated by child protective services, resulting in 679,000 children identified as victims. Of these, 147,462 maltreated children were removed to out-of-home care, as were another 94,457 children who were classified as nonvictims. The rate of victimization was highest for infants and lowest for adolescents.[1]

When children or adolescents are removed from their families of origin by child welfare services, they may be placed in foster family care, kinship care, or group care. Foster and kinship care are intended to be a temporary respite for a family in crisis, and there is an increasing trend toward keeping children with their parents or extended family in lieu of foster care. In most states, kinship care remains a less formal arrangement and includes care by extended family, neighbors, or friends, frequently without the oversight of child welfare services. Although adolescents in out-of-home care frequently enter because of parental inability to cope with their behavioral or emotional issues, they have often experienced abuse and neglect during their childhoods. While this chapter focuses on children and adolescents in out-of-home care, the information applies to the larger population of children and teens who remain in families of origin that are involved with child welfare because these children and teens experience childhood adversities and trauma similar to those experienced in foster and kinship care.

In the United States, on September 30, 2016, approximately 437,465 children and adolescents resided in foster care, approximately 32% in the care of extended family members.[2] Furthermore, estimates suggest that more than 600,000 individual children resided in foster care sometime during the preceding 12 months; approximately 4 times as many children and teens lived in informal, unregulated kinship care.[3,4] These children and teens are, by and large, from indigent households, and 70% have a documented history of child abuse or neglect. However, children enter foster or kinship care after experiencing many other severe childhood adversities and trauma that can result in toxic stress and negatively affect health and well-being. More than 80% have been exposed to high levels of violence in their homes or communities, with more than 40% living in homes with active domestic violence at the time of removal.[5,6] Close to one-half (48%) have a caregiver with a significant mental health impairment, and rates of parental substance and alcohol use are enormous, ranging up to 80% for the youngest children.[7] These children have often had multiple caregivers even before removal and have not experienced the predictable, responsive parenting that promotes well-being.[8]

Despite such high levels of family dysfunction, removal from their families of origin and all that is familiar is emotionally traumatic for almost all children. Placement in foster or kinship care is intended to nurture and heal children while facilitating the rehabilitation of their families. In reality, foster care has become a system of last resort for the most vulnerable children and most challenging families.

Most pediatric clinicians (ie, primary care pediatricians, pediatric subspecialists, and family physicians, internists, nurse practitioners, and physician assistants who provide pediatric care) will encounter children and adolescents in foster or kinship care, or otherwise involved with child welfare, during the course of their practice; thus, it is important to be familiar with the effects and treatment of child abuse and neglect, as well as the effects of early childhood trauma, removal, and placement in foster or kinship care, on children, adolescents, and their families. Early exposure to childhood adversity and trauma often results in toxic stress, which may manifest as mental health problems rooted in early psychosocial deprivation.

Summary of Key Legislation

The foster care system seems to always be in a state of flux, burdened by huge caseloads, birth families with multiple intractable problems, inadequate funding, and complex and often conflicting bureaucratic, legal, and ethical demands. The recognition that separating children and adolescents (henceforth collectively called *children* unless otherwise specified) from their families, only to leave them lingering in foster care without permanency, is harmful to children, together with burgeoning costs, led to several attempts at reforming child welfare. In 1980, the Adoption Assistance and Child Welfare Act (Public Law [PL] 96–272) mandated states to provide preventive services (eg, counseling, child care, parenting education, drug rehabilitation) to avert the removal of children from their birth families. Agencies were also mandated to conduct semiannual case reviews and to develop permanency plans within 18 months of placement. In an effort to move children out of the system, adoption subsidies were funded so that a marginal family income would be less of a hindrance to the adoption of children out of foster care. After enactment of PL 96–272, the size of the foster care population transiently declined until the cocaine epidemic led to a dramatic increase in the number of infants in foster care in the late 1980s and early 1990s. More recent legislative initiatives have focused on reducing admissions to and length of stay in foster care by enabling earlier termination of parental rights (TPR) and promoting adoption, kinship care, and guardianship.

Of particular relevance to pediatric clinicians, the Fostering Connections to Success and Increasing Adoptions Act of 2008, the Child and Family Services Improvement and Innovation Act (PL 112–34), and the Patient Protection and Affordable Care Act (ACA) (PL 111–148) specifically address health care services and resources for children in foster care.[9] Together, these federal laws require states to develop health oversight systems for children in foster care, monitor and treat emotional trauma, coordinate health care, monitor psychotropic medication use, connect children with medical homes, and measure outcomes. The ACA, in particular, grants those who emancipate from foster care at age 18 years or older automatic Medicaid eligibility until age 26 years. Such legislative changes are intended to protect vulnerable young adults during a critical transitional period of their lives when the loss of health care oversight can exacerbate many chronic physical and mental health problems, and these loss of supports may cause homelessness among adolescents leaving the foster care system.[10]

Trends in Out-of-Home Care

Legislative and policy changes that occur in response to scientific studies and advocacy ultimately affect foster care practice. With the emphasis on kinship care, more and more children are entering foster care for very short stays while the child welfare agency attempts to identify and investigate kinship resources. The definition of *kin* has expanded to include familiar nonrelatives. Children residing in kinship homes achieve permanency in these placements at a higher rate than those in foster care, although an unknown percentage of kinship homes disrupt, leading to subsequent foster or other kin care placement.[3]

Adoptions out of foster care peaked in the early part of the millennium. The children who remain in care awaiting adoption are older, are predominantly children of ethnic and racial minorities, are part of large sibling groups, or have disabilities. Parental substance use, combined with neglect or domestic violence, has become an increasingly important reason for removing children. Child welfare has become more focused on the effects of childhood trauma and evidence-based interventions to treat children and families, although resources are often scarce. Foster and kinship parents remain the major therapeutic intervention of the foster care system. Some elegant studies show that specific education and supports for foster parents and birth parents improve outcomes for children, although these studies have yet to be disseminated widely.[11–13] A recent study that looked at child welfare trends over the decade 2001–2011 demonstrated that child maltreatment referrals have increased but foster care admissions have decreased. During this time frame, the complexity associated with health of children in foster care increased, as measured by the larger number of children who had experienced multiple forms of maltreatment and who had been diagnosed as having emotional disturbances.[14] There is anecdotal information from some states that the opioid epidemic has contributed to an increase in out-of-home placements in the past 12 to 24 months, but this information awaits verification.

Risk Factors for Placement

Families whose children reside in foster care are, in general, impoverished and living on the fringes of society, with few social supports. Child neglect, including neglect of basic nutritional needs, educational and medical neglect, and lack of supervision, is the most commonly cited reason for placement.[2] Reports of child physical abuse and sexual abuse have declined in the past

2 decades[15] but remain reasons for placement.[2,16] Reports of multiple forms of maltreatment have increased,[14] although it is unclear whether this increase reflects a true increase or improved reporting. Although child abuse and neglect occur in all socio-demographic groups, young people placed in foster care come from the most economically deprived segments of society; thus, extreme poverty remains a pervasive common factor underlying foster care placement. Parental mental illness, substance use, active domestic violence, and criminal activity permeate the environments in which children have lived before removal. More than 80% of young children entering foster care have a parent who uses drugs, alcohol, or both.[6] Many children come from homes and neighborhoods in which drug sales and the presence of drug paraphernalia are common. National data indicate that 48% of foster children's parents have a mental illness and 10% are cognitively impaired.[16] Before entering foster care, 44% of children were living in homes with active domestic violence, and 84% experienced significant levels of violence in their homes, schools, or neighborhoods.[6] In one national data set, child protective services caseworkers identified 80% of birth parents as having significantly impaired parenting skills at the time of the child protective services investigation.[16] Other social stressors in these families include single parenthood, lack of education, and unemployment. Approximately one-third of birth parents admit to being abused or neglected as children, and approximately the same number spent time in foster care. Removal of a child often occurs after prolonged involvement with social service agencies, including child protective services, when preventive strategies have been exhausted and the child's health and safety are at imminent risk.

Early childhood trauma or multiple adverse childhood experiences and chronic stress have been shown in multiple studies to be associated with very poor long-term mental health, developmental, and physical health outcomes.[9,17–22] Trauma and chronic stress, in the absence of protective factors, alter the neurobiology of the brain, especially in the young child, affecting those areas involved in cognition, rational thought, emotional regulation, activity level, and the relationship between thought and emotion.[18,19] (See Chapter 13, Children Exposed to Adverse Childhood Experiences.) Thus, children entering foster care, with their cumulative and often chronic adverse experiences and early life traumas, are a group with immense emotional, developmental, and physical health needs. Studies on resiliency and recovery from traumatic experiences are just now accumulating, but early data indicate that children need stability in nurturing and responsive families and communities for healing after such experiences.[18,19]

Foster Care System

The foster care system, simple in its conception of providing needy children with nurturing families, is in fact a complex bureaucracy. Federal legislation determines patterns of funding and regulatory guidelines, but responsibility for the structure and implementation of foster care programs resides with state social service agencies, which may delegate daily management to county or private child welfare agencies.

Role of Caseworkers

Each child welfare agency retains the responsibility for hiring and training caseworkers for a demanding job requiring multiple skills. Assigned to the family, caseworkers must make a *diligent effort* to rehabilitate the parent or parents, engage them around the care of their child, and ensure accessibility to whatever educational or service resources are necessary (eg, housing, counseling, medical care, drug and alcohol rehabilitation) for reunification. Meanwhile, they must also coordinate educational, developmental, medical, and mental health services for children and teens. When birth parents are nonadherent or unable to reunify with their children, caseworkers must develop an alternate permanency plan (eg, kinship care, foster care, temporary guardianship, or adoption).

Caseworkers must have a working familiarity with the legal system in their states, particularly the family court and juvenile justice systems. Within 72 hours of removal of the child from the home, the foster care agency's attorney, working with the caseworker, must prepare a petition for the court documenting the reasons for removal. Many children are returned to birth parents or relatives within this time frame if the court finds insufficient basis for the removal. For the child or adolescent who remains in foster care, the caseworker must return to court at intervals to provide ongoing documentation of necessity for the continuation of placement and to detail efforts toward reunification and alternate permanency planning. Children will likely have multiple caseworkers while in foster care, because of both high turnover rates and built-in transitions. Children enter care with a child protective worker, transition to an intake worker, and then transition to a foster home caseworker in the first 90 days. Multiple transitions add to the losses children experience and can be frustrating in terms of case continuity.

The Legal System Surrounding the Child in Foster Care

The legal system surrounding the child in foster care is, by its nature, an adversarial one. Each child in foster care is appointed an attorney who is assigned to protect the child's interests in court. Birth parents and the child welfare agency also each have their own attorneys. Children, in special circumstances, may also have a Court-Appointed Special Advocate (commonly known as CASA) assigned by the judge.

Legally, parents retain guardianship of their children who are residing in the *care and custody* of the state or county commissioner of social services. Guardianship can be terminated only as part of a court process in which it may be transferred to a relative or, more frequently, to the commissioner, when parental rights are terminated. Parents occasionally choose to surrender their parental rights and place their children for adoption, but TPR usually occurs involuntarily, after all efforts at reunification have failed. The TPR process can take years, creating great uncertainty for children and their caregivers.

Children in Foster Care

Entry into foster care is fraught with uncertainty, upheaval, and losses for children and for parents. Family, no matter how dysfunctional, is the center of a child's world, and removal separates the child or adolescent from family and all that is familiar. Removal, by law, is supposed to occur only when there is imminent threat to the child's health and safety because it is an emotionally traumatizing experience for almost all children, save the newborns and young infants.[8,23] However, it is only after removal that some children and teens feel safe for the very first time.

Child protective services are required by federal law to identify kinship resources before placement in nonrelative foster care. However, in emergent removals, agencies may first place children in a shelter or an emergency foster home, pending the availability of a traditional foster home. While most foster parents are kind and welcoming, they are usually unfamiliar to the child. Placement with kin caregivers can be less traumatic if the child already has a meaningful relationship with them. Within the first few days, the child meets a variety of strangers, from child protective service personnel and foster care caseworkers to police officers, health care professionals, and members of the foster home. Little privacy is afforded, and most children, grieving the loss of their homes and families, are uncertain when they will see them again, are afraid to ask questions, and feel alone and isolated. The traumatic grief that accompanies removal and placement is layered on top of the child's previous history of adversity and trauma.[24] Some children will externalize that grief, while others internalize it and seem compliant and passive. As children and teens adjust to their new circumstances, some will act out their anger, frustration, and sadness. Children with severe trauma histories may have developed certain behaviors that were adaptive in their previous environments but are highly maladaptive in their new environments. However, most children are simply overwhelmed and confused by experiences they do not understand and feelings they cannot express in healthier ways or control. Pediatric clinicians can help caregivers understand children's behaviors and grief responses in terms of their trauma experiences.[25] The American Academy of Pediatrics (AAP) has produced a guidebook that can assist with the transition into foster care (*Helping Foster and Adoptive Families Cope With Trauma*).

Children spend varying lengths of time in foster care. Although many children (approximately 50%) cycle through foster care in weeks to months,[1] approximately 10% to 20% remain in care for years, as their families repeatedly fail to meet the goals set for reunification and resist other permanency options. In 2014, 48% of children were in care for fewer than 12 months, but this percentage may not have included, in some states, those who spent a few days in care but never reached the status of court adjudication. The mean length of stay in foster care is about 22 months, but the median is closer to 13 months. In 2014, 17% of children in foster care had been in foster care for more than 3 years and 8% for more than 5 years. The largest determinant of length of stay is the biological family's level of cooperation with the individualized case plan for their child or children, although reports indicate that minorities, older children, and children with severe behavioral and developmental disabilities are almost twice as likely to remain in care.[26]

Longer stays in foster care are associated with a reduced likelihood of reunification and more placements. Changes in foster care placement are almost always traumatic for children,[27] given that each transition involves a loss that reinforces feelings of rejection and worthlessness. Approximately 50% of children and teens in foster care will experience more than 1 placement, with approximately 25% having 3 or more placements. Reasons for disrupted placements vary; however, most frequently, a child's behavioral problems are beyond the skills of a particular foster parent or deteriorate to the point at which the child needs a higher level of care. Less often, placements disrupt because foster parents retire, become ill or die, feel threatened by the birth parent, or move out of the child's community. Some placement changes occur to reunify siblings. Approximately 20% of all foster homes close each year, and about half of this number are closed by child welfare agencies for inadequate care. Stability in placement is a major goal, however, because it is associated with improved outcomes.[26,27]

Disparities in foster care placement remain an issue, and minorities are still overrepresented, despite significant efforts by child welfare to address this issue in the past decade. Overall, the number of children in foster care has declined 25% in the past decade, and the number of black children has declined even more (about 40%), as child welfare has focused on reducing bias in investigation and removal. However, concern persists that the over-representation of minority children in foster care reflects bias in investigation and removal.[28,29] In 2015, 23% of children in foster care were black and non-Hispanic, 20% were Hispanic, 6% were multiracial or of other races, and 45% were white.[1] The average age of a child in foster care in 2014 was 7.3 years, although about 40% were younger than 5 years and another 40% were adolescents. In 2015, placement settings varied, with 53% of children living in nonrelative foster care; 30%, in kinship homes; 4%, in preadoptive homes; and 6%, in group home or residential care. Unaccompanied refugee minors, especially from Central America, Africa, and Haiti, represent a very small proportion of the total foster care population.

Grief, uncertainty, powerlessness, and guilt pervade the life of children in foster care. They often deny awareness of the reason for placement, and some may even blame themselves for the disruption of their families. Most children worry about the well-being of their parents and siblings. Birth parents may make promises they do not or cannot keep, and children live in an uncertain world, where they do not know how long they will be in care, whether their parent will come for visits, or when their parent will get out of jail or rehabilitation. Children are sometimes discharged from foster care or transitioned between placements without preparation. Other children tease them about being in foster care, contributing to their already poor self-regard and sense of alienation. Younger children and infants quickly form attachments to foster parents and may view their less-frequently-seen birth parent as a stranger. Differences in parenting style, as well as outright conflict between birth parents and current caregivers, create confusion for children and teens.

Adolescents in Foster Care

Adolescence is the time during which the individual is supposed to form a stable identity rooted in self-esteem, a sense of autonomy rooted in self-efficacy, and a larger sense of commitment and comfort in relatedness to peers. For young people in foster care, especially minority adolescents, negative self-concept, lack of self-esteem, and a lack of self-efficacy are likely outcomes because of early adverse experiences, the accrual of multiple losses over time, and a sense of helpless dependence developed from living in the uncertain world of foster care. Early abuse and neglect coupled with impaired caregiving, repeated separation and losses, unpredictability, and a lack of role models for healthy relationships results in a high prevalence of young adults who are isolated, alienated, dependent, and prone to distrust.

Adolescents in foster care are a varied group; most enter foster care through juvenile detention or Persons in Need of Supervision (PINS) petitions, although some enter care as a result of being homeless or sexually exploited. Those placed through PINS petitions are placed because they have failed to attend school or have repeatedly run away from home or defied curfew or they have otherwise placed themselves at risk. Occasionally, teens are placed when a parent is unable to manage the teen's behaviors or afford mental health care. Some adolescents have grown up in foster care, and this group is likely to have experienced a variety of foster care settings over time. Some teens are intellectually disabled or developmentally delayed, with or without significant behavioral issues. Some teens linger in care because a suitable adoptive home is never identified. Pregnant or parenting teens are a small group who may be living with their children in foster care or placed separately if they have significant mental health issues or constitute a risk to their offspring. A small group enters foster care as emancipated refugee minors, having immigrated to the United States from a variety of war-torn countries after surviving war, rape, injury, or the death of their families. Some have relatives in the United States with whom they will be placed, while others will remain in care until emancipation.

Most adolescents in foster care reside in group homes or residential treatment facilities where their activities are restricted, their education is structured, and they receive mental health services and substance use disorder treatment, if needed. The outcomes of residential and group home care have not been adequately studied, and little is known about the prevalence of evidence-based treatment in such settings. Some teens in foster care reside in foster families. In general, adolescents in foster care have had adverse life experiences similar to those of younger children entering foster care but have also experienced many transitions and engaged in high-risk behaviors, including substance use, sexual activity, school truancy, and petty criminal mischief.[27,30] A careful history will often reveal a life of frequent adversity and trauma.

Adolescents in foster care are less likely to be adopted than are younger children. When they do leave foster care, they do so to return home or because they "age out" of foster care and need to leave the system. Most states now allow adolescents to remain in care until age 21 years if employed, in job training, or in school. Some choose to leave earlier, run away, or are moved to another agency or placement setting (residential care or group home care, jail, or inpatient mental health or drug and alcohol treatment). Foster care caseworkers are charged with preparing adolescents who are aging out of care for independent living by offering them education regarding finances, job training, and health insurance. However, resources for independent living education are limited, transitional services are few, and adolescents aging out of care often find their way back to their families of origin if they have no sense of belonging elsewhere. Foster or kin families who remain invested in adolescents are their best resource, and adolescents who identify and remain connected to adult mentors seem to fare better.[30] There is evidence suggesting that adolescents in out-of-home care may achieve better social relationships and mental health if they are engaged in structured activities.[31] Enhancing peer networks and focusing on mindfulness skills may help teens in foster care manage stress.[32] A recent study showed that about half of teens can form a stable attachment relationship to a long-term foster caregiver, despite ongoing unstable attachment to their birth parents.[33]

Visitation

Although consistent visitation with the biological family is the best predictor of reunification, visits are laden with difficulty for the child. The tenor of the parent-child relationship is variable. Children who have been abused or severely neglected by their parents may not feel safe, even in a supervised visitation setting. Birth parents may attempt to sabotage the relationship of the child with his or her current caregivers, and vice versa. Parents may visit inconsistently, which is confusing, disappointing, and sometimes frightening for children. When the parent does come, every visit ends with the child reliving the initial separation from his or her parent. When the parent fails to show, feelings of rejection and abandonment are reinforced.

Visitation usually progresses through stages, beginning with visits supervised by caseworkers in a neutral setting. Visits then transition to the parent's home, where they may be monitored before eventually becoming unsupervised. Kinship placement may allow for more frequent contact with the birth parent, but kin caregivers may also be in a particularly difficult situation regarding visitation if they harbor resentment toward the birth parent, are conflicted about visitation, or have to enforce court-ordered restrictions to which the parent and other relatives object.

Evidence is mounting for models of visitation in which a mental health specialist provides child-parent psychotherapy or child-parent interaction therapy.[34] Such models focus on helping the parent identify the child's cues, understand his or her developmental capacities, practice parenting skills learned in court-ordered parenting education, and respond to the child in an appropriate manner. These models are time- and labor-intensive, and expensive, but have increased successful reunification in communities that have adopted them. Another promising but less expensive model is Visitation Coaching, through which trained visitation specialists prepare birth parents for visits, help the parents stay on track during the visit, and debrief with them afterward.

Foster Families

Foster and kinship families are the major therapeutic intervention and the unsung heroes of the foster care system.[35] Most of these families are warm, caring, dedicated individuals who open their homes to society's most fragile and needy children, taking them into their own families and nurturing them through multiple crises. Although foster parents vary in the skills they bring to caring for children, they are generally motivated by religious conviction, altruism, or personal commitment. They tend to be *child centered,* often having raised children of their own, and see foster care as a mission because of their love for children. Some choose fostering as a path to adoption, although a guarantee that a child placed with them will become eligible for adoption seldom exists. Foster parents are usually married, have a middle or lower-middle income, come from tradition-rich backgrounds, are deeply religious, and have a fairly open definition of who constitutes family. A very small percentage of foster parents are same-sex couples. Almost every state now allows same-sex couples to foster and adopt, although at this writing there remains at least one state that allows only one member of a same-sex couple to adopt. Approximately 5% of foster families have specialized training or skills and act as resources for severely emotionally disturbed or medically fragile children. Many states now have designated skilled homes that provide care for children with complex medical problems.

Recruitment, adequate training, and retention of suitable foster families are some of the most compelling tasks facing child welfare agencies. Agencies are supposed to provide potential foster parents with education in the areas of child development, child abuse and neglect, behavioral problems, discipline, safety issues, and their roles in relation to the agency and birth families; however, training is often minimal. Certification occurs only after agencies have conducted successful home visits, criminal background checks, and a review of the state's child abuse registry. Agencies lack adequate staff to scrutinize foster homes carefully, and annual recertification is less rigorous than the original certification process. Foster parents often request increased education and support, but the resources for such intensive efforts are minimal.

Boundaries are blurred in the foster care system in authority, responsibility, and accountability.[35] Foster families retain the bulk of the daily responsibility for children and teens but are accountable to caseworkers, the legal system, and the birth family for the child's or teen's care. Foster parents may feel excluded from planning on the child's behalf, given that birth parents retain legal custody, child welfare agencies have authority to make decisions on behalf of the child and generate permanency plans, and courts make placement decisions. However powerless, foster families often remain the individual child's strongest advocate.

Foster parents usually have only limited information about children in their care, including their health histories. Foster families may be overwhelmed, and placements may fail when foster families feel isolated in dealing with a child's complex behavioral and emotional problems. Because of foster home shortages in many areas, particularly large urban centers, most homes maintain the maximum number of children allowed under regulations, further stressing a family's emotional resources. Documented abuse and neglect are rare in foster or kinship care, but the physician needs to remain alert for signs of inadequate care, such as poor weight gain.

Foster families, like children in foster care, experience multiple separations and losses as children enter and then leave their homes, often for a living situation that the foster parent deems unsuitable. Thus, grief and loss are common. Relationships between foster and birth families range from adversarial to mutually supportive. Foster parents often bear the brunt of a child's anger over a failed visit or a parent's telephone call, or they may be unjustly accused of neglect or abuse by an angry birth parent. They may feel scrutinized, but simultaneously unsupported, by child welfare staff.

Kinship Care

In the past decade, the numbers of children placed in kinship care increased dramatically (>300%). Unofficial placement with kin caregivers is more common than *relative resource care,* defined as care provided by a relative who has become certified as a foster parent. Although driven by a commitment to maintaining a child within their family of origin, kinship care providers have often made this choice under some duress and with the recognition that a member of their own family, who is often their adult child, has neglected or abused the child. Kin caregivers are often older, poorer, and with less access to resources than nonrelative foster caregivers. Unless they have become certified foster parents, they are not subject to the same review or oversight as foster caregivers, nor do they have access to the same supports.

Placement with a relative, however, offers significant advantages to children, the most obvious of which is that it maintains their ties with their larger families of origin, their communities, and their cultures.[3,26] A few studies have also shown that kinship care is associated with fewer placement disruptions and, in one study, a reduced incidence of abuse or neglect, compared with placement with a nonrelative. Compared with nonrelative foster parents, relative caregivers report that children have fewer behavioral problems.[36,37] Kin caregivers with marginal incomes have the option of applying for foster care certification in many states, making them eligible for foster care stipends, with all the oversight of foster care.[37]

Birth Families

Removal of a child is also a traumatic event for the birth parent. For some, the shock of the removal is sufficient to precipitate cooperation with child welfare, family court, and prescribed therapies, resulting in speedy reunification. Approximately one-half of children in foster care are returned to their birth families within the first 6 months. For other families, even the removal of a child does not alter ingrained patterns of substance use, violence, and child neglect.

Parents, while battling addiction, mental illness, and poverty, often have to contend with feelings of guilt, powerlessness, inadequacy, anger, frustration, and resentment when children are removed. Even though they retain legal custody, their contact with their children is constrained, with only several hours of supervised visitation per week initially. Parents may fail to show up for visitation, whether because of substance use, mental illness, guilt, the pain of separation, fear of confronting their child or children, or barriers such as transportation.

Even though one of the goals of the foster care system is reunification and caseworkers are mandated to provide a range of services supporting this goal, some birth parents become locked in an adversarial relationship with child welfare staff, resentfully refusing all help offered. In the past, some parents effectively abandoned their children to the system, maintaining contact just sufficient to prevent termination of their rights. Many of these same parents refused to surrender their children for adoption, even when reunification was clearly not an option. Federal legislation has made the TPR easier in such situations, while supporting open adoption, which is thought to benefit the child by providing some ongoing limited supervised contact with the family of origin.

Health Needs of Foster Children

Children in foster care represent a highly vulnerable population of children with special health care needs, as they have high rates of chronic medical illness, developmental disabilities, educational disorders, dental problems, and behavioral, emotional, and mental health problems.[17,38-47] In general, for older children and adolescents, these conditions predate placement and are rooted in their experiences of childhood trauma and loss. Prenatal drug exposure, poor maternal nutrition, genetic risks for mental health problems, and poor prenatal care lead to an increased incidence of preterm and small-for-gestational-age infants. Postnatally, psychosocial deprivation, poor nutrition, maltreatment, and failure to attend to the child's health and developmental needs exacerbate problems. Limited use of preventive health services, fragmentation of health care, and under-immunization are typical of children entering foster care. Children also enter foster care with a history of complex trauma, including child maltreatment, and toxic stress that adversely affects their physical, emotional, and developmental well-being.[17-19,24]

Medical and Dental Issues

Approximately 45% of foster children have at least 1 chronic medical condition, with approximately one-fourth of all children in care having 3 or more chronic problems.[42,45-47] The most commonly encountered diagnoses include asthma, respiratory problems, dermatologic problems, anemia and hematologic problems, gastroesophageal problems, growth abnormalities (failure to thrive or obesity), neurological problems, and parasitic infections.[41,46] Hematologic disorders, mostly attributable to anemia, are present in approximately 20% of children. Burn scars or scars from physical abuse are encountered in 10% to 15% of children younger than 12 years. Visual and hearing loss and neurological disorders (varying from mild motor delay to seizures and cerebral palsy) are more prevalent in this population and may be the result of prior physical abuse or medical neglect, or they may be the reason for voluntary placement in foster care. Congenital anomalies occur at higher rates than in the general pediatric population. Sexually transmitted infections (STIs) and other infectious diseases, whether vertically or horizontally transmitted, are more frequent. Approximately 8% of children in foster care are high-cost patients because they depend on technology, have multiple disabilities, or heavily use ancillary services.[41]

It is common to find children in foster care experiencing a high prevalence of dental problems, especially dental caries and malocclusion. Changes in placement may result in lapses in dental care, further exacerbating dental problems.

Mental Health and Substance Use Issues

Professionals experienced in foster care recognize that the prevalence and severity of mental health disabilities have increased dramatically in the past decade, although some of this increase may be attributed to heightened awareness among child welfare, pediatric, and mental health specialists. The burden of early childhood trauma and toxic stress predating foster care placement is enormous.[24,46] Entry into foster care and placement in a good home environment may remediate emotional disorders or may exacerbate them because of the trauma of separation from families and the emotional turmoil of living as a child in an uncertain world.

Mental health care is the greatest health care need of most children in foster care and is rooted in childhood trauma and adversity. The prevalence of severe disturbance ranges from 35% to 85%.[38,39,46,48] Children in foster care use inpatient and outpatient mental health services at rates 15 to 20 times those of other children of similar backgrounds but are still thought to be underserved. Oppositional defiant disorder, attention-deficit/hyperactivity disorder (ADHD), attachment disorder, and anxiety disorders are the most commonly cited mental health diagnoses for children in foster care. Longitudinal studies of young adults formerly in foster care have recommended that young adults and adults receive increased access to evidence-based medical and mental health treatment.

One study in the Midwest reported that 45% of teens in foster care used alcohol or illicit substances in the prior 6 months, whereas 49% acknowledged past use and 35% met criteria for a substance use disorder. Those at highest risk are those with conduct disorder or post-traumatic stress disorder and those residing in independent living situations. This study may not reflect actual use because teens may have underreported or the reporting population may not have been adequately representative of all teens in foster care. What is known about the effect of childhood trauma suggests that substance use is often a form of self-treatment. Although marijuana is the most commonly used drug among those in foster care, teens using addictive substances may experience acute withdrawal from addictive substances at entry into foster care.

Multiple studies have shown that approximately 60% of young children entering foster care have developmental delays, especially in the areas of communication, social-emotional, and cognitive skills. Before foster care placement, school-aged children and teens experience high rates of absenteeism, suspension, school failure, grade retention, and multiple school transitions.[49] Children and teens in foster care are an educationally vulnerable population that continues to perform below grade level (75%), perform poorly on standardized testing, and exhibit significant behavioral issues.[49] Forty-four percent of children and teens in foster care are in special education settings, one-half for behavioral concerns. Of seniors in high school who were also in foster care, 65% said that a parent or guardian had never attended a parent-teacher conference.

Outcomes for Children in Foster Care

The outcomes for children in foster care remain mixed. Young children have been shown to benefit from placement in a nurturing foster home and receipt of early intervention services.[50] Stable placement in foster care has also been shown to result in improved school attendance and is often accompanied by improved academic performance for younger children.[50]

On the other hand, after children enter foster care, their overall health does not seem to improve significantly. A recent study[51] in New York State reported that less than 30% of children in foster care had access to preventive health services before foster care and had minimally improved access while in foster care. The high mobility of this population contributes to poor preventive health care access.

Recent government data show that just more than 60% of children exiting foster care are reunited with a parent or relative, 19% are adopted, 10% age out, and the remaining either elope or transfer to the care of other agencies. The overall recidivism (return to foster care) rate is 20% during the first year after reunification but approaches 30% for infants.[1]

Children in foster care who are eventually adopted are usually adopted by their foster parents (56%) or by a member of their extended families (30%).[1] Almost all adoptions out of foster care involve some subsidy, reflecting the child's physical health, mental health, and developmental needs. Many children also retain their Medicaid insurance, although this retention depends on laws in individual states. An adoption subsidy, once granted, continues until the child reaches 18 years of age. Only half the children freed for adoption have an adoptive home identified. Those awaiting adoptive placement are mostly children considered difficult to adopt by virtue of their significant medical or behavioral problems, older minority children, or those who are part of large sibling groups.

More than 20,000 teens and young adults age out of foster care's independent living programs annually, often without family connections, although some maintain contact with their families of origin or foster families. Current child welfare practice dictates that agencies assist these young people in identifying meaningful adult resources as part of the emancipation process. Under the ACA, young people leaving care can retain their Medicaid eligibility until age 26 years. As noted previously, the outcomes of adolescents leaving foster care for independent living are very poor.[10,48,50]

What is known about the outcomes of young people who age out of foster care is discouraging. A national study of 20,000 young adults who aged out of foster care in 1998 showed that only 35% graduated from high school and only 11% went on to college or vocational school; 37% of foster teens in another study dropped out of high school.[49] Teens in foster care are as likely to drop out or attain a general education degree as to graduate from high school.[49] The 1% to 2% of young people who go onto higher education are far less likely than their peers to graduate.

In the few small prevalence studies available, young adults a decade removed from foster care were underemployed and undereducated, had difficulty with trust in intimate relationships, and blamed the child welfare system for the disruption of their families. As young people age out of foster care, their access to mental health care also decreases.[50] In other prevalence studies, adults with a history of foster care are overrepresented among the homeless and the incarcerated.[27] It is not known, in general, whether young adults who were adopted fare better than those who remained in foster care or reunified or lived with kinship caregivers.

Adoption

The foster family is most often the party to whom the system turns for adoption when reunification is no longer considered an option. Long-term foster care placement is no longer an option under federal law, although some foster families make a long-term commitment to one or several of the children and teens who have been freed for adoption but for whom belonging in a *forever family* remains an elusive goal. Termination of rights severs children's legal ties to their birth families, but not their emotional ones, and these children may be torn between conflicting loyalties to birth and adoptive families. Behavioral problems may escalate or resurface around termination or as adoption nears, as the child reexperiences rejection and loss of his or her original family.

Health Care Recommendations for Children in Foster and Kinship Care

Initial Care

Children entering foster care should have a series of health care encounters over the first 3 months (Box 15-1). Some communities have developed special clinics and unique health care models dedicated to providing health care and systems management for children in foster care.[52] Adherence to national guidelines that have been developed specifically for children in foster care,[53–54] is helpful in maintaining quality of care, regardless of whether a child is seen in a dedicated foster care clinic or general health care setting. Multiple encounters during this transitional phase often reveal more than one isolated evaluation and are useful in monitoring the child's adjustment to care and in

Box 15-1. Guidelines for Health Care of Children and Adolescents Entering Foster or Kinship Care

Children and adolescents entering foster care should have an admission health evaluation, which includes the following steps:

❶ Newborns, infants and preverbal children and those with chronic or acute medical problems or on medication should be seen within the first 24 h whenever possible. All other children and adolescents should undergo a health screening within 72 h of placement to assess and document

   a. Symptoms or signs of child abuse and neglect, with referral as needed

   b. Growth parameters

   c. Symptoms or signs of acute illness and use of any over-the-counter or prescribed medications

   d. Symptoms or signs of chronic illness and use of any over-the-counter or prescribed medications

   e. Developmental screening and referral for evaluation

   f. Behavioral and mental health screening (focusing on suicidal or homicidal ideation or intent, history of aggressive behaviors, and substance use) and referral for evaluation

   g. Appropriate referral for emergent health issues or sexual abuse evaluation

   h. Appropriate treatment of identified issues

   i. Health education of foster or kinship caregiver

❷ Health information gathering: an ongoing process that begins at admission to foster care

Box 15-1. Guidelines for Health Care of Children and Adolescents Entering Foster or Kinship Care (*continued*)

❸ Comprehensive health evaluation within 30 d of placement to

   a. Review all available health history.

   b. Address health concerns.

   c. Assess adjustment to foster or kinship care, child care, school, and visitation.

   d. Address behavior concerns and daily schedule.

   e. Assess growth parameters.

   f. Review systems.

   g. Perform a developmental or an educational evaluation, or review of evaluation or referral for evaluation, if not previously completed.

   h. Perform a mental health evaluation, or review of evaluation or referral for evaluation, if not previously completed.

   i. Perform a complete physical examination.

   j. Screen for signs and symptoms of child abuse and neglect.

   k. Undertake all recommended screening tests (hearing, vision, lead, CBC and differential, purified protein derivative tuberculin, rapid plasma reagin, hepatitis B and C, and HIV).

   l. Administer immunizations (consider catch-up immunizations if no history is available).

   m. Provide age-appropriate anticipatory guidance, focusing on transition issues.

   n. Provide appropriate or indicated treatment and referrals, including dental treatment.

   o. Provide communication in writing of health plan to foster care agency.

❹ Follow-up admission assessment within 60–90 d of placement to

   a. Review all available health history, including results of mental health assessment, developmental and educational evaluations, and dental assessment.

   b. Address interval concerns.

   c. Document growth parameters.

   d. Assess adjustment to foster care, child care, school, and visitation.

   e. Conduct behavioral screening.

   f. Conduct developmental screening and review.

   g. Perform a focused physical examination.

   h. Screen for child abuse and neglect.

   i. Administer immunizations as indicated.

   j. Ensure that all referrals and recommended treatments are in process or have been completed.

   k. Schedule or plan next visit.

Abbreviation: CBC, complete blood cell count.

identifying emerging issues.[55-56] Approximately 70% of children and adolescents entering foster care have been physically abused, sexually abused, or neglected. Clinicians should be familiar with the signs and symptoms of abuse and neglect and should screen all children and teens at the time of admission to care. Children and teens with suspected sexual abuse should be referred to a center specializing in child sexual abuse, if one is available, to prevent the trauma of repeated interviews and examinations.

Optimizing Ongoing Health Care for Children in Foster Care

Ideally, children in foster care receive their health care in the context of a medical home. For the child in foster care, the medical home ideally includes a foster care–friendly office with providers who understand the effect of childhood trauma and loss on health, development, and well-being; education and support for caregivers in the context of such trauma; and collaboration and communication with child welfare personnel around a child's needs. The AAP Task Force on Foster Care has developed many resources for clinicians regarding health care for children in foster care. Resources, including *Fostering Health: Health Care Standards for Children and Adolescents in Foster Care,* are now available on a Web site, Healthy Foster Care America (HFCA) (www.aap.org/en-us/advocacy-and-policy/aap-health-initiatives/healthy-foster-care-america). *Fostering Health* was designed for use by interdisciplinary professionals, health care professionals, and families and children.[54] The National Resource Center for Permanency and Family Connections also hosts a Web site, Fostering Connections, at http://nrcpfc.org/fostering_connections. Because many states have only broad guidelines governing the provision of health services to children in foster care, these detailed standards may be helpful to health care professionals advocating with foster care agencies for improved care. Unfortunately, multiple barriers still prevent translation of these guidelines into accessible, effective, and efficient health care. The barriers include inadequate funding, insufficient caseworker and foster family knowledge, limited understanding of the foster care experience by health care professionals, and blurred boundaries of responsibility for the health care management of this complex population.

Preventive Care

Routine primary preventive health care should be scheduled according to AAP guidelines, although experts recommend that children in foster care have more frequent monitoring visits because of their health needs and high mobility. Ideally, newborns and infants in foster care should receive monthly visits until age 6 months. Toddlers should receive a health visit at

21 months to monitor development and emerging behavior concerns. After age 2 years, children should have a health encounter between annual preventive health visits until they exit foster care.

Every preventive health visit with a child in foster care ideally includes anticipatory guidance around issues specific to foster care: transition issues, visitation issues, the need for routines and reasonable expectations, the effect of prior trauma on emotional and developmental well-being, and appropriate discipline, among others.

Extended appointment slots and a tracking system are strongly suggested. Ideally, the caseworker should inform the pediatric clinician about changes in placement and casework assignment and about any referrals made by the caseworker. The clinician, in turn, can provide the caseworker with periodic updates around health care encounters to keep the health plan current.

Monitoring for abuse or neglect at every health encounter is part of the pediatric clinician's responsibility and includes addressing concerns about the adequacy of parenting in a foster home. Some red flags for poor care include inadequate weight gain in a foster home (often the first sign of neglect), lack of warmth between the child and the caregiver, hypervigilance by the child around the caregiver, and caregiver reluctance to allow a private conversation between the child and the clinician. In addition, ancillary office staff may sometimes witness and should be encouraged to report concerning caregiver-child interactions to the clinician. Although poor adherence to recommended health visits may represent scheduling difficulties, it may be a sign of poor overall care in a foster home.

Because of the high prevalence of developmental (60% of children <6 years) and educational (45% of children >6 years) problems, screening with the use of standardized instruments is recommended at the time of the comprehensive admission visit, with periodic reassessments at preventive and monitoring visits. See Appendix 2 for a description of instruments useful for psychosocial assessment. Ideally, all children receive a full developmental-educational evaluation within 3 months of placement, but lack of resources usually precludes this evaluation. With services and an appropriate home environment, many children make developmental strides in foster care. For children who are undereducated because of a lack of schooling, catch-up can be dramatic with increased school attendance, although learning disabilities, behavioral disorders, and limited cognitive ability remain major challenges. Upward of 40% of children in foster care qualify for special education services or an educational plan. Some children in foster care qualify for special education for emotional rather than cognitive concerns, given that attentional difficulties, poor impulse control, and aggressive behaviors often preclude placement in a regular classroom.[55] The high prevalence of language disorders (50%–60%) of preschool children implies that universal hearing and speech evaluations of toddlers and preschool children may be beneficial in identifying children who would benefit from such services.[56,57] The primary care clinician and caseworker ideally maintain contact with the case manager for developmental-educational services and receive copies of all evaluations.

Because of the high likelihood of mental health problems in foster children, pediatric clinicians should screen for emotional and behavioral issues using standardized instruments at admission and at each preventive health and monitoring of care visit.[55,57] (See Appendix 2.) Obtaining some information about a child's trauma history, whether from child welfare personnel or by screening, can provide helpful insight into a child's emotional and behavioral symptoms. Every child in foster care should ideally have a full mental health evaluation by 2 years of age or within 3 months of placement. Children with newly identified mental health or behavioral issues should be referred to appropriate mental health services, ideally with pediatric mental health specialists who use evidence-based, trauma-informed practice.[52,58] The mental health treatment plan for children previously involved in the mental health system, including those for whom psychotropic medications have been prescribed, should be thoroughly reviewed, ideally through direct contact with the mental health specialists who previously assessed the child and who prescribed the medication.

All children in foster care have to deal with ongoing separation and loss issues as well as feelings of anger, sadness, rejection, powerlessness, alienation, and guilt. Even children who do not initially seem to need mental health services should be rescreened at intervals to assess for changes in their emotional well-being. Some of the common stressors that upend the lives of children in foster care include inconsistent visitation, resumption of regular visits after a prolonged lapse, cessation of visitation, incarceration of a parent, illness of a foster parent, and being freed for adoption. These critical junctures are times at which resumption of lapsed counseling or increased frequency of counseling visits is beneficial. It may also be challenging for mental health specialists to know which of a child's parents (foster, birth, or kin) should be involved in therapy with the child. The California Evidence-Based Clearinghouse for Child Welfare maintains a list of trauma-informed, evidence-based therapies for children in foster care and their caregivers (www.cebc4cw.org).

Psychotropic Medication

The use of psychotropic medication has become controversial in the foster care population. Studies show that children and teens in foster care are more likely than peers not in foster care to be on psychotropic medications. They are also more likely to be on multiple medications and sometimes on multiple medications from the same class.[59–61] Studies also indicate that psychotropic medications may not match the major symptom of concern or diagnosis. At least 2 states, Texas and New York,[62–63] have developed comprehensive guidelines regarding the prescription and management of psychotropic medications in the foster care population, and the reader is directed to these states for further information.

In general, psychotropic medications should be used only as part of a comprehensive mental health treatment plan and are best prescribed for patients in foster care by a qualified pediatric mental health specialist. Childhood trauma underlies many of the behavioral and mental health issues of this population, which are best treated with evidence-based mental health psychosocial therapies. A detailed health history, including mental health, behavior, development, trauma history, medication use, social and family history, and a full mental health evaluation, should be obtained before deciding on a course of treatment. When psychotropic medication is indicated, it should be specific to the diagnosis, initiated with a single agent in the lowest dose, and increased gradually, with close monitoring for efficacy and unintended side effects. Single-agent therapy should be used whenever possible. Close monitoring is the essence of good care for children and teens who are prescribed psychotropic medication.[54,59–66]

Pediatric clinicians also need to be acutely aware that not every child in foster care who presents with school or parent concerns of hyperactivity and inattention has ADHD, because such behaviors may be a manifestation of early childhood trauma experiences, depression, anxiety, or other psychiatric diagnoses. Referral to mental health specialists for evidence-based, trauma-informed mental health evaluation and services is the ideal initial intervention for the child or teen in foster care presenting with emotional and behavioral problems.

Counseling Foster Families

Many foster families have a wealth of child-rearing experiences, but the clinician should not presume that knowledge about child development, behavior, discipline, or safety or about parenting a traumatized child is adequate. Anticipatory guidance should be a routine part of child health supervision care and should include issues specific to foster care, such as trauma-related behavioral problems (including sleep disruption), visitation and the permanency planning process, confused loyalties, attachment issues, violence, and coercion. Adolescents should be counseled not only about safe behaviors but also about healthy activities, planning for their futures, healthy peer relationships, and connecting with adult mentors. Many teens in foster care, fearing yet another disappointment, have exhausted their capacities to attach to a parental figure, and families need to be offered guidance in promoting attachment relationships with teens in foster care. Pediatric clinicians can help foster parents understand the teen's emotional world while supporting an authoritative parenting style. Support for foster families and older children in foster care around transitions and other stressors can stabilize a foster care placement for a child.

Other Guidance

Other recommendations for optimizing health care in the medical home and promoting healing for children and adolescents in foster care (Box 15-2) are available on the HFCA Web site (www.aap.org/en-us/advocacy-and-policy/aap-health-initiatives/healthy-foster-care-america) and include the following guidance:

▶ The pediatric clinician ideally has a relationship with the foster care agency (Box 15-3) through which established methods of communication and information exchange facilitate the child's care.

Box 15-2. Special Considerations in Caring for Children and Adolescents in Foster Care

Every health encounter in foster care requires extra diligence on the part of the clinician, including the following care:

- Children and adolescents in foster care should be screened for abuse and neglect and monitored for inadequate weight gain.

- Children entering foster care should ideally undergo a full mental health (ideally, including trauma history) and behavioral health evaluation performed by trauma-informed pediatric mental health specialists within 60–90 d of entry into foster care. Periodic monitoring of mental health is encouraged with all patients, but especially with those for whom adverse experiences continue to accumulate. (See the AAP mental health toolkit at www.aap.org/en-us/advocacy-and-policy/aap-health-initiatives/Mental-Health/Pages/Addressing-Mental-Health-Concerns-in-Primary-Care-A-Clinicians-Toolkit.aspx.)

Box 15-2. Special Considerations in Caring for Children and Adolescents in Foster Care (*continued*)

- Children entering foster care should ideally undergo a full developmental or educational evaluation performed by professionals in the field within 60–90 d of entry into foster care.

- Children in foster care should be referred for dental care at the first health encounter or by 1 year of age.

- The clinician should attend to the quality of the interaction between caregivers and children.

- The clinician is encouraged to review recent changes in the child's visitation and contact with birth family, school attendance and performance, and participation in normalizing activities, among other issues.

- Every encounter should be considered an opportunity to immunize the child.

- The clinician should maintain a well-documented health record for the child in foster care.

- The clinician ideally has a foster care–friendly office and offers anticipatory guidance with an additional focus on normalizing activities, predictable routines, positive parenting strategies, helping children deal with transitions such as visitation, and the effect of trauma and separation on emotional and developmental well-being, among other issues. (See www.aap.org/en-us/advocacy-and-policy/aap-health-initiatives/healthy-foster-care-america.)

- A system for tracking health care use and adherence for children in foster care is useful for ensuring that children's needs are met.

- Referrals should be made promptly when an issue is identified.

- Children leaving foster care and adolescents and young adults "aging out" of care benefit from a discharge health visit, summarizing health information to share with a new health care provider or caregiver. This visit is an opportunity to transfer health information to the new health care provider and caregiver or to the patient who is aging out of foster care. Discharge planning is also advisable for youths emancipating from care.

- Systems for information exchange is encouraged to improve coordination of care between the foster care agency and the clinician.

- Up-to-date health summaries that include diagnoses, recommended treatment, and follow-up should be provided to enable the caseworker to keep the health plan current.

- The foster care agency should provide the clinician with as complete a health history as is available for the child, copies of appropriate consents and releases, notification of changes in placement or caseworker assignment, and notification of referrals made by the agency shortly after the child enters foster care.

Abbreviation: AAP, American Academy of Pediatrics.

Box 15-3. Pediatric Clinician's Roles in Caring for Children in Foster Care

This list is intended to show 2 possible separate, but overlapping, roles for pediatric clinicians. Of course, the clinician in the medical home may choose to serve any or all of the consulting roles.

Consultant Role for Child Welfare Agency Regarding Children in Foster Care

- Ensure that the foster care agency understands all AAP standards for health care.

- Help the foster care agency ensure that each child has a medical home with access, insurance, consents, continuity, and other avenues of support.

- Develop systems for communication and information exchange among caseworkers, mental health specialists, the court system, other health care providers, and school personnel.

- Provide or refer to health education resources for foster parents, caseworkers, the court system, attorneys, and school personnel.

- Develop systems for merging health information and planning into child welfare permanency plan.

- Develop systems for transitioning health care when the child or teen transitions or leaves foster care.

- Develop systems for tracking patients that include information on their health needs and data, monitoring outcomes, and any other information.

Medical Home Provider Role for Children in Foster Care

- Deliver care by the AAP foster care standards. Identify and attend to the child's health care needs.

- Accept patients in foster care and provide a medical home for them.

- Communicate and coordinate with caseworker, foster parents, school personnel, subspecialists, and the court system regarding individual patients in foster care.

- Educate the foster parents, caseworkers, or anyone else involved regarding the child's health care needs.

- Advocate on behalf of patients in foster care to ensure that health care needs are met.

- Share health information and plan for the child with the caseworkers, foster parents, court system, and older children in foster care.

- Ensure that information on the patient is transmitted to the appropriate professionals when the patient transitions out of foster care or from one foster care placement to another.

- Monitor and track the patient's health needs and care.

Abbreviation: AAP, American Academy of Pediatrics.

▶ The caseworker is the case manager, whose responsibilities include the child's health. The caseworker is responsible for obtaining appropriate releases of information and medical consents from the birth family and sharing copies with health care providers, including the pediatrician. The pediatric clinician may wish to become familiar with the foster care agency's guidelines regarding consent and confidentiality. The foster care agency should have the authority to provide consent in the absence of the birth parent. Certain adolescent health issues, such as pregnancy, STIs, birth control, and substance use, are governed by separate confidentiality laws in most states.

▶ All medical information, unless specifically prohibited by law, should be shared with the child's caseworker and foster parent and, when allowed, with birth parents in appropriate lay language. The caseworker has the responsibility for communicating the information to the birth parent in the likely event that the parent was not present at the medical visit. If possible, the clinician should provide a written summary of each health encounter, including the assessment, the treatment plan, and any scheduled follow-up. Caseworkers are required to conduct at least semiannual *Child and Family Service Reviews,* during which health information can be incorporated into planning for the child. Gathering health information is a challenging task. The caseworkers, who should have contact with the birth parents, are invaluable in this respect, although they may also be stymied by a dearth of contact and of records. A standardized health information form can help with information collection.

▶ The pediatric clinician may have access to information from prior health care providers, schools, regional health information organizations, and immunization registries. In addition to the usual health history, information that should be sought includes prenatal and perinatal history; developmental history; history of early intervention; mental health history, including the use of psychotropic medications; growth curves; immunization records; risk factors for HIV; accounts of other vertically transmitted infections; allergies; chronic illnesses; and medications. Adherence to guidelines for children with special health care needs can serve as a template for monitoring.[67] For older children, additional information should also include any educational or mental health problems. A paucity of such information may exist because the child may not have received adequate services before foster care or may have had multiple providers.

▶ Monitoring of dentition and reminders to foster parents about the importance of routine dental care and dental hygiene are important. Referral for dental care should begin at age 1 year.

▶ Children entering foster care tend to be under-immunized, even compared with other poor children, and every health encounter should be viewed as an opportunity to immunize a child in foster care.

▶ The underuse of routine preventive health care services before foster care placement implies a deficiency of screening for lead, iron-deficiency anemia, and tuberculosis exposure. Many children in foster care reside in or have resided in older housing stock, and pica is a commonly encountered behavioral issue in this population, increasing the risk for elevated plasma lead levels. Poor nutrition before foster care places children at risk for iron-deficiency anemia and other micronutrient deficiencies; thus, clinicians should obtain plasma lead levels and screen all children younger than 6 years for anemia at least annually. Obesity is now a prevalent form of disordered nutrition, and appropriate diet and exercise should be addressed with caregivers and children. Children entering foster care have an overall obesity rate of 27%. Of obese children who remain in foster care for at least 1 year, only 12% lose weight in care, whereas 7% gain weight. Children residing in congregate care have higher rates of obesity than other children in care do.[68] Menstruating adolescent girls should have annual hemoglobin screening. Universal tuberculosis screening is recommended using the purified protein derivative tuberculin test at admission and every 3 to 5 years thereafter because children may have had high-risk exposures before foster care and visit in high-risk situations (eg, jail) while in foster care. Hemoglobin electrophoresis should be considered in at-risk children with no documentation of sickle cell screening at birth.

▶ Maternal lifestyles during pregnancy, including substance use and promiscuity, place children in foster care at increased risk for a variety of vertically transmitted infectious diseases, including HIV, hepatitis B and C, congenital syphilis, and herpes. Every child placed in foster care should be screened for these infections early in placement. Up to 80% of young children placed into foster care are at high risk for vertically transmitted HIV infection, but fewer than 10% are screened because of the complexities of risk assessment, obtaining informed consent, and confidentiality barriers.[69] Guidelines for HIV risk assessment and screening of children in foster care vary from state to state. Some agencies use risk-assessment tools to determine a child's risk for HIV infection, although the accuracy of such tools depends on the birth parent's availability and truthfulness. In general, the biological parent retains the right to consent to testing or not, unless the child has been freed for adoption or parental rights have been terminated. Agencies vary in their policies regarding consent procedures when a parent declines screening but the child meets high-risk criteria. Identifying children who are HIV positive is critical to appropriate medical management, including pneumocystis pneumonia prophylaxis, modification of the immunization schedule, and early antiretroviral therapy. Pediatric clinicians may wish to become familiar with the HIV policies in their states and promote appropriate risk assessment and screening for the individual child.

▶ Adolescents in foster care also represent a high-risk group for HIV and other STIs, because of either unprotected sex with multiple partners or prior sexual abuse.[65] In general, adolescents in foster care are allowed by law to give consent for HIV testing, unless they are cognitively impaired. Confidentiality laws vary, however. In some states, the adolescent has the right to designate who has access to HIV-related information, whereas in others, social service agencies and their representatives have access to such data on any child in their care and custody, including adolescents. Obviously, pediatric clinicians need to provide detailed anticipatory guidance around healthy and safe sexuality. Screening for gonorrhea and chlamydia is recommended at admission and at each preventive health care visit. Testing for other STIs should be considered on the basis of history and local epidemiology. In caring for a child in foster care, the primary care clinician might sometimes need to assume the role of advocate for appropriate health care for the child.

Advocacy

Children and adolescents in foster care access high-cost services, such as the emergency department and inpatient medical and psychiatric services, at very high rates. Health information on admission is almost universally lacking, and it can be difficult to identify who previously provided medical care. Neither caseworkers nor foster parents have the level of knowledge necessary to serve as the health care manager, yet the system relies on them to perform this complex task.[23] The Fostering Connections to Success and Increasing Adoptions Act of 2008 now requires states to develop health care systems for children in foster care, to work with pediatric clinicians to accomplish this development, and to promote the medical home as a source of care. This process is, however, in its infancy in most states. Health systems are essential because inadequate health care management underlies the pattern of inadequate, fragmented, and occasionally redundant care received.[53] Medicaid programs in some states limit access to health care because of inadequate financing, delays in payment, and limited numbers of medical subspecialists willing to accept payment. Some Medicaid managed care programs increase access to medical subspecialists for children in foster care but significantly reduce access to mental health care, although this care is the most significant health care need of the foster care population. Complex consent and confidentiality procedures required by the foster care system often limit access to health care, delay evaluations and treatment, and confound communication among professionals. Failure to support and educate foster parents about a child's medical, developmental, and mental health needs and failure to secure appropriate treatment can lead to disruptions in placement when foster parents are overwhelmed.[54] As states move toward the implementation of recent legislation to adopt health systems in foster care, pediatric clinicians may have the opportunity to engage state and county officials to improve outcomes for children in foster care. The AAP has a number of resources to help clinicians in this role (see Box 15-1; see also www.aap.org/en-us/advocacy-and-policy/aap-health-initiatives/healthy-foster-care-america).

Summary

Children and adolescents removed from their families for reasons of health and safety enter foster or kinship care having experienced multiple adversities and trauma that negatively affect their health and well-being. As a result, these children and adolescents have a high prevalence of medical, mental health, developmental, educational, and dental conditions. Pediatric clinicians should use foster care as a window of opportunity in which the child or teen can heal. The clinician can provide the medical home while the child or teen is in foster care, following recommended standards of health care to identify and treat all the child's or teen's health needs. The clinician should be proactive in engaging child welfare agencies to ensure that health planning is integrated into the child's permanency plan in a meaningful way. Pediatric clinicians also have a role in educating child welfare professionals, foster and kinship parents, birth parents, and adolescents and young adults about health issues and in advocating for and coordinating health care to this vulnerable population.

Acknowledgment: The authors gratefully acknowledge the children and families they serve for their inspiration and the staffs of Starlight Pediatrics and child welfare services for their compassion, dedication, and caring.

AAP Policy

American Academy of Pediatrics Committee on Pediatric AIDS. Identification and care of HIV-exposed and HIV-infected infants, children, and adolescents in foster care. *Pediatrics.* 2000;106(1):149–153. Reaffirmed December 2016 (pediatrics. aappublications.org/content/106/1/149)

American Academy of Pediatrics Committee on Psychosocial Aspects of Child and Family Health; Committee on Early Childhood, Adoption, and Dependent Care; and Section on Developmental and Behavioral Pediatrics. Early childhood adversity, toxic stress, and the role of the pediatrician: translating developmental science into lifelong health. *Pediatrics.* 2012;129(1):e224–e231. Reaffirmed July 2016 (pediatrics. aappublications.org/content/129/1/e224)

American Academy of Pediatrics Council on Children With Disabilities, Section on Developmental and Behavioral Pediatrics, Bright Futures Steering Committee, and Medical Home Initiatives for Children With Special Needs Project Advisory Committee. Identifying infants and young children with developmental disorders in the medical home: an algorithm for developmental surveillance and screening. *Pediatrics.* 2006;118(1):405–420. Reaffirmed August 2014 (pediatrics.aappublications.org/content/118/1/405)

Shonkoff JP, Garner AS; American Academy of Pediatrics Committee on Psychosocial Aspects of Child and Family Health; Committee on Early Childhood, Adoption, and Dependent Care; and Section on Developmental and Behavioral Pediatrics. The lifelong effects of early childhood adversity and toxic stress. *Pediatrics.* 2012;129(1): e232–e246. Reaffirmed July 2016 (pediatrics.aappublications.org/content/129/1/e232)

References

1. Children's Bureau. *Child Maltreatment 2014.* Washington, DC: Children's Bureau, Administration for Children and Families, US Dept of Health and Human Services; 2016. http://www.acf.hhs.gov/programs/cb/research-data-technology/statistics-research/child-maltreatment. Accessed January 24, 2018
2. Children's Bureau, Administration for Children and Families, US Department of Health and Human Services. AFCARS report #23. Children's Bureau Web site. http://www.acf.hhs.gov/programs/cb/resource/afcars-report-23. Published June 30, 2016. Accessed January 24, 2018
3. Barth RP, Green R, Guo S. Kinship care and foster care: informing the new debate. In: Haskins R, Wulczyn F, Bruce Webb M, eds. *Child Protection: Using Research to Improve Policy and Practice.* Washington, DC: Brookings Institution Press; 2007
4. Children's Bureau. *Trends in Foster Care and Adoption: FFY 2002-FFY 2013.* Washington, DC: Children's Bureau, Administration for Children and Families, US Dept of Health and Human Services; 2014. http://www.acf.hhs.gov/sites/default/files/cb/trends_fostercare_adoption2013. pdf. Accessed January 24, 2018
5. Barbell K, Freundlich M. *Foster Care Today.* Washington, DC: Casey Family Programs, National Center for Resource Family Support; 2001
6. Stein BD, Zima BT, Elliott MN, et al. Violence exposure among school-age children in foster care: relationship to distress symptoms. *J Am Acad Child Adolesc Psychiatry.* 2001;40(5): 588–594
7. Leslie LK, Landsverk J, Ezzet-Lofstrom R, Tschann JM, Slymen DJ, Garland AF. Children in foster care: factors influencing outpatient mental health service use. *Child Abuse Negl.* 2000;24(4):465–476

8. American Academy of Pediatrics Committee on Early Childhood and Adoption and Dependent Care. Developmental issues for young children in foster care. *Pediatrics*. 2000; 106(5):1145–1150

9. Children's Bureau, Administration for Children and Families, US Department of Health and Human Services. Major federal legislation index and search. Child Welfare Information Gateway Web site. https://www.childwelfare.gov/topics/systemwide/laws-policies/federal/search. Accessed January 24, 2018

10. Fowler PJ, Toro PA, Miles BW. Pathways to and from homelessness and associated psychosocial outcomes among adolescents leaving the foster care system. *Am J Public Health*. 2009;99(8):1453–1458

11. Dozier M, Lindhiem O, Lewis E, Bick J, Bernard K, Peloso E. Effects of a foster parent training program on young children's attachment behaviors: preliminary evidence from a randomized clinical trial. *Child Adolesc Social Work J*. 2009;26(4):321–332

12. Dozier M, Bick J, Bernard K. Intervening with foster parents to enhance biobehavioral outcomes among infants and toddlers. *Zero Three*. 2011;31(3):17–22

13. Dorsey S, Farmer EM, Barth RP, Greene K, Reid J, Landsverk J. Current status and evidence base of training for foster and treatment foster parents. *Child Youth Serv Rev*. 2008;30(12): 1403–1416

14. Conn AM, Szilagyi MA, Franke TM, et al. Trends in child protection and out-of-home care. *Pediatrics*. 2013;132(4):712–719

15. Jones LM, Finkelhor D, Halter S. Child maltreatment trends in the 1990s: why does neglect differ from sexual and physical abuse? *Child Maltreat*. 2006;11(2):107–120

16. Szilagyi MA, Jee S, Nilsen W, et al. Under-utilization of specialty mental health services by young children in foster and kinship care. Abstract presented at: Pediatric Academic Society Meetings; May 1, 2006; San Francisco, CA

17. Flaherty EG, Thompson R, Litrownik AJ, et al. Adverse childhood exposures and reported child health at age 12. *Acad Pediatr*. 2009;9(3):150–156

18. Shonkoff JP, Levitt P. Neuroscience and the future of early childhood policy: moving from why to what and how. *Neuron*. 2010;67(5):689–691

19. Gunnar MR, Fisher PA; Early Experience, Stress, and Prevention Network. Bringing basic research on early experience and stress neurobiology to bear on preventive interventions for neglected and maltreated children. *Dev Psychopathol*. 2006;18(3):651–677

20. Anda RF, Felitti VJ, Bremner JD, et al. The enduring effects of abuse and related adverse experiences in childhood: a convergence of evidence from neurobiology and epidemiology. *Eur Arch Psychiatry Clin Neurosci*. 2006;256(3):174–186

21. Felitti VJ. Adverse childhood experiences and adult health. *Acad Pediatr*. 2009;9(3):131–132

22. Shonkoff JP, Garner AS; American Academy of Pediatrics Committee on Psychosocial Aspects of Child and Family Health; Committee on Early Childhood, Adoption, and Dependent Care; and Section on Developmental and Behavioral Pediatrics. The lifelong effects of early childhood adversity and toxic stress. *Pediatrics*. 2012;129(1):e232–e246

23. Szilagyi M. The pediatrician and the child in foster care. *Pediatr Rev*. 1998;19(2):39–50

24. Walker JS, Weaver A, Gowen LK, Aue N. Traumatic stress/child welfare. *Focal Point Res Policy Pract Child Ment Health*. 2007;21(1):1–32. http://eric.ed.gov/?id=ED501744. Accessed January 24, 2018

25. Brown EJ, Amaya-Jackson L, Cohen J, et al. Childhood traumatic grief: a multi-site empirical examination of the construct and its correlates. *Death Stud*. 2008;32(10):899–923

26. Rubin DM, O'Reilly AL, Luan X, Localio AR. The impact of placement stability on behavioral well-being for children in foster care. *Pediatrics*. 2007;119(2):336–344

27. Reilly T. Transition from care: status and outcomes of youth who age out of foster care. *Child Welfare*. 2003;82(6):727–746

28. Hill RB. *Synthesis of Research on Disproportionality in the Child Welfare System: An Update*. Washington, DC: Casey-CSSP Alliance for Racial Equity in Child Welfare; 2006. http://www.cssp.org/reform/child-welfare/other-resources/synthesis-of-research-on-disproportionality-robert-hill.pdf. Accessed January 24, 2018

29. Drake B, Jolley JM, Lanier P, et al. Racial bias in child protection? A comparison of competing explanations using national data. *Pediatrics.* 2011;127(3):471–478

30. Ahrens KR, DuBois DL, Richardson LP, Fan MY, Lozano P. Youth in foster care with adult mentors during adolescence have improved adult outcomes. *Pediatrics.* 2008;121(2):e246–e252

31. Conn AM, Calais C, Szilagyi M, Baldwin C, Jee SH. Youth in out-of-home care: relation of engagement in structured group activities with social and mental health measures. *Child Youth Serv Rev.* 2014;36:201–205

32. Jee SH, Couderc JP, Swanson D, et al. A pilot randomized trial teaching mindfulness-based stress reduction to traumatized youth in foster care. *Complement Ther Clin Pract.* 2015;21(3):201–209

33. Joseph MA, O'Connor TG, Briskman JA, Maughan B, Scott S. The formation of secure new attachments by children who were maltreated: an observational study of adolescents in foster care. *Dev Psychopathol.* 2014;26(1):67–80

34. Mersky JP, Topitzes J, Janczewski CE, McNeil CB. Enhancing foster parent training with parent-child interaction therapy: evidence from a randomized field experiment. *J Soc Social Work Res.* 2015;6(4):591–616

35. Simms MD. Foster children and the foster care system, part I: history and legal structure. *Curr Probl Pediatr.* 1991;21(7):297–321

36. Winokur M, Crawford G, Longobardi R, Valentine D. Matched comparison of children in kinship care and foster care on child welfare outcomes. *Fam Soc.* 2008;89(3):338–346

37. Rubin DM, Downes KJ, O'Reilly AL, et al. Impact of kinship care on behavioral well-being for children in out-of-home care. *Arch Pediatr Adolesc Med.* 2008;162(2):550–556

38. Jee SH, Conn AM, Blumkin A, Szilagyi PG, Baldwin CD, Szilagyi MA. Identification of social-emotional problems among young children in foster care. *J Child Psychol Psychiatry.* 2010;51(12):1351–1358

39. Jee SH, Halterman JS, Szilagyi MA, Conn AM, Alpert-Gillis L, Szilagyi PG. Enhanced detection of social-emotional problems among youth in foster care. *Acad Pediatr.* 2011;11(5):409–413

40. American Academy of Pediatrics Committee on Early Childhood, Adoption, and Dependent Care. Health care of children in foster care. *Pediatrics.* 1994;93(2):335–338

41. Halfon N, Mendonca A, Berkowitz G. Health status of children in foster care. The experience of the Center for the Vulnerable Child. *Arch Pediatr Adolesc Med.* 1995;149(4):386–392

42. Jee SH, Simms MD. Health and well-being of children in foster care placement. *Pediatr Rev.* 2006;27(1):34–36

43. Leslie LK, Hurlburt MS, Landsverk J, Rolls JA, Wood PA, Kelleher KJ. Comprehensive assessments for children entering foster care: a national perspective. *Pediatrics.* 2003;112(1, pt 1):134–142

44. Ringeisen H, Casanueva C, Urato M, Cross T. Special health care needs among children in the child welfare system. *Pediatrics.* 2008;122(1):e232–e241

45. Simms MD, Dubowitz H, Szilagyi MA. Health care needs of children in the foster care system. *Pediatrics.* 2000;106(4)(suppl):909–918

46. Steele JS, Buchi KF. Medical and mental health of children entering the Utah foster care system. *Pediatrics.* 2008;122(3):e703–e709

47. Jee SH, Barth RP, Szilagyi MA, Szilagyi PG, Aida M, Davis MM. Factors associated with chronic conditions among children in foster care. *J Health Care Poor Underserved.* 2006;17(2):328–341

48. McMillen JC, Zima BT, Scott LD Jr, et al. Prevalence of psychiatric disorders among older youths in the foster care system. *J Am Acad Child Adolesc Psychiatry.* 2005;44(1):88–95

49. Smithgall C, Gladden RM, Yang D, et al. *Behavior Problems and Educational Disruptions Among Children in Out-Of-Home Care.* Chicago, IL: Chapin Hall Center for Children, University of Chicago; 2005

50. Horwitz SM, Balestracci KM, Simms MD. Foster care placement improves children's functioning. *Arch Pediatr Adolesc Med.* 2001;155(11):1255–1260

51. Johnson C, Silver P, Wulczyn F. *Raising the Bar for Health and Mental Health Services for Children in Foster Care: Developing a Model of Managed Care.* New York, NY: Council of Family and Child Caring Agencies; 2013. http://www.cofcca.org/current-newstrending-now/1384. Accessed January 24, 2018

52. Jee SH, Szilagyi M, Schriefer J, et al. Quality improvement learning collaborative to examine foster care guidelines. *Child Youth Serv Rev.* 2015;59:84–88

53. Child Welfare League of America. *Standards of Excellence for Health Care Services for Children in Out-of-Home Care.* Washington, DC: Child Welfare League of America; 1988

54. American Academy of Pediatrics Task Force on Health Care for Children in Foster Care and District II, New York State. *Fostering Health: Health Care for Children and Adolescents in Foster Care.* 2nd ed. Elk Grove Village, IL: American Academy of Pediatrics; 2005

55. Simms MD, Freundlich M, Battistelli ES, Kaufman ND. Delivering health and mental health care services to children in family foster care after welfare and health care reform. *Child Welfare.* 1999;78(1):166–183

56. Leslie LK, Gordon JN, Meneken L, Premji K, Michelmore KL, Ganger W. The physical, developmental, and mental health needs of young children in child welfare by initial placement type. *J Dev Behav Pediatr.* 2005;26(3):177–185

57. Jee SH, Szilagyi M, Ovenshire C, et al. Improved detection of developmental delays among young children in foster care. *Pediatrics.* 2010;125(2):282–289

58. Taussig HN, Clyman RB, Landsverk J. Children who return home from foster care: a 6-year prospective study of behavioral health outcomes in adolescence. *Pediatrics.* 2001;108(1):E10

59. Rubin DM, Feudtner C, Localio R, Mandell DS. State variation in psychotropic medication use by foster care children with autism spectrum disorder. *Pediatrics.* 2009;124(2):e305–e312

60. Zito JM, Safer DJ, Sai D, et al. Psychotropic medication patterns among youth in foster care. *Pediatrics.* 2008;121(1):e157–e163

61. Coyle JT. Psychotropic drug use in very young children. *JAMA.* 2000;283(8):1025–1030

62. Malkin M. *Psychotropic Medication for Children and Adolescents.* Los Angeles, CA: Juvenile Court Mental Health Services, Los Angeles County Dept of Mental Health; 2005

63. Texas Department of Family and Protective Services, University of Texas at Austin College of Pharmacy. Psychotropic medication utilization parameters for children and youth in foster care. Texas Department of Family and Protective Services Web site. https://www.dfps.state.tx.us/Child_Protection/Medical_Services/documents/reports/2016-03_Psychotropic_Medication_Utilization_Parameters_for_Foster_Children.pdf. Published March 2016. Accessed January 24, 2018

64. Stambaugh LF, Leslie LK, Ringeisen H, Smith K, Hodgkin D. *Psychotropic Medication Use by Children in Child Welfare.* Washington, DC: Office of Planning, Research and Evaluation; Administration for Children and Families; US Dept of Health and Human Services; 2012. OPRE report 2012-33. http://www.acf.hhs.gov/sites/default/files/opre/psych_med.pdf. Accessed January 24, 2018

65. Irwin M. *Understanding the Use of Psychiatric Medication in Foster Care and Residential Treatment.* Saratoga Springs, NY: New York Public Welfare Association Summer Conference; 2004

66. American Academy of Child and Adolescent Psychiatry. *AACAP Position Statement on Oversight of Psychotropic Medication Use for Children in State Custody: A Best Principles Guideline.* Washington, DC: American Academy of Child and Adolescent Psychiatry; 2003. http://www.aacap.org/App_Themes/AACAP/docs/clinical_practice_center/systems_of_care/FosterCare_BestPrinciples_FINAL.pdf. Accessed January 24, 2018

67. American Academy of Pediatrics Council on Children With Disabilities, Section on Developmental Behavioral Pediatrics, Bright Futures Steering Committee, and Medical Home Initiatives for Children With Special Needs Project Advisory Committee. Identifying infants and young children with developmental disorders in the medical home: an algorithm for developmental surveillance and screening. *Pediatrics.* 2006;118(1):405–420

68. Schneiderman JU, Smith C, Arnold-Clark JS, Fuentes J, Duan L, Palinkas LA. Overweight and obesity among Hispanic children entering foster care: a preliminary examination of polyvictimization. *Child Maltreat.* 2013;18(4):264–273

69. American Academy of Pediatrics Committee on Pediatric AIDS. Identification and care of HIV-exposed and HIV-infected infants, children, and adolescents in foster care. *Pediatrics.* 2000;106(1, pt 1):149–153

Adopted Children

Sarah H. Springer, MD

"Today, adopted children come with a history of
life before their adoptions, and this history
has a tremendous effect on their needs
and outcomes, both in the short-term and
over time."

Who Are the Children?

Most children adopted in the United States today are not adopted as
newborns. With easy availability of family planning and general acceptance
of single motherhood, fewer newborns are placed for adoption than in
generations past. Instead, most adopted children join their families after
being in the domestic child welfare system or in foster or institutional care
overseas. Many children with medical or developmental disabilities who
were, in previous times, considered unadoptable are now being successfully
placed with adoptive families. Today, adopted children come with a history
of life before their adoptions, and this history has a tremendous effect on
their needs and outcomes, both in the short-term and over time.

Some children adopted from the domestic foster care system come to
their adoptive families as newborns or young infants, placed first as foster
children and then later adopted by their foster parents. These children have
the benefits of nurturing care from infancy but may still experience the
long-term sequelae of prenatal adversity, particularly substance exposure.
More commonly, children adopted from foster care are older and have experienced significant abuse, neglect, and other trauma before adoption. Their
long-term physical, mental, developmental, and behavioral health risks and
needs are determined by the specifics of these traumas and are frequently
complex. (See Chapter 15, Children in Foster or Kinship Care or Involved
With Child Welfare.)

Child care circumstances vary tremendously among the countries from which children are adopted internationally.[1] Some children are cared for in high-quality, family-setting foster care, whereas others are cared for in institutional settings that can vary from small group homes with reasonable resources to large, extremely resource-poor orphanages. Some children enter care as newborns because of poverty, social adversity, or political circumstances; others enter as older children after experiencing the same sorts of trauma that place children into the foster care system in the United States.

More international children than ever before are being adopted with identified special health care needs. These needs can range from fairly simple problems such as orthopedic deformities, isolated cleft lip and palate, or ventricular septal defects; to chronic infectious illnesses such as hepatitis B and HIV infection; to complex syndromes with multiple medical and developmental disabilities. Health care for these needs may or may not have been available before adoption, and medical procedures may have been traumatic for the child who experienced them without the love or support of a parent.

With or without identified special needs, most children are at least older infants or toddlers before they are eligible for international adoptive placement. Knowing how and why a child came into care is important, as is knowing the type of care a child experienced, because the history before adoption often sheds light on the physical, mental, and developmental health issues a child might be expected to face immediately and over the long-term.

Children come to the United States from many different countries through adoption. Although some countries have sent substantial numbers of children for many years, the list of sending countries is continually changing because of political and social circumstances both in the United States and abroad. The US Department of State listing of adoption visa types issued provides a concise listing of the numbers of children adopted from countries around the world each year.[2]

The reasons children are eligible for adoption in all countries include severe poverty, social adversity (eg, maternal drug or alcohol use, incarceration, homelessness, mental health disabilities), and child abuse and neglect, with government termination of parental rights. The specific details for any given child are often unknown, but these early life experiences frequently have significant long-term implications for the child's mental health.

Other common adoptions today include kinship placements and second- or co-parent adoptions. Current child welfare practice emphasizes finding permanency for children and adolescents (referred to as *children* throughout the remainder of this chapter unless otherwise specified) more quickly than in the past and keeping children within their communities and cultures of origin whenever possible. Estimates indicate that approximately 120,000 children, or approximately 29% of those in foster care, are placed in foster care with extended family members.[3] If they are not able to return to the custody of their birth parents, many of these children are adopted by their extended family members or cared for in permanent legal guardianship relationships. This approach allows children to maintain family connections but can pose unique challenges to the adopting parents, who must negotiate complicated relationships among the children, the birth parents, and other extended family members. Second-parent adoptions refer to the adoption of a child who already has one legal parent by the spouse or partner of that parent. Co-parent adoption is the adoption of a child by 2 unmarried adults.

Understanding the Adoption Process: An Opportunity to Provide Proactive Support

Pediatric clinicians (ie, primary care pediatricians, pediatric subspecialists, and family physicians, internists, nurse practitioners, and physician assistants who provide pediatric care) can be most helpful to adopting parents if they are knowledgeable about the processes and types of adoptions.[4,5] Adoption laws vary by state, but the basic legal requirements are the same. Adopting parents must undergo a social work evaluation (commonly referred to as the *home study* or *family assessment*) to verify that they are minimally fit to be parents, have minimal resources to support a child, and do not have records of child abuse or significant criminal records. Families do not have to be wealthy or highly educated; they simply have to prove that they would be able to love and nurture a child. The home study must typically be provided by a social worker licensed to work in a particular state, who produces a written document verifying the adults' suitability for parenthood, which becomes part of the legal record of the adoption. Families adopting across state lines must satisfy the requirements of both states, and families adopting internationally must meet all requirements of the state and federal governments as well as those of the child's birth country.

Adoption placements can be arranged and carried out by licensed agencies or independent facilitators, depending on the laws of individual states and countries. Adoption agencies may be public agencies acting as an arm of the public child welfare system or may be licensed private agencies. Facilitators may be of any training background but are commonly social workers or attorneys who specialize in connecting would-be adoptive parents with available children. For international adoptions, most countries of origin require that their children be placed by a licensed nonprofit agency. In addition, the Hague Convention on Intercountry Adoption (a multinational treaty that was signed by the United States in 1994 and entered into force in 2008) requires that all child placements between participating countries be governed by a strict set of ethical guidelines and be carried out by licensed and accredited agencies that have enforceable government oversight.[6,7] Approximately 95 countries have signed on to the convention so far, meaning that adoptions between these countries must meet ethical and procedural guidelines that provide greater protections for children, birth parents, and adopting parents.

Families adopting newborns are often in touch with the child's birth parents before the adoption because most birth parents today participate in the choosing of their child's adoptive parents. Many adoptive parents travel to be at their child's delivery and often participate in ongoing, open relationships with the child's birth parents. Some adoptions are finalized very quickly, whereas others take significantly longer, depending on the laws of the state where the child was born and of the state where the adoptive parent or parents live. Financial costs for domestic newborn adoptions are extremely variable and can be significant when all the individual services performed are tallied. Costs may include legal and social work fees, travel expenses, and, in some states, payment of room and board or health care expenses for the birth mother before the delivery.

Families adopting children from the child welfare system may be the child's foster parents from birth, but they become eligible to adopt only after the child's birth parents are unable to resume custody. Other children come into the child welfare system later, after experiencing abuse or neglect. If birth parent rights are later terminated (see Chapter 15, Children in Foster or Kinship Care or Involved With Child Welfare), the child may be adopted by his or her foster parents or by another family. Adoptive families have ongoing contact with birth parents less frequently in this kind of adoption, although some adoptions, especially kinship placements, do maintain ongoing contact with birth parents. Many of the children who are waiting in the child welfare system for adoptive families are older, are part of sibling groups, and have significant psychological scars from their earlier traumatic life experiences. Travel is less often a part of adopting from the public system because most communities have more children in care who are in need of permanent homes than families waiting to adopt them. Adoptions from the public child welfare system are often finalized months, or even years, after the child is placed in the home as due process is carried out to protect the rights of birth parents. Financial costs for this type of adoption are typically much more modest, with many of the services provided free of charge to the adopting family by the public agency, its mission being to find the best home for each child on behalf of the state or local government.

Parents adopting internationally most often travel to adopt their child, with adoptions from some countries requiring 2 or 3 trips. Although this process can be stressful and financially costly, it offers adopting parents the opportunity to get to know the people and culture of their child's birth country. In addition to having a valid home study, families are required to pass criminal record clearance from the Federal Bureau of Investigation, document that the child meets the US definition of an adoptable child, and complete a detailed immigration application for the child. Families adopting from Hague Convention countries must also complete at least 10 hours of training on the needs of internationally adopted children, and the child must be deemed eligible for international placement by the sending country after reasonable efforts to place the child in-country have been documented.

On finalization of the adoption by US citizen parents, the child is automatically granted US citizenship, although parents must complete the last portions of the immigration application to claim this legal status for the child. It is critical that parents complete this process to ensure the child's full legal rights as a US citizen.[8] Reports of deportation of international adoptees whose citizenship had never been completed highlight the importance of this final step, and pediatric clinicians can help prevent future trauma by encouraging families to complete this final step in the process.[9,10]

Roles of the Pediatric Clinician in Preadoption Care

Unless the clinician has a special interest in adoption medicine, a family adopting its first child might not meet the clinician until the parent or parents receive information about a specific child or even until the child is home with the parents. Most pediatric clinicians, however, will have families already in their practices who decide to adopt, and these clinicians can play an important role in helping the entire process to be a success. Pediatric clinicians should be familiar with common adoption concerns[11-13] and can contact members of the American Academy of Pediatrics (AAP) Council on Foster Care, Adoption, and Kinship Care for help (www.aap.org/en-us/about-the-aap/Committees-Councils-Sections/Council-on-Foster-Care-Adoption-Kinship/Pages/Foster-Care-Adoption-Kinship.aspx). Resources such as *Talking With Families About Adoption, Foster Care, and Kinship*

Care in the Pediatric Office, available at www.aap.org/en-us/Documents/ TalkingWithFamilies.pdf, may be useful in conducting office visits.

Parents who are wondering what type of adoption to pursue should consider the potential needs of the children. By looking at the intersection of 3 variables, families and their pediatric clinicians can anticipate at least some of the needs a child might be expected to have and some of the adoption process issues. Carefully assessing their own capacities to handle different issues *before* a child is placed can help families thrive, even through very difficult long-term needs.

First, families need to consider the age of a child: while even newborns may have experienced prenatal adversity, children placed beyond the newborn period bring with them psychological, physical, and social consequences from previous life experiences and traumas. In addition to developmental and educational supports, professional mental health care is often needed to allow a child to reach full potential. The second variable is whether a child is of the same or another race as the adopting parent or parents, and the third variable is whether the child is from the same or a different country or culture. Although transracial, transcultural, and international adoptions are not associated with poor outcomes, helping a child develop a strong sense of racial and cultural identity is important to the child's self-esteem and psychological well-being. This identity building can be challenging, especially in communities with little racial or cultural diversity.[14]

Parents may also request help in deciding on an agency or a facilitator to conduct the adoption. In general, parents should be encouraged to use agencies that are licensed (and therefore subject to minimal ethical and practice standards) and that have a mission to promote the welfare of children. Agencies with the mission of finding the right family for each child often cost more and require more of adopting parents, but they will also provide appropriate education and long-term support for families. Agencies with the mission of conducting an adoption rapidly may seem appealing at first glance, but they often do not share the complexities or risks of the children with adopting parents and may not be there for the long-term support that many families need.

Pediatric clinicians may also be asked to review the information a family receives about a particular child whom they are considering adopting. Reviewing this information with a family is not to screen out children but rather to help the prospective family understand the information given to them, know what additional information they need to gather, and, finally, make a well-informed decision as to their ability to be the best parents for the child, given the predictable needs or risks.[13] This service is often best performed by clinicians familiar with all the types of adoptions, the information available for children coming from different countries, and the common risks seen among different groups of available children. Many agencies provide families with lists of clinicians specializing in adoption medicine, and a list can also be found through the AAP Council on Foster Care, Adoption, and Kinship Care Web site (www.aap.org/en-us/about-the-aap/Committees-Councils-Sections/Council-on-Foster-Care-Adoption-Kinship/Pages/Foster-Care-Adoption-Kinship.aspx).

Finally, pediatric clinicians need to know the infectious diseases and travel health issues involved for families traveling internationally to adopt.[15] A discussion of these issues is beyond the scope of this book but can be found in Chapter 70, Adoption, in the *American Academy of Pediatrics Textbook of Pediatric Care,* 2nd Edition, and Chapter 4, Pre-adoption Considerations for Pediatricians, of *Adoption Medicine: Caring for Children and Families.*

New-Arrival Issues

Social and Adjustment Concerns

The arrival of a newly adopted child into a family brings joys and stresses similar to those that accompany the birth of a child. In addition, however, all the circumstances that led to the adoption must be managed by adopting parents, birth parents, siblings, extended family, and the child. Adopting parents who have experienced infertility or the loss of previous children may have unresolved grief, which can complicate the feelings of joy accompanying the arrival of this child. In addition, long waits for parenthood can create unrealistic expectations, which are often in stark contrast with the reality of parenting any child, let alone one who has lived through trauma and adversity and whose whole world has just changed. Postadoption depression is as real an entity as postpartum depression, and pediatric clinicians should be prepared to identify and refer affected parents.[16–18]

For children adopted outside the immediate newborn period, the transition into the new adoptive family is often bewildering, frightening, and full of loss. Ideally, children should be given as much preparation as possible, with older children even participating in the decision to join a particular family. In reality, however, many children are simply taken one day from everything that is familiar and handed to strangers. Children who have been in foster care or who have developed strong attachments to orphanage caregivers will usually grieve the loss of these significant people, and older children may worry about their well-being or wonder if the caregivers are searching for them. Even children who have not been treated well by previous caregivers still have connections to them and may still grieve their loss. Adoptive parents and clinicians need to understand this process, comfort the grieving child, and help the child develop a strong sense of connection and security with the new parents. Allowing the child to talk about the previous caregivers, to look at pictures of them, and even to telephone or write to them can help the child process this grief. Parents may need encouragement to allow children to share their grief, given that not talking about it may seem easier. Allowing children to share these strong feelings can help build strong bonds of new attachment.[16,19–21]

All children have to adjust to the arrival of a new sibling, but an adopted sibling brings challenges that a newborn does not. Most often, the new child is not a helpless newborn but rather a mobile, demanding competitor for not only parental time and attention but also toys, food, and space. Extra love, understanding, and attention from parents are in order, which can be hard to attain when the demands of the newly transitioning adoptee are high.

Extended family members also have a significant effect on the new-arrival period. Some may be eager to shower love and attention on the bewildered, overwhelmed, grieving child, whereas others may not accept the child as a true member of the family. Sharing information about adoption and the child's expected transition needs with extended family members before the adoption can help create a nurturing acceptance into a warm extended family without overwhelming the child.

Adopting parents should plan for plenty of quiet, uninterrupted time with their newly adopted child, regardless of the age of the child at arrival. Helping the child develop a strong attachment to the parents is of utmost importance because this groundwork is the foundation of healthy parent-child relationships and, ultimately, of all human relationships. Parents should think of their child as a newborn emotionally in an older child's body. Parents should be the ones to meet physical needs and to provide comfort so the child learns to use them as a secure base in the world. Some parents are granted parenting leave by employers, whereas others must fight for it, given that many employers finance parenting leave through medical disability coverage, which does not apply when a woman has not given birth. Clinicians should work with parents to convince employers that time at home with their newly adopted child is vital to the child's long-term physical and emotional health, and parents should be encouraged to use as much leave time as possible.

Medical Issues

The physical health needs of newly adopted children can be significant. Some children are adopted with known special health care needs, while others' health concerns are discovered after placement. Whether the child was adopted domestically as a newborn, from the foster care system, or internationally, the social and medical risk factors of the child's birth parents and prior circumstances should guide medical and developmental assessments.

All newly adopted children, regardless of the type of adoption, should undergo a thorough assessment of development, including hearing and vision.[22] For newborns, this assessment will be the same as for any other routine child health supervision care, with special attention to any known long-term risk factors. Children adopted after the newborn period should undergo a careful assessment of all domains of development soon after placement. Most children make rapid developmental progress after they are in a nurturing family environment. Children whose delays are profound or persist beyond the first 2 to 3 months after adoption should be referred to formal developmental support services.

Balancing Priorities

As noted in the previous paragraphs, many children have significant medical needs upon their arrival to their new families, some of which are known before the adoption and some of which will be revealed by the new-arrival evaluation. Further diagnostic workup and treatment of these medical needs should be planned carefully, balancing medical urgency with the child and family's need for quiet nesting time in the early days of the adoption. Simple treatments, such as antibiotics or iron supplements, can begin right away. Potentially transmissible infections, such as intestinal parasites, hepatitis, and tuberculosis, should also be treated quickly. Urgent, time-sensitive, or potentially life-threatening medical conditions must be treated immediately (eg, congestive heart failure, dehydration, extremely high lead levels, untreated syphilis, dense cataracts). Treatment of nonurgent medical concerns, however, can and should be deferred until the family has had some time together and the child has begun to learn to use the parents for comfort and support. Common problems in this category include repair of cleft lip and palate, orthopedic conditions, nonurgent congenital heart defects, dental work, and strabismus surgery. Truly elective procedures, such as circumcision or repair of minor anomalies, should always be deferred until the child has developed a secure bond with the new family.[20]

The First Year Home: An Important Transition Time for the New Family

The first months in the adoptive home represent a transition time for the adopted child and the rest of the family, during which the groundwork is laid for the long-term success of the adoption.[16,20,23] Regardless of age, the child should be seen at least several times over the first year home to monitor catch-up in growth and development, child and family mental health needs, and the developing attachment of the child to the new family. All children should undergo age-appropriate hearing and vision screenings, given that children adopted from foster care or orphanages have high rates of auditory and visual impairments.[22] These visits can be timed to accommodate catch-up on immunizations and follow-up of identified medical needs.

Perhaps most important, careful attention should be paid to attachment-related behaviors in newly adopted children. Children who have always had loving, nurturing care understand how to use an adult as a secure base in the world and will transfer this designation to a new parent quickly, usually within several weeks. Children who have never experienced one-on-one, emotionally attuned caregiving, however, have often learned to cope with life's hardships on their own, without relying on an adult. These children need to be overtly taught to use their new parents as their base in the world because secure attachments are the foundation of healthy long-term relationships.[24] Parents may be impressed with the child's self-sufficiency, but they should be encouraged to intervene frequently, teaching the child to see the parent as the active provider of food, comfort, and nurturing. Pediatric clinicians should closely monitor newly adopted children for signs of developing strong attachments. If, after several months, the child does not preferentially use the parent or parents as a source of safety, security, and joy, the clinician should refer the family to a therapist experienced in attachment and early childhood adversity.[16,20,21,24,25]

Developmental Catch-up

Most children adopted out of foster care or internationally have significant developmental delays at the time of placement.[19,26–31] These delays usually resolve rapidly after the child is in the care of loving, nurturing parents; therefore, delays that persist beyond the first 2 to 3 months after adoption should be carefully evaluated. Young children learn new languages very quickly; thus, language delays that persist should not be presumed to be the result of learning a new language but rather should be carefully investigated, with early initiation of speech and language therapy.[32–34] Younger children qualify in most states for Early Intervention services, and older children can be evaluated and treated through local school districts or privately. For internationally adopted school-aged children, having academic assessments performed in the native language can be advantageous within the first 1 to 2 months home, before fluency in that language is lost, given that full fluency in the new language may take several years.[35,36]

Deciding when to start a newly adopted school-aged child in school can be difficult and needs to be an individual decision for each child, balancing the need for family bonding time with the child's academic needs and social desires. Children who have never been to or have missed substantial portions of school may need to work on academic basics typically taught to younger children, while being afforded social opportunities and enrichment classes with same-aged peers. Many children do well to start school part-time, gradually working up to full-time attendance as they develop greater comfort with all their new surroundings. Some children do well starting at a lower grade level to be taught academic basics and then move rapidly through several grade levels as they acquire skills and catch up to their same-aged peers. School-aged international children will qualify for ELL (English language learner) or ESL (English as a second language) services, in addition to any learning supports that they may need. Parents and clinicians should not let schools opt out of learning supports because a child is not a native English speaker; internationally adopted school-aged children frequently have *both* learning support needs and second-language needs.[37]

Routines of Daily Living

Most newly adopted children struggle in some way with the routines of daily living, including eating, sleeping, bathing, and toileting, among other routines. Even a child placed as a newborn may have these issues if exposures were encountered prenatally from which the child experiences withdrawal symptoms. Children who have not had enough food (particularly those cared for in institutional settings where, in addition to inadequate volumes, food is almost never available to satisfy individual hunger) often eat huge volumes of food and may hoard food, alarming parents and clinicians alike. This circumstance should be recognized as an adaptive survival behavior from the prior life circumstances and should be not restricted or punished. When children are allowed unlimited access to healthy, age-appropriate food, most will learn within several months that enough is now available and that they can have it whenever they need it, and they will slow down to more typical levels of intake. If, on the other hand, the child's intake is restricted, the previously learned strategy of taking all that is available whenever it is available will continue, often developing into more secretive food-hoarding behaviors and other long-term eating disorders.[16,19,20,38] Given all the information currently targeted at parents around preventing childhood obesity, pediatric clinicians may need to help parents understand this seemingly paradoxical advice and realize that the healthy eating habits of the family will prevail after the child truly believes that there will always be enough food.

Sleep problems are obviously a common concern for all children but are almost universal among newly adopted children. Many newly adopted children have never slept alone, in a dark room, or with any notion of safety at night, and internationally adopted children may have traveled through many time zones to arrive at their new homes. Sleep deprivation quickly takes its toll on parents and children alike, complicating all the other new-arrival transitions. Until a child has developed strong attachments to the parent or parents, however, sleep strategies that encourage parents to leave a child alone are inappropriate and may create more long-term anxiety. Until the child has thoroughly internalized the notion that the parent or parents will always be available when the child needs them, parents should be encouraged to be as physically and emotionally present at nighttime as the child needs to feel safe and secure. This task can be accomplished, however, in the child's room and bed, using the desired long-term sleep routines so parents can wean themselves out of the child's bedtime routine as the child develops a sense of safety and security. Older children, especially those who have experienced trauma or abuse, may need explanations from parents of nighttime noises before they will feel safe enough to sleep. By balancing these short- and long-term goals from the beginning, most children can be helped to sleep peacefully all night in their own beds within several months.[16,18,20,38]

Sensory-seeking or avoiding behaviors, as well as autism spectrum disorder–like repetitive behaviors, are common among children who have experienced severe deprivation before adoption. As with overeating mentioned earlier, these are adaptive behaviors in a setting with little or no stimulation,[19,39] and they usually resolve quickly when more stimulation and human interaction are made available. Many children revert to these behaviors when tired, stressed, or bored, and parents can learn to read these behaviors as cues to these feelings. Reverting to self-stimulating behaviors to cope with fatigue or stress may continue for years after adoption, with no other pathological behavioral concerns. On the other hand, children who do not respond to nurturing parenting, but instead continue to self-stimulate regularly rather than interact with the world, should have a full developmental and behavioral evaluation.[16,20,40,41]

Unknown Date of Birth

Another common dilemma, particularly for internationally adopted children, is an uncertain date of birth. Many children come into care after being born at home, with no official record of the birth or, more commonly, after being abandoned. Assigned birth dates may or may not be accurate, particularly for older children, given that the growth and developmental delays that result from malnutrition and neglect make children seem to be younger than they really are. Older children are occasionally deliberately assigned a younger age for well-intended reasons, such as increasing the child's chances of being adopted or enabling an oldest child to remain with younger siblings. As previously reviewed, most children are significantly delayed in their growth and development on arrival, and these delays, combined with knowledge of an assigned birthday, often tempt new parents and clinicians to consider changing the child's date of birth. Because these delays usually quickly resolve, however, the notion to consider legally changing the child's birth date in the first or second year after arrival is rarely advisable. Bone age testing or dental age assessments are not helpful early on, given that both malnutrition and neglect cause delays in bone and dental age as they do in the rest of the child's development and should thus not be used as justification for changing a birth date. When concerns about age discrepancy persist a year or more after adoption, parents and clinicians should carefully consider what would be gained and lost for the child if the date were to be changed. While an assigned birth date may seem meaningless to a parent, it may be seen by the child as an important connection to his or her past, either now or in the future. The situation of a meaningful age discrepancy is obviously more common for children adopted at older ages and as such, children should be included in the decision-making about this important piece of their identity.[20,23,42]

Long-term Needs

In addition to any issues identified before or immediately after adoption, long-term mental and physical health issues common to adopted children should be considered. Recognizing these risk factors in a child's history can help pediatric clinicians maintain appropriate surveillance above and beyond the usual child health supervision care routine and provide referrals and support proactively.

Most important, the long-term effects of early adversity cannot be forgotten. Early malnutrition, abuse, neglect, or trauma can cause significant long-term cognitive, developmental, behavioral, and mental health struggles, even after years in a warm, nurturing adoptive family. Developmental disabilities, mental health problems, and substance use struggles of birth parents are not uncommon factors in unplanned pregnancies or inability to care for their children in the first place, leaving adopted children as a group with a higher frequency of genetic predispositions to these diagnoses than among the general population.[35,43–45] Prenatal substance exposure, especially to alcohol, also carries significant long-term risks.[46–49] Teasing out which of these factors is responsible for a given child's struggles is often difficult or impossible; but, for most adopted children, it is a safe assumption that any of these predisposing issues might be a contributing factor.

Many children experience significant struggles as they enter school age. Difficulties with attention and impulse control often lead to the diagnosis of attention-deficit/hyperactivity disorder (ADHD), although this diagnosis is frequently just a portion of a far more complex learning profile. Children should undergo a thorough psychoeducational or neuropsychological evaluation to tease out complex visual, auditory, language, and sensory processing differences, difficulties with executive functioning, and specific learning disabilities before being assumed to have simple, uncomplicated ADHD.[36,37,43,50–52] In addition, many children who spent their early lives in institutional care, lacking much direct human contact, have difficulties reading nonverbal social cues. As a result, they often have great difficulties with peer relationships and can benefit from direct teaching on social skills and reading body language.

Children who experience serious malnutrition, followed by significant catch-up growth, have a significantly higher risk for precocious puberty compared with the general population.[53] In addition to having a young age of onset, these children typically proceed through the stages of puberty at a very rapid rate, making early recognition and treatment imperative to both physical health and mental health. Uncertainty about a child's true age can further complicate the evaluation.[54,55]

Many adoptees have little or no knowledge of their biological family medical histories, and those who do often have only the information that was available at the time of their births. This missing history can be a source of social and emotional distress to adolescents and their families, but for children of any age, it can also be a significant impediment to providing appropriate health care, particularly in the case of serious illness. Some states now provide registries of birth parent and adoptee information, with access granted by mutual consent. (See "Access to Adoption Records," the

Child Welfare Information Gateway, at www.childwelfare.gov/topics/
systemwide/laws-policies/statutes/infoaccessap.) Laws vary from state to
state regarding who may have access to this information and under what
circumstances. Some adoption agencies also maintain and update health
records of birth parents whose children they have placed, and some will
help families locate birth parents. Children who were adopted from overseas
generally have little or no information about birth family medical history,
and records may or may not be maintained, thus making further investigation difficult or impossible. Children who were abandoned have no way to
know any family medical history. Lack of birth family medical history
should be considered when determining risk factors for routine screening
(eg, for hypercholesterolemia).[56]

Issues Unique to Adoptive Families

Adoptive families come in all shapes and sizes. These families may include
children by birth and adoption, children and parents of different races, single
parents, parents who are gay or lesbian, grandparents and other relatives raising children, and stepparents adopting a new spouse's children, just to name a
few. Depending on the size and diversity of the community, some of these
families may be conspicuous, and parents and children will need to learn how
to handle questions from strangers and acquaintances. Parents and clinicians
need to help children learn to interpret which questions are ill intended vs
simply curious, what information is appropriate to share (with whom, when,
and where), and what information is private.[57] Children can and do thrive in
all these varieties of families, especially when parents are open and honest
with children about these topics that are unique to adoptive families.[14,58–62]

All pediatric clinicians should be familiar with basic issues that are
common to all adopted children and should ensure that they and the entire
office staff use language that reflects respect for adopted children and their
birth and adoptive families (Box 16-1).

Clinicians should help and encourage adoptive parents to talk with
their children about adoption from a very young age, given that all available research has shown that children do far better when they come to
understand adoption over time, rather than as a single, bombshell discussion.[63] Adoptive parents often struggle with how to begin these discussions
and how to handle children's questions, fearing that they might jeopardize
the child's sense of security or belonging in the family or that they might
overwhelm the child with difficult-to-comprehend details. Just as with any
other complicated matter, however, children come to understand the

Box 16-1. Respectful Ways to Talk About Adoption: A List of Dos and Don'ts

Do: Use the words *birth child* and *adopted child* only when they are relevant to the discussion; otherwise, simply use *child*.
Don't: Refer to a child born to his parents as the parents' "real child," "own child," or "natural child." A child who was adopted is very real and not at all unnatural; she is very much her parents' "own child."

Do: Use the words *birth parents* or *biological parents* only when asking about them is relevant.
Don't: Refer to the child's birth parents as his "real parents" or "natural parents." Adoptive parents are very real and not at all unnatural.

Do: Treat siblings who joined families by birth or adoption equally. They are loved equally by their parents and experience all of the joys and trials of any sibling relationship.
Don't: Distinguish between children who were adopted into the family and children who were born into the family unless it's relevant.

Do: Describe birth parents as choosing "to make an adoption plan for the child" or "to place the child for adoption."
Don't: Refer to a child as being "put up" or "given up" for adoption. Most birth parents have thought long and hard about their decision to place a child for adoption. It is very important to a child's self-esteem to know that her birth parents loved her and worked hard to reach a decision that they felt to be in her best interest. Even when birth parent rights are terminated involuntarily, the child needs to know that it wasn't her fault that her birth parents could not take care of her at the time and that other adults are looking out for her best interests.

Do: Recognize that families come in all shapes and sizes. Some families may have a single adoptive parent or permanent legal guardian and no other legal parent. Other families have same-sex parents.
Don't: Assume that the child has two opposite-sex parents.

Do: Refer to birth parents as "choosing not to parent" their child. This implies to the child who was adopted that birth parents made their decisions based on what they felt was in the best interest of each child when they made their decision.
Don't: Refer to birth parents as "choosing not to keep" their child. This implies to a child who was adopted that he was "not worth keeping."

Do: Talk with a family about how it celebrates the intercultural and/or interracial nature of the family. Many families make special efforts to include their children's culture and heritage in daily routines and traditions. Available research shows that children clearly benefit from this practice.
Don't: Ignore a child's birth country, race, or genetic heritage. Especially in communities where there is limited ethnic diversity, children from racial or ethnic minorities need family and physician support to overcome racism and develop a strong, positive racial identity.

Do: Recognize that a child understands adoption gradually as she grows, just as with all other developmental tasks.
Don't: Ask, "Are you going to tell your son that he's adopted?" Adoptive parents are encouraged to talk freely and honestly about adoption from the time their child is very young so that there is never a time in the child's life when this information comes as shocking news.

Box 16-1. Respectful Ways to Talk About Adoption: A List of Dos and Don'ts (*continued*)

Do: Be sympathetic with the long and sometimes arduous path that parents have traveled to become parents. Some may be experiencing significant financial stresses after the adoption, some may still be grieving infertility losses, and some may be coping with extended family members who do not accept the new member of the family. Recognize that even though the child may not be a newborn, the adults may be new parents. Recognize that post-adoption depression exists and is similar to post-partum depression.

Don't: Ask, "How much did you pay for your daughter?" Children are not bought. Fees go to pay social workers and attorneys, to complete court and government paperwork, and to cover travel, medical, foster/orphanage care, and other expenses, not to "buy children."

From American Academy of Pediatrics Council on Foster Care, Adoption, and Kinship Care. Respectful ways to talk about adoption: a list of do's and dont's. HealthyChildren.org Web site. https://www.healthychildren.org/English/family-life/family-dynamics/adoption-and-foster-care/Pages/Respectful-Ways-to-Talk-about-Adoption-A-List-of-Dos-Donts.aspx. Updated November 21, 2015. Accessed January 24, 2018

complexities of adoption over time and in more detail as they progress developmentally. Young children simply need to learn the language and can begin to understand that, "I didn't grow inside Mommy's tummy." Preschoolers ask many questions, and adoptive parents who respond openly to their inquiries are setting the stage for more in-depth, open dialogue as time goes on. School-aged children begin to understand that they have 2 sets of parents and spend a great deal of time thinking about their birth parents. They often fear talking about this subject with their adoptive parents, worrying that these questions will hurt the feelings of or minimize their love for their adoptive parents. Parents need to offer many opportunities for children to talk and clearly show them that this topic of conversation is acceptable. Teens begin to incorporate what they know about their birth parents and their own stories into their developing identity and may experiment with lifestyles that they know or imagine their birth parents to be living. Anticipatory guidance for adopted children should include encouraging parents to talk openly and honestly in simple, direct, developmentally appropriate language to help the children understand and deal with the specific details of their own life stories.[60] Resources are available to help parents, professionals, and children negotiate the complexities of grief, loss, and joy that come when a child is placed for adoption by one set of parents and adopted by another (Box 16-2).

Many adoptions, particularly domestic adoptions, include some degree of openness or ongoing contact between children and their birth parents.

Box 16-2. Online Resources for Clinicians and Families

- *Adoption Disruption/Dissolution* (booklet), Child Welfare Information Gateway (www.childwelfare.gov/topics/adoption/adopt-parenting/disruption)

- Fostering Connections (Web site), National Resource Center for Permanency and Family Connections (www.nrcpfc.org/fostering_connections)

- "International Adoption: Health Guidance and the Immigration Process" (Web page), Centers for Disease Control and Prevention (www.cdc.gov/immigrantrefugeehealth/adoption)

- NCTSN Learning Center (Web site), National Child Traumatic Stress Network (https://learn.nctsn.org)

- "The Resilience Project: Clinical Assessment Tools" (Web page), American Academy of Pediatrics (www.aap.org/en-us/advocacy-and-policy/aap-health-initiatives/resilience/Pages/Clinical-Assessment-Tools.aspx)

- "Trauma Guide" (Web page), American Academy of Pediatrics (www.aap.org/en-us/advocacy-and-policy/aap-health-initiatives/healthy-foster-care-america/Pages/Trauma-Guide.aspx)

Although this idea is frightening at first to many prospective adoptive parents and might seem harmful to those unfamiliar with adoption, research and experience have shown that children thrive when birth and adoptive parents carefully and lovingly maintain relationships over time. Although these relationships can at times be complicated, the benefit to children of being able to know exactly why their birth parents chose not to raise them and of knowing details such as who they resemble, whose musical talent or crooked toes they inherited, and how their birth parents are doing today is beyond measure.

Children who do not have ongoing contact with their birth parents often choose to search for them as they become adolescents or adults. Many adoption agencies and therapists offer help and support to adopted persons and their families as they proceed through this process. The emotional and legal complexities of this process vary from family to family and state to state, with some states allowing adoptees full access to records, some having mutual consent registries, and some allowing limited or no information to be obtained from sealed records. In the age of social media, adopted persons and birth family members are often able to find each other, circumventing formal supports or legal boundaries. This contact may be welcomed by and helpful to the adoptee, or it may cause significant upheaval. As in every other area of life, adoptive parents should monitor their child's social media use and be available for support and guidance if unexpected contacts occur.

Pediatric clinicians can help parents understand that the desire to search does not imply a rejection of the adoptive parents but rather a need for the adopted person to fully understand himself or herself. Some adoptees find and develop good relationships with their birth families, some find them but do not develop strong relationships, and others are never able to locate biological relatives. Clinicians need to support families as they negotiate all these possibilities.

Although most adoptive placements generate positive outcomes for both children and their families, not all adoptive placements achieve permanency for children or happy long-term outcomes. Although exact numbers are unclear because of variable state reporting systems, estimates indicate that between 10% and 25% of adoptive placements are disrupted (ended before the adoption is finalized), and 1% to 10% are dissolved (legally reversed, similar to a divorce, after the adoption was final).[64] Most commonly, this event happens with children who are older, with a complicated, traumatic history and complex behavioral and mental health needs, who were placed with families who were either unaware of these needs or inadequately prepared to meet them. Such occurrences are traumatic for everyone involved, especially the child, and are best avoided by full disclosure of information before the adoption and long-term, ongoing support for the family after the adoption is finalized. Families who are considering or pursuing a disruption or dissolution of their adoption should be referred to an experienced adoption professional.[17,58] These same stresses, combined with unrealistic expectations, can also leave children at risk for abuse or neglect in their adoptive homes, just as can occur in any other family. Pediatric clinicians should maintain the same surveillance for these possibilities as they would for any other child and family.

Conclusion

Caring for adopted children and their families can be among the most rewarding experiences of a pediatric clinician's career. By working closely with parents to address the special needs of their adopted children, clinicians can help ensure a bright future for children whose futures might otherwise have been bleak.

AAP Policy

American Academy of Pediatrics Council on Foster Care, Adoption, and Kinship Care; Committee on Adolescence; and Council on Early Childhood. Health care issues for children and adolescents in foster care and kinship care. *Pediatrics.* 2015;136(4):e1131–e1140 (pediatrics.aappublications.org/content/136/4/e1131)

Jones VF; American Academy of Pediatrics Committee on Early Childhood, Adoption, and Dependent Care. Comprehensive health evaluation of the newly adopted child. *Pediatrics*. 2012;129(1):e214–e223. Reaffirmed September 2015 (pediatrics. aappublications.org/content/129/1/e214)

Jones VF, Schulte EE; American Academy of Pediatrics Committee on Early Childhood and Council on Foster Care, Adoption, and Kinship Care. The pediatrician's role in supporting adoptive families. *Pediatrics*. 2012;130(4):e1040–e1049. Reaffirmed December 2016 (pediatrics.aappublications.org/content/130/4/e1040)

Rubin D, Springer SH, Zlotnik S, Kang-Yi CD; American Academy of Pediatrics Council on Foster Care, Adoption, and Kinship Care. Needs of kinship care families and pediatric practice. *Pediatrics*. 2017;139(4):e20170099 (pediatrics.aappublications. org/content/139/4/e20170099)

References

1. Intercounty Adoption. US Department of State Web site. https://travel.state.gov/content/travel/en/Intercountry-Adoption.html. Accessed January 24, 2018
2. Bureau of Consular Affairs, US Department of State. Intercountry adoption: adoption reference; adoption statistics. Travel.State.Gov Web site. https://travel.state.gov/content/adoptionsabroad/en/about-us/statistics.html. Accessed January 24, 2018
3. Child Welfare Information Gateway. *Foster Care Statistics 2015*. Washington, DC: Children's Bureau, US Dept of Health and Human Services; 2017. https://www.childwelfare.gov/pubs/factsheets/foster. Accessed January 24, 2018
4. Peterson V, Ames HW. The process of adoption in the United States. In: Mason PW, Johnson DE, Prock LA, eds. *Adoption Medicine: Caring for Children and Families*. Elk Grove Village, IL: American Academy of Pediatrics; 2014:25–43
5. Freundlich M. Legal considerations in adoption. In: Mason PW, Johnson DE, Prock LA, eds. *Adoption Medicine: Caring for Children and Families*. Elk Grove Village, IL: American Academy of Pediatrics; 2014:45–72
6. Bureau of Consular Affairs, US Department of State. Intercounty adoption: adoption process; understanding the Hague Convention. Travel.State.Gov Web site. https://travel.state.gov/content/adoptionsabroad/en/hague-convention/understanding-the-hague-convention.html. Updated March 23, 2017. Accessed January 24, 2018
7. Callahan NF, Johnson C. Intercountry adoption under the Hague Convention. In: Mason PW, Johnson DE, Prock LA, eds. *Adoption Medicine: Caring for Children and Families*. Elk Grove Village, IL: American Academy of Pediatrics; 2014:411–417
8. Bureau of Consular Affairs, US Department of State. Intercounty adoption: adoption process; acquiring U.S. citizenship for your child. Travel.State.Gov Web site. https://travel.state.gov/content/adoptionsabroad/en/us-visa-for-your-child/acquiring-us-citizenship-for-your-child.html. Accessed January 24, 2018
9. Domonoske C. South Korean adopted at age 3 is to be deported nearly 40 years later. *Two-Way: Breaking News From NPR*. October 27, 2016. http://www.npr.org/sections/thetwo-way/2016/10/27/499573378/south-korean-adopted-at-age-3-is-to-be-deported-37-years-later. Accessed January 24, 2018
10. Bahrampour T. They grew up as American citizens, then learned that they weren't. *Washington Post*. September 2, 2016. https://www.washingtonpost.com/local/social-issues/thousands-of-adoptees-thought-they-were-us-citizens-but-learned-they-are-not/2016/09/02/7924014c-6bc1-11e6-99bf-f0cf3a6449a6_story.html?utm_term=.c52330ea2eaf. Accessed January 24, 2018
11. Chambers J. Preadoption opportunities for pediatric providers. *Pediatr Clin North Am*. 2005;52(5):1247–1269

12. Miller LC. Pre-adoption counseling and evaluation of the referral. In: Miller LC, ed. *The Handbook of International Adoption Medicine: A Guide for Pediatricians, Parents, and Providers*. New York, NY: Oxford University Press; 2005

13. Lee PJ, Sagor LD. Pre-adoption considerations for pediatricians. In: Mason PW, Johnson DE, Prock LA, eds. *Adoption Medicine: Caring for Children and Families*. Elk Grove Village, IL: American Academy of Pediatrics; 2014:73–96

14. Steinberg G, Hall B. *Inside Transracial Adoption*. Indianapolis, IN: Perspectives Press; 2000

15. Division of Global Migration and Quarantine, National Center for Emerging and Zoonotic Infectious Diseases, Centers for Disease Control and Prevention. Travelers' Health Web site. https://wwwnc.cdc.gov/travel. Accessed January 24, 2018

16. Miller LC. Immediate behavioral and developmental considerations for internationally adopted children transitioning to families. *Pediatr Clin North Am*. 2005;52(5):1311–1330

17. Miller LC. After the adoption: unspoken problems. In: Miller LC, ed. *The Handbook of International Adoption Medicine: A Guide for Pediatricians, Parents, and Providers*. New York, NY: Oxford University Press; 2005

18. Fields ES, Meuchel JM, Jaffe CJ, Jha M, Payne JL. Post adoption depression. *Arch Womens Ment Health*. 2010;13(2):147–151

19. Miller LC. Immediate developmental and behavioral challenges post-adoption. In: Mason PW, Johnson DE, Prock LA, eds. *Adoption Medicine: Caring for Children and Families*. Elk Grove Village, IL: American Academy of Pediatrics; 2014:177–192

20. Schulte EE, Springer SH. Health care in the first year after international adoption. *Pediatr Clin North Am*. 2005;52(5):1331–1349

21. Miller LC. Attachment. In: Miller LC, ed. *The Handbook of International Adoption Medicine: A Guide for Pediatricians, Parents, and Providers*. New York, NY: Oxford University Press; 2005

22. Knauf L, Iverson S, Johnson D. International adoptees are at high risk for vision and hearing problems. Paper presented at: Pediatric Academic Societies Meeting; May 1–4, 2004; San Francisco, CA. Abstract 1382

23. Schulte EE, Springer SH. Post-adoptive evaluation for the health care professional. In: Mason PW, Johnson DE, Prock LA, eds. *Adoption Medicine: Caring for Children and Families*. Elk Grove Village, IL: American Academy of Pediatrics; 2014:163–175

24. Mason CN, Alvarado SB, Mason PW. Attachment and the adopted child. In: Mason PW, Johnson DE, Prock LA, eds. *Adoption Medicine: Caring for Children and Families*. Elk Grove Village, IL: American Academy of Pediatrics; 2014:257–281

25. Association for Treatment and Training in the Attachment of Children Web site. http://www.attach.org. Accessed January 24, 2018

26. Johnson DE, Dole K. International adoptions: implications for early intervention. *Infants Young Child*. 1999;11(4):34–45

27. Miller LC, Hendrie NW. Health of children adopted from China. *Pediatrics*. 2000;105(6):E76

28. Albers LH, Johnson DE, Hostetter MK, Iverson S, Miller LC. Health of children adopted from the former Soviet Union and Eastern Europe. Comparison with preadoptive medical records. *JAMA*. 1997;278(11):922–924

29. Miller LC. Developmental delay. In: Miller LC, ed. *The Handbook of International Adoption Medicine: A Guide for Pediatricians, Parents, and Providers*. New York, NY: Oxford University Press; 2005

30. Simms MD, Dubowitz H, Szilagyi MA. Health care needs of children in the foster care system. *Pediatrics*. 2000;106(4)(suppl):909–918

31. Jee SH, Szilagyi M, Ovenshire C, et al. Improved detection of developmental delays among young children in foster care. *Pediatrics*. 2010;125(2):282–289

32. Glennen SL. Predicting language outcomes for internationally adopted children. *J Speech Lang Hear Res*. 2007;50(2):529–548

33. Glennen S. New arrivals: speech and language assessment for internationally adopted infants and toddlers within the first months home. *Semin Speech Lang*. 2005;26(1):10–21

34. Glennen S. Speech and language outcomes after international adoption. In: Mason PW, Johnson DE, Prock LA, eds. *Adoption Medicine: Caring for Children and Families.* Elk Grove Village, IL: American Academy of Pediatrics; 2014:283–315

35. Weitzman C, Albers L. Long-term developmental, behavioral, and attachment outcomes after international adoption. *Pediatr Clin North Am.* 2005;52(5):1395–1419

36. Dole KN. Education and internationally adopted children: working collaboratively with schools. *Pediatr Clin North Am.* 2005;52(5):1445–1461

37. Prock LA. Working with schools: considerations for adopted children and their families. In: Mason PW, Johnson DE, Prock LA, eds. *Adoption Medicine: Caring for Children and Families.* Elk Grove Village, IL: American Academy of Pediatrics; 2014:355–365

38. Miller LC. Travel and transition to the adoptive family. In: Miller LC, ed. *The Handbook of International Adoption Medicine: A Guide for Pediatricians, Parents, and Providers.* New York, NY: Oxford University Press; 2005

39. Tirella LG, Chan W, Cermak SA, Litvinova A, Salas KC, Miller LC. Time use in Russian baby homes. *Child Care Health Dev.* 2008;34(1):77–86

40. Miller LC. Dysfunction of sensory integration. In: Miller LC, ed. *The Handbook of International Adoption Medicine: A Guide for Pediatricians, Parents, and Providers.* New York, NY: Oxford University Press; 2005

41. Costello E. Complementary and alternative therapies: considerations for families after international adoption. *Pediatr Clin North Am.* 2005;52(5):1463–1478

42. Miller LC. Uncertain age. In: Miller LC, ed. *The Handbook of International Adoption Medicine: A Guide for Pediatricians, Parents, and Providers.* New York, NY: Oxford University Press; 2005

43. Prock LA. Long-term developmental and behavioral issues following adoption. In: Mason PW, Johnson DE, Prock LA, eds. *Adoption Medicine: Caring for Children and Families.* Elk Grove Village, IL: American Academy of Pediatrics; 2014:217–237

44. Nalven L. Strategies for addressing long-term issues after institutionalization. *Pediatr Clin North Am.* 2005;52(2):1421–1444

45. Deye KP, Hymel KP. The long-term consequences of child maltreatment in adopted children. In: Mason PW, Johnson DE, Prock LA, eds. *Adoption Medicine: Caring for Children and Families.* Elk Grove Village, IL: American Academy of Pediatrics; 2014:193–216

46. Davies JK, Bledsoe JM. Prenatal alcohol and drug exposures in adoption. *Pediatr Clin North Am.* 2005;52(5):1369–1393

47. Miller LC. Fetal alcohol syndrome. In: Miller LC, ed. *The Handbook of International Adoption Medicine: A Guide for Physicians, Parents, and Providers.* New York, NY: Oxford University Press; 2005

48. Miller LC. Prenatal drug exposure. In: Miller LC, ed. *The Handbook of International Adoption Medicine: A Guide for Physicians, Parents, and Providers.* New York, NY: Oxford University Press; 2005

49. Coles CD. Prenatal substance exposure: alcohol and other substances—implications for adoption. In: Mason PW, Johnson DE, Prock LA, eds. *Adoption Medicine: Caring for Children and Families.* Elk Grove Village, IL: American Academy of Pediatrics; 2014:97–122

50. Miller LC. School issues. In: Miller LC, ed. *The Handbook of International Adoption Medicine: A Guide for Physicians, Parents, and Providers.* New York, NY: Oxford University Press; 2005

51. Meese RL. *Children of Intercountry Adoption in School: A Primer for Parents and Professionals.* Westport, CT: Bergin and Garvey; 2002

52. Nalven L. Identifying and accessing supports: strategies for addressing long-term issues in adopted children. In: Mason PW, Johnson DE, Prock LA, eds. *Adoption Medicine: Caring for Children and Families.* Elk Grove Village, IL: American Academy of Pediatrics; 2014:317–353

53. Teilmann G, Pedersen CB, Skakkebaek NE, Jensen TK. Increased risk of precocious puberty in internationally adopted children in Denmark. *Pediatrics.* 2006;118(2):e391–e399

54. Mason P, Narad C. Long-term growth and puberty concerns in international adoptees. *Pediatr Clin North Am.* 2005;52(5):1351–1368

55. Mason PW. Long-term growth and puberty concerns for adopted children. In: Mason PW, Johnson DE, Prock LA, eds. *Adoption Medicine: Caring for Children and Families.* Elk Grove Village, IL: American Academy of Pediatrics; 2014:239–256

56. Daniels SR, Greer FR; American Academy of Pediatrics Committee on Nutrition. Lipid screening and cardiovascular health in childhood. *Pediatrics.* 2008;122(1):198–208

57. Paveo JM. Working with adoptive families: what every professional should know. In: Mason PW, Johnson DE, Prock LA, eds. *Adoption Medicine: Caring for Children and Families.* Elk Grove Village, IL: American Academy of Pediatrics; 2014:395–410

58. Jenista JA. Special topics in international adoption. *Pediatr Clin North Am.* 2005;52(5):1479–1494

59. Cox SS, Lieberthal J. Intercountry adoption: young adult issues and transition to adulthood. *Pediatr Clin North Am.* 2005;52(5):1495–1506

60. Kang JE. International adoption: a personal perspective. *Pediatr Clin North Am.* 2005;52(5):1507–1515

61. American Academy of Pediatrics Committee on Psychosocial Aspects of Child and Family Health. Coparent or second-parent adoption by same-sex parents. *Pediatrics.* 2002;109(2):339–340

62. Pawelski JG, Perrin EC, Foy JM, et al. The effects of marriage, civil union, and domestic partnership laws on the health and well-being of children. *Pediatrics.* 2006;118(1):349–364

63. Riley D, Meeks J. *Beneath the Mask: Understanding Adopted Teens.* Silver Spring, MD: CASE Publications; 2005

64. Child Welfare Information Gateway. *Adoption Disruption and Dissolution: Numbers and Trends.* Washington, DC: Children's Bureau/Administration on Children, Youth, and Families, US Dept of Health and Human Services; 2012. https://www.childwelfare.gov/pubPDFs/s_disrup.pdf. Accessed January 24, 2018

Children in Poverty

Renée R. Jenkins, MD; Earnestine Willis, MD, MPH; and
Sheryl Allen, MD, MS

"Although children living in poverty and
low-income environments are at greater risk
than their peers for adverse health and
educational outcomes, a number of home,
clinic, school, community, and government
interventions have been shown to mitigate
these risks successfully."

Introduction

Poverty, a social determinant of health, is a major contributor to adverse
physical, developmental, social-emotional, and mental health outcomes. The
negative effects of poverty and low income on health are seen across all
populations; however, they disproportionately affect racial and ethnic
minority groups and children (defined in this chapter as people from birth
to age 18 years unless otherwise specified), resulting in significant racial and
ethnic health disparities (Figure 17-1).[1]

Defining Poverty and Low-Income Status

Family income, although not the only measure of poverty, is the measure
most commonly used in defining poverty in the United States. Poverty
guidelines are issued each year by the US Department of Health and
Human Services (HHS) for administrative use in determining family eligibility for certain federal and state-administered programs. The same
guidelines apply across the 48 contiguous states, with separate, slightly
higher guidelines for Hawaii and Alaska. Since 1963, when the poverty
thresholds were developed, 100% of the federal poverty threshold (FPT)
has been calculated by multiplying the cost of an economy food plan by

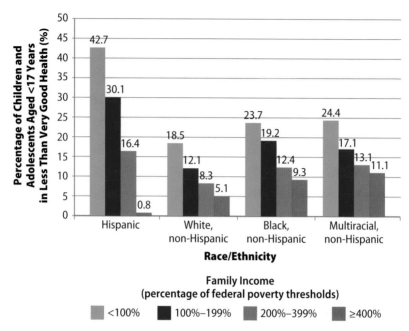

Figure 17-1. Across every racial and ethnic group, children's health varies according to family income.

Data compiled from 2011/12 National Survey of Children's Health. Child and Adolescent Health Measurement Initiative (CAHMI), "2011-2012 NSCH: Child Health Indicator and Subgroups SAS Codebook, Version 1.0" 2013, Data Resource Center for Child and Adolescent Health, sponsored by the Maternal and Child Health Bureau. www.childhealthdata.org. Accessed April 11, 2018.

3 and adjusting for family size; however, the food share used to develop these thresholds does not represent today's consumption pattern for either the general population or the poverty population.[2] Today, given the comparatively greater cost of housing and other basic needs, families are estimated to need an annual income of about twice the FPT to meet their basic requirements; hence, families living between 100% and 200% of the FPT are identified as low-income or near-poor families.[3] Other definitions follow suit: families who are extremely poor are those below 50% of the FPT, families who are poor are those between 50% and 100% of the FPT, low-income are families between 100% and 199% of the FPT, and nonpoor are families living at or above 200% of the FPT. Less stigmatizing language refers to lower-income families as *families living in poor and near-poor circumstances.*

Determination of poverty levels based only on annual household income suggests homogeneity of resources across families and denies the effects of other socioeconomic factors, such as total wealth (including all assets), investments and liabilities, occupational status, neighborhood conditions, and other socioeconomic measures. For racial and ethnic minority populations, discrimination, at the institutional or personal level, may interact with poverty in ways that increase negative effects. (See Chapter 25, Children Affected by Racism.) Child development experts generally support the opinion that multiple risk or protective factors (eg, economic resources, nutrition, education, social stimulation, home stability) affect health and social-emotional development and a person's subjective sense of well-being.[4] Table 17-1 summarizes children affected by poverty in the United States by age, race and ethnicity, living locations, and levels according to the US Census data estimation, 2015. To view current federal poverty guidelines, see https://aspe.hhs.gov/2017-poverty-guidelines.

The percentage of children in poor families is almost twice that of adults aged 18 to 64 years and 2.5 times that of seniors 65 years and older. Young children are more likely to be poor or live in low-income conditions, as are children from racial and ethnic minority populations, children of parents who did not complete high school, and children with unemployed

Table 17-1. Child and Adolescent Poverty Rates by Age, Race/Ethnicity, and Income Ranges, July 2015

Children and Adolescents	Total Population	<50% FPT (Extremely Poor) (%)	50%–99% FPT (Poor) (%)	100%–199% FPT (Low-Income) (%)	≥200% FPT (Nonpoor) (%)
Age					
<18 y	73,647	8.9	10.8	22.1	58.2
Birth–5 y	19,735	10.4	10.9	22.1	55.5
5–17 y	53,912	8.3	10.8	21.7	59.3
Race and Ethnicity					
All races	73,647	8.9	10.8	22.1	58.2
Asian	3,786	5.8	6.5	14.4	73.3
Black	11,087	15.8	17.1	27.6	39.4
Hispanic	18,231	11.5	17.4	31.9	39.2
White	37,859	5.8	6.3	16.9	71.1
Other	2,684	10.5	10.3	16.3	62.9

Abbreviation: FPT, federal poverty threshold.
Data compiled from US Census Bureau. 2011-2015 ACS 5-year estimates. US Census Bureau Web site. https://www.census.gov/programs-surveys/acs/technical-documentation/table-and-geography-changes/2015/5-year.html. Updated December 8, 2016. Accessed May 18, 2018.

or part-time working parents. Contrary to the traditional stereotypes, 72% of children with at least one parent who works part-time or part-year and 48% of children living with married parents are low-income children.[3]

Poverty and Place of Residence

Place of residence is also associated with poverty rates. Figure 17-2 demonstrates the rates of childhood poverty in metro vs nonmetro residential areas. Children in nonmetro areas have higher levels of poverty than children in metro areas do, across all age cohorts. Accordingly, parents in nonmetro areas are more likely than parents in metro areas to have less education and greater underemployment. In 2015, nonmetro children in female-headed households with no spouse present were estimated to have

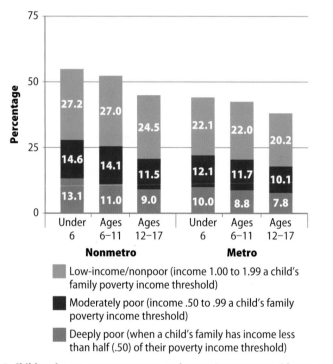

Figure 17-2. Children by age, poverty status, and metro/nonmetro residence, 2015.

Note: Children are defined as all persons under 18 years old. Nonmetro/metro status is based on 2013 Office of Management and Budget designations.

Source: USDA, Economic Research Service using data from U.S. Census Bureau, American Community Survey, 2015.

From Farrigan T. Children by age, poverty status, and metro/nonmetro residence, 2015. US Department of Agriculture Economic Research Service Web site. https://www.ers.usda.gov/data-products/chart-gallery/gallery/chart-detail/?chartId=82278. Updated March 2, 2017. Accessed January 24, 2018.

poverty rates of 52.5%, compared with 44.9% for metro children in similar families; rates of poverty for children with married parents were 12.3% for nonmetro children and 9.6% for metro children.[5]

Why Income Matters: Poverty and Child Health and Development

Based on an eco-bio-developmental framework, the multidisciplinary science of human development has shown that adult health conditions begin in early life, when brain structure is vulnerable to adverse environmental circumstances such as poverty and its associated stress, limited stimulation, and poor nutrition.[6] An analysis of poverty, overall health status, and activity limitation using the National Health Interview Status (NHIS) survey demonstrated, among children in poverty, a higher prevalence of chronic conditions, a higher incidence of low birth weight, and a lower percentage of mothers rating their children's health as excellent or very good. Measures of unmet mental health needs also disproportionately affected poor children. Low-income parents were almost twice as likely to identify their children as having difficulties with serious emotional and behavioral difficulties compared with families in more affluent families. Table 17-2 summarizes data from the NHIS demonstrating the adverse health effects of poverty on children in poor and low-income families from the perinatal period through adolescence. The negative effect on child health status occurred across the income gradients: the lower the income, the greater the effect.[7] Figure 17-3, also derived from NHIS data, summarizes rates of severe emotional or behavioral difficulties in children and adolescents aged 4 to 17 years by poverty status and sex.

Children in families that experience food hardship or housing insecurity are also more likely than other children to have health problems.[8] In 2000, food insecurity was present in 10.5% of households and reached a peak of 14.9% (17.9 million) by 2011. In 2015, the rate of households experiencing food insecurity trended downward to 12.7%.[9]

Studies have shown that neonates and infants of mothers with depression are at risk for multiple social-emotional developmental and medical problems, and disadvantaged mothers experience depression well beyond the postpartum period. If treated, the mother's symptoms improve, as does her perception of her child's behavior.[10] Furthermore, mothers of poor children were more likely to perceive their children as being progressively limited over time because of chronic conditions when compared with nonpoor children. This finding points to the potentially enhanced benefit of early intervention (EI) and intervention for poor children with chronic conditions.[11]

Table 17-2. Health Status of US Children According to Family Income Level

(%)	Sample Size (N)[a]	Below 100% FPL	100%– 199% FPL	200%– 299% FPL	300%– 399% FPL	400% FPL or Greater	Linear Trend[b]	Deviation From Linearity[b]
Physical Health								
Good/fair/poor health[c]	90,601	33.0	19.0	11.3	7.8	6.2	$P < .05$	$P < .05$
Activity limitations	90,491	9.3	6.8	4.8	4.1	3.3	$P < .05$	NS
Good/fair/poor teeth[d]	84,788	51.3	39.6	27.4	22.0	17.1	$P < .05$	$P < .05$
Overweight/obese	73,852	32.8	29.8	25.0	20.9	17.6	$P < .05$	NS
Diabetes	90,564	0.4	0.3	0.3	0.4	0.2	NS	—
Bone, joint, muscle problems	90,532	3.8	3.4	2.8	3.0	3.2	NS	—
Vision/hearing problems	79,796	4.0	2.9	2.6	2.2	2.3	$P < .05$	$P < .05$
Asthma	90,443	13.8	13.0	12.4	12.2	11.3	$P < .05$	NS
Moderate/severe asthma[e]	7,653	54.2	36.6	34.5	22.5	21.3	$P < .05$	$P < .05$
Severe headaches	75,512	8.1	6.0	4.9	5.2	4.3	$P < .05$	$P < .05$
Ear infections	75,502	7.5	5.4	4.8	3.9	3.5	$P < .05$	NS
Allergies								
Respiratory/hay fever	90,371	12.8	13.7	15.7	16.4	17.2	$P < .05$	NS
Digestive/food	90,477	3.5	3.2	3.6	3.7	3.9	$P < .05$	NS
Skin	90,492	9.1	9.8	9.4	9.6	11.1	$P < .05$	NS

Emotional, Developmental, Behavioral Health								
Problems with emotions, concentration, behavior	75,414	24.5	21.3	17.3	14.2	13.2	$P<.05$	NS
Learning disabilities	75,426	14.8	11.0	9.4	7.4	6.8	$P<.05$	$P<.05$
Autism	90,530	0.5	0.4	0.4	0.6	0.5	NS	—
ADHD	79,620	8.2	7.0	7.3	5.9	6.4	$P<.05$	$P<.05$
Behavior/conduct problems	79,823	9.6	6.2	4.5	3.6	2.8	$P<.05$	$P<.05$
Depression/anxiety	79,777	5.8	4.3	3.9	3.8	3.4	$P<.05$	NS
Speech problems	75,545	5.8	3.8	3.3	2.9	2.5	$P<.05$	NS

Abbreviations: ADHD, attention-deficit/hyperactivity disorder; FPT, federal poverty threshold; NS, not significant.

Note: Children are defined as all persons under 18 years old. Nonmetro/metro status is based on 2013 Office of Management and Budget designations.

Source: USDA, Economic Research Service using data from U.S. Census Bureau, American Community Survey, 2015.

[a] The sample size (N) is limited to only those individuals with no missing data on the covariates for the logistic regression models. The age range of the sample is 0 to 17 years, although some questions were not relevant and not asked of infants or very young children. There is variability in sample size across all outcomes due to differences in age and missing data on the outcome variables.

[b] Results from linear polynomial statistical test. A significant linear component indicates a trend of increasing (or decreasing) health across categories of family income. A significant deviation from linearity (quadratic/cubic trend) indicates that the change is not constant across all five given categories of family income (e.g., gradient may be steeper at lower end of income distribution).

[c] Good/fair/poor health vs excellent/very good.

[d] Good/fair/poor teeth vs excellent/very good.

[e] Only among those with asthma.

From Larson K, Halfon N. Family income gradients in the health and health care access of US children. *Matern Child Health J.* 2010;14(3):332–342. Distributed under a Creative Commons License. https://www.ncbi.nlm.nih.gov/pmc/articles/PMC2862175/. Accessed June 1, 2018.

Promoting Mental Health in Children and Adolescents: Primary Care Practice and Advocacy

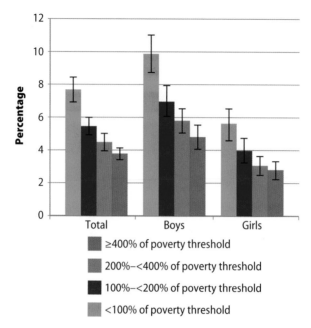

Figure 17-3. QuickStats: Percentage[a] of children and adolescents aged 4-17 years with serious emotional or behavioral difficulties,[b] by poverty status[c] and sex—National Health Interview Survey, 2011–2014.[d]

[a] With 95% confidence intervals indicated with error bars.

[b] Emotional or behavioral difficulties of children were based on parents' responses to the following question: "Overall, do you think that (child) has any difficulties in one or more of the following areas: emotions, concentration, behavior, or being able to get along with other people?" Response options were 1) "no"; 2) "yes, minor difficulties"; 3) "yes, definite difficulties"; and 4) "yes, severe difficulties." Children whose parents responded "yes, definite difficulties" or "yes, severe difficulties" were defined as having serious emotional or behavioral difficulties. These difficulties may be similar to but do not equate with the federal definition of serious emotional disturbance.

[c] Poverty status is based on family income and family size using the annually updated U.S. Census Bureau poverty thresholds. Family income was imputed when missing.

[d] Estimates are based on household interviews of a sample of the civilian noninstitutionalized U.S. population and are derived from the National Health Interview Survey's Sample Child component.

From QuickStats: percentage of children and adolescents aged 4-17 years with serious emotional or behavioral difficulties, by poverty status and sex—National Health Interview Survey, 2011–2014. *MMWR Morb Mortal Wkly Rep.* 2015;64(46):1303.

Morris and colleagues proposed a conceptual framework to explain the vulnerability of child health and social-emotional development in poor and low-income families.[8] They cited 2 mechanisms: the effect of family stress and parenting practices and the inability to invest in material (eg, food, housing) and nonmonetary (eg, time) resources. The family stress model proposes that instability of income raises parental stressors (eg, hardships such as utility shutoffs, missed rent or mortgage payments, unstable housing with high risk of evictions, no primary care physician, and inconsistent child care arrangements) and results in a more punitive and inconsistent style of parenting. The inadequate resource model aligns with findings of poorer educational outcomes for children experiencing limited cognitive stimulation in their home environments, insufficient nutritional foods, less active parental engagement, and unavailability of books.

Children living in poverty and low-income environments are not homogenous in their resources, either personally or materially. Family structure and dynamics, resilience, gender roles and expectations, education, duration and depth of poverty, and access to health insurance and health care are among the factors associating poverty with health status.[3,7,11–13]

Mitigating Poverty's Effects

Resilience

Resilience is defined as "exhibiting a better-than-expected outcome in the face of adversity." The concept of resilience is useful in explaining variations among health and educational outcomes of children in low-income families.[14,15] Positive interactions between a child's biology and environment, particularly her relational environment, contribute to healthy development by building the child's resilience (ie, her ability to cope with stress and overcome adversity). Conversely, prolonged periods of toxic stress exposure without a supportive relational environment put the child at risk for negative developmental outcomes. (See Chapter 13, Children Exposed to Adverse Childhood Experiences.) Poverty creates chronic stress for families. In fact, poverty is strongly associated with lower educational attainment, more frequent traumatic and stressful life events, and higher prevalence of learning disabilities, social-emotional problems, and behavioral and mental disorders in children.[16,17]

Families living in poverty are described as resilient when their beliefs about the social world or the spiritual world or both nourish them, when they know how to take steps to control their destinies, and when they are good at seeking, receiving, and giving support and building interconnectedness. Examples of resilience in surveys show that low-income parents who rate their children as having excellent health are more likely to maintain more structured home environments around meals, follow safety practices, and practice routine dental hygiene.[18–21] Family resiliency is fostered through protective factors: individual factors (eg, belief systems, effective coping skills), family factors (eg, family cohesion, supportive parent-child interactions), and community factors (eg, adequate housing, access to *quality* child care and school setting).[22] Foundational factors that positively affect child development and promote resilience in response to adversity are providing supportive adult-child relationships, building a sense of self-efficacy and perceived control, providing opportunities to strengthen adaptive skills and self-regulatory capacities, and mobilizing sources of faith, hope, and cultural traditions.[23]

Family and Parenting Supports

Health Insurance

Fortunately, most poor and low-income children are covered by publicly funded health insurance (Medicaid or their state's Children Health Insurance Program [CHIP]); however, gaps persist between the numbers of children eligible and those enrolled. Noncitizen children residing in the United States are less likely to be insured than children who are citizens.[24]

Children with public health insurance are more likely than uninsured children to receive preventive health care in the primary care setting, and they have rates for child health supervision visits similar to those of children with private insurance.[25] Uninsured children are 6 times more likely to have unmet medical needs and twice as likely to have unmet dental needs than are children covered by Medicaid or CHIP.[26] Being insured provides significant opportunity for children to have positive health outcomes.

Food Supplemental Programs

Food supplemental programs, such as the Special Supplemental Nutrition Program for Women, Infants, and Children (WIC) (described later in this chapter), have been shown to reduce rates of low birth weight[27] and iron deficiency.[28]

Although there is a decline in iron-deficiency prevalence among 1-year-old, black, and poor children, overall iron-deficiency prevalence in US toddlers has persisted over the past 3 decades, and, despite the decline, it remains disproportionately elevated in certain high-risk populations: being higher among children living below the poverty threshold and certain racial and ethnic groups such as Hispanic toddlers, 1 to 3 years of age, and recently immigrated Asian children. Other risk factors include overweight toddlers, low birth weight infants, and preterm infants.

Child Support

Child support enforcement occurs at the state level and involves the collection of court-ordered child support payments. More than 60% of child support collected each year occurs by the court-ordered direct withholding of money from the noncustodial parent. If child support monies are not collected from the noncustodial parent, serious penalties can occur, including the retention of federal and state tax refunds, liens on property, freezing of bank accounts, and suspension of driver, occupational, or operation license.[29]

Home Visitation

Home visiting programs, although variable in content and outcome measures, have shown accumulating evidence that mothers with the fewest resources (ie, low-income) often benefit most from the services. Home visiting has been shown to reduce rates of childhood injury, to reduce family welfare dependency, and to improve school readiness in at-risk families.[30]

Housing Subsidies

Understanding of housing conditions, quality, affordability, and choice is essential, as poverty is a major factor that contributes to the homelessness epidemic in America. Increasingly, the federal government relies on portable housing subsidies, which provide lower-income households with vouchers to make housing more affordable in higher-quality neighborhoods. These housing subsidies have resulted in improved neighborhood safety and reduced exposure to violence, most successfully in black households, with limited effectiveness in Hispanic and white households.[31] Housing assistance programs are administered by the US Department of Housing and Urban Development (HUD). The largest program is the Housing Choice Voucher program, commonly referred to as *Section 8* or *Tenant-Based Rental Assistance,* which is operated by local public housing agencies (PHAs). Voucher amounts are based on a standard rental rate in localities of PHAs and adjusted to limit a family's rental expense to 30% of their monthly income. To qualify, a tenant must have an income below 50% of the median income for the county or metropolitan area in which the tenant resides. According to the American Housing Survey of 2013, two-thirds of people who live in poor circumstances do not benefit from federal housing programs, and long waiting periods are common.[32] The numbers of units a local housing authority can subsidize under its Section 8 programs is determined by Congressional annual funding appropriations. HUD and PHAs also manage the Project-Based Rental Assistance Program, through which apartment owners can acquire subsidies for low-income tenants. Each program has its own regulations, qualifications, and benefit structure, adapted to local conditions and policies. HUD also administers block-grant funds such as the Community Planning and Development Program for unique community development needs such as homeless shelters, returning citizens programs, and other community development purposes.

Quality Preschool

Early childhood interventions, such as Head Start and Early Head Start, that address health and educational needs comprehensively have demonstrated positive health and behavioral outcomes. Head Start's mission acknowledges the influence of positive health care practices on multiple aspects of a child's early social-emotional development. Healthy preschoolers from low-income families served by Head Start have shown consistently to improve vocabulary, early writing, and early mathematics scores.[33] Parents of children in Head Start are more likely to report having health insurance and regular dental care visits for their children. Reductions in mortality among children aged 5 to 9 years have been reported in examined long-term effects of Head Start since its introduction in the 1960s.[11]

Clinical Care of the Poor and Low-Income Child

Expanded Social History

The traditional social history obtained in the primary care office is not structured to assess basic needs of poor and low-income families. For these families, the history should include more detailed information and encompass actual contributors to poor health, such as risk for hunger and substandard housing. Other social history probes that can augment assessment of a family's social-economic status include identification of social stressors and support networks, recent change in physical environment, health threats, the ability to control events in one's life, and literacy development. It is important to recognize a child and family's assets, along with income-related risk factors, as part of the assessment.

Five tools are described on the American Academy of Pediatrics (AAP) Poverty and Child Health Web site (www.aap.org/poverty) under Practice Tips. The first tool, the Hunger Vital Sign, is a validated 2-question tool that assesses food insecurity. Parents are asked whether either or both of the following 2 statements are "often true" or "sometimes true" vs "never true": "Within the past 12 months we worried whether our food would run out before we got money to buy more" and "Within the past 12 months the food we bought just didn't last and we didn't have money to get more." An answer of "often true" or "sometimes true" identifies a family at risk for food insecurity. See Appendix 2 for more information about this and other useful tools.

Clinicians can also use a tool like the IHELLP mnemonic described in Table 17-3 to assess whether the family's basic needs are being met.

Health Promotion

Low-income children are at greater risk than their peers for overall poor health and conditions such as overweight or obesity, asthma, vision and hearing problems, severe headaches, and ear infections (see Table 17-2). In day-to-day practice, pediatric primary care clinicians (PCCs) (ie, pediatricians, family physicians, internists, nurse practitioners, and physician assistants who provide frontline pediatric care) can promote optimal nutrition,

Table 17-3. Examples of Potential Social History Questions (Using the "IHELLP" Mnemonic) to Address Basic Needs

Domain/Area	Examples of Questions
Income	
General	Do you ever have trouble making ends meet?
Food income	Do you ever have a time when you don't have enough food? Do you have WIC? Food stamps?
Housing	
Housing	Is your housing ever a problem for you?
Utilities	Do you ever have trouble paying your electric/heat/telephone bill?
Education	
Appropriate education placement	How is your child doing in school? Is he/she getting the help to learn what he/she needs?
Early childhood program	Is your child in Head Start, preschool, or other early childhood enrichment?
Legal Status	
Immigration	Do you have questions about immigration status? Do you need help accessing benefits or services for your family?
Literacy	
Child literacy	Do you read to your child every night?
Parent literacy	How happy are you with how you read?
Personal Safety	
Domestic violence	Have you ever taken out a restraining order? Do you feel safe in your relationship?
General safety	Do you feel safe in your home? In your neighborhood?

Abbreviation: WIC, Special Supplemental Nutrition Program for Women, Infants, and Children.
From Kenyon C, Sandel SM, Silverstein M, Shakir A, Zuckerman B. Revisiting the social history of child health. *Pediatrics.* 2007;120(3):e734–e738.

growth, and physical and social-emotional development as part of health supervision, including provision of immunizations and anticipatory guidance. When psychosocial assessment reveals health-promoting behaviors in the child and family, PCCs can provide positive feedback and encouragement to continue and expand the practices. Guidance regarding developmental and behavioral concerns can be aimed at enhancing parents' nurturing relationships with their children. Chapter 1, Healthy Child Development, describes a process for integrating this guidance into primary care practice.

There are many examples of health promotional programs that can be offered to low-income families. Reach Out and Read is an evidence-based program that stimulates early brain development by promoting early literacy. This program emphasizes the 5 Rs of early language skill development: **reading** together as a daily family activity; **rhyming,** playing, and cuddling together often; **routines** and regular times for meals, play, and sleeping, which help children know what they can expect and what is expected from them; **reward** with praise for everyday successes; and **reciprocal and nurturing relationships,** which are foundational actions through which parents and caregivers can foster healthy child development.[34] Evidence-based parenting programs such as the Triple P – Positive Parenting Program, home visiting programs, and Nurturing Parenting Programs have been shown to provide numerous benefits, including prevention of child maltreatment.

Risk Assessment and Screening

Bright Futures: Guidelines for Health Supervision of Infants, Children, and Adolescents, 4th Edition, and the AAP recommend that low-income children with environmental risk, including limited access to food, should undergo a risk assessment for anemia at the 15- and 18-month visits; at the 2- and 2½-year visits; and at annual visits thereafter, in addition to an initial universal screening at 12 months of age and periodic screening of adolescent girls. *Bright Futures,* 4th Edition, recommends universal blood lead screening at the 12-month visit, with consideration of a repeat screening at 2 years of age; the AAP recommends that children exposed to old housing and children in communities with identified lead exposure receive additional lead screening between 12 months and 2 years of age. *Bright Futures,* 4th Edition, recommends that immigrant children born in high-risk countries be screened for tuberculosis[35] and that PCCs follow guidelines for dyslipidemia screening of children who are overweight living in low-income circumstances.

Research on children living in poverty has determined that poverty has a profound impact on early childhood development, resulting in poorer cognitive outcomes and school performance. Primary care clinicians can improve identification of children with developmental delays by integrating regular, systematic, developmental screening and surveillance into their practice settings. See Appendix 2 for a description of tools to assist. Children identified as having developmental delays and children at risk for delays can be referred to community-based services, such as the EI program, quality child care, home visiting programs, Head Start and Early Head Start, and special education programs available through public schools.[36]

Referral to Safety Net Programs

Safety net programs offer low-income families opportunities to become more economically stable. Primary care clinicians need to become knowledgeable about the basics of such programs specific to their respective communities of practice, to advocate for them and to consider them as a resource for low-income and poor families in their care. Safety net programs may be sponsored by nonprofit or faith-based organizations or local, state, or federal government. Several federally funded programs (Temporary Assistance for Needy Families [TANF], Earned Income Tax Credit [EITC], child support, child care subsidies, WIC, National School Nutrition Programs, and Supplemental Nutrition Assistance Program [SNAP] [Food Stamps]) are discussed in the following text.

Not detailed in this chapter are several other safety net programs beneficial to economically disadvantaged populations. Primary care clinicians should familiarize themselves with those programs, which include Supplemental Security Income, Social Security Disability Insurance, and Unemployment Insurance. Many low-income families depend on the National School Lunch Program and the School Breakfast Program to provide food for their school-aged children; these programs provide free and reduced-priced, nutritionally balanced meals to eligible children living below 130% and below 185% of the FPT, respectively, so children can meet their daily food requirements.

An appropriate response to identified socioeconomic stressors is to offer potential problem-solving strategies, pose further questions for clarification, and offer referral to one or more of the safety net programs described in the following text or to the mental health services listed in Appendix 3 or to both. Primary care clinicians can monitor children's participation and progress as a result of these referrals.[34] When making these referrals, PCCs can apply "common factors" communication techniques to identify and address barriers to family participation. See Chapter 2, Family-Centered Care: Applying Behavior Change Science, for more information about this approach.

Temporary Assistance for Needy Families

In 1996, welfare reform legislation replaced the existing welfare programs (Aid to Families with Dependent Children, Job Opportunities and Basic Skills Training, and Emergency Assistance) with TANF. The Personal Responsibility and Work Opportunity Reconciliation Act released the federal government from responsibility to provide direct financial support based on entitlement and instead provided funds for administration of public assistance at the state level. To receive TANF, adults with dependent children must pursue job opportunities and training. After the benefits begin, the adult has up to 60 months of support, which can be terminated if the state determines the individual is capable of obtaining an entry-level position. Of the 12 million people who receive TANF, most are single mothers.[37,38]

Earned Income Tax Credit

The EITC is a refundable income tax credit for low- to moderate-income working individuals and families, usually for those whose annual income is between $35,000 and $48,000. The structure of the federal EITC program and the 24 state-level EITCs allow families to receive money back, on the basis of income, marital status, and number of children. To qualify, an individual must meet certain requirements and file a tax return, even if he does not owe any taxes. Congress approved this tax credit legislation in 1975 with the goal of rewarding and encouraging working, in addition to helping families offset the burden of Social Security taxes. Many families use EITC refunds to pay for necessities, make repairs to homes or vehicles, or continue with higher education and training.[39]

Child Care Subsidy

The Child Care and Development Fund (CCDF) is the key resource through which the federal government funds child care subsidies to support work among low-income families. It is administered by the Administration for Children and Families (commonly known as ACF) in the HHS. Annually, each state has an allocation of funds for child care subsidies consisting of separate mandatory, matching, and discretionary funds. Child care subsidies provided through the CCDF and associated state funding assist nearly 1 million families and 1.6 million children in an average month.[40]

Supplemental Nutrition Assistance Program (Food Stamps)

The national SNAP, historically known as the Food Stamps program, provides more than 46 million poor and low-income Americans with a mechanism to acquire nutritionally adequate food. Since 2004, all states use an Electronic Benefits Transfer (debit card) for all food stamp benefits. Eligibility for food stamps is based on the following rules: (1) A household's gross monthly income must be at or below 130% of the FPL, and (2) household and vehicle assets must be below $2,000 to $3,250 (on the basis of different circumstances), consistent with TANF rules. There is some variability, however, in how states handle the vehicle assets: some exclude the entire value of vehicles, some count the value of vehicles, and some exclude the value of 1 vehicle per household. Each state designates the application process for food stamps, although most have a centralized location and most require able-bodied adults between 16 and 60 years of age to register for work, accept suitable employment, and take part in an employment and training program to receive the nutrition benefit.[41,42] Figure 17-4 illustrates the proportion of households with children receiving food stamps by working status from 1990 to 2013.[41]

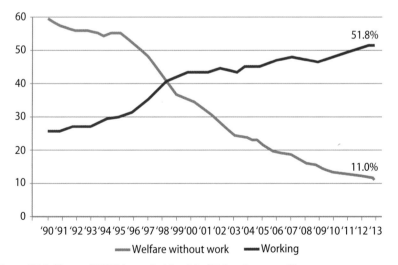

Figure 17-4. Share of SNAP households with children by type of income.

Abbreviation: SNAP, Supplemental Nutrition Assistance Program.

From Greenstein R. Testimony of Robert Greenstein, president, Center on Budget and Policy Priorities before the House Committee on Agriculture. Center on Budget and Policy Priorities Web site. https://www.cbpp.org/testimony-of-robert-greenstein-president-center-on-budget-and-policy-priorities-before-the-house. Published February 25, 2015. Accessed January 24, 2018. Reproduced with permission.

Special Supplemental Nutrition Program for Women, Infants, and Children

WIC is a federally funded program administered by the states for low-income pregnant women, breastfeeding mothers, neonates, infants and children up to the age of 5 years. Families receive monthly checks or vouchers redeemable for baby formula, infant cereal, iron-fortified adult cereal, milk, vitamin C–rich fresh fruit, fruit juices or vegetable juices or both, eggs, cheese, and certain other foods for their consumption. Soy-based beverages, tofu, baby foods, whole-wheat bread, and other whole-grain options were recently added to the program. A few state agencies distribute WIC foods through warehouses or deliver the food to participants' homes. In addition to making nutritious foods more accessible to families, WIC provides nutrition education, breastfeeding support, health and social service referral, and referrals for health care. The WIC eligible food list is available at www.federalregister.gov/documents/2014/03/04/2014-04105/special-supplemental-nutrition-program-for-women-infants-and-children-wic-revisions-in-the-wic-food. The nutritional foods supplied by WIC vouchers provide families with access to a balanced diet of specific items.

A study in 2008 found that families participating in WIC who had access to a weekly voucher for fresh foods from either a farmers' market or a supermarket were more likely to increase their daily intake of fruits and vegetables and maintain that increase.[43,44] Beginning in 2009, WIC participants began receiving vouchers for farmers' market and supermarket use, covering fresh, frozen, and canned fruits and vegetables (minus potatoes and foods provided by their respective state commodity supplement programs). WIC also covers many unprepared foods, whole grains, and brown rice, all of which are high in protein, calcium, iron, vitamin A, or vitamin C.[45] Additional foods are available for women who are breastfeeding, until their infant turns 12 months of age. If a woman chooses not to breastfeed, infant formula is included with WIC program vouchers, along with infant solid foods.[46]

The medical benefits of providing foods with strong nutritional value include higher birth weights, lower infant mortality rates, lower numbers of preterm births, and a higher rate of preventive health service use. Women enrolled in WIC tend to have healthier pregnancies and deliveries. These women deliver fewer preterm newborns than women not enrolled in WIC do.[47] In fact, these women generally tend to have babies of healthy birth weight.[48] Khanani and colleagues demonstrated that WIC participation significantly reduced the disparity in infant mortality rates between black infants and white infants compared with infants whose families were not participating in WIC.[49] In addition to food vouchers, the

WIC program provides some nutritionally at-risk women and children with social service referrals.

Cautionary Note: Limited Coordination of Safety Net Programs

Unfortunately, lack of coordination among safety net programs has limited their impact. For example, as wages increase to elevate a family's income, the family may lose benefits such as child care subsidy and have, effectively, less cash than before the wage increase. This fragmentation of safety net programs might be remedied by allowing families to phase out, rather than immediately lose, government-sponsored benefits such as EITC, child care, or food stamps as their income rises, preventing them from slipping back into poverty. To minimize the poverty burden on children and families, policy makers must examine the consequences of lack of coordination of programs that were originally designed to lift families out of poverty.

Public Policy Options for Child Advocates

Most low-income children have parents who work at low-wage jobs, bringing in insufficient income to pay for basic family expenses, with employment benefits that are inadequate and difficult to access. Limitations in social and political power result from low-income status. Primary care clinicians, who serve as frontline guardians of healthy child development, are strategically positioned as community leaders to build foundations for economic productivity, educational achievements, responsible citizenship, and lifelong health.[50]

Primary care clinicians and other child advocates can collaborate with policy makers to reframe social and health policies to support low-income families and promote the healthy growth and development of their children. Examples of such policy reframes might include a reduction or elimination of asset tests for major means-tested benefit programs. Many states have chosen to reduce or eliminate asset tests in work support programs as a means to assist recipients in achieving self-sufficiency. Other states, such as California, Colorado, and Illinois, have restructured their programs by increasing the amount of cash resources and exemptions allowed for certain forms of assets.[51]

Primary care clinicians have opportunities to affect their communities through AAP grant programs, educational resources, and federal and state advocacy strategies. Grants for projects that increase access to health care, preventive health care, and service coordination are just a few of the services funded through the CATCH (Coordinated Approach to Child Health) and Healthy Tomorrows programs. The AAP Council on Community Pediatrics is a source of ongoing direction to PCCs about poverty and child health. Box 17-1 summarizes public policy options that the 2016 AAP position statement recommends as opportunities to mitigate economic insecurity for children of low-income families.[52] Recommendations to enhance the care of children living in poverty are also outlined in the statement and include medical home resources, screening for social determinants of health, and referral to community services. Practice tips for incorporating interventions such as these are available at www.aap.org/poverty.

In addition, collaboration between PCCs and lawyers can ensure that the basic needs of families are met. A national model called "medical-legal partnerships" has emerged as an effective intervention to ensure that low-income families benefit from government-sponsored programs for which they are eligible. In this model, a lawyer on-site at a medical practice offers families assistance in advocating for legal and social services, especially those with outcomes that affect health status, such as housing and special education programs.[53]

Box 17-1. Public Policies to Mitigate Economic Insecurity

- Invest in young children and make healthy development of young children a national priority.
- Protect and expand funding for essential benefits program that assist children living in low-income and poor circumstances.
- Support 2-generation strategies that focus on helping children and parents simultaneously.
- Support and expand strategies that promote employment and increase parental income.
- Support policy measures that improve community infrastructure, including affordable housing and public spaces.
- Improve access to quality health care and create incentive to improve population health.
- Enhance health care financing to support comprehensive care for at-risk families.
- Make a national commitment to fully fund nurse home visiting programs for low-income and poor children and quality early childhood education.
- Support integrated modes of care in the medical home that promote effective parenting and school readiness.
- Improve national poverty definitions and measures.
- Support a comprehensive research agenda to improve understanding of the effects of poverty on children.

Adapted from American Academy of Pediatrics Council on Community Pediatrics. Poverty and child health in the United States. *Pediatrics.* 2016;137(4):e20160339.

Summary

Although children living in poverty and low-income environments are at greater risk than their peers for adverse health and educational outcomes, a number of home, clinic, school, community, and government interventions have been shown to mitigate these risks successfully. Pediatric PCCs and other pediatric health care professionals have opportunities to nurture resilience in low-income children and families, identify and address the health problems they face, and connect them to community services and safety net programs that are likely to improve their health and educational outcomes. Pediatric health care professionals can also serve as advocates for enactment of public policies that support children in low-income environments. These roles build on an eco-bio-developmental framework to incorporate growing evidence of the impact of toxic stress on the developing brain, to inform a deeper understanding of the early life origins of both educational failure and adult disease, and to underscore the need for collaborative efforts to prevent the long-term consequences of early adversity[51]: "We need to find ways to look beyond what seems hopeless and to provide resources and support so that the hopes placed in us by poor children and their families are not futile but are fulfilled."[54]

AAP Policy

American Academy of Pediatrics Council on Community Pediatrics. Poverty and child health in the United States. *Pediatrics*. 2016;137(4):e20160339 (pediatrics. aappublications.org/content/137/4/e20160339)

American Academy of Pediatrics Council on Community Pediatrics and Committee on Native American Child Health. Health equity and children's rights. *Pediatrics*. 2010;125(4):838–849. Reaffirmed October 2013 (pediatrics.aappublications.org/content/125/4/838)

Milteer RM, Ginsburg KR; American Academy of Pediatrics Council on Communications and Media and Committee on Psychosocial Aspects of Child and Family Health. The importance of play in promoting healthy child development and maintaining strong parent-child bond: focus on children in poverty. *Pediatrics*. 2012; 129(1):e204–e213. Reaffirmed September 2015 (pediatrics.aappublications.org/content/129/1/e204)

Pascoe JM, Wood DL, Duffee JH, Kuo A; American Academy of Pediatrics Committee on Psychosocial Aspects of Child and Family Health and Council on Community Pediatrics. Mediators and adverse effects of child poverty in the United States. *Pediatrics*. 2016;137(4):e20160340 (pediatrics.aappublications.org/content/137/4/e20160340)

References

1. Braveman P, Barclay C. Health disparities beginning in childhood: a life-course perspective. *Pediatrics.* 2009;124(suppl 3):S163–S175

2. Office of the Assistant Secretary for Planning and Evaluation, US Department of Health and Human Services. US federal poverty guidelines used to determine financial eligibility for certain federal programs. ASPE Web site. https://aspe.hhs.gov/poverty-guidelines. Accessed January 24, 2018

3. Jiang Y, Ekono M, Skinner C. *Basic Facts About Low-Income Children: Children Under 18 Years, 2014.* New York, NY: National Center for Children in Poverty, Mailman School of Public Health, Columbia University; 2016

4. Grantham-McGregor S, Cheung YB, Cueto S, Glewwe P, Richter L, Strupp B; International Child Development Steering Group. Developmental potential in the first 5 years for children in developing countries. *Lancet.* 2007;369(9555):60–70

5. Bishaw A, Benson C. Poverty: 2015 and 2016. *Am Community Survey Briefs.* 2017:1–14

6. Hair NL, Hanson JL, Wolfe BL, Pollak SD. Association of child poverty, brain development, and academic achievement. *JAMA Pediatr.* 2015;169(9):822–829

7. Larson K, Halfon N. Family income gradients in the health and health care access of US children. *Matern Child Health J.* 2010;14(3):332–342

8. Morris P, Gennetian LA, Duncan GJ, Huston AC. How welfare policies affect child and adolescent school performance: investigating pathways of influence with experimental data. In: *Welfare Reform and Its Long-term Consequences for America's Poor.* New York, NY: Cambridge University Press; 2009:255–289

9. Coleman-Jensen A, Rabbitt MP, Gregory CA, Singh A. *Household Food Security in the United States in 2015.* Washington, DC: Economic Research Service, US Dept of Agriculture; 2016. ERR-215

10. O'Keefe L. Each year 400,000 infants are born to depressed mothers: how you can help. *AAP News.* 2010;31(11):29

11. Currie J, Lin W. Chipping away at health: more on the relationship between income and child health. *Health Aff (Millwood).* 2007;26(2):331–344

12. Gennetian LA, Castells N, Morris P. Meeting the basic needs of children: does income matter? *Child Youth Serv Rev.* 2010;32(9):1138–1148

13. Denburg A, Daneman D. The link between social inequality and child health outcomes. *Healthc Q.* 2010;14(1):21–31

14. McCubbin MA, McCubbin HI. Families coping with illness: the resiliency model of family stress, adjustment, and adaptation. In: Danielson CB, Hamel-Bissel B, Winstead-Fry P, eds. *Families, Health, and Illness: Perspectives on Coping and Intervention.* St Louis, MO: Mosby; 1989

15. Allen MT. *Traditional Parenting and Childrearing: Promoting Harmony and Beauty for Life.* Flagstaff, AZ: Navajo Parenting Workshop, Northern Arizona Museum; 1998

16. Carneiro PM, Heckman JJ. Human capital policy. In: Heckman JJ, Krueger AB, Friedman BM, eds. *Inequality in America: What Role for Human Capital Policies?* Cambridge, MA: MIT Press; 2003

17. Brooks-Gunn J, Duncan GJ. The effects of poverty on children. *Future Child.* 1997;7(2):55–71

18. Patterson J. The role of family means in adaptation to chronic illness and disability. In: Turnbull AP, Patterson JM, Behr SK, et al, eds. *Cognitive Coping Research and Developmental Disabilities.* Baltimore, MD: Paul H. Brookes Publishing Co Inc; 1933:221–238

19. Patterson J. A family stress model: the family adjustment and adaptation response. In: Ramsey C, ed. *The Science of Family Medicine.* New York, NY: Guilford Press; 1989:95–118

20. Patterson J. Families experiencing stress: I. The Family Adjustment and Adaptation Response Model; II. applying the FAAR Model to health-related issues for intervention and research. *Fam Syst Med.* 1988;6(2):202–237

21. Patterson JM. Understanding family resilience. *J Clin Psychol.* 2002;58(3):233–246

22. Benzies K, Mychasiuk R. Fostering family resiliency: a review of key protective factors. *Child Fam Soc Work.* 2009;14(1):103–114

23. Resilience. Center on the Developing Child at Harvard University Web site. https://developingchild.harvard.edu/science/key-concepts/resilience. Accessed January 24, 2018

24. Key facts on health coverage for low-income immigrants today and under the Affordable Care Act. The Henry J. Kaiser Family Foundation Web site. https://www.kff.org/uninsured/upload/8279-02.pdf. Published March 4, 2013. Accessed January 24, 2018

25. Federal advocacy. American Academy of Pediatrics Web site. https://www.aap.org/en-us/advocacy-and-policy/federal-advocacy/Pages/Poverty.aspx. Accessed January 24, 2018

26. Ku L, Lin M, Broaddus M. *Chartbook: Improving Children's Health—The Roles of Medicaid and SCHIP.* Washington, DC: Center on Budget and Policy Priorities; 2007. https://www.cbpp.org/sites/default/files/atoms/files/schip-chartbook-section3.pdf. Accessed January 24, 2018

27. Devaney B. *Very Low Birthweight Among Medicaid Newborns in Five States: The Effects of Prenatal WIC Participation.* Alexandria, VA: US Dept of Agriculture; 1992

28. Miller V, Swaney S, Deinard A. Impact of the WIC program on the iron status of infants. *Pediatrics.* 1985;75(1):100–105

29. Koball H, Douglas-Hall A. State policy choices. National Center for Children in Poverty Web site. http://www.nccp.org/publications/pub_539.html. Published September 2004. Accessed January 24, 2018

30. Kitzman HJ. Effective early childhood development programs for low-income families: home visiting interventions during pregnancy and early childhood. Encyclopedia on Early Childhood Development Web site. http://www.child-encyclopedia.com/documents/KitzmanANGxp-Low_income.pdf. Published 2004. Updated August 2007. Accessed January 24, 2018

31. Lens MC, Ellen IG, O'Regan K; Office of Policy Development and Research. *Neighborhood Crime Exposure Among Housing Choice Voucher Households.* Washington, DC: US Dept of Housing and Urban Development; 2011. https://www.huduser.gov/portal/publications/pdf/Lens_NeighborhoodCrime_AssistedHousingRCR08.pdf. Accessed January 24, 2018

32. Desmond M. Unaffordable America: poverty, housing, and eviction. *Fast Focus.* 2015;22:1–6

33. Office of Planning, Research and Evaluation; Administration for Children and Families. *"Friendly FACES" - FACES Findings: New Research on Head Start Outcomes and Program Quality.* Washington, DC: US Dept of Health and Human Services; 2006. http://www.acf.hhs.gov/programs/opre/hs/faces/#reports. Accessed January 24, 2018

34. High PC; American Academy of Pediatrics Committee on Early Childhood, Adoption, and Dependent Care and Council on School Health. School readiness. *Pediatrics.* 2008;121(4):e1008–e1015

35. Hagan JF Jr, Shaw JS, Duncan PM, eds. *Bright Futures: Guidelines for Health Supervision of Infants, Children, and Adolescents.* 4th ed. Elk Grove Village, IL: American Academy of Pediatrics; 2017

36. American Academy of Pediatrics Council on Children With Disabilities, Section on Developmental Behavioral Pediatrics, Bright Futures Steering Committee, and Medical Home Initiatives for Children With Special Needs Project Advisory Committee. Identifying infants and young children with developmental disorders in the medical home: an algorithm for developmental surveillance and screening. *Pediatrics.* 2006;118(1):405–420

37. Hildebrandt E, Stevens P. Impoverished women with children and no welfare benefits: the urgency of researching failures of the Temporary Assistance for Needy Families program. *Am J Public Health.* 2009;99(5):793–801

38. Hildebrandt E, Ford SL. Justice and impoverished women: the ethical implications of work-based welfare. *Policy Polit Nurs Pract.* 2009;10(4):295–302

39. Policy basics: the Earned Income Tax Credit. Center on Budget and Policy Priorities Web site. http://www.cbpp.org/cms/index.cfm?fa=view&id=2505. Updated October 21, 2016. Accessed January 24, 2018

40. *Child Care: Multiple Factors Could Have Contributed to the Recent Decline in the Number of Children Whose Families Receive Subsidies.* Washington, DC: US Government Accountability Office; 2010. GAO-10-344. http://www.gao.gov/products/GAO-10-344. Accessed January 24, 2018

41. Policy basics: introduction to the Supplemental Nutrition Assistance Program (SNAP). Center on Budget and Policy Priorities Web site. http://www.cbpp.org/cms/index. cfm?fa=view&id=2226. Updated October 3, 2017. Accessed January 24, 2018

42. Supplemental Nutrition Assistance Program (SNAP). US Department of Agriculture Food and Nutrition Service Web site. https://www.fns.usda.gov/snap. Updated January 30, 2017. Accessed January 24, 2018

43. WIC food packages - regulatory requirements for WIC-eligible foods. US Department of Agriculture Food and Nutrition Service Web site. https://www.fns.usda.gov/wic/wic-food-packages-regulatory-requirements-wic-eligible-foods. Updated January 24, 2018. Accessed January 24, 2018

44. Herman DR, Harrison GG, Afifi AA, Jenks E. Effect of a targeted subsidy on intake of fruits and vegetables among low-income women in the Special Supplemental Nutrition Program for Women, Infants, and Children. *Am J Public Health.* 2008;98(1):98–105

45. Committee to Review WIC Food Packages; Food and Nutrition Board; Health and Medicine Division; National Academies of Sciences, Engineering, and Medicine. Table 1-4, substitutions allowed by WIC state agencies, fiscal year 2015. In: *Review of WIC Food Packages: Improving Balance and Choice; Final Report.* Washington, DC: National Academies Press; 2017. https://www.ncbi.nlm.nih.gov/books/NBK435927/table/tab_1-4. Accessed January 24, 2018

46. Jacknowitz A, Novillo D, Tiehen L. Special Supplemental Nutrition Program for Women, Infants, and Children and infant feeding practices. *Pediatrics.* 2007;119(2):281–289

47. El-Bastawissi AY, Peters R, Sasseen K, Bell T, Manolopoulos R. Effect of the Washington Special Supplemental Nutrition Program for Women, Infants and Children (WIC) on pregnancy outcomes. *Matern Child Health J.* 2007;11(6):611–621

48. Kowaleski-Jones L, Duncan GJ. Effects of participation in the WIC program on birthweight: evidence from the National Longitudinal Survey of Youth. Special Supplemental Nutrition Program for Women, Infants, and Children. *Am J Public Health.* 2002;92(5):799–804

49. Khanani I, Elam J, Hearn R, Jones C, Maseru N. The impact of prenatal WIC participation on infant mortality and racial disparities. *Am J Public Health.* 2010;100(suppl 1):S204–S209

50. Garner AS; Shonkoff JP; American Academy of Pediatrics Committee on Psychosocial Aspects of Child and Family Health; Committee on Early Childhood, Adoption, and Dependent Care; and Section on Developmental and Behavioral Pediatrics. Early childhood adversity, toxic stress, and the role of the pediatrician: translating developmental science into lifelong health. *Pediatrics.* 2012;129(1):e224–e231

51. Vallas R, Valenti J. Asset limits are a barrier to economic security and mobility. Center for American Progress Web site. https://www.americanprogress.org/issues/poverty/reports/2014/09/10/96754/asset-limits-are-a-barrier-to-economic-security-and-mobility. Published September 10, 2014. Accessed January 24, 2018

52. American Academy of Pediatrics Council on Community Pediatrics. Poverty and child health in the United States. *Pediatrics.* 2016;137(4):e20160339

53. Kenney GM, Coyer C. National findings on access to health care and service use for children enrolled in Medicaid or CHIP. MACPAC Web site. https://www.macpac.gov/wp-content/uploads/2015/01/Contractor-Report-No_1.pdf. Published March 2012. Accessed January 24, 2018

54. Maholmes V. *Fostering Resilience and Well-being in Children and Families in Poverty: Why Hope Still Matters.* New York, NY: Oxford University Press; 2014

Children of Divorce

Rhonda Graves Acholonu, MD, and Lori Legano, MD

> "Divorce should never be viewed...as an isolated event but rather as a process that significantly affects both the parents and the children. Thoughtful and timely intervention coupled with practical guidance by primary care clinicians...can aid in the anticipation, prevention, and alleviation of many potential conflicts."

Approximately 1 million children experience divorce or separation of their parents in the United States each year.[1] In the early 1960s, almost 90% of children spent their childhood and adolescence with 2 biological parents. Now, that number has decreased to 69%.[2] For adults, divorce is second only to the death of a spouse or a parent in its intensity as a stressor and the length of time required to adjust to it.[3] Children's mental health and their ability to adjust after divorce has been a significant topic for debate over the years with 2 extreme positions: the notion that the long-term effects on their mental health and relationships are profoundly crippling vs the notion that the long-term effects are minimal. Moreover, some have noted that it is not the divorce itself that is damaging to children and their adjustment but rather the exposure to such high levels of conflict between the parents.[4]

Many researchers concur that divorce often produces anger and a sense of failure for parents; conflicted loyalties, guilt, grief, and anxiety for children and adolescents (collectively called *children* in this chapter); and concern on the part of all about whether the children will experience long-term harm. Most children of divorce experience, at the least, a potent transient stress. The Adverse Childhood Experiences Study revealed that 23.3% of participants had dealt with divorce, leading to impaired health in adulthood.[5] It should never be viewed, therefore, as an isolated event but rather as a process that significantly affects both the parents and the children.[6] Thoughtful and timely intervention coupled with practical guidance by primary care clinicians (PCCs) (ie, pediatricians, family physicians, internists, nurse practitioners, and physician assistants in longitudinal relationships with children and families) can aid in the anticipation, prevention, and alleviation of many potential conflicts.

Family Changes Precipitated by Divorce

In most cases, both parents are awarded joint legal custody, but the children's primary physical residence is with their mother in more than 80% of cases.[1] It should be noted that throughout this article, the parenting model referenced is primarily that of a mother and father, although the effects described could result from breakup of the relationship between any 2 co-parenting adults, regardless of gender identity, sexual orientation, or biological relationship to the child.[7]

Divorce often has devastating financial consequences for these children and their mothers. Children living in households headed by single mothers are more than 5 times as likely to live in poverty compared with children in households with married parents.[8] A significant number of divorced mothers have few financial and personal resources to direct toward the children, and many take on new employment arrangements. This circumstance may result in new child care arrangements for younger children, older children taking care of themselves or siblings for greater parts of the day, and curtailment of certain activities because of expense or parental time constraints.

For parents who do not reside with their children, who are most often fathers, problems range from what to do with children on visiting days to profound concern about the emotional consequences for their children. Bernet et al review the struggles experienced by children, which may range from loyalty conflicts to parental alienation, manifested as a child's refusal to maintain a good relationship with a parent.[5] Some parents have unrealistic expectations about the kind of relationship they will have with their children, while others believe divorce deprives them of the right to exercise authority and to discipline the children. Much public attention has focused on issues of failed child support, nonresidential fathers who do not visit, and the economic plight of single-parent households. The importance of the mental health of children affected by divorce and other relational stressors is now reflected in a new term in the fifth edition of the *Diagnostic and Statistical Manual of Mental Disorders* (commonly known as *DSM-5*), *child affected by parental relationship distress* (commonly known as CAPRD).[5,9]

Phases of Divorce

Families progress through different stages after divorce.[10] The period immediately before and after the separation is referred to as the *acute stage;* it is characterized by maximal turmoil and generally lasts up to 2 years. The family then moves into the *transitional stage,* which is characterized by more controlled changes. The final stage is the *postdivorce stage* (long-term adaptation stage), when major family restructuring ceases. The child's age and developmental stage and the parent's coping abilities are among the many factors affecting children's manifestations at each stage of the divorce process.

Acute

During the acute stage, all family members are confronted with disruptions of their expectations, relationships, and support systems. Parents may be depressed, may be preoccupied with personal concerns, and may exhibit diminished parenting abilities. During this stage, 2 events seem to be most stressful to most children: learning about the divorce and the actual departure of a parent. The first year after divorce is the year of maximal negative behavior by children and the poorest parenting by parents. The apparent intensity of a child's reaction to this stage, however, does not predict long-term adjustment. Initially, many parents make fewer demands on the children, communicate less effectively, are less affectionate, and have difficulty disciplining children. For some divorces, the troubled relationship between parents continues indefinitely. In these cases, children have the greatest incidence of postdivorce maladjustment.[1,11-15] This observation is consistent with the research finding that conflict surrounding the divorce is equally, if not more, detrimental than the divorce itself.

Transitional

The transitional stage is marked by new undertakings for the single-parent household and more stability than that of the acute stage. Children must accommodate to their parents' new relationship with each other, to new friends, and often to new romantic partners of one parent or both parents. During this stage, children are often concerned about the well-being of, and their relationship with, the nonresidential parent. Visitation patterns tend to have become more stable, whether they are acceptable to all parties or not. The major exception to the general pattern of increased stability is the family in which the parents are still actively in conflict, either informally with each other and the children or formally through the legal system.

Postdivorce (Long-term Adaptation)

In the postdivorce stage, relative stability is achieved via adaptation. The family may still be headed by one parent, or a stepparent may now be present. Remarriage does not convey automatic stability but rather requires new adjustments because of the reawakening of unresolved issues and new roles in the new family.

Effects of Divorce on Children's Adjustment

On average, small but detectable negative emotional, cognitive, social, and physical effects, both short-term and long-term, are found among children of divorce. Of course, these effects vary greatly and depend on many factors.

Initial Effects

Initial responses are greatly influenced by the developmental stage and age of the child, the child's temperament,[16] the level of parental conflict, and the emotional, cognitive, and economic support available to the child. Gender differences have been explored, and no consistent pattern has been found regarding adverse effects of divorce on boys vs girls.[4]

Newborns, infants, and toddlers have minimal to no comprehension that divorce has occurred and may not have a direct reaction to the divorce.[17] Preschoolers, aged 2 to 5 years, initially tend to display regressive behaviors that can be highly stressful for parents, such as sleep disturbances, tantrums, separation anxiety, loss of bowel and bladder control, and increased need for parental attention.[17] School-aged children, 5½ to 12 years of age, may experience sadness, grief, or intense anger at one parent or both parents. School performance and peer relationships may deteriorate, and phobias may emerge among both early and late school-aged children.[17] Children may demonstrate difficulty with reading comprehension both before and after the separation or divorce.[18]

Adolescents of divorcing parents find themselves without the expected home base from which to move away. This situation may result in insecurity, loneliness, decreased self-esteem,[19] and depression. These feelings may be overtly or covertly expressed in diminished school performance; school failure; truancy; violent and nonviolent criminal behavior; substance use, including earlier initiation of alcohol use[20]; eating disorders; or sexual promiscuity. Children of any age may exhibit psychosomatic symptoms as a reaction to the stressors placed on them by the divorce.[21]

Long-term Effects

Prior studies revealed long-lasting effects of parental divorce in some cases.[1,11-15] Adults who experienced divorce as children tend to score lower on a variety of indicators of psychological, interpersonal, and socio-economic well-being. Although most adults who experienced divorce as children seem to do well, as a group overall they have higher rates of depression, job changes, premarital pregnancies, and divorce. The degree of marital conflict before the divorce has been shown to be a stronger predictor of adjustment than the divorce itself or the conflicts after the divorce.[22]

A 25-year follow-up study confirmed that children of divorced parents are less likely to marry and when they do marry are more likely to divorce.[23] They are also less likely to enter and complete college.[16] The gap between children of divorced and married parents with respect to academic achievement, psychological well-being, self-concept, and social relations was small in both the 1980s and the 1990s, although a trend for a wider gap began in the 1990s.[24] The differences in outcomes between children of married parents and children of divorced parents may be influenced by ethnicity, with smaller differences seen in black families than in European American families.[25] The long-term negative effects of divorce are mitigated by a variety of social factors: support of parents[26] and grandparents,[27] social support in adulthood,[26] educational attainment by the child[26] and mother,[28] and socioeconomic status of the family.[28]

Not all effects of divorce are negative, however. Children from divorced families demonstrate less stereotyped sexual behavior, greater maturity, and greater independence.[29]

Tasks for the Children and Parents of Divorce

Children of divorce have several specific tasks on which they work simultaneously and with varying degrees of success.[30] Because divorce is a process and not a discrete event, it is important for parents to recognize that these tasks greatly depend on the child's development and age and may therefore change throughout the course. Mastery of these tasks is facilitated by support and cooperation of both parents. Parents can better help children cope with divorce if they are aware of the child's developmental age and respond to the child accordingly.

Understanding the Meaning of Divorce and Custody

Toddlers and preschoolers may have a difficult time understanding the meaning of divorce. Because these children view their worlds very concretely, they may not be able to comprehend the changes in relationships and the alterations within their households. Confusion about the actual meaning of divorce is the rule rather than the exception.[31] Parents should provide simple explanations about the meaning of divorce and custody and should never avoid the subject. Parents should maintain routines so that the child does not equate divorce with instability or loss of normalcy.

Accepting the Permanency of Divorce

The task of acceptance requires the child to accept the reality of the divorce despite tendencies to deny the dissolution of the family and fears of abandonment. The stigmatization of divorce may also play a role in the child's adjustment, although some data have shown these effects to be decreasing over time.[4] These tendencies and fears may persist, leading to repeated efforts by children to persuade their parents to reconcile, even after one or more has remarried. Young school-aged children fantasize about being able to reunite their parents. Parents need to recognize that their children have these fantasies and that they will try to get them to interact with each other in any way and as often as possible. Older children and adolescents who have lived in persistent high-conflict or violent marriages, however, are more likely to be relieved about parental separation and are less likely to wish for parental reunion.[32]

Regaining and Maintaining a Sense of Normalcy

Immediately after divorce, many children experience emotional and behavioral difficulties, and many seem to lose interest in school, friends, and leisure-time activities. Approximately one-third of adolescents, particularly boys, in divorced and remarried families separate from the family unit, spend little time at home, and avoid interactions with family members.[4] Generally, the return to more typical activities for the child takes approximately 1 year. If this transition has not occurred within this period, referral of the child or family for psychotherapy may be indicated. During this time, parents must maintain discipline and avoid allowing their own emotions surrounding the divorce to cloud their judgment and authority. If a child is having a particularly difficult time adjusting in one home, parents may then consider a trial of living with the noncustodial parent. Children who are better adjusted before the marital breakup, those who are not enmeshed in a prolonged battle between the parents, and those who are supported in their efforts to understand their feelings are better able to accomplish this task.

Dealing With Painful Feelings

Departure of a parent through divorce is experienced by some children as a major assault on the child's self-esteem and sense of security. Because of preschoolers' egocentric thinking, they may believe that they are responsible for the divorce, must therefore be bad, and consequently are at risk for further abandonment by the other parent. Older children, appreciating that the departing parent is exercising a choice to leave, often feel anger as well as other negative aspects of grief. These feelings result in a complex interplay of negative emotions and their consequences. Parents should explain the situation to their children in simple, age-appropriate language and assure them that they are not the cause of the divorce. Despite parents' best efforts, however, long-term follow-up studies indicate that divorce may leave children feeling that they were the cause of their parents' conflicts, may pose a risk to future parent-child relationships, and may impair their responses to psychological interventions.[30]

Not Choosing Sides

Children, especially school-aged children, may see divorce as posing a problem of conflicting loyalties. Divided loyalties are more likely to occur in situations of high, persistent parental conflict.[5] Parents must consistently reassure children that they are equally loved by both of them and that divorce is not going to change these feelings. Parents should refrain from pressuring their children to support one parent's side over another and should also avoid both buying excessive gifts to prove their affection and using the child as message bearer to the other parent.

Remaining a Child

Divorce leads to many changes, but one of the most obvious is the physical absence of one parent in the home. Older adolescents often feel responsible for the happiness of their parents and the well-being of their younger siblings. They may make attempts to comfort and console their parents. Parents should avoid treating their children as adults, and children should be reassured that they do not need to take on adult roles.[33] Children's lives will undergo enough changes without also relinquishing their childhood.

Forgiving the Parents

Forgiving the parents is often a task for older children. Adolescents often struggle with chaos in their own lives and are often angered by having to deal with their parents' lives. Forgiving their parents therefore requires their ability to appreciate the parents' need to separate as being more important than any reason to stay together, including the desires of the children. Children must then overcome grief over the loss of the intact family as well as the anger and resentment generated by the resulting changes in their lives. Some children may refuse to have a relationship with one parent without a plausible explanation. This parental alienation is usually observed in cases of high-conflict relationships.[5] Parents should be flexible and understanding of the adolescent's need for space as well as available for comfort and maintenance of discipline.

Resolving Issues of Relationship

As Judith Wallerstein has observed, divorce often leaves children fearful and unable "to reach, sustain, and support the personal vision that love, mutual understanding, and constancy are expectable components of human relationships. Perhaps the major developmental task posed by divorce is this: to achieve realistic hope regarding future relationships and the enduring ability to love and be loved."[3] "At young adulthood, when love, sexual intimacy, commitment and marriage take center stage, children of divorce are haunted by the ghosts of their parents' divorce and are frightened that the same fate awaits them."[23] This task is difficult for a significant number of adults who experienced divorce as children. As children get older, parents should discuss the reasons for the divorce so that the young person learns to view the divorce "not as inevitable but as a result of avoidable human error."[33]

Custody

If the noncustodial or nonresidential parent has not abandoned the family and wants to remain involved with the children, the custodial or residential parent must not attempt to sabotage this relationship. Shared parenting has been linked to better outcomes in emotional, behavioral, and physical health for children of all ages.[34] Shared parenting conducted with cooperation and agreement has been significantly associated with children's overall mental health, self-esteem, and academic performance.[7]

Remarriage and Stepfamilies

Within 4 years, 50% of divorced adults remarry, and one-third of American children will eventually become members of a stepfamily. More than 80% of these stepfamilies are composed of a biological mother and a stepfather.[4] In many cases, remarriage restores a secure, 2-parent environment, and it may provide children with a model of a loving, caring adult relationship. Despite the wicked stepmother figure portrayed in fairy tales, most stepchildren like their stepparents and report that they get along with them well. Most studies have shown that stepchildren do not appear to differ from other children in personality characteristics or in cognitive or intellectual accomplishments.[35]

Remarriage, however, has the potential of creating new tensions and stresses for both the parent and the child. When one parent remarries, the other may fear that the children will abandon them for the new stepparent. Lutz's interviews of preadolescents, adolescents, and young adults between 12 and 18 years of age living in stepfamilies revealed that the areas causing the most difficulty are those of divided loyalty and adjusting to and accepting discipline from stepparents. Many children may feel conflicted about loving their stepparent and may even see it as a source of betrayal of their biological parent. In addition, many children may continue to wish for parental reunion. Regarding discipline, stepparents are often unsure of their roles and may feel awkward in these situations. Discussing these issues with the custodial biological parent and conforming to that parent's approaches is important for stepparents.[36]

Adults can help children adapt to remarriage. Children adjust better to remarriage with decreased conflict among family members and a supportive residential parent and stepparent. The stepparent should not exert authority immediately but instead be supportive of the residential parent. Social support from peers, grandparents,[27] and school personnel may positively influence the child's adjustment.[37]

Two other factors may play significant roles in the adjustment of children within stepfamilies. First, the child's age is an important aspect to consider in the evaluation. Although a toddler may not fully understand the implications of a stepparent, the school-aged child has been found to be the most vulnerable to the stresses associated with the remarriage. Second, timing is equally important to the overall adjustment. If the remarriage occurs abruptly or before the child is ready to accept a new parent into the child's life, the stress may be magnified. Unfortunately, the divorce rate of second marriages is still higher than that of first marriages.[17]

Preventive Interventions for Divorcing Families

Different interventions have been attempted to help alleviate the deleterious effects of divorce on families. Court-connected divorce education programs have been developed to inform parents of how children respond to divorce and to help parents respond to the child's needs. Evaluations of these programs are sparse.[24] Mediation of divorce and custody issues before the court hearing promotes higher levels of agreement among parents than does the adversarial process without prior mediation.[17] Therapy for the mother and child can reduce symptoms of mental disorders; reduce marijuana, alcohol, and other drug use; and reduce sexual promiscuity.[38] An intervention to improve the quality of the mother-child relationship was shown to improve long-term coping in children.[39] An online coping skills program to prevent mental health problems was found to be effective, especially in children and adolescents aged 11 to 16 years identified to be at higher risk for development of mental health problems[40] according to a parent-report risk index that predicts child and adolescent mental health problems up to 6 years following divorce.[41]

The Primary Care Clinician's Role

The PCC can help the family anticipate, prevent, or address problems that frequently accompany divorce by providing anticipatory guidance to divorcing parents about their children's needs during each phase of the divorce process, counseling for problems as they arise, and assessing and referring children and family members for more extensive or detailed psychosocial intervention when needed. Examples of resource materials to assist PCCs include *Divorce and Children,* available at https://patiented. solutions.aap.org; "How to Support Children After Their Parents Separate or Divorce," available at www.healthychildren.org/English/family-life/family-dynamics/types-of-families/Pages/Making-the-Divorce-Livable-for-Your-Child.aspx; and *Little Children, Big Challenges: Divorce,* available at https:// cdn.sesamestreet.org/sites/default/files/media_folders/Images/Divorce_ CaregiverGuide.pdf. Parents and courts may also ask that PCCs offer expert witness testimony when custody is questioned.[42]

The first year after divorce is often the worst; parents often feel depressed and angry. If the parents are not otherwise receiving counseling, the PCC may offer to meet with one or preferably both of them to facilitate cooperation regarding child-related issues, such as helping the parents formulate an approach to informing the children about the divorce. Primary care clinicians need to be the advocate for the child. They should avoid taking sides between parents.[21]

Parents should be encouraged to avoid placing the children in the difficult position of choosing which parent to believe or side with when the 2 most significant adults in their lives have widely differing views. They should also be informed that behind many of their questions, children are asking, "Do you still love me, and can I trust you?" Parents should explain the divorce process to children in a developmentally appropriate manner. Also suggested is that parents be *concrete* about the children's future: where they will live, who will care for them, where the nonresidential parent will live, and how often he or she will visit. Parents should be encouraged to maintain children's routines, including going to school and taking on responsibilities inside and outside the home. Parents should maintain consistent discipline strategies.

Before and after the divorce, children need reassurance that they are not unique as offspring of divorced parents. They may find comfort in discovering that many other children have divorced parents, live in step-families, and have the feelings they are having and that nothing is wrong with feeling this way. They should also be encouraged to ask questions and express feelings, and they should be brought to realize that hoping their parents will be reunited will expend a great amount of energy, as it is unlikely that their parents will reunite. Visitation with the nonresidential parent may be court mediated. PCCs need to be aware of the visitation agreement that is permitted; the clinician can then offer guidance about how to make visits more comfortable for the child. Suggestions that can be given to make this visitation easier include allowing the child to bring a friend along so that the child will not be bored, setting up the child's room as it was in the original home, spending time with the child, and not expecting the child to fit into the noncustodial parent's new world.

If a child does not wish to visit, parents should be informed that the child should not be made to feel guilty, and the offer to visit soon should be extended. The nonresidential parent should be counseled to avoid forcing visitation if the child refuses. Persistent refusals to visit the nonresidential parent may suggest that the child is enmeshed in parental difficulties or is siding with the residential parent or that the residential parent may be using the child to hurt the nonresidential parent.

Primary care clinicians should work with both parents; if abuse by a parent is thought to exist, however, the appropriate action should be taken. Clinicians should be knowledgeable about confidentiality laws; sharing medical information with any party during a divorce proceeding requires written permission by both parents or a court order.[43] Clinicians should maintain an accurate record of the custody arrangements.

Visits for child health supervision care and for acute illnesses can be used routinely to assess children's adjustment, to screen for mental health symptoms or functional impairment, and to determine the need for further counseling by the PCC or for referral for individual or family therapy.

AAP Policy

Cohen GJ, Weitzman CC; American Academy of Pediatrics Committee on Psychosocial Aspects of Child and Family Health and Section on Developmental and Behavioral
Pediatrics. Helping children and families deal with divorce and separation. *Pediatrics.*
2016;138(6):e20163020 (pediatrics.aappublications.org/content/138/6/e20163020)

References

1. Shiono P, Quinn L. Epidemiology of divorce. *Future Child.* 1994;4(1):15–28
2. The majority of children live with two parents, Census Bureau reports [press release].
   Washington, DC: US Census Bureau; November 17, 2016. https://www.census.gov/newsroom/
   press-releases/2016/cb16-192.html. Accessed January 24, 2018
3. Wallerstein JS. Children in divorce: stress and developmental tasks. In: Garmezy N, Rutter
   M, eds. *Stress, Coping, and Development in Children.* New York, NY: McGraw-Hill Book Co;
   1983:265–302
4. Lansford JE. Parental divorce and children's adjustment. *Perspect Psychol Sci.* 2009;4(2):140–152
5. Bernet W, Wamboldt MZ, Narrow WE. Child affected by parental relationship distress. *J Am
   Acad Child Adolesc Psychiatry.* 2016;55(7):571–579
6. Hetherington EM. Divorce and the adjustment of children. *Pediatr Rev.* 2005;26(5):163–169
7. Lamela D, Figueiredo B. Coparenting after marital dissolution and children's mental health: a
   systematic review. *J Pediatr (Rio J).* 2016;92(4):331–342
8. Semega JL, Fontenot KR, Kollar MA. *Income and Poverty in the United States: 2016.*
   Washington, DC: US Census Bureau; 2017. *Current Population Reports;* P60-259
9. American Psychiatric Association. *Diagnostic and Statistical Manual of Mental Disorders.*
   5th ed. Arlington, VA: American Psychiatric Association; 2013:716
10. Trozzi M. *Talking With Children About Loss: Words, Strategies, and Wisdom to Help Children
    Cope With Death, Divorce, and Other Difficult Times.* New York, NY: Berkley Publishing
    Group; 1999
11. Amato PR. Life-span adjustment of children to their parents' divorce. *Future Child.* 1994;4(1):
    143–164
12. Amato PR, Keith B. Parental divorce and the well-being of children: a meta-analysis. *Psychol
    Bull.* 1991;110(1):26–46
13. Chase-Lansdale PL, Cherlin AJ, Kiernan KE. The long-term effects of parental divorce on the
    mental health of young adults: a developmental perspective. *Child Dev.* 1995;66(6):1614–1634
14. Emery R, Forehand R. Parental divorce and children's well-being: a focus on resilience. In:
    Haggerty RJ, Sherrod LR, Garmezy N, et al, eds. *Risk and Resilience in Children.* London, UK:
    Cambridge University Press; 1994:64–99
15. Fincham FD. Child development and marital relations. *Child Dev.* 1998;69(2):543–574
16. Lengua LJ, Sandler IN, West SG, Wolchik SA, Curran PJ. Emotionality and self-regulation,
    threat appraisal, and coping in children of divorce. *Dev Psychopathol.* 1999;11(1):15–37
17. Bryner CL Jr. Children of divorce. *J Am Board Fam Pract.* 2001;14(3):201–210
18. Arkes J. The temporal effects of divorces and separations on children's academic achievement
    and problem behavior. *J Divorce Remarriage.* 2015;56(1):25–42
19. Emery RE, Laumann-Billings L. Practical and emotional consequences of parental divorce.
    Adolesc Med. 1998;9(2):271–282
20. Jackson K, Rogers M, Sartor C. Parental divorce and initiation of alcohol use in early
    adolescence. *Psychol Addict Behav.* 2016;30(4):450–461
21. Cohen GJ, Weitzman CC; American Academy of Pediatrics Committee on Psychosocial
    Aspects of Child and Family Health and Section on Developmental and Behavioral
    Pediatrics. Helping children and families deal with divorce and separation. *Pediatrics.*
    2016;138(6):e20163020

22. Kelly JB. Children's adjustment in conflicted marriage and divorce: a decade review of research. *J Am Acad Child Adolesc Psychiatry.* 2000;39(8):963–973

23. Wallerstein J, Lewis J, Blakeslee S. *The Unexpected Legacy of Divorce: Report of a 25-Year Landmark Study.* New York, NY: Hyperion Press; 2000

24. Amato PR. Children of divorce in the 1990s: an update of the Amato and Keith (1991) meta-analysis. *J Fam Psychol.* 2001;15(3):355–370

25. Shaw DS, Winslow EB, Flanagan C. A prospective study of the effects of marital status and family relations on young children's adjustment among African American and European American families. *Child Dev.* 1999;70(3):742–755

26. O'Connor TG, Thorpe K, Dunn J, et al. Parental divorce and adjustment in adulthood: findings from a community sample. The ALSPAC Study Team. Avon Longitudinal Study of Pregnancy and Childhood. *J Child Psychol Psychiatry.* 1999;40(5):777–789

27. Lussier G, Deater-Deckard K, Dunn J, Davies L. Support across two generations: children's closeness to grandparents following parental divorce and remarriage. *J Fam Psychol.* 2002; 16(3):363–376

28. DeGarmo DS, Forgatch MS, Martinez CR Jr. Parenting of divorced mothers as a link between social status and boys' academic outcomes: unpacking the effects of socioeconomic status. *Child Dev.* 1999;70(5):1231–1245

29. Emery RE, Coiro MJ. Divorce: consequences for children. *Pediatr Rev.* 1995;16(8):306–310

30. Zill N, Morrison DR, Coiro MJ. Long-term effects of parental divorce on parent-child relationships, adjustment, and achievement in young adulthood. *J Fam Psychol.* 1993;7(1): 91–103

31. Pruett KD, Pruett MK. "Only God decides": young children's perceptions of divorce and the legal system. *J Am Acad Child Adolesc Psychiatry.* 1999;38(12):1544–1550

32. Kelly JB. Marital conflict, divorce, and children's adjustment. *Child Adolesc Psychiatr Clin N Am.* 1998;7(2):259–271

33. Wallerstein JS, Blakeslee S. *What About the Kids? Raising Your Children Before, During, and After Divorce.* New York, NY: Hyperion; 2003

34. Vezzetti VC. New approaches to divorce with children: a problem of public health. *Health Psychol Open.* 2016;3(2):2055102916678105

35. Dubowitz H, Newberger CM, Melnicoe LH, Newberger EH. The changing American family. *Pediatr Clin North Am.* 1988;35(6):1291–1311

36. Lutz P. The step-family: an adolescent perspective. *Fam Relat.* 1983;32(3):367–375

37. Isaacs A. Children's adjustment to their divorced parents' new relationships. *J Paediatr Child Health.* 2002;38(4):329–331

38. Wolchik SA, Sandler IN, Millsap RE, et al. Six-year follow-up of preventive interventions for children of divorce: a randomized controlled trial. *JAMA.* 2002;288(15):1874–1881

39. Vélez CE, Wolchik SA, Tein JY, et al. Protecting children from the consequences of divorce: a longitudinal study of the effects of parenting on children's coping processes. *Child Dev.* 2011;82(1):244–257

40. Boring JL, Sandler IN, Tein JY, Horan JJ, Vélez CE. Children of divorce—coping with divorce: a randomized control trial of an online prevention program for youth experiencing parental divorce. *J Consult Clin Psychol.* 2015;83(5):999–1005

41. Tein JY, Sandler IN, Braver SL, Wolchik SA. Development of a brief parent-report risk index for children following parental divorce. *J Fam Psychol.* 2013;27(6):925–936

42. Emery RE. *Renegotiating Family Relationships: Divorce, Child Custody, and Mediation.* New York, NY: Guilford Press; 1994

43. Wolraich ML, Aceves J, Feldman HM, et al; American Academy of Pediatrics Committee on Psychosocial Aspects of Child and Family Health. The child in court: a subject review. *Pediatrics.* 1999;104(5, pt 1):1145–1148

Children in Military Families

Timothy Wilks, MD, MHA, and
Beth Ellen Davis, MD, MPH (COL, MC, USA, Retired)

"Children who have supportive caregivers,
school environments, and adults who
understand their military situation are
more able to effectively recruit coping skills
that augment family supports."

Background

The military family is a modern experience. Before the Vietnam War, US service members were discouraged from having families. Entry into the armed services was primarily through conscription at a young age. When military service became voluntary in 1973, the number of individuals looking for a career increased, and with them came their families. Currently supporting a population of families larger than its serving force, the Department of Defense (DoD) is responding to a stressor affecting service members and their families more than any other in the new millennium: the need to understand the effects of lengthy, recurrent, and dangerous wartime deployments. With 2.2% of all US births, and more than 2 million children,[1] military families and their unique issues are not confined to the mission of the DoD but rather extend to local communities, schools, child care, and health care systems. All pediatric primary care clinicians (PCCs) (ie, pediatricians, family physicians, internists, nurse practitioners, and physician assistants who provide frontline, longitudinal health care to pediatric patients) need to be aware of the physical and mental health needs of children and adolescents (collectively called *children* in this chapter) in military families and the supports available to them.

In the past, the image of military families evoked a stereotypical profile, sometimes referred to as the "military family syndrome,"[2] which described a rigid, authoritarian active-duty father, a stay-at-home submissive mother and wife, and "out-of-control" children with rootless identities exhibiting severe psychological problems. Subsequent research, including prospective studies of military vs nonmilitary children, failed to validate this profile and found no inherent psychosocial differences between military and nonmilitary children.[3-5] In fact, one study of Navy families, for whom routine 6-month sea-duty deployments have been a way of life for years, indicated that children demonstrated increased responsibility, independence, and confidence compared with their peers without deployment experiences,[6] suggesting that children develop a different and often beneficial parent-child relationship during parental deployment. Despite its varied components, the US military is a unified community with a strong sense of patriotism, pride, and self-sufficiency. Uniform attitudes and values, rank hierarchy, dress, and customs support a robust and resilient military culture.

Military Life

Although military families experience matters common in all US families, many aspects of military family life are extraordinary: its diversity, frequent geographic relocations, opportunities to live in foreign countries, forced adaptations to new communities and schools, use of the largest single-payer health entitlement program (TRICARE) in the country, peacetime separations, remote unaccompanied assignments of service members, and dangerous, lengthy combat deployments. The DoD has 3.6 million members serving on active duty (AD) or selected reserve (SR), including the National Guard. Nearly half of these service members have children. Most children in AD households are younger than 6 years, whereas more than 60% of children in SR families are of school age.[1] Geographically, AD families typically live within military communities where resources and support systems for young children are readily available. Selected reserve service members may be activated for service from civilian jobs in geographic areas quite remote from military resources and often have individual and family unmet needs in their communities during service member activation. Of the service members with children, 5% (AD) to 9% (SR) are single parents. In 7% of families, both parents serve on AD.[1] These families have additional needs when the military mission requires them to step away from parenting responsibilities. Thirty percent of the service members identify as nonwhite, non-Hispanic minorities. The diversity of US military families can be compared with that of other American families, and appreciation of various cultural contexts will help enhance understanding of family needs and provision of care.

Relocation

Frequent relocations are commonplace for the military family and can present significant challenges. At least 60% of military families have relocated at least once in the past 3 years.[7] In a 2009 survey of AD families with deployed service members, 47% reported 3 or more moves in the past 5 years,[8] significantly higher than SR families and the general US population. Frequent relocations affect spouse employment, school continuity, and child care, not to mention services needed for children with special health care needs. To help ease the economic burden of renting or owning a home, the AD service member is provided a housing allowance. Additionally, most military installations have housing available. Housing on military bases can provide a significant source of community and social supports for both adults and children.[9] Military housing neighborhoods are often filled with families and children in similar life stages, and neighbors take on the role of extended family members. Assignment to installation housing is determined by availability. Many times, families must live in the local community for several months before moving to installation housing, which can result in additional school relocations. Overseas assignments are also a common experience for service members and their families. At any given time, approximately 13% of AD members are stationed outside the United States and its territories.[1] The military family can move overseas with the service member in many locations, but some assignments require the AD member to be separated from his or her family for a 1- or 2-year unaccompanied assignment. For foreign locations that do allow families, the experience can be enriching. Families have the opportunity to travel and learn about new cultures. Often, overseas military installations provide many services (eg, housing, schools, supermarkets, department stores, restaurants) to families, and they can choose how involved in the local culture they want to be. Previously, communication with families back in the United States was difficult and expensive, but in the current digital age, the largest barrier is the time differences between countries.

Schooling

Children in military families, on average, attend 6 to 9 different school systems between kindergarten and 12th grade. Many will change high schools more than twice.[10] Traditionally, this has led to less academic success[11] and difficulties participating in competitive interscholastic activities. All 50 states and the District of Columbia, however, have now adopted the Interstate Compact on Educational Opportunities for Military Children to ensure "uniform treatment of military children transferring between school districts and states." This interstate compact addresses issues of enrollment, eligibility, and graduation parity between states. Many military families are unaware of the agreement, and many students resign themselves to less or fragmented school participation.

Deployment

One aspect of military life that is well-known and accepted among all service members is the needs of the "military mission," which often require the service member to spend time away from home and his or her regular assigned workplace. Deployment is defined as a temporary, 3- to 15-month movement of an individual or military unit away from his or her local work site, resources, and family to accomplish a task or mission. Deployments can occur as a peacetime activity or to support wartime operations. Peacetime deployments (separations other than war) include humanitarian missions such as when activated service members were sent to assist following Hurricane Katrina in 2005 or when more than 12,000 US service members were involved in the global response to the 2010 earthquake in Haiti. Operations other than war usually mean travel to safe locations, short duration, and interludes of rest and recovery between absences, and most military families cope well with these separations. Military families may also expect 3- to 6-month annual separations from their family service member for specialized schooling or training. Traditionally, unaccompanied tours of 1-year remote overseas assignments, when the family remains stateside, have not been defined as deployments. Wartime combat deployments, on the other hand, represent separation from family to an area with hostile, dangerous conditions for variable durations.

Before the wars in Iraq and Afghanistan, combat deployment was a rare occurrence for most military forces. Most families had never experienced the separation of a loved one to a hostile environment prior to 2001. Since then, families have experienced the most prolonged and repeated combat deployments in American history.[12] Deployments have 3 main phases, each with predictable dynamics: predeployment, deployment, and postdeployment (or redeployment) (Table 19-1).

Effects of Deployment

The years since 2001 have provided most of the research on responses to war by US service members, their spouses, and their children.[13–16] Complications related to war-combat stress disorder, traumatic brain injury, development of psychiatric illness, and increase in health risk behaviors can complicate family life for a child. Postdeployment emotional and behavioral responses by a service member can range from typical short-term distress responses, such as change in sleep, decreased sense of safety, or social isolation, to the development of more serious psychiatric conditions such as post-traumatic stress disorder (PTSD) or depression. It is estimated that more than 30% of returning service members have experienced PTSD, depression, or traumatic brain injury.[12] Comorbidities, such as aggression and alcohol use, are prevalent in up to half of those with impairment.[13] Studies of spouses of service members indicate that deployment affects their well-being and marital relationships. In a review of more than 250,000 Army wives, Mansfield and colleagues found that soldier length of deployment was associated with elevated symptoms of depression, sleep problems, anxiety, acute stress reactions, and adjustment disorders in their wives.[17] It is not surprising that the toll of lengthy and recurrent deployments has been reflected in marital discord. In 2008, an Army Mental Health Advisory Team reported that the number of months deployed has a statistically significant linear relationship with married soldier reports on plans for divorce or separation, especially among the junior enlisted ranks.[18] There is well-established literature across a range of populations to inform pediatricians about the effects of parental psychopathology and marital discord on child well-being, separate from the challenges faced by deployed service members and their spouses. Recognizing the increased vulnerability of children in these circumstances is a role PCCs have assumed for decades.[19]

Coping With Deployment

Over the past decade, researchers have compiled a few dozen studies to create the current profile of military children and their families coping with parental combat deployments.[20] Recent systematic reviews consolidate the evidence associating parental deployment with increased risk for childhood emotional and behavioral problems, poorer academic achievement, and risk-taking behaviors. At all ages studied, parental wartime deployments exposed children to developmental and behavioral challenges in a "dose-dependent" manner, according to the number and duration of parental deployments.[21-24] Very little is known about military infants and toddlers. There is evidence of increased maternal stress related to pregnancy and childbirth when a service member partner is deployed.[25] In 2008, Chartrand and colleagues studied preschool-aged children with and without a deployed parent and found increased behavioral symptoms in the preschoolers experiencing parental deployment.[26] Flake and colleagues found increased rates of psychosocial morbidity among more than one-third of school-aged children with a deployed parent. At-home parental

Table 19-1. Phases of Deployment and the Role of the Primary Care Clinician

Stages of Deployment	Characteristics	Primary Care Clinician Assessment	Primary Care Clinician Anticipatory Guidance
Predeployment: from notification of deployment to actual departure	• Often intense preparation of military units; requires extensive time away from family. • Decisions made about careers, financial adjustments, legal issues, and child care. • Experience with previous deployments may interfere with preparation for new deployment. • Can be confusing to children, who may not understand why separation is necessary and have no concept of what this change means. • Children at various developmental ages experience excitement, denial, worry, fear, and anger. Emotional withdrawal is not uncommon immediately before deployment. • Last-minute or recurrent goodbyes often increase tension. • Teens can be angry at the "selfish" nature of a service member's job that takes the adult away from his or her role as parent, coach, and supporter.	Assess for preexisting • Family dysfunction • Mental health issues in parent • Children with special health care needs • Recent family relocation • Recent divorce or remarriage • Previous problems during a deployment	• Discuss responsibilities and expectations of each family member during upcoming deployment. • Make plans and goals for family rather than "put lives on hold." • Decrease likelihood of misperception and distortion. • Prepare for communication strategies and expectations, perhaps avoiding everyday contact. • Plan to maintain rules, rituals, and routines.

Deployment: typically lasts between 3 and 15 mo	• Usually begins with a tearful going-away ceremony, followed by a period (usually 1–6 wk) of emptiness and loss.
	• The intensity leading up to a goodbye can be overwhelming.
	• The sense of relief that the deployment has actually started can be confusing.
	• After about 6 wk, most families try to establish and settle into a new routine.
	• The "midtour" R & R leave
	  – Is when the deployed service member can come home for 2 wk
	  – Is often a difficult time for children
	  – May occur during the school year
	  – Is when children are often distracted by anticipation, excitement, and a short period of visitation and then have to say goodbye all over again
	• Many families describe deployment as "surviving, not thriving" despite trying to find resilience and strength.
	• For the month or two before homecoming,
	  – There may be worry as well as excitement as new independence or self-reliance may have emerged into a "new normal."
	  – Family members are unsure of how to reintegrate a deployed parent.
		• Assess at-home parent and children for
		  – Adjustment (1–6 wk after deployment)
		  – Sleep regularity
		  – School attendance
		  – Mood problems
		• Spend time in private conversation with adolescents to assess
		  – Adjustment
		  – School performance
		  – Mood
		  – Risk-taking
		  – Role in family
		• Offer free deployment video for youths.
			• Discuss responsibilities and expectations of each family member during upcoming deployment.
			• Make plans and goals for family rather than "put lives on hold."
			• Decrease likelihood of misperception and distortion.
			• Prepare for communication strategies and expectations, perhaps avoiding everyday contact.
			• Plan to maintain rules, rituals, and routines.

Postdeployment (redeployment)	• Often begins with "honeymoon" period of happiness and putting off the chores of the day.
	• Happiness of reuniting is mixed with needing to get reacquainted and deciding how to share the time lost.
	• "Block leave" is 30 d of vacation time given to the postdeployment unit, sometimes delayed after the actual return.
	  – May not coincide with when family members have availability to leave school or work.
	  – At-home spouse often wants some much-needed respite after a year of "full-time" parenting.
		Assess family for
		• Readjustment (1–6 wk)
		• Parental mood
		• PTSD
		• Substance use
		• Marital discord
			• Take time to communicate and to get to know each other.
			• Spend time talking with each other.
			• Take time to make decisions and to discuss changes in routine.
			• Lower holiday expectations.
			• Keep plans simple and flexible.
			• Don't try to schedule too many things during the first few weeks.
			• Let absent parent "back into" the family circle.

Abbreviations: R & R, rest and recuperation; PTSD, post-traumatic stress disorder.

stress was reported to be very high in this group.[8] Aranda et al queried adolescents in military families with and without a deployed parent, and both the teen self-reports and the parental reports revealed increased levels of stress in the deployed subgroup.[27] Lester and colleagues and Barker and Berry each provide evidence of the cumulative effects of deployment experiences, as well as risk to children, associated with psychological stress of either parent.[28,29] Mansfield and colleagues studied the electronic medical record data of more than 300,000 Army children and observed a "dose-response" pattern between deployment of a parent and increased rates of child mental health diagnoses.[30] At a population level, Gorman and colleagues found that rates of mental health, behavioral, and stress problems in children increased by 11% during parental deployment.[31] A similar increase in psychiatric hospitalizations when a parent was deployed was found by Millegan and colleagues.[32] Two studies of youths, one in Washington state[33] and another in Iowa,[34] showed that those with a parent in the military had higher rates of risk-taking behaviors, including substance use and school-based violence. One study, by interviewing youths, associated parental deployment with suicidal ideation as well as reports of depressed mood and lower quality of life compared with nondeployed and civilian peers.[35]

Other Stressors

Although no specific or consistent pediatric diagnoses have emerged as indicators of the severity of chronic wartime stress,[36] there are examples of significant distress: in testimony to Congress, there is evidence of increases in military preteen inpatient mental health stays,[37] and 2 studies suggested military families experiencing repeated or prolonged deployments, especially in young marriages with young children, were at risk for child maltreatment, specifically neglectful home environments.[38,39] Another study confirmed the increased risk of child maltreatment during deployment and also found a high-risk period for the 6 months postdeployment.[40] While studies have traditionally reported child maltreatment rates less than half of civilian counterparts, new data indicate an under-ascertainment of child maltreatment by the program responsible for ensuring child safety in the Army.[41] Another stressor, perhaps underappreciated, includes food insecurity. Nearly 1 in 7 families at a large military installation with a child younger than 6 years enrolled in the child care center system reported food insecurity. Few families reported enrollment in government supplemental food programs.[42] These examples remind PCCs not to assume deployment stressors are sole contributors to military children's emotional and behavioral problems; rather, they should remain vigilant to other possible contributing stressors.

To help understand the generational and life course effects of deployment, 3 longitudinal studies are underway, one of which (Millennium Cohort Study, www.millenniumcohort.org) is a 20-year prospective study and will substantially enhance our understanding of risks among and resilience of military children during and after parental deployments. The Deployment Life Study, a large representative sample of deployable married service members and their spouses across all services, is allowing RAND researchers the ability to assess predeployment planning and preparation strategies and to track active coping of families postdeployment.[43]

When a Parent Dies

The death of a parent or significant parenting figure during war is a catastrophically disorganizing event for a child, the surviving parent, and the family. It is one of the unspoken fears that family members endure during wartime deployments. Helping children understand parental injury or death requires a developmentally unique sensitivity.[44,45] The PCC should assess the social-emotional reaction of the child in relationship to his or her developmental stage, follow the child over time, and support the remaining parent or life partner. The severity of parental injury is not directly related to the degree of child distress.[45] It is important to consider not *how* the child is acting, reacting, or overreacting but for *how long*. It is common for children to demonstrate their grief for 4 to 6 weeks. Because of the devastating nature of parental disfigurement or death, most spouses or partners should be referred for social-emotional assessment and therapy to support their personal grief and to understand how to support their children. A specific resource for military families is the Tragedy Assistance Program for Survivors (www.taps.org; Box 19-1). The PCC can encourage a surviving parent to seek military support through Decedent Affairs, the Chaplains' Office, or commanders of the military unit. This support is usually made available at the time the spouse or partner is notified of the death of her or his loved one.

Resilience

Resilience seems to play a major factor in all phases of deployment as well as military life. Protective factors include family readiness, "meaning making" of a situation, receipt of community and social support, acceptance of the military lifestyle, ability of the at-home parent to develop self-reliant coping skills (Box 19-1), and adoption of flexible gender roles. Children who have supportive caregivers, school environments, and adults who understand their military situation are more able to effectively recruit

Box 19-1. Resources for Primary Care Clinicians to Support Military Families

- For PCC
  - AAP *Addressing Mental Health Concerns in Primary Care: A Clinician's Toolkit* (https://shop.aap.org)
  - AAP "Mental Health Initiatives" (www.aap.org/en-us/advocacy-and-policy/ aap-health-initiatives/Mental-Health/Pages/default.aspx)
  - AAP Section on Uniformed Services (www.aap.org/en-us/about-the-aap/ Committees-Councils-Sections/Section-on-Uniformed-Services/Pages/ default.aspx)
  - Center for the Study of Traumatic Stress (www.centerforthestudyoftraumaticstress.org)
  - Military OneSource (www.militaryonesource.com)
  - TAPS (www.taps.org)
  - TRICARE Online (www.tricare.mil)

- For parent
  - American Red Cross (www.redcross.org)
  - Ginsburg KR, Jablow MM. *Building Resilience in Children and Teens: Giving Kids Roots and Wings.* 3rd ed. Elk Grove Village, IL: American Academy of Pediatrics; 2014 (https://shop.aap.org)
  - Military OneSource (www.militaryonesource.com)
  - National Military Family Association (www.militaryfamily.org)
  - Zero to Three "Military Family Projects" (www.zerotothree.org/about-us/funded-projects/military-families)

- For child
  - Operation Purple (through the National Military Family Association) (www.militaryfamily.org)

- Education
  - DoDEA Partnership (www.dodea.edu/Partnership/index.cfm)
  - Military Child Education Coalition (www.militarychild.org)
  - Military Interstate Children's Compact Commission (www.mic3.net)
  - Military Parent Technical Assistance Center (https://branchta.org)

- Service related
  - Air Force (www.af.mil)
  - Air Force Reserve Command (www.afrc.af.mil)
  - Army Family Readiness Group (www.armyfrg.org)
  - Army Reserve Family Programs (www.arfp.org)
  - Coast Guard (www.uscg.mil/mwr)
  - Marine Corps Family Team Building (www.mccscp.com/mcftb)
  - Marine Forces Reserve "MFR Family Readiness" (www.marforres.marines.mil/FamilyReadinessOffice.aspx)
  - National Guard Family Program (www.jointservicessupport.org/fp)
  - Naval Services FamilyLine (www.cnic.navy.mil/FamilyLine)

Abbreviations: AAP, American Academy of Pediatrics; DoDEA, Department of Defense Education Activity; K–12, kindergarten through 12th grade; PCC, primary care clinician; TAPS, Tragedy Assistance Program for Survivors.

coping skills that augment family supports. Evolving understanding of these factors supports the role of systematic approaches to prevention and care of the military-connected child. As programs to support children and families are developed, it is important that they are evaluated for their effectiveness. As an example, a family-centered, preventive care program developed by Lester and colleagues[46] showed a statistically significant decrease in anxiety and depression measures and led directly to increases in healthy family functioning.

Benefits of Military Service

Even in the midst of ongoing deployments, military families, regardless of service or component, appreciate the advantages of military life, including adequate free housing, an "on post" community with shopping; accessible child care and schools; low cost or free medical care; community services, including free financial and behavioral counseling; emphasis on recreational facilities; subsidized educational opportunities; relatively stable family income; shared identity and mission with peers as well as senior leaders; and a feeling of patriotism and national contribution.

Mental Health Care in the Military

The AD service members and their families receive significant health care entitlements under TRICARE, including inpatient, outpatient, primary, and subspecialty care; therapies; medications; and equipment. The administrative agent for TRICARE is contracted regionally (ie, east, west) and includes both military treatment facility (MTF) or "direct care" and a network "purchased care" component. There are 149 MTFs in the United States and around the world, accounting for 63% of DoD pediatric beneficiary care and supporting Army, Navy, and Air Force military pediatric residencies, subspecialty pediatrics, pharmacy, behavioral health, and ancillary care services.[47] The medical coverage exclusions are regulated by Congress and implemented by the regional administrative agents. The Defense Health Agency recently concluded that the Military Health System is generally meeting the needs of pediatric beneficiaries, but it also outlined several opportunities for improvement. Recognized gaps were noted in several areas, including transferring care when children move between regions, using preventive care programs, and providing habilitative care.

Several options are given to military families regarding their medical entitlements. TRICARE Prime requires the assignment of a primary care manager (PCM). Perhaps one of the most significant benefits under TRICARE is the mental health option or Behavioral Health Portal. Family members can be seen up to 8 times by any mental health provider in the TRICARE network without a consultation from a PCM. This benefit allows for improved access to mental health services for all military family members. Interested providers should consult Web site references listed in Box 19-1 for the most current information regarding TRICARE benefits.

To prevent moving a family with a dependent who requires significant medical, mental health, or educational services to a medically underserved area, the military requires AD service members and their families to enroll in the Exceptional Family Member Program (EFMP). The EFMP is designed to help select appropriate service member duty assignments and continue to meet family members' health care needs without detriment to the service member's career and military mission. Dependents enrolled in the EFMP are potentially eligible for services under the Extended Care Health Option (ECHO). Habilitative equipment and skilled nursing care are provided as part of the ECHO program. The Comprehensive Autism Care Demonstration project provides intensive autism spectrum disorder (ASD) supports, such as applied behavioral analysis for children with ASD who are TRICARE eligible.

Children of military members require an identification card at age 10 years and are eligible for care up to age 23 if they remain full-time students. TRICARE Young Adult (commonly known as TYA) is a premium-based program available for young adults 23 to 26 years of age. For children with chronic lifelong medical issues resulting in diminished capacity to live independently, the AD or retired service member has the opportunity to request indefinite medical support for that family member. After a service member retires, the family continues to be eligible for TRICARE retired medical benefits.

Recommendations for Primary Care Clinicians

To support children of military families, a nondeployed parent needs to feel in control and to have support. The PCC can encourage the at-home parent to stay healthy and connected, including sharing experiences and finding opportunities for personal growth, respite, and spiritual wellness. If needed, the PCC can support and help the parent find a mental health professional. One resource, www.militaryonesource.com, is available for PCCs and military spouses to access adult mental health services regardless of location or service. Primary care clinicians should be familiar with this Web site to help family caregivers with their own emotional needs. Many of the deployment-specific resources available to AD families can be accessed on this Web site for activated National Guard and Reserve families, including Military Family Life Consultants, chaplains, legal assistance, social work services, and New Parent Support Program services. In addition to requesting direct contact with a case manager or mental health locator, at-home parents can request free parenting and support books from the OneSource library, and they can find parent support groups in their local areas.

The needs and concerns of the military family vary depending on the specific phase of deployment. Table 19-1 shows the phases of deployment and the role of the PCC in providing appropriate anticipatory guidance. Primary care clinicians can connect a family struggling with deployment to resources available in the military community. Some military bases have deployment-related respite or child care services available. School-aged children can participate in Operation Purple Camp (a free summer camp for military children), which uses peer relationships to build resiliency.

Understanding military culture and asking initial questions of a child or teen who has a military parent can help unveil etiologies of academic problems, poor peer interactions, or risk-taking behaviors. Primary care clinicians need to be able to access a "virtual toolbox" containing health and mental health screening tools to help identify children in need of additional services. Appendix 2 lists tools useful in primary care, including "Cover the Bases," a mental health screening tool that combines the Pediatric Symptom Checklist with 4 questions specifically for military children. Box 19-2 contains guidelines for PCCs to consider referral to a mental health professional.

Box 19-2. Indications for Referral of Military Families to Mental Health Professionals

Primary care clinicians should consider referral of a child or the child's family (or both) to a mental health professional when

- They have tried reassurance and helping the parent cope using a psychoeducational intervention or generally supportive counseling, which is not working after 2 visits.

- They feel uncomfortable about their own counseling and psychoeducational skills.

- Child behavior has become more extreme or continues for up to 3 mo after the deployed parent has returned home.

- There is a significant change in behavior or a drop in school performance.

- There has been an injury or death of a deployed parent.

Primary care clinicians are on the front line in meeting the needs of military families. By understanding the strengths and challenges of living in a military family, clinicians can recognize opportunities to respond within the context of the pediatric medical home.

Disclaimers: The views expressed in this chapter are those of the authors and do not necessarily reflect the official policy or position of the Department of the Army, the Department of the Navy, the Department of Defense, or the US Government.

Manuscript preparation was supported by the Health Resources and Services Administration (HRSA) of the US Department of Health and Human Services (HHS) under grant T73MC00041, Excellence in Comprehensive Interdisciplinary Leadership Education: Enabling Children and Youth with Neurodevelopmental Disabilities to Achieve Their Dreams (UW LEND).

AAP Policy

Siegel BS, Davis BE; American Academy of Pediatrics Committee on Psychosocial Aspects of Child and Family Health and Section on Uniformed Services. Health and mental health needs of children in US military families. *Pediatrics.* 2013;131(6): e2002–e2015 (pediatrics.aappublications.org/content/131/6/e2002)

References

1. US Department of Defense. *2009 Demographics: Profile of the Military Community.* Washington, DC: Office of the Deputy Under Secretary of Defense (Military Community and Family Policy). http://download.militaryonesource.mil/12038/MOS/Reports/2009-Demographics-Report.pdf. Accessed January 25, 2018
2. Lagrone DM. The military family syndrome. *Am J Psychiatry.* 1978;135(9):1040–1043
3. Jensen PS, Lewis RL, Xenakis SN. The military family in review: context, risk, and prevention. *J Am Acad Child Psychiatry.* 1986;25(2):225–234
4. Jensen PS, Xenakis SN, Wolf P, Bain MW. The "military family syndrome" revisited: "by the numbers". *J Nerv Ment Dis.* 1991;179(2):102–107
5. Ryan-Wenger NA. Impact of the threat of war on children in military families. *Am J Orthopsychiatry.* 2001;71(2):236–244
6. Nice DS. *A Longitudinal Analysis of Navy Family Separation.* San Diego, CA: Navy Personnel Research and Development Center; 1981. http://www.dtic.mil/cgi-bin/GetTRDoc?AD=ADA108381. Accessed January 25, 2018
7. Burrell LM, Adams GA, Durand DB, Castro CA. The impact of military lifestyle demands on well-being, Army, and family outcomes. *Armed Forces Soc.* 2006;33(1):43–58
8. Flake EM, Davis BE, Johnson PL, Middleton LS. The psychosocial effects of deployment on military children. *J Dev Behav Pediatr.* 2009;30(4):271–278
9. Chandra A, Lara-Cinisomo S, Jaycox LH, et al. Children on the homefront: the experience of children from military families. *Pediatrics.* 2010;125(1):16–25
10. Military Interstate Children's Compact Commission Web site. http://www.mic3.net. Accessed January 25, 2018

11. Temple JA, Reynolds AJ. School mobility and achievement: longitudinal findings from an urban cohort. *J School Psychol.* 1999;37(4):355–377

12. Tanielian T, Jaycox LH. *Invisible Wounds of War: Psychological and Cognitive Injuries, Their Consequences, and Services to Assist Recovery.* Santa Monica, CA: Rand Corporation; 2008. http://www.rand.org/pubs/monographs/MG720.html. Accessed January 25, 2018

13. Thomas JL, Wilk JE, Riviere LA, McGurk D, Castro CA, Hoge CW. Prevalence of mental health problems and functional impairment among active component and National Guard soldiers 3 and 12 months following combat in Iraq. *Arch Gen Psychiatry.* 2010;67(6):614–623

14. Milliken CS, Auchterlonie JL, Hoge CW. Longitudinal assessment of mental health problems among active and reserve component soldiers returning from the Iraq war. *JAMA.* 2007;298(18):2141–2148

15. Hoge CW, Castro CA, Messer SC, McGurk D, Cotting DI, Koffman RL. Combat duty in Iraq and Afghanistan, mental health problems, and barriers to care. *N Engl J Med.* 2004;351(1): 13–22

16. Hoge CW, McGurk D, Thomas JL, Cox AL, Engel CC, Castro CA. Mild traumatic brain injury in U.S. Soldiers returning from Iraq. *N Engl J Med.* 2008;358(5):453–463

17. Mansfield AJ, Kaufman JS, Marshall SW, Gaynes BN, Morrissey JP, Engel CC. Deployment and the use of mental health services among U.S. Army wives. *N Engl J Med.* 2010;362(2): 101–109

18. Mental Health Advisory Team (MHAT) V. Operation Iraqi Freedom 2006-2008. Army Medicine Web site. https://armymedicine.health.mil/~/media/.../Redacted1MHATV 4FEB2008Overview.ashx. Published February 14, 2008. Accessed March 20, 2018

19. Woolston JL. A child's reactions to parents' problems. *Pediatr Rev.* 1986;8(6):169–176

20. Chandra A, London AS. Unlocking insights about military children and families. *Future Child.* 2013;23(2):187–198

21. White CJ, de Burgh HT, Fear NT, Iversen AC. The impact of deployment to Iraq or Afghanistan on military children: a review of the literature. *Int Rev Psychiatry.* 2011;23(2): 210–217

22. Bello-Utu CF, DeSocio JE. Military deployment and reintegration: a systematic review of child coping. *J Child Adolesc Psychiatr Nurs.* 2015;28(1):23–34

23. Creech SK, Hadley W, Borsari B. The impact of military deployment and reintegration on children and parenting: a systematic review. *Prof Psychol Res Pr.* 2014;45(6):452–464

24. Trautmann J, Alhusen J, Gross D. Impact of deployment on military families with young children: a systematic review. *Nurs Outlook.* 2015;63(6):656–679

25. Haas DM, Pazdernik LA. Partner deployment and stress in pregnant women. *J Reprod Med.* 2007;52(10):901–906

26. Chartrand MM, Frank DA, White LF, Shope TR. Effect of parents' wartime deployment on the behavior of young children in military families. *Arch Pediatr Adolesc Med.* 2008;162(11): 1009–1014

27. Aranda MC, Middleton LS, Flake E, Davis BE. Psychosocial screening in children with wartime-deployed parents. *Mil Med.* 2011;176(4):402–407

28. Lester P, Peterson K, Reeves J, et al. The long war and parental combat deployment: effects on military children and at-home spouses. *J Am Acad Child Adolesc Psychiatry.* 2010;49(4): 310–320

29. Barker LH, Berry KD. Developmental issues impacting military families with young children during single and multiple deployments. *Mil Med.* 2009;174(10):1033–1040

30. Mansfield AJ, Kaufman JS, Engel CC, Gaynes BN. Deployment and mental health diagnoses among children of US Army personnel. *Arch Pediatr Adolesc Med.* 2011;165(11):999–1005

31. Gorman GH, Eide M, Hisle-Gorman E. Wartime military deployment and increased pediatric mental and behavioral health complaints. *Pediatrics.* 2010;126(6):1058–1066

32. Millegan J, Engel C, Liu X, Dinneen M. Parental Iraq/Afghanistan deployment and child psychiatric hospitalization in the U.S. military. *Gen Hosp Psychiatry.* 2013;35(5):556–560

33. Reed SC, Bell JF, Edwards TC. Adolescent well-being in Washington state military families. *Am J Public Health.* 2011;101(9):1676–1682

34. Acion L, Ramirez MR, Jorge RE, Arndt S. Increased risk of alcohol and drug use among children from deployed military families. *Addiction.* 2013;108(8):1418–1425

35. Reed SC, Bell JF, Edwards TC. Weapon carrying, physical fighting and gang membership among youth in Washington state military families. *Matern Child Health J.* 2014;18(8): 1863–1872

36. Card NA, Bosch L, Casper DM, et al. A meta-analytic review of internalizing, externalizing, and academic adjustment among children of deployed military service members. *J Fam Psychol.* 2011;25(4):508–520

37. National Military Family Association. *Testimony Before the Subcommittee on Personnel of the US Senate Committee on Armed Forces, June 3, 2009.* Alexandria, VA: National Military Family Association; 2009

38. Gibbs DA, Martin SL, Kupper LL, Johnson RE. Child maltreatment in enlisted soldiers' families during combat-related deployments. *JAMA.* 2007;298(5):528–535

39. Rentz ED, Marshall SW, Loomis D, Casteel C, Martin SL, Gibbs DA. Effect of deployment on the occurrence of child maltreatment in military and nonmilitary families. *Am J Epidemiol.* 2007;165(10):1199–1206

40. Taylor CM, Ross ME, Wood JN, et al. Differential child maltreatment risk across deployment periods of US army soldiers. *Am J Public Health.* 2016;106(1):153–158

41. Wood JN, Griffis HM, Taylor CM, et al. Under-ascertainment from healthcare settings of child abuse events among children of soldiers by the U.S. Army Family Advocacy Program. *Child Abuse Negl.* 2017;63:202–210

42. Wax SG, Stankorb SM. Prevalence of food insecurity among military households with children 5 years of age and younger. *Public Health Nutr.* 2016;19(13):2458–2466

43. Troxel WM, Trail TE, Jaycox LH, Chandra A. Preparing for deployment: examining family- and individual-level factors. *Mil Psychol.* 2016;28(3):134–146

44. Wessel MA. The primary pediatrician's role when a death occurs in a family in one's practice. *Pediatr Rev.* 2003;24(6):183–185

45. Cozza SJ, Guimond JM, McKibben JB, et al. Combat-injured service members and their families: the relationship of child distress and spouse-perceived family distress and disruption. *J Trauma Stress.* 2010;23(1):112–115

46. Lester P, Saltzman WR, Woodward K, et al. Evaluation of a family-centered prevention intervention for military children and families facing wartime deployments. *Am J Public Health.* 2012;102(suppl 1):S48–S54

47. Office of the Secretary of Defense. *Report to Congressional Defense Committees: Study on Health Care and Related Support for Children of Members of the Armed Forces.* Washington, DC; Dept of Defense; 2014

Chapter

Lesbian, Gay, and Bisexual Youths

Robert J. Bidwell, MD

"The major health challenges faced by lesbian,
gay, and bisexual youths...are related to
achieving optimal physical and mental health
while growing up in the context of
an often disapproving family and
community environment."

In 2004, the American Academy of Pediatrics (AAP) issued its clinical report on sexual orientation and adolescents.[1] This report was followed, in 2013, by an AAP policy statement titled "Office-Based Care for Lesbian, Gay, Bisexual, Transgender, and Questioning Youth"[2] and a Society for Adolescent Health and Medicine position paper titled "Recommendations for Promoting the Health and Well-Being of Lesbian, Gay, Bisexual, and Transgender Adolescents."[3] Together, these publications affirm the responsibility of pediatric clinicians (ie, primary care pediatricians, pediatric subspecialists, and family physicians, internists, nurse practitioners, and physician assistants who provide care to children and adolescents) to provide supportive and comprehensive health care to all young people, including those who are lesbian, gay, bisexual, transgender, or questioning (LGBTQ). They also provide clinicians with the understanding and tools to do so in a respectful and relevant manner. The major health challenges faced by LGBTQ youths (ie, those in preadolescence through young adulthood) are related to achieving optimal physical and mental health while growing up in the context of an often disapproving family and community environment. Lesbian, gay, bisexual, transgender, and questioning youths are present in every pediatric setting. Therefore, an understanding of sexual orientation and gender identity and the unique experiences and needs of LGBTQ youths is essential to the practice of pediatrics, with specific attention paid to their developmental, social, and psychological well-being.

Definitions

Sexual orientation is an integral part of human sexuality; it refers to an individual's pattern of affectional, romantic, or sexual attractions to the same sex (homosexual), opposite sex (heterosexual), or both sexes (bisexual). Homosexual men are generally referred to as *gay;* homosexual women, as *lesbian* (or *gay*); and heterosexual individuals, as *straight;* bisexual individuals are sometimes referred to as *bi.* Sexual orientation is generally represented as a continuum from completely homosexual to completely heterosexual, with many individuals finding themselves somewhere in between. Some individuals describe themselves as *asexual,* attracted to neither sex. Some youths are not yet certain of their sexual orientation or gender identity and are referred to as *questioning.* Others may engage in same-gender sexual behavior but may not describe themselves as lesbian, gay, or bisexual (LGB). They are sometimes referred to as *men who have sex with men* (commonly known as MSM) or *women who have sex with women* (commonly known as WSW). *Gender identity* is another important aspect of human sexuality, distinct from sexual orientation; it refers to a person's inner sense of being female, male, or another gender. Although too simplistic a definition, *transgender* individuals are generally described as those whose genetic and anatomic sex may be female or male but whose inner identity is of another gender. *Transgender* may also be used as an umbrella term encompassing the many forms of gender identity and gender expression that are anything other than *cisgender* (the term used to describe people whose birth gender and experienced or expressed gender are the same). When a child displays behaviors, attitudes, or interests outside the cultural norm for the child's biological (genetic or anatomic) sex, the terms *gender nonconforming* or *gender variant expression* may be used to describe these behaviors, attitudes, or interests. More-recent terms include *gender creative* and *gender expansive expression.* The experiences and needs of transgender youths are discussed in Chapter 21, Children With Gender Expression and Identity Issues, which refers to the growing number of clinical guidelines that address these issues.[4,5] Although the term *queer* historically has been considered pejorative, an increasing number of LGBTQ and other individuals across the broad spectrum of gender and sexuality are claiming this term, along with *genderqueer,* as more accurate and positive descriptors of their identity.

Prevalence

The percentage of youths who recognize or eventually will recognize their LGB identities is uncertain. Estimates for gay and lesbian individuals within adult populations range from approximately 3% to 10%, with an even larger percentage being bisexual.[6,7] Whatever the exact percentage, LGB youths are present in all pediatric practices. They exist within all ethnic, religious, and socioeconomic groups and may be more highly represented among youths facing homelessness and youths who have run away and those in the juvenile justice and child welfare systems.[8,9] However, LGB youths are often unrecognized, because they do not fit LGB stereotypes, because they have not yet labeled their orientation as LGB, or because they are reluctant to reveal in health care settings their sexual orientation for fear of clinician disapproval or lack of confidentiality. Many of these individuals likely remain unrecognized because clinicians do not routinely address sexual orientation with their adolescent patients.

Development

The process of LGB identity acquisition is long, complex, and often difficult because of the generally negative societal stance toward nonheterosexual orientations. Several models of LGB identity formation have been proposed, each citing stigma as a major factor influencing development. Troiden[10] and Cass[11] offered early models of identity acquisition, proposing stages of increasing self-acceptance as an individual moves from childhood through adolescence into adulthood. Later research suggests that these models were perhaps too linear, requiring an individual to pass through one stage to the next on the path to full self-acceptance. More recent models suggest more complex and varied developmental paths. They take into account the many factors involved in sexual identity development, which, in addition to biology, include ethnicity, gender, social class, geography, degree of family and community acceptance, life experiences, and personality traits. The clinician should therefore not assume a predefined developmental trajectory for any given patient.[12]

As reflected in the 2004 AAP clinical report and 2013 AAP policy statement, the pediatric profession views heterosexuality, homosexuality, and bisexuality as equally valid and healthy developmental outcomes for youths. This view is consistent with the American Psychiatric Association position that homosexuality is part of the spectrum of normal human sexuality.[13] Homosexuality and bisexuality seem to be well established by early childhood and are not a choice or a matter of something gone wrong. Sexual orientation is likely shaped by biological, genetic, and environmental factors, and these influences may differ for individuals.[12,14] Biological theories have received the strongest research support in recent years. Despite supportive AAP statements and a growing understanding of the biological underpinnings of sexual orientation, significant sectors of American and other societies do not accept the normalcy of homosexuality and bisexuality, seeing them as shameful, sinful, or pathological. This negative view has significant adverse implications for the development of LGB youths.

Environmental Effects

Lesbian, gay, and bisexual youths are ordinary adolescents in every regard except that most grow up in environments that are deeply disapproving of their sexual orientation, a fundamental part of who they are. Research strongly suggests that societal stigma and the resultant stress, victimization, and discrimination under which LGB youths grow up are the primary reasons for the unique physical, emotional, and social problems they face.[7,15–19] While more LGB youths are finding support within their families and communities, many still experience an adolescence of profound isolation, believing they are absolutely alone in their feelings of same-sex attraction. They have little or no access to accurate information about sexual orientation, yet they may be surrounded by a multitude of negative messages about homosexuality coming from their families, schools, churches, and communities and often from people they love and respect. Many LGB youths have little or no access to LGB-supportive clinicians, counselors, or community programs. Some grow up in families and communities where prejudice, discrimination, and violence against LGB individuals are approved or tolerated. Home and school can be especially dangerous places for LGB youths whose sexual orientation is known or presumed. Gender variant youths, whether LGB or straight, seem to be especially vulnerable to victimization and risk for suicidal symptoms.[20,21]

Given the stigma related to homosexuality and their own fears about their emerging same-sex attractions, many LGB youths repress their same-sex feelings or decide to keep them hidden from others, some expending great energy attempting to pass as heterosexual. They may avoid any exploration of their LGB orientation, thereby delaying an essential part of their identity development. Most LGB youths are denied socially approved dating rituals through which adolescents begin to explore, understand, and become comfortable with their sexuality. Many LGB youths have never had sex with another person; others have been only heterosexually active. Some LGB youths realize that the only way to begin exploring their same-sex attractions is through secretive or anonymous sexual encounters; such encounters are likely increasingly facilitated through the Internet. Although these situations are understandable, given the lack of opportunities for sexual socialization enjoyed by heterosexual youths, they are potentially dangerous and may engender feelings of anxiety, guilt, and self-hatred. Some LGB youths are fortunate to live in communities where schools and agencies have begun to provide safe, healthy, and accepting venues, such as school-based gay-straight alliance (commonly known as GSA) clubs, support groups, drop-in centers, dances, and leadership retreats, for LGB adolescents to meet one another and engage in a process of healthy peer socialization.

Lesbian, gay, and bisexual youths of color; LGB youths who immigrated to the United States; LGB youths with a disability; LGB youths who live in a rural area; and LGB youths belonging to a conservative religious faith group may have an especially difficult time understanding and accepting their sexual orientation. This intersection of multiple, often stigmatized or conflicting, identities is thought to place these youths at even greater risk than their LGB peers. In many instances, they have few LGB-supportive resources within their communities and risk rejection if they openly acknowledge or explore their LGB identity.

Some LGB youths, as with other young people who are alone, fearful, and stigmatized, respond in predictable ways, by dropping out of school, running away from home, engaging in risky sex, using drugs, and turning to street life and prostitution.[6,7,22–25] People struggling for survival on the streets often encounter violence and sexual exploitation, with the attendant risks of sexually transmitted infections (STIs) and pregnancy. A significant percentage of LGB youths consider suicide to be their only choice.[26–29] Clinicians should realize that these risky behaviors are not a necessary part of the script for growing up LGB. Research has shown that vulnerable adolescents who grow up in stigmatizing or risky environments thrive when they are connected to safe and supportive families, friends, and communities.[26,30,31] One of the most important roles for clinicians in working with LGB youths is to participate in creating safe environments and supportive networks of family, peers, teachers, counselors, clergy, clinicians, and others to buffer the often hostile society in which LGB youths grow up. An equally important role of the clinician is to remind LGB youths and their families of the positive social changes that are occurring. These changes are evidenced by the expansion of civil rights on many fronts, including same-sex marriage, the increased presence of respected and openly LGB people in media and across many occupations, and the growing acceptance of LGB people across many sectors of American society, including communities of faith.

Evaluation

The 2013 AAP policy statement on office-based care of LGBTQ youths, together with its accompanying technical report as well as *Bright Futures: Guidelines for Health Supervision of Infants, Children, and Adolescents* and other guidelines for health supervision, provides detailed guidance on providing respectful and relevant care to LGBTQ youths.[2,5,32,33] Clinicians should not presume a youth's sexual orientation on the basis of stereotypes or reported sexual behaviors. One of the greatest barriers LGB youths face in receiving appropriate health care is clinicians' belief that they have no LGB youths in their practices. Many LGB youths will deny same-sex attractions or behaviors, even when directly asked. This tendency may result from fear of clinicians' disapproval or lack of confidentiality or of their own uncertainty about their sexual feelings. Fortunately, the goal of pediatric practice is not to identify all LGB youths. Instead, the objective is to create a safe and comfortable clinical setting in which youths can discuss sexual orientation issues when they are ready to do so. This task can be accomplished indirectly through posters, brochures, health questionnaires, and other clinic forms that demonstrate respect for diversity, including diversity of sexual orientation and gender identity. More direct messages come from office staff and clinicians who model respectful attitudes and make no assumptions about sexual orientation or gender identity in their interactions with patients.

Perhaps the strongest message that would allow an LGB youth to open up and discuss these issues is that these issues are raised routinely, in a genuinely interested and nonjudgmental manner, at all teen health supervision visits and any visit suggestive of a youth in distress. It is important that the clinician open the door to discussion, because youths, uncertain of how their clinician may respond, will seldom raise these issues on their own. A candid discussion of sexuality and other personal issues is facilitated further by meeting with the youth alone, without parents or friends present, and accompanied by appropriate assurances of confidentiality. Revealing a youth's LGB orientation to others, including parents, without the youth's consent is unethical and potentially dangerous. If issues of LGB orientation arise, youths should be asked whether they are comfortable with the clinician recording these issues in the medical record. Although there are increasingly frequent recommendations to record sexual orientation and gender identity in the medical record to provide optimal care, LGB youths in particular may have concerns about confidentiality that are justifiable and should be respected. Even with permission, these notations should be made carefully and perhaps indirectly, because parents often have the ability to obtain or review the patient's medical record, including specific parts that should remain confidential.

Clinicians must reflect on their own attitudes and comfort around issues of sexual orientation and consider how their personal biases might affect their ability to provide quality care. Research has shown that many pediatric clinicians are uncomfortable in discussing sexuality, including sexual orientation, with their patients, and this discomfort limits their ability to provide appropriate care.[34,35] Studies of LGB youths reveal that only some of them have ever been asked about or discussed sexual orientation with their pediatricians.[36,37] Research has also demonstrated that many clinicians disapprove of homosexuality.[7] This disapproval makes the provision of appropriate health care and counseling to LGB youths nearly impossible. The failure of clinicians to discuss relevant health issues knowledgeably, comfortably, and nonjudgmentally has been a major barrier to accessing health care for LGB youths. Only when issues of sexual orientation are addressed openly and supportively can appropriate medical screening, treatment, education, counseling, and advocacy be provided. Clinicians who recognize their discomfort or disapproval around issues of sexual orientation should refer youths who may be dealing with these issues to accepting and supportive clinicians.

History

Every annual youth health supervision visit should include a sexual history.[38] Sexual activity, sexual orientation, and sexual decision-making skills should be routinely assessed at these visits.[39,40] Sexual orientation should also be addressed with youths having chronic or recurring somatic concerns or at any acute care visit suggestive of a youth in distress (eg, parent-teen conflict, school problems, substance use, increased heterosexual or homosexual activity, depression, self-harm, unusual displays of anger or frustration). Signs and symptoms of STIs should also prompt an inquiry into sexual practices and orientation.

In addressing sexuality with a patient, the clinician should begin by using gender-neutral language, letting the patient know that no assumptions are made about the patient's sexual orientation or practices. For example, the use of terms such as *partner* rather than *boyfriend* or *girl-friend* and *protection* rather than *birth control* is important until a more complete history has been obtained. The clinician can approach the issue of sexuality first by asking if a youth has ever been in a dating or romantic relationship with another person. If yes, have these relationships been with girls, boys, or both girls and boys? To learn whether a youth has been in a dating or romantic relationship, the clinician also should ask, "Have you ever had sex with another person, including just kissing or touching?" If the answer is yes, again, the clinician should ask, "Has this been with girls, boys, or both boys and girls?" An important point to remember is that the question "Have you ever had sexual intercourse?" may be interpreted as meaning only vaginal intercourse and may not identify youths who have engaged only in petting, oral sex, or anal intercourse.

Clinicians should remember that many LGB youths may have been only heterosexually active or not sexually active with others at all. Youths who have been homosexually active may be afraid to acknowledge same-sex behaviors. Therefore, the clinician should search beyond dating relationships and sexual behaviors and ask all youths whether their feelings of attraction are generally to girls, boys, or both boys and girls. The clinician should also ask about their comfort around these feelings. Many LGB youths have not yet labeled their sexual feelings; therefore, asking patients early in the interview whether they consider themselves gay, lesbian, or bisexual is usually an ineffective and sometimes frightening screening approach for LGB youths. However, as part of a broader discussion over time, asking a youth in a supportive and nonjudgmental manner, "Have you ever wondered if you might be lesbian (or gay or bisexual)?" may be appropriate at some point. Finally, use of the word *homosexual* as a label ("Are you a homosexual?") is thought to be stigmatizing by many LGB people and should be avoided.

In interviewing youths who acknowledge same-sex behaviors or attractions, the clinician should not focus only or even primarily on their sexual practices and the degree to which they use safer sex. Because most of the health risks faced by LGB youths are related not to their sexual behavior but to growing up in a hostile environment, the clinician should address these latter issues in depth before engaging in a detailed discussion of sexual behaviors. For example, the clinician should ask how comfortable LGB youths feel about their same-sex attractions and relationships. How do family background, religion, ethnicity, and community norms play a role in their degree of self-acceptance? The clinician should also ask whether the patient has told others of his or her LGB orientation and whether family members, friends, school counselors, and others have been supportive or rejecting in their responses. In other words, knowing whether an LGB youth is isolated or has a network of supportive family, friends, and adults already in place is important. Another area to explore with LGB youths is the degree to which they think their sexual orientation will limit or enhance their future career, relationships, or acceptance in the community. Can they envision themselves as happy, healthy, and productive LGB adults? What are their concerns or fears, if any? What are their hopes and dreams?

Because some LGB youths respond to stigmatization and rejection by engaging in risky behaviors, the clinician should inquire directly about the possibility of parent-teen conflict, school problems, runaway behavior and street life, sexual exploitation, substance use, eating disorders, depression, suicidal ideation or behavior, and involvement in the child welfare or juvenile justice systems. Because many LGB youths grow up in nonaccepting or even hostile environments, the clinician should ask specifically about their experience of violence in the home, school, and community. When providing care to LGB youths in the child welfare or juvenile justice systems, clinicians should be aware that although there are standards of care recommending respectful and supportive treatment of LGB youths in foster care and other out-of-home settings, they are not always met.[8,9] Therefore, clinicians should respect the confidentiality of LGB youths in these systems, recognizing that disclosure of sexual orientation and gender identity through verbal and written communications and documentation could put these youths at greater risk related to safety and the receipt of appropriate care.

As when treating other sexually active youths, the clinician should ask sexually active LGB youths how comfortable they are with their sexual behaviors and relationships. Specifically, have these behaviors and relationships been healthy and fulfilling or unpleasant and exploitative in nature? A comprehensive health history should also include a detailed sexual history. It should be preceded by an explanation from the clinician that obtaining personal information about sexuality is helpful in providing patients quality care that meets their specific needs. At the same time, patients should be assured that they have a right to answer only specific questions they are comfortable answering. The sexual history should include a discussion of specific sexual behaviors in which the youth is engaged, frequency of activity, consensual and nonconsensual encounters, safer-sex practices, number and nature of partners (age and boyfriend or girlfriend vs acquaintance or anonymous), and how contact with potential partners is made (eg, school, church, malls, parties, the Internet). Few sexual practices exist that are unique to LGB youths; thus, history taking related to this specific issue is similar for both LGB youths and heterosexual youths. Symptoms of STIs should also be elicited, as should any history of combining substance use and sexual activity or exchanging sex for money, drugs, or shelter.

Physical Examination and Laboratory Evaluation

The physical examination and laboratory evaluation of LGB youths, whether sexually active or not, does not differ from that of heterosexual youths.[6] At the same time, clinicians should remember that many LGB youths are *invisible,* so any adolescent may have a history of same-sex activity, although it may not always be acknowledged. Clinicians should also remember that some gay and lesbian youths have been heterosexually active. The content of the physical examination and laboratory evaluation should be determined by a comprehensive health history, including sexual and other risk behaviors, and not by sexual orientation.

Management

As stated in the 2004 AAP clinical guidelines, the goal of care in working with LGB youths is "to promote normal adolescent development, social and emotional well-being, and physical health."[1] Clinicians can help realize this goal not only by focusing on the risks that LGB youths face but also by identifying specific strengths that have allowed them to survive and often thrive in the face of often hostile environments. Historically, because of the serious risks faced by LGB youths, clinicians and allied youth service providers have employed a *risk-reduction model* in addressing the experience and needs of these young people. This model focuses on the vulnerabilities of LGB youths and the need to ameliorate the risks and manage the problems they face. Under this model, healthy adolescent development often seemed to be defined primarily as an avoidance of risk and an absence of negative activities, such as substance use, unsafe sex, dropping out of school, running away from home, or suicidal behavior. Unfortunately, this approach tended to underestimate the strength and resiliency of LGB youths, many of whom presented to their clinicians after having overcome enormous obstacles, including parental rejection, bullying, and internalized homophobia. In working with LGB youths, clinicians should adopt an approach that recognizes and builds on the developmental potential of most LGB youths to overcome the risks and obstacles they encounter. This approach is reflected in the Youth Empowerment and Positive Youth Development models of supporting healthy adolescent development.[41] These approaches seek to support youths in recognizing their strengths and gaining the self-confidence and skills needed to address challenges and create change in their own lives and in the world around them. Clinicians can use this approach in their counseling and encouragement of individual patients. They can also join with others in providing opportunities for LGB youths to assume a leading role in sharing the stories of their lives with others, in creating LGB youth support activities, in achieving leadership skills, and in engaging in civic affairs that address their specific experience and needs. This approach is directly related to risk reduction, but it also transcends this narrow goal by providing opportunities for LGB youths not just to survive but to achieve their full developmental potential and thrive.

Physical Well-being

Lesbian, gay, and bisexual youths face the same kinds of health issues as other youths. Therefore, clinicians should follow AAP policy and *Bright Futures*, 4th Edition, guidelines in providing prevention and screening services to LGB youths.[6,32] The health screening, immunizations, and treatment provided to LGB youths should not be based on sexual orientation but rather on information obtained from an accurate history, physical examination, and evaluative studies. Appendix 2, Mental Health Tools for Pediatrics, lists tools to assist PCCs at various stages in the flow of primary care practice. Nevertheless, many LGB youths face increased risks to health because of societal nonacceptance. Patients who show evidence of substance use, eating disorders, depression, anxiety, and other mental health concerns should be referred to appropriate LGB-supportive community resources. As an LGB youth approaches adulthood, discussions about transition to an LGB-supportive adult health care professional should begin.

Developmental, Social, and Emotional Well-being

Although providing appropriate health care is important, for many LGB youths, the most important role a clinician can play is that of supportive counselor. Youths who acknowledge same-sex or bisexual attractions exhibit varying levels of self-acceptance and differing issues of concern. Therefore, a first step in counseling LGB youths is to listen carefully to their stories, because these will help shape the content of issues to be discussed during the present and subsequent visits. In general, the counseling of LGB youths addresses the following 6 areas: self-acceptance and validation of same-sex attractions; safety; connectedness to supportive others;

self-disclosure, or coming out; healthy relationships and sexual decision-making; and optimism for the future. Clinicians often focus their counseling of LGB youths only on sexual activity, risk for STIs, and safer-sex practices. However, addressing each of the 6 areas is important in ensuring the healthy development of LGB youths.

Self-acceptance and Validation

Most youths grow up surrounded by negative messages about LGB sexual orientation and the presumption that heterosexuality is the only acceptable orientation. These messages often come from people they love and respect and have a negative effect on the health and development of LGB youths. Lesbian, gay, and bisexual youths often think they are sick or sinful because of their emerging sexual feelings and are filled with shame and self-hatred. The clinician should try to determine the degree of comfort each LGB youth has with emerging sexual feelings and discuss the youth's specific concerns or fears. While acknowledging that some cultures and communities may view LGB orientation as unhealthy or wrong, the clinician should state clearly that the pediatric profession considers homosexuality and bisexuality to be healthy and normal. They are not a choice and do not represent something gone wrong. This emphatic reassurance of normalcy from the pediatric perspective is perhaps the most powerful and important statement that a clinician can make to an LGB youth. The clinician should also determine a youth's accuracy of knowledge about sexual orientation and correct any misconceptions. Some LGB youths are frightened by LGB stereotypes, thinking these somehow represent who they are as a person. The clinician should remind LGB youths that the stereotypes do not define who they are; rather, they, in their own individuality, help define what it means to be LGB. Lesbian, gay, and bisexual youths of an ethnic or another minority may have an especially difficult time as they try to manage more than 1 type of stigma. The clinician should recognize and discuss this difficult reality with the patient. Letting the LGB youth know that growing self-acceptance of a person's sexual orientation is an evolutionary process is helpful. The uncertainty and discomfort this youth may experience now will likely diminish or disappear as he or she moves into adulthood.

If a youth denies same-sex attractions, yet the clinician or others think that it is an issue that may emerge later in the youth's life, the clinician can simply say, "This may or may not ever be a part of your life, and I hear you telling me clearly today that it is not. I just want you to know that, as your clinician, I will always be here for you and available to discuss any issues that come up in your life as you grow older."

For youths who express uncertainty about their sexual orientation, the clinician can say, "It's not my place to tell you if you are gay, lesbian, bisexual, or straight; only you can discover this for yourself. What I can do is provide you information and support and let you know that whoever you finally discover you are is all right. The most important thing is that you are happy and comfortable with who you are, no matter what your sexual orientation might be." It is not unusual for some youths to go through stages during which they think they are gay, then straight, then bisexual, and then gay again. This uncertainty is part of the normal process of self-discovery and will eventually be resolved, although not necessarily during adolescence. The clinician should not tell youths who are experiencing same-sex attractions that they are "just going through a phase." For a significant percentage of youths, these feelings do, in fact, represent an emerging LGB identity, and false reassurances to the contrary can be harmful. Clinicians should be ready to link youths who are LGB or questioning with supportive national organizations that maintain Web sites providing accurate and validating information and resources for young people. In addition to examples mentioned in the Isolation and Optimism for the Future sections that follow, the Centers for Disease Control and Prevention offer resources for LGBT youths at www.cdc.gov/lgbthealth/youth-resources.htm. Other organizations provide tools for clinicians to help them engage LGB youths and their families.

Safety

Many LGB youths grow up in environments that are potentially harmful to their physical, emotional, and developmental health. Many of these individuals endure harassment and bullying, discrimination, or social rejection; at the very least, many are surrounded by negative messages about LGB orientation. These dangers may arise at home, school, or church and within the peer group or the broader community. Clinicians should ask LGB youths about their safety in each of these settings. If a youth acknowledges teasing, harassment, or other harmful treatment, the clinician should work with the youth to identify and implement appropriate strategies to end the violence. Unfortunately, many LGB youths are filled with shame and are afraid to advocate for their own safety. They may feel that reporting harassment will only make the situation worse. They often think that they deserve the harm inflicted on them, or they simply accept the situation as normal. The clinician should tell youths clearly that they have done nothing to deserve such treatment and that they should expect and demand safety and respect from everyone in their lives and in all settings. Because LGB youths have so few advocates, the clinician should offer to join with the youth in approaching every venue in which the youth experiences violence, including the home and school, to work out a plan to end violence immediately and completely. If necessary, the clinician should call on the state child protective services or advocacy organizations such as the American Civil Liberties Union to join in the effort to keep the youth safe.

Isolation

Lesbian, gay, and bisexual youths are among the most isolated of youths. Although societal changes in attitude toward homosexuality have been significant, many LGB youths continue to have little or no access to accurate and supportive information about sexual orientation, and many know of no accepting and supportive counselors in their schools or communities. At a time when they should begin exploring their sexuality, most LGB youths have no safe venues in which to meet other LGB youths. Many of them have distanced themselves emotionally or become estranged from their parents and siblings. Many LGB youths believe they are the only ones they know who are experiencing same-sex attractions. Few of them have visible LGB adult role models in their communities to provide reassurance that a happy and rewarding adulthood is attainable. As with any other young people, isolation and loneliness can lead to compromised physical and emotional health, including increased risk for anxiety and depression. Clinicians should routinely screen for these possibilities and address the issue of isolation by giving accurate information about sexual orientation. They should provide supportive and reassuring counseling, or they should refer the youth to LGB-supportive colleagues who have the time, comfort, and expertise to do so. They should connect LGB youths to local community resources, such as support groups and other youth programs for LGB youths. Lesbian, gay, and bisexual youths who do not have access to local programs should be informed about Web sites created for LGB youths, such as The Trevor Project at www.thetrevorproject.org, from which they can receive accurate information and communicate with other LGB youths in a safe, monitored setting. Clinicians can also point out positive LGB youth and adult role models in the community or nationally. In certain circumstances, for LGB clinicians to present themselves openly as role models to LGB youths and their families is also appropriate. Such disclosure should be done only after careful consideration of the clinician's own confidentiality needs and how sharing such information might affect, either positively or negatively, the clinician-patient/family relationship.

Self-disclosure, or Coming Out

Lesbian, gay, and bisexual youths often reach a point in their development at which they feel a strong urge to disclose their sexual orientation to others, referred to as *coming out*. The process of disclosure to family and friends is often emotional and frequently traumatic. Youths who come out risk condemnation and rejection by family and peers. Disclosure can also result in physical violence at home and at school. Therefore, coming out should be considered carefully, weighing the risks and benefits. If a youth expects a negative response from his or her parents, the youth should wait to disclose until legally and financially independent. However, many youths think that continuing to live a lie is intolerable and harmful to their self-esteem; therefore, they come out to their parents much earlier. Under no circumstances should a clinician reveal a youth's orientation to parents without permission. A clinician can play an important role in the process of disclosure by helping young people decide whether they are ready to come out to family or friends and helping them choose an appropriate time, place, and approach for disclosure.

Healthy Relationships and Sexual Decision-making

Although some LGB youths manage to meet other LGB youths and establish friendships and dating relationships, most do not. Clinicians should help connect LGB youths to local LGB youth support groups and LGB-supportive programs in the community if they exist. This task can be accomplished ethically without parental notification. Clinicians can suggest national telephone hotlines or Web sites from which LGB youths can receive accurate information and supportive counseling and communicate with other LGB youths. If these options are not available, the clinician can serve as a supportive and reassuring lifeline until the young person is old enough to become independent and possibly move away to work or go to school in a community more accepting of LGB people.

Lesbian, gay, and bisexual youths who are in relationships face many of the same questions as their heterosexual peers. "Am I in love?" "What do I want from a relationship?" "Do I really want to be in this relationship?" "How do I know if this is a good relationship?" "How do I get out of this relationship?" An LGB-supportive clinician or counselor can help youths reflect on and find answers to these questions.

As with other youths, many LGB youths know little about sexuality and how to make healthy sexual choices. Abstinence is always the appropriate option for young people who do not feel ready for a sexual relationship.

Lesbian, gay, and bisexual youths should understand that when they are ready for a sexual relationship, they can expect to lead healthy and fulfilling sexual lives. All youths who have decided that they are ready for a sexual relationship should be advised to limit their number of sexual partners and avoid mixing sex and alcohol or drugs so as to reduce their risk for infection, trauma, and sexual assault. Safer-sex practices related to oral, vaginal, and anal sex should be reviewed in detail. Lesbian, gay, and bisexual youths should also be aware that *no always means no* in negotiating sex, and any forced or coerced sexual experience represents sexual assault. Lesbian, gay, and bisexual youths should also understand that no set LGB repertoire of sexual behaviors exists and that they should engage only in sexual practices with which they are comfortable.

Optimism for the Future

Clinicians should challenge the belief of many LGB youths that their futures will be significantly limited by their sexual orientation. Referral of LGB youths to the It Gets Better Project Web site (www.itgetsbetter.org) can be especially helpful. Although some communities are clearly more accepting of LGB people than others, most LGB adults lead happy, healthy, and productive lives. Lesbian, gay, and bisexual youths should be encouraged to pursue any career they wish. They should expect to have deep, long-lasting, and fulfilling relationships throughout their lives. They should expect to be respected and valued members of their communities. They should also understand that marriage and parenthood are enhancing the lives of thousands of LGB adults across the United States. They may also be enhancing the well-being of LGB youths. A recent study based on Youth Risk Behavior Surveillance System (commonly known as YRBSS) data found that state same-sex marriage policies were associated with a reduction in adolescent suicide attempts, especially among LGB youths.[42] Although growing up LGB is often challenging, the future should be seen as hopeful and exciting.

Parents

Parents who learn of their son or daughter's LGB orientation often experience an intense mix of emotions. Some respond to this new understanding of their child with ready support and expressions of love. Many others feel varying degrees of guilt, shame, fear, anger, repulsion, and profound sadness. Many parents go through a deep mourning period, feeling as if they have lost the child they knew and loved. Some parents will reject or physically and emotionally abuse an LGB youth. Parents are often as isolated from accurate information and supportive resources as are their children. Clinicians should listen patiently and respectfully to parents' concerns and fears, acknowledging their pain and sense of loss. The clinician should emphasize the importance of their continued expressions of love for their child, especially at this time when many youths think that they will lose their parents' love and support. At the same time, the clinician can acknowledge that understanding and acceptance of their child's sexual orientation is an evolutionary process and will take time. Nevertheless, parents should be informed of the growing research-based understanding that parental rejection is a predictor of negative health outcomes for LGBTQ youths, including substance use, risky sexual behaviors, suicidal ideation, and limited hopes for a happy future.[43] Therefore, while acknowledging that negative responses to a youth's disclosure of LGB identity may come from a place of genuine concern and love, it is essential that clinicians engage families in supporting their LGB youths through increased acceptance. Parents should be reassured that they did nothing wrong and that the pediatric profession has come to accept homosexuality and bisexuality as normal and healthy developmental outcomes. To decrease their isolation, parents can be referred to the online AAP patient education Web page titled "Gay, Lesbian, and Bisexual Teens: Information for Teens and Parents" at www.healthychildren.org/English/ages-stages/teen/dating-sex/Pages/Gay-Lesbian-and-Bisexual-Teens-Facts-for-Teens-and-Their-Parents.aspx. They should be referred to relevant books, Web sites, and support programs for parents and families of LGB youths such as the Family Acceptance Project at http://familyproject.sfsu.edu. One of the most prominent national parent support organizations is PFLAG (www.pflag.org), which has many local affiliate groups across the country. Parents should be reassured that American society as a whole is becoming increasingly accepting of LGB people. By providing love, support, and protection, parents should expect their adolescent to achieve a happy, healthy, and rewarding adulthood.

The clinician should discourage any parental search for treatment that is directed at changing their son's or daughter's sexual orientation. Such *reparative therapy* or similar religion-based *transformational ministries* are considered by the pediatric profession to be both unethical and dangerous. Finally, clinicians who think that they are unable to give LGB-supportive counseling to families should refer them to colleagues who have the time, comfort, and expertise to provide such support.

Mental Health Advocacy

One of the most important roles that clinicians can play in ensuring the optimal mental health and safety of LGB youths is that of advocate. The advocacy role is essential, even lifesaving, because many LGB youths grow up in extremely hostile environments and have few, if any, advocates in their families or communities. Clinicians' expertise is respected, and their offering of visible and confident support for LGB youths can promote increased community awareness, understanding, and acceptance, which are essential for the healthy development of these youths.

Advocacy can take place on many levels. On an individual patient level, clinicians can meet with families, school officials, social welfare agency staff, mental health care providers, and others to ensure that their patient is safe and accepted in the home, school, and community. They should also ensure that clinic and hospital policies and practices reflect respect for LGB patients. At a community level, clinicians can participate in educational forums that present the pediatric perspective that LGB orientations are normal and healthy. Clinicians should be willing to go to schools and school boards, child welfare agencies, juvenile detention and correctional institutions, city councils, legislatures, and faith communities to advocate for policies and programs that specifically ensure the respectful treatment and address the special needs of LGB youths. National guidelines have been developed addressing these issues.[8,9]

In addition, clinicians can advocate for school curricula, extracurricular programs, and library holdings that reflect the diversity of students and their families, including diversity of sexual orientation and gender identity. Furthermore, they should advocate for the development and implementation of robust medical school, residency training, and continuing medical education curricula that include an in-depth consideration of the development, life experiences, and health needs of LGB youths and adults and provide the skills to work with these populations respectfully and effectively. This effort is especially important because, for many LGB youths, a supportive clinician may be the only lifeline they have ensuring safe passage into a happy, healthy, and rewarding adulthood.

When to Refer

► When a youth has acute or recurrent suicidal ideation
► When a youth is engaged in high-risk behaviors
► When the clinician decides that time, expertise, or comfort is insufficient to provide LGB-supportive care and counseling
► When a youth's physical, emotional, or developmental well-being and safety may be at risk because of family nonacceptance

Referral should be made only to pediatric, adolescent medicine, adult medical, or mental health specialists who have experience in working with LGB youths and who accept same-sex attractions as normal and healthy. Referrals for reparative therapy or to transformational ministries are unethical and potentially dangerous.

AAP Policy

American Academy of Pediatrics Committee on Adolescence. Office-based care for lesbian, gay, bisexual, transgender, and questioning youth. *Pediatrics.* 2013;132(1):198–203 (pediatrics.aappublications.org/content/132/1/198)

References

1. Frankowski BL; American Academy of Pediatrics Committee on Adolescence. Sexual orientation and adolescents. *Pediatrics.* 2004;113(6):1827–1832
2. American Academy of Pediatrics Committee on Adolescence. Office-based care for lesbian, gay, bisexual, transgender, and questioning youth. *Pediatrics.* 2013;132(1):198–203
3. Society for Adolescent Health and Medicine. Recommendations for promoting the health and well-being of lesbian, gay, bisexual, and transgender adolescents: a position paper of the Society for Adolescent Health and Medicine. *J Adolesc Health.* 2013;52(4):506–510
4. Makadon HJ, Mayer KH, Potter J, Goldhammer H, eds. *The Fenway Guide to Lesbian, Gay, Bisexual, and Transgender Health.* Philadelphia, PA: American College of Physicians; 2008
5. Gay and Lesbian Medical Association. *Guidelines for Care of Lesbian, Gay, Bisexual, and Transgender Patients.* San Francisco, CA: Gay and Lesbian Medical Association; 2006. http://glma.org/_data/n_0001/resources/live/GLMA%20guidelines%202006%20FINAL.pdf. Accessed January 25, 2018
6. Levine DA; American Academy of Pediatrics Committee on Adolescence. Office-based care for lesbian, gay, bisexual, transgender, and questioning youth. *Pediatrics.* 2013;132(1): e297–e313
7. Institute of Medicine. *The Health of Lesbian, Gay, Bisexual, and Transgender People: Building a Foundation for Better Understanding.* Washington, DC: National Academies Press; 2011
8. Wilber S, Ryan C, Marksamer J. *CWLA Best Practice Guidelines: Serving LGBT Youth in Out-of-Home Care.* Washington, DC: Child Welfare League of America; 2006
9. Majd K, Marksamer J, Reyes C. *Hidden Injustice: Lesbian, Gay, Bisexual, and Transgender Youth in Juvenile Courts.* San Francisco, CA: National Center for Lesbian Rights; 2009
10. Troiden RR. Homosexual identity development. *J Adolesc Health Care.* 1988;9(2):105–113
11. Cass VC. Homosexual identity formation: a theoretical model. *J Homosex.* 1979;4(3):219–235

12. Adelson SL; American Academy of Child and Adolescent Psychiatry Committee on Quality Issues. Practice parameter on gay, lesbian, or bisexual sexual orientation, gender nonconformity, and gender discordance in childhood and adolescence. *J Am Acad Child Adolesc Psychiatry*. 2012;51(9):957–974

13. American Psychiatric Association. *Diagnostic and Statistical Manual of Mental Disorders*. 5th ed. Washington, DC: American Psychiatric Association; 2013

14. Savin-Williams RC, Cohen KM. Homoerotic development during childhood and adolescence. *Child Adolesc Psychiatr Clin N Am*. 2004;13(3):529–549

15. Bontempo DE, D'Augelli AR. Effects of at-school victimization and sexual orientation on lesbian, gay, or bisexual youths' health risk behavior. *J Adolesc Health*. 2002;30(5):364–374

16. Ryan C, Rivers I. Lesbian, gay, bisexual and transgender youth: victimization and its correlates in the USA and UK. *Cult Health Sex*. 2003;5(2):103–119

17. Pilkington NW, D'Augelli AR. Victimization of lesbian, gay, and bisexual youth in community settings. *J Community Psychol*. 1995;23:34–56

18. Berlan ED, Corliss HL, Field AE, Goodman E, Austin SB. Sexual orientation and bullying among adolescents in the Growing Up Today study. *J Adolesc Health*. 2010;46(4):366–371

19. Hatzenbuehler ML, Pachankis JE. Stigma and minority stress as social determinants of health among lesbian, gay, bisexual, and transgender youth: research evidence and clinical implications. *Pediatr Clin North Am*. 2016;63(6):985–997

20. Friedman MS, Koeske GF, Silvestre AJ, Korr WS, Sites EW. The impact of gender-role nonconforming behavior, bullying, and social support on suicidality among gay male youth. *J Adolesc Health*. 2006;38(5):621–623

21. Fitzpatrick KK, Euton SJ, Jones JN, Schmidt NB. Gender role, sexual orientation and suicide risk. *J Affect Disord*. 2005;87(1):35–42

22. Marshal MP, Friedman MS, Stall R, et al. Sexual orientation and adolescent substance use: a meta-analysis and methodological review. *Addiction*. 2008;103(4):546–556

23. Kann L, Olsen EO, McManus T, et al. Sexual identity, sex of sexual contacts, and health-risk behaviors among students in grades 9–12–youth risk behavior surveillance, selected sites, United States, 2001–2009. *MMWR Surveill Summ*. 2011;60(7):1–133

24. Rice E, Barman-Adhikari A, Rhoades H, et al. Homelessness experiences, sexual orientation, and sexual risk taking among high school students in Los Angeles. *J Adolesc Health*. 2013;52(6):773–778

25. Tornello SL, Riskind RG, Patterson CJ. Sexual orientation and sexual and reproductive health among adolescent young women in the United States. *J Adolesc Health*. 2014;54(2):160–168

26. Eisenberg ME, Resnick MD. Suicidality among gay, lesbian and bisexual youth: the role of protective factors. *J Adolesc Health*. 2006;39(5):662–668

27. Hatzenbuehler ML. The social environment and suicide attempts in lesbian, gay, and bisexual youth. *Pediatrics*. 2011;127(5):896–903

28. Liu RT, Mustanski B. Suicidal ideation and self-harm in lesbian, gay, bisexual, and transgender youth. *Am J Prev Med*. 2012;42(3):221–228

29. Silenzio VM, Pena JB, Duberstein PR, Cerel J, Knox KL. Sexual orientation risk factors for suicidal ideation and suicide attempts among adolescents and young adults. *Am J Public Health*. 2007;97(11):2017–2019

30. Blum RW, McNeely C, Nonnemaker J. Vulnerability, risk, and protection. *J Adolesc Health*. 2002;31(1)(suppl):28–39

31. Saewyc EM, Homma Y, Skay CL, et al. Protective factors in the lives of bisexual adolescents in North America. *Am J Public Health*. 2009;99(1):110–117

32. Hagan JF Jr, Shaw JS, Duncan PM, eds. *Bright Futures: Guidelines for Health Supervision of Infants, Children, and Adolescents*. 4th ed. Elk Grove Village, IL: American Academy of Pediatrics; 2017

33. Coker TR, Austin SB, Schuster MA. The health and health care of lesbian, gay, and bisexual adolescents. *Annu Rev Public Health*. 2010;31:457–477

34. East JA, El Rayess F. Pediatricians' approach to the health care of lesbian, gay, and bisexual youth. *J Adolesc Health*. 1998;23(4):191–193

35. Lena SM, Wiebe T, Ingram S, Jabbour M. Pediatricians' knowledge, perceptions, and attitudes towards providing health care for lesbian, gay, and bisexual adolescents. *Ann R Coll Physicians Surg Can*. 2002;35(7):406–410

36. Allen LB, Glicken AD, Beach RK, Naylor KE. Adolescent health care experience of gay, lesbian, and bisexual young adults. *J Adolesc Health*. 1998;23(4):212–220

37. Meckler GD, Elliott MN, Kanouse DE, Beals KP, Schuster MA. Nondisclosure of sexual orientation to a physician among a sample of gay, lesbian, and bisexual youth. *Arch Pediatr Adolesc Med*. 2006;160(12):1248–1254

38. Goldenring JM, Rosen DS. Getting into adolescent heads: an essential update. *Contemp Pediatr*. 2004;21:64–90

39. Garofalo R, Harper GW. Not all adolescents are the same: addressing the unique needs of gay and bisexual male youth. *Adolesc Med*. 2003;14(3):595–611

40. Catallozzi M, Rudy BJ. Lesbian, gay, bisexual, transgendered, and questioning youth: the importance of a sensitive and confidential sexual history in identifying the risk and implementing treatment for sexually transmitted infections. *Adolesc Med Clin*. 2004;15(2): 353–367

41. Russel ST, Muraco A, Subramanium A, Laub C. Youth empowerment and high school Gay-Straight Alliances. *J Youth Adolesc*. 2009;38(7):891–903

42. Raifman J, Moscoe E, Austin SB, McConnell M. Difference-in-differences analysis of the association between state same-sex marriage policies and adolescent suicide attempts. *JAMA Pediatr*. 2017;171(4):350–356

43. Ryan C, Huebner D, Diaz RM, Sanchez J. Family rejection as a predictor of negative health outcomes in white and Latino lesbian, gay, and bisexual young adults. *Pediatrics*. 2009;123(1):346–352

Children With Gender Expression and Identity Issues

Robert J. Bidwell, MD

"The goal of pediatric clinicians is not to identify every child with gender variant behaviors or transgender identity; instead, it is to create a safe and accepting clinical setting in which children, youths, and their families know they can discuss any topic of concern, including gender identity and expression, without discomfort or disapproval on the part of the clinician."

Introduction

Throughout history and across many cultures, children and adolescents have, through their gender expression and gender identity, transcended cultural expectations about the meaning of being a girl or a boy.[1-4] In some times and places, as these children and adolescents grew into adulthood, they became respected and even revered members of their societies. In others, including the current culture in many parts of the United States, they have been seen as legitimate targets of discrimination and persecution. Issues related to gender expression and gender identity are often highly controversial, and the understanding of them is evolving on the basis of increased research and societal changes. In 2013, the American Academy of Pediatrics (AAP) issued a policy statement and accompanying technical report on office-based care of youths who are lesbian, gay, bisexual, transgender, or questioning (commonly known as LGBTQ).[5,6] These publications give pediatric clinicians (ie, primary care pediatricians, pediatric subspecialists, and family physicians, internists, nurse practitioners, and physician assistants who provide care to children and adolescents) the basic understanding and skills to work in a respectful and relevant manner with young people facing issues related to sexual orientation and gender identity. A similar position paper has been issued by the Society for Adolescent Health and Medicine.[7] Both statements emphasize that among the most important challenges facing gender variant and transgender children and *youths* (a term used in this chapter to encompass preadolescents through young adults) are achieving optimal physical and mental health while growing up in the context of often disapproving family and community environments. They also stress the essential role that clinicians can play in facilitating the physical, social, and psychological well-being of these children and youths.

Definitions

A consideration of gender expression and identity in childhood requires a brief examination of commonly used terms and concepts (Table 21-1). While sex and gender are often conflated in popular usage, they are, in fact, distinct concepts. An individual's *sex* is usually assigned at birth (*birth-assigned sex*) as female or male, and this is usually done on the basis of a child's genital anatomy. If the anatomy is ambiguous, gender may be determined on the basis of other biological indicators, such as chromosomes. In contrast to sex, which is a biological attribute, *gender* is a social construct, varying among cultures. It may reflect a binary conceptualization of what it means to be female or male, but it may also include a more expansive nonbinary view of various gender possibilities, with distinct roles, responsibilities, expression, and behaviors associated with each. Assigning sex at birth on the basis of anatomy usually leads to assumptions about a child's gender (*birth-assigned gender*), but since it is impossible to consult infants on their personal sense of gender identity or predict their future expression of gender, these assumptions are sometimes later discovered to be incorrect.

Gender expression represents the ways in which individuals express their gender in dress, grooming, speech, mannerisms, interests, and other gendered characteristics as defined by a particular culture. Gender expression is not intrinsically tied to biological sex, gender identity, or sexual orientation. In contrast, *gender identity* is an individual's deep inner sense of being female or male, somewhere in between, or another gender.

Different cultures have varying expectations related to appropriate roles, responsibilities, expression, and behaviors related to gender. Traditionally, in Western cultures there has been a binary division of gender into female and male, with strict culturally defined expectations for each, which are often rigorously enforced. Yet, clearly there have always been individuals

Table 21-1. Definition of Terms Related to Sex, Gender, and Sexual Orientation

Term	Definition
Sex	The combination of chromosomes, hormones, reproductive anatomy, and secondary sexual characteristics, often divided into male, female, and a variety of intersex conditions
Birth-assigned sex	The sex assigned to an individual at birth, usually based on the child's genital anatomy
Gender identity	The deep inner sense of being male or female, somewhere in between, or another gender. It may or may not be congruent with others' assumptions of an individual's gender based on birth-assigned sex.
Gender expression	The ways in which an individual expresses her/his gender (in dress, grooming, mannerisms, speech, interests, and other gendered characteristics), regardless of biological sex, sexual orientation, or gender identity
Gender variant	Having characteristics or expression that does not conform to culturally defined expectations around male and female appearance, behavior, or identity. Sometimes referred to as *gender nonconforming, gender diverse, gender expansive, gender creative,* or *gender atypical.*
Transgender	Having an inner gender identity that is culturally considered incongruent with one's birth-assigned sex
Cisgender	Having an inner gender identity that is culturally considered congruent with one's birth-assigned sex
Gender dysphoria	Distress or discomfort related to the perceived incongruence between one's inner gender identity and one's birth-assigned sex
Transition	The process of physical, emotional, social, legal, psychological, and physical change experienced by transgender individuals to increasingly embrace and reflect their inner gender identity
Sexual orientation	A person's enduring pattern of sexual, romantic, and emotional attraction to people of the same or different sex

who transcend this gender binary by expressing their gender and professing a gender identity outside the cultural norm. These individuals, including children and adolescents, have been referred to as *gender variant* (the term used in this chapter), *gender diverse, gender expansive, gender creative, gender nonconforming,* and *gender atypical*—all synonymous.

Among gender variant children and youths are those who self-identify as *transgender.* These are individuals who come to recognize that their inner gender identity differs from the cultural gender expectations associated with their birth-assigned sex. People whose gender identity is congruent with these cultural expectations are referred to as *cisgender.* Transgender individuals, including children and youths, prefer that others refer to them on the basis of their gender identity, not their birth-assigned sex. Thus, female-to-male (FTM) transgender individuals should be referred to as *transgender* (or *trans*) *boys or men,* and male-to-female (MTF) transgender individuals should be referred to as *transgender* (or *trans*) *girls or women,* even if legal documents or medical registration information do not yet reflect this reality. Some transgender youths may alternatively describe themselves as *transfeminine* (MTF) or *transmasculine* (FTM). Understandably, like their cisgender peers, many transgender youths prefer to be referred to simply as a *boy* or a *girl,* on the basis of their gender identity.

More and more non-cisgender individuals describe themselves using terms other than *transgender,* which they feel has binary implications and limits their ability to describe their gender as anything other than female or male. Instead, they may refer to themselves as *gender nonbinary, genderqueer, genderfluid, agender,* or *pangender* or in other ways that transcend the binary female-male view of gender.

Some, but not all, transgender individuals experience *gender dysphoria.* This can be described as significant discomfort or distress related to a perceived noncongruence between a person's gender identity and birth-assigned sex. Dysphoria may be related to a person's gendered physical attributes reflecting birth-assigned sex. It may also be related to growing up in a society enforcing a strict gender binary and unaccepting of gender variance.

Most transgender individuals experience a process of *transition,* often beginning in childhood and extending through adolescence into adulthood. It can take many forms and often involves social, emotional, psychological, legal, and physical changes through which transgender individuals increasingly embrace and reflect to the world their inner gender identity. Transition may, but does not necessarily, include gender-affirming hormonal and surgical treatments. (See Understanding the Choices Ahead section later in this chapter.)

Clinicians should be careful not to conflate gender identity with *sexual orientation.* Sexual orientation refers to a person's pattern of sexual, romantic, and emotional attraction to people of the same or another sex. Both transgender people and cisgender people may be lesbian, gay, or bisexual (LGB); asexual; or straight. Conversely, an individual who is LGB, asexual, or straight may be transgender or cisgender.

Prevalence of Gender Variance

The prevalence of gender variant expression and identity among children and youths is uncertain. In a 2011 population-based survey of middle school students in San Francisco, 1.3% self-identified as transgender.[8] Several recent studies looking at clinical samples of children referred to gender clinics have suggested that about 2% to 6% of boys and 5% to 12% of girls display gender variant behavior.[9] Most gender variant children and youths do not experience gender dysphoria and, in the absence of population-based surveys, the prevalence of gender dysphoria in childhood and adolescence is unknown. Research has demonstrated, however, that referrals of children and youths to gender clinics have increased over recent years.[10] Also, the prevalence of gender variant expression seems to decrease with age from childhood into adolescence, likely because of a variety of factors including the increasing social pressure to conform to cultural gender norms as a child grows older.[9]

The prevalence of transgenderism within the adult population is somewhat better understood. A recent meta-analysis of research surveys reports that about 1 in 250 adults in the United States is transgender.[11] This is considered an underestimate of actual prevalence because studies included in the analysis relied on clinical samples of adults seeking hormonal or surgical transition treatments. Not all transgender adults desire such treatments, or they may seek care outside the usual health care system. Others may not be able to access these treatments because of financial, geographic, medical, or other barriers. Another reason that adult data cannot be extrapolated to children and youths is the findings of research showing that a significant number of children diagnosed as having gender dysphoria in childhood no longer fit criteria for gender dysphoria as adolescents or adults.[10,12]

Historical Perspective

Until 2013, transgenderism appeared in the American Psychiatric Association (APA) *Diagnostic and Statistical Manual of Mental Disorders* (*DSM*) under the rubric "Gender Identity Disorder"(GID).[13] Its appearance in the *DSM* had long been controversial, as a growing body of research supported an increased professional understanding that the issue of concern was not gender identity per se, but rather *dysphoria* related to gender identity. In preparation for the publication of the *DSM-5* in 2013, an APA working group conducted a rigorous review of this research and recommended that issues related to transgenderism should henceforth be addressed under the rubric "Gender Dysphoria," as it now appears in the current *DSM*.[14] New research-based diagnostic criteria were established both for children and for adolescents and adults. Both sets of criteria require a marked difference between an individual's experienced or expressed gender and the gender assigned at birth. They also require that this gender incongruence must have persisted for at least 6 months and resulted in significant distress or impairment in social, school, occupational, or other important areas of functioning.

It is important for clinicians to recognize that, per the *DSM-5*, simply being transgender, gender nonbinary, or gender variant is not a concern. The issue of concern is *dysphoria* related to gender, which may have varying sources for transgender individuals. For some, distress and impairment may derive from a perceived deep incongruence between their inner gender identity and the physical realities associated with their birth-assigned sex. However, research has shown that distress may also be the predictable result of stigmatization, discrimination, and violence that often accompanies being gender variant in a society that espouses and strictly enforces a binary view of gender. Evidence suggests that transgender individuals who grow up in accepting and supportive environments experience less distress and impairment,[15] supporting an understanding that these are not innate characteristics of being transgender.

Developmental Trajectories of Gender Variant Children

The developmental trajectories of gender variant and gender dysphoric children are diverse and unpredictable.[16] Studies in this area have relied on clinical rather than population-based samples, and sometimes reflect a conflation of behaviors with identity, as well as cross-gender identity with gender dysphoria. Not all children expressing a cross-gender identity experience distress or impairment, especially when raised in safe and affirming environments.

Children generally have a sense of their own gender at about age 2 years, and the appearance of behaviors not generally considered typical of a child's birth-assigned sex can also appear around this time.[9] Only a small percentage of these gender variant children will also express having a cross-gender identity or meet the diagnostic criteria for childhood gender dysphoria. Research has shown that most gender dysphoric children will no longer meet criteria for gender dysphoria in adolescence and adulthood.[10,17,18] These children are referred to as *desisters* in the research literature. A significant percentage will eventually self-identify as cisgender as adolescents and adults, with many eventually reporting a gay, lesbian, or bisexual orientation. About 12% to 27% of children with gender dysphoria will continue to meet criteria for gender dysphoria in adolescence (referred to as *persisters*), and most will eventually self-identify as transgender or gender nonbinary.[19] Youths likeliest to persist in their expression of cross-gender identity beyond childhood, whether gender dysphoric or not, include those who have a greater number and intensity of gender variant behaviors in childhood, who exhibit these at a younger age, who have expressed "being" the other gender rather than simply "wishing" to be the other gender, and who have been persistent, insistent, and consistent in asserting their cross-gender identity throughout childhood and into adolescence.[10,19,20]

For some individuals, gender dysphoria does not appear until adolescence or adulthood.[19]

Etiology of Gender Variance

Considerable controversy exists around possible causes for the development of persistent gender variant expression, cross-gender identity, and gender dysphoria, which are related yet distinct phenomena.[21] Theories proposed have suggested psychosocial, biological, and genetic factors, or varying combinations thereof. However, research data are very limited, often narrowly focused, and sometimes contradictory. Nevertheless, among all theories offered, those suggesting a biological or genetic basis for cross-gender expression and identity are gathering the most robust scientific interest and support. Recent reviews have documented what little is known and how much still needs to be learned about the origins of gender identity and expression and the developmental trajectories experienced by gender variant and gender dysphoric children and youths.[16]

Psychosocial theories seeking to explain gender variant expression and gender dysphoria often focus on familial, and particularly parental psychopathology, and aberrant parenting practices that may interact with biological factors and predispose a child to gender dysphoria.[19,22] Zucker, for example, posits that some children may experience subtle biologically or genetically related prenatal events affecting areas of the brain that lead to gender variant behavior or personality traits.[23] These theories suggest that brain effects may in turn interact with parenting styles or psychopathology that encourages persistent gender variant behaviors and possibly the development of gender dysphoria. Much of the controversy around such theories, in addition to a lack of robust scientific evidence to support them, is that many feel they are similar to earlier theories related to the origins of homosexuality, later discredited, that saw aberrant parenting and familial psychopathology as probable etiologies. An understanding of this controversy is especially important because research demonstrates that many gender variant and gender dysphoric children later come to recognize a cisgender identity and LGB orientation in adolescence or adulthood. Psychosocial theories are no longer widely accepted as primary causal explanations for variances in gender expression and identity, while their role in informing the treatment approach to gender dysphoria remains highly controversial.[24–26] Some have suggested that a likelier route to gender dysphoria for some children is growing up in a home and community that pathologizes their gender expression and identity,[26] although this theory, like all others, lacks robust research support at this time.

Most recent scientific attention has focused on possible biological, genetic, and neurological explanations for gender variant expression, cross-gender identity, and gender dysphoria.[27] No clear unequivocal biological markers for these have been identified, but early limited findings are intriguing and invite further research. Recent research provides incomplete but increasing evidence for a genetic component to gender variance and cross-gender identity.[28–30] Another focus of biomedical inquiry has been comparison studies of transgender and cisgender individuals looking at sex-related anatomic dimorphism of brain structure and functioning.[31–33]

Given the complexity of gender as a concept, and the diverse ways in which it is experienced and expressed within a population, continuing research may reveal that the origins of gender expression and identity are multifactorial, with genetic factors, biological factors, and environment each playing a role in varying combinations and degrees of influence. Because gender variance and cross-gender identity do not appear in the *DSM-5* and may therefore be considered part of the normal spectrum of human experience, the most valuable research likely will be that which examines the factors contributing to gender dysphoria among children and youths. With this increased understanding, pediatric clinicians will be better able to prevent the onset of dysphoria or to ameliorate its effects in the child or youth in whom it already exists.

Preventive Health Care of Gender Variant Children and Transgender Youths

Identifying Strengths and Health Risks

In large part because of the experience of societal stigma and ostracism, gender variant and transgender youths may be at high risk on many fronts, as outlined in the paragraphs that follow. Nevertheless, there are reasons for immense optimism because these young people are coming of age on the cusp of enormous and positive societal change. This change is marked by an increased understanding and celebration of the diversity of gender expression and identity and an awareness of how this diversity can enrich families, schools, workplaces, and the broader community. In many parts of the

United States, clinicians have begun to recognize the amazing creativity and resilience of these youths as they navigate changing societal currents. They have met parents who love their children unconditionally and who confidently and passionately work to make the world a safer, more accepting place for them. They have joined with educators, social workers, mental health professionals, and others to create empowering transgender youth programs, including youth leadership workshops; mentorship programs; music, poetry, and art events; speakers' panels; and many others. Such programs help develop important life skills but, just as important, validate the rightful place of gender variant and transgender youths among other happy, healthy, and hopeful young people. These exciting changes have not yet arrived in many parts of the United States, but they are on the horizon. The clinician can use each clinical encounter to acknowledge the strengths and assets she or he recognizes in the patient, the family, and their environment and to express optimism about the future.

The risks described in the next 5 paragraphs are still very real for many gender variant children and youths. But it is important to recognize that they are an aberration, a result of living in the presence of stigma and ostracism. They are not part of the natural history of being gender variant or transgender. In communities in which the societal change described earlier in this section has not yet arrived, transgender youths often experience a profound isolation that intensifies their feelings of confusion and distress. They and most people in their lives, including parents, teachers, counselors, clergy, and physicians, often know little about gender identity or what it means to be transgender. In many instances, gender identity is confused with sexual orientation, a much different concept. Many clinicians and counselors were trained at a time when gender variant behaviors and transgender identity were seen as aberrant or pathological, and some continue to conduct their practices accordingly. Many transgender youths have few adult role models or mentors for support or validation, and many know no other transgender youths. When transgender youths have little access to accurate information, supportive counselors, or clinicians, and when they have no opportunity for healthy interactions with transgender peers and adults, the negative messages that surround them in their daily lives go unchallenged. Although this situation continues to be true in many communities across the United States, over the past decade there have been major advances in increasing the understanding of families, health and social service providers, educators, and others about the importance of recognizing, validating, and empowering gender variant and transgender youths.[21,34] Clinicians have often been at the forefront of the movement to increase public awareness, developing creative programs for youths and their families and providing needed advocacy on their behalves. With the growing love and support of families and communities, more and more gender variant and transgender youths no longer struggle under the burden of stigma and ostracism.

For the many children and youths who grow up in families and communities still untouched by this societal change, the most harmful reality they face is society's disapproval of who they are and how they present themselves to the world. Social stigma, and the violence and discrimination it engenders, often permeates their daily lives. It makes completing the expected developmental tasks of childhood and adolescence related to identity and self-esteem enormously difficult. Many of these children and youths are viewed by their families with shame and disgust. They are often forced to change their behaviors and renounce their declared inner sense of gender. Many of them are taken to therapists for the express purpose of changing their gender expression or identity. Many transgender youths and adults recall being ridiculed, ostracized, or beaten for being true to who they were, including within their own families. Many gender variant and transgender youths drop out of school and run away or are thrown out of their homes; some seek survival on the streets; many contemplate or attempt suicide. In fact, multiple research studies document the exceptionally high rates of suicidality among transgender and gender variant youths as compared with their cisgender and gender nonvariant peers.[35-39] Given these youths' experience of rejection, victimization, and risk for self-harm, it is not surprising that they are greatly overrepresented in the child welfare or juvenile justice system.[40-42] The harassment and abuse against gender variant and transgender young people often continues in these settings, perpetrated both by other youths and by staff members. Fortunately, state judiciaries across the country as well as organizations such as the Child Welfare League of America and The Equity Project, with the active involvement of pediatric clinicians and other advocates, have developed training curricula, model policies, and other tools to meet the needs of transgender youths in out-of-home care and address the societal antecedents that bring them into these systems.

Schools are often especially dangerous places for gender variant children and transgender youths.[43-45] Many of them experience daily verbal, physical, and sexual harassment on the playground and in the classroom. Often this harassment is not addressed by teachers, counselors, or other school staff, or it is dealt with by blaming the harassed child or youth. Sometimes, disapproving teachers and other school staff members engage in harassing behaviors themselves. Many schools have no specific policies prohibiting harassment or bullying based on gender identity or expression, even though these, along with sexual orientation, are among the most common targets of harassment on school campuses. More and more school systems, however, are adopting rigorous anti-bullying programs and anti-harassment policies that specifically include harassment based on gender identity and expression. Many have included transgender issues in regular teacher trainings and have worked with national organizations such as GLSEN to ensure that school campuses are safe places for transgender students. Many school systems have encouraged the establishment of gay-straight alliances (GSAs) in schools to support students who are lesbian, gay, bisexual, or transgender (LGBT) and their friends. Many schools also routinely invite pediatric clinicians to join in the development of Individualized Education Programs and participate in other discussions related to addressing the needs of individual gender variant and transgender students.

Societal stigma and the experience of minority stress also have a deep impact on the health and well-being of gender variant and transgender children and youths.[46] These factors may be reflected in the daily discrimination experienced by some children and youths. Children may be admonished for playing with toys or displaying interests that are considered inappropriate for their presumed gender. They are told by what names they will be called and by what pronouns they will be referred to, in spite of their protests that these names and pronouns do not reflect who they really are. Their genitalia rather than their inner identity as female, male, or another gender are referenced in assigning them to bathrooms, lockers, physical education classes, athletic teams, graduation ceremonies, and other school activities in which gender is still considered relevant. School dress codes often limit transgender students' ability to wear clothes that are consistent with their gender identity. Many clinicians have begun to work with individual schools on behalf of their gender variant and transgender patients, advocating policies and accommodations that ensure safety, affirmation, and respect for their patients in the school setting.

As transgender youths grow older, they begin to experience broader societal forms of discrimination. Their birth certificates, driver's licenses, and other forms of identification, as well as their school, employment, and health records, usually reflect their biological sex rather than their gender identity. Because fear, embarrassment, and potential humiliation accompany the presentation of these documents to others, many transgender adolescents may avoid applying for school or college admission or a job, and they may avoid accessing health care. Transgender individuals have been denied access to educational opportunities, community programs, social services, and health care simply because of their gender identity. Fortunately, each year more states and municipalities enact laws and ordinances that prohibit discrimination based on gender identity and expression in the areas of housing, employment, public accommodations, and health care, providing transgender individuals, including youths, legal recourse when faced with discrimination. In addition, LGBT communities have made great strides in recognizing that LGBT social and health services should be as welcoming and accessible to transgender individuals as they are to members of the LGB communities.

The risks described are not inherent in being a gender variant child or transgender youth. They are the common experience of any young person who is stigmatized, fearful, and alone. The genuine distress experienced by children and youths diagnosed as having gender dysphoria related to the perceived dissonance between their biological sex and their gender identity should not be dismissed or minimized. Nevertheless, evidence from other cultures and a growing body of research suggests that when provided love, support, and validation, these young people thrive and can expect to grow into happy, healthy, and productive adults. Perhaps the most important role that pediatric clinicians can play in the lives of gender variant children and transgender youths is to go beyond the confines of their offices and engage with schools, social service agencies, faith communities, legislatures, and others to ensure that these young people grow up in safe and nurturing environments.

Routine Health Supervision (RHS)

The AAP, the American Academy of Child and Adolescent Psychiatry, and the Society for Adolescent Health and Medicine have each issued official guidelines related to providing supportive care to children and youths facing issues of gender identity and gender expression.[5,7,21] In addition, several resources are available to clinicians on providing culturally sensitive and relevant care to gender variant children and transgender youths and adults.[47-50]

Clinicians should not presume the sexual orientation or gender identity of any patient. Children with gender variant behaviors, many of whom will later identify as LGB, have often learned or have been pressured to change their behaviors, particularly in public settings such as schools and health clinics. Many transgender youths will also hide their true gender identity. Even when asked in a sensitive and nonjudgmental manner about their inner feelings of being female, male, or another gender, they will often deny these feelings because they are fearful of clinician disapproval, uncertain about confidentiality, or still confused about the meaning of their emerging feelings. Perhaps one of the greatest barriers to appropriate health care for gender variant and gender dysphoric children and transgender youths is clinicians' assumption that they have no patients in their practices who are dealing with issues of gender identity and expression. Another mistaken assumption is that significant gender variant behavior in childhood accurately predicts sexual orientation. Although some children with persistent gender variant behaviors will later identify as LGB, many will not. Few clinicians may consider that some may also later identify as transgender. Many transgender youths are thought by their clinicians, and sometimes by themselves, to be LGB. However, the distinction between sexual orientation and gender identity is important for the provision of care because the different issues related to each require different responses from a clinician. In addition, transgender identity does not predict sexual orientation. Transgender youths may be gay, lesbian, heterosexual, bisexual, or asexual. For example, an MTF-transgender adolescent who is attracted to boys may be considered heterosexual, if she so considers herself. Some, however, may describe themselves as gay, either because it feels like the appropriate term to them or because it is easier for others to understand.

The goal of pediatric clinicians is not to identify every child with gender variant behaviors or transgender identity; instead, it is to create a safe and accepting clinical setting in which children, youths, and their families know they can discuss any topic of concern, including gender identity and expression, without discomfort or disapproval on the part of the clinician. Some patients and parents do not know that pediatric clinicians may have expertise in discussing issues of sexual and gender development. Specific messages can be provided through clinic posters and displayed brochures informing patients that these issues are appropriate topics of discussion. The most important signal that these topics are a natural part of pediatric practice is the clinician's own history taking and anticipatory guidance, in which issues of child and adolescent sexuality and gender are routinely discussed.

After patients have identified themselves as transgender, the clinician should create an accepting and supportive clinical environment by using pronouns consistent with the patient's gender identity and asking by what name the patient would like to be called by clinic staff. Although medical records must retain the patient's legal name, the notice "also known as [preferred name]" can be added to the medical record, and all clinic staff members should use this name in personal encounters with the patient. Patients should be invited to use either a unisex restroom or a restroom consistent with their gender identity while in the clinic. As with all adolescents, transgender patients should be seen alone for at least part of each visit and their confidentiality should be respected. A youth's gender identity should not be revealed to parents without the patient's permission. Patients should also be asked how they would like their gender identity recorded in the medical record, if at all, because medical records containing confidential information are sometimes accessible to parents.

Clinicians should reflect on their own feelings about gender variant behaviors and gender identity issues. As products of their own society, many clinicians may initially approach these issues with discomfort or disapproval. However, such an approach to gender variant children or transgender youths will diminish the clinician's ability to care for these patients and may likely cause harm. Many transgender patients have had profoundly negative experiences with the health care system.[48,51,52] In the past, these patients have been labeled as disordered and were often treated accordingly. Transgender patients report how staff in clinical settings often display fear or open disapproval of them or joke about them, even within earshot of the patient. At times, these patients have been refused medical care. Clinicians who receive little training about transgender health issues often do not understand the transgender youth's unique life experiences and needs. Most clinicians are unfamiliar with community resources that might help their transgender patients. Some health insurance companies refuse to pay for transition treatments, including hormone therapy, surgery, and the laboratory studies needed to monitor treatment. The decision by insurance companies not to cover these services is not a neutral one, since impeding access to necessary transition care can have profoundly negative impact on the physical and mental well-being of transgender individuals.[53] Conversely, the provision of appropriate and timely transition care has been shown to significantly decrease anxiety and depression in many transgender individuals,[10,21,54–57] and it can therefore be literally lifesaving. Fortunately, this refusal of payment for necessary care is changing quickly across the United States.

Clinicians are in a position of power relative to their transgender patients. As gatekeepers, clinicians decide who is eligible for transition treatments. Many, often through lack of knowledge or disapproval, have barred transgender patients from passing through that gate, preventing them from receiving necessary transition treatment and care. Clinicians must understand the history of tension between the transgender community and the medical community. Clinicians can improve this strained relationship by listening carefully and respectfully to their patients' life stories and expressions of need and by providing care that addresses these needs in an informed, respectful, and timely manner.

Surveillance and Screening as Part of RHS

Gender and sexuality are important parts of a child's life. At each child health supervision visit, as part of routine surveillance of the child's well-being beginning in early childhood, the clinician should ask parents how they think their child is developing compared with other children. Parents and child should be asked how the child is getting along with siblings and peers. Does their child seem happy? Is their child teased or harassed by other children and over what issues? All parents should be asked if they have any concerns over their child's sexual development or gender expression. Many parents who have such concerns are hesitant to bring them up on their own but are often relieved when the clinician does so. If a child with gender nonconforming behavior is happy and safe from teasing and parents have no concerns about these behaviors, no reason exists for the clinician to question further. However, as a child grows older and has more social contacts beyond the family, issues will likely arise related to being gender variant or transgender in a society that is often nonaccepting. Clinicians should remain attuned to this likelihood and reopen the door to discussion of these issues in future visits.

If parents express concerns about their child's gender expression or gender identity, the clinician should ask what they have noticed or heard from their child and what their concerns or fears might be. Parents' concerns are often related to their own embarrassment because of their child's behavior; they may also fear for their child's safety in a nonaccepting world. Many of them fear that their child's behavior or verbal expressions of wanting to be the opposite gender signal an eventual lesbian or gay sexual orientation or transgender identity. Clinicians may gently question gender variant children if they feel safe from teasing at home and school and about their feelings of being more like a girl, a boy, or another gender inside. Care must be taken to avoid conveying the message that anything is wrong with the child because of the child's gender variance. At the same time, it must be remembered that growing up gender variant in an unaccepting home or community carries with it significant risks. The clinician, therefore, should screen for the possibility of undue anxiety and depression or suicidality at each child health supervision visit. Also, any visit suggesting an unhappy child or a child in distress should lead the clinician to consider discussing issues of gender variant expression and gender identity with the parents and child.

Almost all pediatric practices have youths facing personal issues of gender identity. Many transgender youths hide any evidence of their inner gender identity; others are presumed, perhaps even by themselves, to be lesbian or gay. Clinicians should initiate discussion of sexuality and gender with all youths at each health supervision visit. Although many clinicians routinely discuss sexual activity and safer-sex practices, fewer discuss sexual orientation, and almost none of them address gender identity. It is important that clinicians open the door to discussion of gender to reduce the turmoil and dangers that these youths face, including the possibility of rejection or harassment by others as well as thoughts of self-harm, including suicidality.

A good way to begin a discussion of gender is in the context of a HEADSSS (home/environment, education and employment, activities, drugs, sexuality, suicide/depression, and safety) interview.[58] Throughout the HEADSSS interview, it is essential that the clinician make no assumptions about a youth's sexual orientation or gender identity. To address gender identity within a broader sexual history, the clinician might say, "Sexuality and sexual feelings can be confusing sometimes. During puberty, bodies change in lots of different ways. Sexual feelings are changing too. Some of my patients are not sure if they are attracted to boys or to girls or maybe to both, and some of my patients even wonder whether they're more like a girl or a boy inside. All of this is completely normal but can be really confusing. So I'm wondering what it's been like for you." After asking about attractions (sexual orientation), the clinician can simply ask, "And how about inside? Do you feel more like a girl or a boy or maybe something else?" For the patient who is not dealing with gender identity issues, these questions may seem odd. This discomfort can be addressed by a simple statement such as "These are questions I ask all my patients, and for some they're really important." For transgender youths, the questions may be lifesaving.

As a demonstration of understanding and respect, if youths acknowledge a transgender or another-gendered identity, the clinician should ask about preferred name and pronouns and use these through the remainder of the interview and subsequent visits. Patients should be reassured that the discussion of gender identity will remain confidential unless they give permission to share it with others or unless a risk of danger to someone exists.

It is appropriate to inquire about a youth's path to recognizing the youth's transgender identity. When did these youths first become aware of their gender identity and what is their present comfort with their identity?

What is their degree of understanding of what it means to be transgender? Are they hopeful about their future as a transgender person? Have they told others about their gender identity and how have those people responded? Have they met other youths or adults who are transgender and have they been supportive? Have they been in relationships and have they been healthy ones? As with all youths, transgender youths should be asked about their sexual activity, the gender of their sexual partners, and any experiences of pregnancy, sexually transmitted infections (STIs), or being forced or coerced to have sex without their permission.

Because transgender youths face an increased risk of rejection and violence at home, at school, and in the broader community, the clinician should ask about their treatment in these settings and whether they have ever run away from home or dropped out of school. Have they needed to sell their bodies, deal drugs, or engage in other illegal activities to survive on the streets? Have they been involved with the child welfare or juvenile justice system? Have they ever used drugs or contemplated suicide? What do they know about gender transitions, and in what ways have they begun the transition process? Have they begun to cross-dress? Have they begun puberty blockers or cross-gender hormone therapy, and, if so, where have they obtained their treatment? Have they thought about gender-affirmation surgery or other transition-related procedures in the future?

Many of these topics can be explored over several visits. If the clinician is not comfortable with the depth of interviewing suggested, she or he has a responsibility to refer the youth to someone else who can have this conversation. One of the most important aspects of history taking with transgender youths is that it provides an opportunity for the clinician to interact with the patient in a comfortable, respectful, and caring manner that validates who the youth is as a human being. Many transgender youths have never experienced such acceptance before, and providing it is among the most important things a clinician can do.

Screening—that is, systematically testing with a validated instrument for an undiagnosed condition in patients who do not have signs or symptoms of that condition—may be useful in identifying children and youths who have occult mental health concerns and symptoms. The AAP/Bright Futures *Recommendations for Preventive Pediatric Health Care* (available at www.aap.org/en-us/Documents/periodicity_schedule.pdf) recommends that primary care clinicians use a validated screening tool to screen all adolescents annually for depression, beginning at 12 years of age, and perform a risk assessment for substance use annually, with "appropriate action to follow" (in this case, formal screening) if positive, beginning at

11 years of age. Because of the psychosocial stresses experienced by many gender variant children, it is also reasonable (some would say advisable) to screen gender variant children routinely for psychosocial problems at each routine health supervision visit from the time their gender variance is evident. Clinicians can use a general screening tool such as the Pediatric Symptom Checklist or the Strengths and Difficulties Questionnaires, followed by secondary screening (eg, the Patient Health Questionnaire for Adolescents depression screening, the Screen for Childhood Anxiety Related Emotional Disorders) and, if indicated, full diagnostic assessment when concerns are identified by screenings. (See Appendix 2 for descriptions of these tools.) Any patient of any age with findings that suggest depression should be assessed for suicidality. (Appendix 2 includes descriptions of tools useful for this purpose.) The AAP also recommends annual risk assessment for STIs, with appropriate action to follow if positive (in this case, laboratory tests), for all adolescents beginning at age 11. This recommendation is regardless of gender identity or sexual orientation.

Physical Examination as Part of RHS

All children, including those who are gender variant in their expression, should have a complete physical examination at each health supervision visit. The clinician should be aware that children who dress, behave, or show interests that might be considered as gender variant may or may not be gender variant in their gender identity. The physical examination of transgender youths is similar to that of cisgender youths. It is comprehensive and additionally guided by specific information gathered through the history-taking process. It also takes into account the sensitivities young transgender people may have about gendered aspects of their bodies and the steps possibly taken to present themselves physically in a way that reflects their inner sense of gender. In considering possible signs related to pregnancy, STIs, or other aspects of sexual activity, clinicians should keep in mind that transgender youths may be heterosexually, homosexually, or bisexually active or not sexually active at all. Some transgender youths hide all public expressions of their gender identity. Some will already have begun their social transition, with their clothing, grooming, mannerisms, and speech reflecting to varying degrees their gender identity. Occasionally, transgender patients may wear non–gender-defining street clothes but underwear consistent with their gender identity. If patients have begun pubertal suppression, they will generally remain at Tanner stage 2 or 3. Depending on the duration of suppression, they may eventually show delay in pubertal development relative to their peers. If patients have already begun gender-affirmation hormone therapy, they may show evidence of breast development (MTF), appearance of facial hair (FTM), and other expected changes of estrogen and testosterone treatment. Few transgender youths younger than 18 will show signs of gender-affirmation surgical treatment. If they have had such treatment, the most common procedure for those younger than 18 is mastectomy (FTM).

In conducting a physical examination, clinicians should keep in mind the significant distress that many transgender youths experience related to their biologically determined pubertal changes, such as development of penile and testicular enlargement, facial hair, deepening of the voice, breast development, erections, and menstrual periods, which often feel like deep betrayals of their gender identity. Some MTF-transgender youths may tuck their genitalia, placing their penis and testes between their legs so they are less visible. Some FTM-transgender youths may wear chest binders or baggy tops to make their breasts less visible. Some may also wear a "packer," which is padding or a phallic-shaped object worn in the front of the underwear or pants to give the appearance of having a penis. Because transgender youths are at high risk for physical and sexual violence, clinicians should look for signs of trauma and, if found, should be prepared to initiate a discussion of safety both in the home and in the community.

Clinicians should remember that a physical examination is done only with a youth's consent, with assurance that the patient has a right to refuse any part of the examination. This is particularly relevant for transgender youths given the often elevated degree of discomfort they have about the gendered parts of their bodies. In preparing for the examination, the clinician should discuss the rationale for suggesting the parts of the examination that might be particularly uncomfortable for a transgender youth, especially the breast and genital examinations. Clinicians should explain that their intention is to make the examination as comfortable as possible for the patient and to elicit the patient's guidance in how best to accomplish this task. The clinician should ask transgender youths what words they would like used in referring to various body parts, for example, *genitalia* instead of *penis* or *vagina*. An FTM-transgender patient may prefer the term *chest* rather than *breast*. An MTF-transgender patient should be treated the same as other female patients and an FTM-transgender patient like other male patients by being gowned and draped appropriately. At the same time, patients understand that their bodies still reflect the realities of their birth-assigned sex. They also understand that certain gendered procedures, such as breast, testicular, or pelvic examinations, might be recommended. For example, suggesting a pelvic examination for an FTM adolescent with unexplained vaginal bleeding or a testicular examination of an MTF youth with groin pain would be appropriate. Most transgender patients will agree to a recommended procedure if the medical rationale is presented in a factual and respectful manner, inviting the patient's questions and input on how to make the examination as comfortable as possible.

All aspects of the physical examination should be for the purpose of medical necessity, not to satisfy clinician curiosity about possible genital or breast changes related to hormone or surgical transition therapy. As for all youths, a chaperone should be present during any breast, genital, or anorectal examination. The gender of the chaperone should be based on patient preference.

Anticipatory Guidance as Part of RHS

Many gender variant children and youths grow up in homes and communities where gender variance in expression and identity is not accepted and is often punished. The clinician's challenge, therefore, is to support these young people in a way that prevents or minimizes dysphoria, assures safety, and promotes optimal physical, developmental, psychological, and social well-being.

Prepubertal Children: Controversy and Consensus

In the past, clinicians often found it challenging to support gender variant and gender dysphoric children and youths with any degree of confidence. In large part, this was because there were competing schools of thought about "best practices" in defining and addressing the needs of these young people, particularly prepubertal children whose gender variance appeared during early and middle childhood.[16] For these younger children, 3 basic approaches to intervention were proposed, each with a distinct theoretical base and philosophical stance, but none of which were supported by a robust body of research.[10,59–61]

The first approach sought actively to discourage gender variant behavior and identity, often focusing on perceived psychopathology in a child, a parent, or family dynamics either as a cause for gender variance or as a factor that allowed gender variance to persist in a child.[59] This approach viewed significant gender variance as less desirable than gender conformity and a cause for concern. It was predicated on the belief that it was possible to influence the trajectory of a child's gender development toward a more normative outcome, which, in turn, would result in less stigma and trauma related to growing up gender variant in a nonaccepting society. The second approach adopted a more gender-affirming "wait and see" stance, understanding that many children with gender dysphoria are no longer gender dysphoric as they enter adolescence. This approach allowed for a certain degree of gender exploration during childhood, but usually only within certain defined parameters (eg, "only at home"), ostensibly out of safety concerns for the child. In contrast, the third approach was fully "gender affirmative" in its outlook, encouraging children to explore and express their gender freely and authentically while actively working to assure they could do so, as much as possible, in a safe and affirming environment. It is this third gender-affirmative model of care that has become ascendant relative to the others, supported by an increasingly robust body of research.[10,62]

Supporting Gender Variant and Gender Dysphoric Children

As discussed earlier in this chapter (see Developmental Trajectories of Gender Variant Children section), some children with variant gender identity are gender dysphoric in childhood but no longer meet criteria for gender dysphoria as they approach adolescence (sometimes referred to as *desisters*). Others who are gender variant in identity, and possibly dysphoric, during childhood will continue to be so into adolescence and adulthood (*persisters*). Since it is impossible to predict if a child will desist or persist in a gender variance (and since the *DSM-5* does not consider variant gender identity per se to be an issue of concern), the approaches to supporting gender variant children, whether gender dysphoric or not, are similar, following a gender-affirmative model of care.

Until recently, it was often advised that social transition into living full-time as a child of a gender other than that assigned at birth, including the use of name and pronouns consistent with inner gender identity, should probably be deferred until adolescence. However, a recent research study examined the experience of prepubertal children who identify as the gender opposite from that assigned at birth and who were supported in living openly as that gender.[63] Where previous studies of children with GID often show significantly increased levels of depression and anxiety, children in this study, who were supported in their expression of gender consistent with their gender identity, showed no elevations in depression and only a slight elevation in anxiety compared to a cisgender peer population. Although further research is needed to define the factors underlying these children's apparent emotional well-being, this study suggests that supporting these children in their social transition appears to do no harm and may, in fact, have a positive effect on their psychological well-being. This understanding has led to an increased willingness of clinicians to support the full social transition of prepubertal children who clearly and consistently assert a cross-gender identity and whose families are prepared to fully support their children in this endeavor.

Another area of general agreement is that support and counseling should be provided to gender dysphoric children and their families by a multidisciplinary team ideally consisting of a primary care clinician, a pediatric endocrinologist, a psychiatrist or another mental health professional, and a social worker. These professionals can be valuable additions to the treatment plan in exploring a child's or youth's sense of gender identity, social and academic functioning, family relationships, cultural expectations, and self-esteem. Contemporary gender-affirmative treatment approaches explicitly emphasize that their goal is not to prevent cross-gender identity or homosexuality. Instead, the stated goal is to prevent or ameliorate gender dysphoria, support resilience in the face of challenges, and ensure optimal physical, developmental, and emotional well-being. Another area of agreement is that medical transition treatments, including cross-hormone therapy, should not be initiated in childhood before the onset of puberty.

The most accepted approach in working with gender variant children and their families is to validate and celebrate the unique gender expression and identity of each child, respecting children's right to express their gender as they wish, while working actively to keep them safe in an often nonaccepting and sometimes hostile world.[54,64,65] Unlike previous intervention approaches, gender-affirmative approaches do not focus on looking for sources of psychopathology as factors contributing to a child's gender variance or dysphoria. Instead, there should be a focus on environmental factors related to home, school, peers, and community that may contribute to a gender variant child's dysphoria. A good measure of the distress experienced by many gender dysphoric children and youths is thought to come from the stigma society attaches to gender variance and the resultant negative responses of family, peers, and community to their cross-gender identity and expression. Therefore, an important aspect of providing support for a gender variant child is to determine how safe and affirming that child's environment is and to work with families, schools, places of worship, and other settings to ensure that a child is safe and validated in all areas of that child's life.

Parents should be provided information about childhood gender variance and its possible developmental trajectories in gender identity and sexual orientation. Parental misconceptions about gender and sexuality should be corrected. They should know that the pediatric profession recognizes both cisgender identities and transgender identities as well as LGB and straight (heterosexual) sexual orientations to be equally valid and healthy developmental outcomes for children and youths. A family's ability to embrace a diversity of gender possibilities predicts a child's ability to experience and express gender in a way that is personally authentic and fulfilling for that child.

Specific guidance for parents will include a discussion of the pros and cons of supporting a child's social transition. While an authentic expression of gender is felt to be the healthiest option for many gender variant children, this will depend in part on a family's readiness to fully support a child in this endeavor. Parents also need to consider the imperative of keeping their child safe from harm in an often unaccepting world. The clinician can help parents identify real and present dangers that might await their child inside and outside the home, if social transition is considered appropriate. Just as importantly, there must be a consideration of the very real risks to a child's well-being if the child is not permitted to express gender authentically. These are likely to include an increased risk of anxiety, an increased risk of depression, and their many significant sequelae.[10,54,55] Clinicians can offer to work with parents and children to find ways to make the home, the school, the neighborhood, the faith community, and other social settings safer for the child. At times, it may be necessary to modify a child's ability to express gender authentically when clear and present danger exists in specific settings (eg, allowing a child to cross-dress at home and during certain social outings, but not at school if safety concerns in that setting have not yet been resolved). Nevertheless, the goal should be to actively work to reduce these dangers so the child might be free to live authentically in terms of gender, as this is thought to result in optimal well-being if allowed to take place in a safe and supportive setting.

Clinicians or other team members should provide the opportunity for a discussion of parental concerns, fears, and degree of comfort related to their child's gender identity and expression. Parents can be referred to Web sites, books, brochures, and media resources geared to parents of gender variant children and youths. See Box 21-1.

Parents should be assured that with love, validation, and support their children should grow up to be happy, healthy, and productive adults, no matter what their gender expression, gender identity, or sexual orientation might be. They should also be made aware of the significant risks associated with parental disapproval or rejection, which in older children and youths may include the possibility of suicidal ideation or attempt.[66]

Parents should also be asked what their hopes and expectations around treatment might be. Parents should be informed clearly that the goals of treatment are to prevent or diminish a child's distress around gender but not to change a child's gender identity or sexual orientation.

Box 21-1. Resources for Parents of Gender Variant Children and Transgender Youths

- Brill S, Kenney L. *The Transgender Teen: A Handbook for Parents and Professionals Supporting Transgender and Non-binary Teens.* San Francisco, CA: Cleis Press Inc; 2016

- Brill S, Pepper R. *The Transgender Child: A Handbook for Families and Professionals.* San Francisco, CA: Cleis Press Inc; 2008

- Gender Spectrum. Resources: parenting and family. Gender Spectrum Web site. https://www.genderspectrum.org/resources/parenting-and-family-2/#more-432. Accessed May 8, 2018

- Marian Wright Edelman Institute, San Francisco State University. Family Acceptance Project Web site. http://familyproject.sfsu.edu. Accessed May 8, 2018

- Outreach Program for Children with Gender-Variant Behaviors and Their Families. *If You Are Concerned About Your Child's Gender Behaviors: A Guide for Parents.* Washington, DC: Children's National Medical Center; 2003. https://www. rainbowhealthontario.ca/wp-content/uploads/woocommerce_uploads/2014/ 08/PARENT%20FLYER.pdf. Accessed May 8, 2018

- The Trevor Project Web site. https://www.thetrevorproject.org. Accessed May 8, 2018

Adapted from Bidwell RJ. Gender expression and identity. In: Foy JM, ed. *Mental Health Care of Children and Adolescents: A Guide for Primary Care Clinicians.* Itasca, IL: American Academy of Pediatrics; 2018:561.

As a gender variant child approaches adolescence, clinicians should be watchful for the persistence or desistence of gender dysphoria. The clinician should also screen for the possibility of new-onset or worsening gender dysphoria as the child approaches puberty and its often distressing physical changes. This is a time when it is especially important for the clinician to screen once again for the presence of depression or suicidality. If dysphoria persists or newly appears at the onset of puberty, discussions with parents and child about approaching transition choices should take place (eg, the initiation of pubertal suppression treatment at the onset of puberty). If a child's gender dysphoria is no longer present at the onset of puberty, it will be important to discuss the possibility that, although the child may be less likely to self-identify as transgender, he or she may be likelier to eventually affirm a gay, lesbian, or bisexual orientation.

Parents should be encouraged to acknowledge and support their child's gender identity and expression, no matter what it might be. They should also be provided the skills and resources to do so effectively. The Children's National Medical Center has developed guidelines to help parents in their provision of support for their children (Box 21-2), and Box 21-3 lists pitfalls parents should try to avoid.

Box 21-2. Children's National Medical Center Outreach Program Guidelines for Parents of Gender Variant and Transgender Youths

- Love your child for who your child is. Love, acceptance, understanding, and support are especially important when peers and society are often intolerant of difference.

- Question traditional assumptions about gender roles and sexual orientation. Do not allow societal expectations to come between you and your child.

- Create a safe space for your child, allowing your child to always be who the child is, especially in the child's own home.

- Seek out socially accepted activities (eg, sports, arts, hobbies) that respect your child's interests while helping your child fit in socially.

- Validate your child and your child's interests, supporting the idea that more than one way exists to be a girl or boy. Speak openly and calmly about gender variance with your child. Talk about these subjects in positive terms, and listen as your child expresses feelings of being different.

- Seek out supportive resources (eg, books, videos, Web sites, support groups) for parents, families, and children.

- Talk about gender variance with other significant people in your child's life, including siblings, extended family members, babysitters, and family friends.

- Prepare your child to deal with bullying. Let your child know that a child does not deserve to be hurt. Be aware of behaviors that suggest bullying and may be occurring, such as school refusal, crying excessively, and reporting aches and pains.

- Be your child's advocate. Expect and insist on acceptance, respect, and safety wherever your child is. Parents may need to educate school staff and others about the special experience and needs of gender variant children.

From Bidwell RJ. Gender expression and identity. In: Foy JM, ed. *Mental Health Care of Children and Adolescents: A Guide for Primary Care Clinicians.* Itasca, IL: American Academy of Pediatrics; 2018:580.

Box 21-3. Children's National Medical Center Pitfalls to Avoid as Parents of Gender Variant and Transgender Youths

- Avoid finding fault. No blame exists. Your child's gender variance came from within, not from you as parents. Blame will get in the way of enjoying your child.

- Do not pressure your child to change, because doing so will cause much pain and harm.

- Do not blame your child. Do not accept bullying as *just the way things are.* No one has the right to torment or criticize others because they are different.

From Bidwell RJ. Gender expression and identity. In: Foy JM, ed. *Mental Health Care of Children and Adolescents: A Guide for Primary Care Clinicians.* Itasca, IL: American Academy of Pediatrics; 2018:580.

Importantly, they should have the skills necessary to address any instances of disapproval, harassment, or discrimination their child might face in the extended family, school, and broader community. Above all, clinicians should remind parents of the importance of expressing their unconditional love for their child and refraining from comments or actions that demonstrate disapproval of their child's gender expression or identity. The Family Acceptance Project at San Francisco University has conducted research demonstrating the important role that parents play in keeping their LGBT children healthy and safe through the provision of acceptance and love.[67] It has also documented the significant harm that results from parental rejection.[66] The clinician should share this understanding with all families.

Supporting Transgender Youths
Physical Well-being
Transgender and other gender variant youths face the same health issues as other young people. The health care they receive should be based on a comprehensive history, physical examination, and evaluative studies, not on their gender expression or identity. It is important to keep in mind, however, that these youths often grow up in very unaccepting and sometimes virulently hostile environments that may have a negative effect on their physical well-being. These negative effects may include the physical sequelae of substance use, poor nutrition caused by homelessness or disordered eating, unprotected sexual behaviors, self-harm, injuries from physical and sexual victimization, and hormone or surgical transition treatments accessed outside of health care settings.

Developmental, Social, and Emotional Well-being
In most ways, gender variant and transgender youths are exactly the same as their peers. They have the same needs for protection, nurturance, and love and the same hopes and dreams for the future. They grow up in the same families and communities and attend the same schools and places of worship. Similar to other children, they face the fundamental task of achieving a sense of identity that integrates all aspects of who they are, including their sexual orientation and gender identity. This integration of sexual and gender identity, accompanied by a growing sense of comfort with that identity, is essential for the optimal health and well-being of each child and youth.

However, the experience of growing up as a youth with gender variant expression or as a transgender youth is different in several important ways.[34,68,69] Unlike their peers, these young people face an often lonely and sometimes frightening journey of self-discovery, attempting to understand one of the most fundamental aspects of who they are as human beings: their gender identity. Some youths accommodate themselves easily to this growing awareness. Many, however, experience significant confusion and distress, feeling different and alone and wondering what their feelings mean in terms of their sense of self and their place in the world. Growing up in a society that believes that a person is either male or female and that gender expression and identity must strictly reflect biological sex undoubtedly intensifies their sense that something inside them has gone wrong. Many of these youths become filled with an overwhelming mix of confusion, shame, anger, self-hatred, and despair.

The clinician's role as educator and counselor is as important as that of medical provider in caring for gender variant and transgender youths. The clinician should avoid assumptions based on cultural stereotypes and listen carefully to understand each patient's unique experience and needs. In general, the counseling of gender variant and transgender youths will address 7 areas: self-acceptance and validation of gender expression and identity; safety; isolation; self-disclosure, or coming out; healthy relationships and sexual decision-making; understanding future choices related to transition; and optimism for the future. Addressing each of these areas is essential in ensuring their healthy development. These should be addressed over time and not all at an initial presentation or single visit.

Self-acceptance and validation. The clinician can play an important role in countering the effects of disapproval and the pathologizing of gender variant expression and identity. Clinicians should present being transgender as part of the tapestry of normal human identity. They should clarify that the issue of concern is not variant gender identity, but instead is the distress that transgender individuals may experience, caused by a perceived incongruence between identity and birth-assigned sex or by having a transgender identity in a society that is unaccepting. This validating reassurance of healthiness and normalcy is perhaps the most powerful statement a clinician can make to transgender youths and their families.

More and more gender variant and transgender youths know a significant amount about gender, gender identity, and gender expression. Many have done extensive research on the Internet, accessing YouTube videos and Web sites that are easily searchable or connecting with other gender variant and transgender youths through social media. Others, however, continue to be very isolated and know little or nothing about the nature and meaning of their emerging sense of identity. Therefore, the clinician should conduct an initial inquiry into what the youth has seen, heard, or read about gender variance and focus on correcting misconceptions, providing validation, and supporting empowerment. Transgender youths should be provided information on gender identity and what it means to be transgender. Some of these youths may go through a period of confusion, not knowing whether they are gay, lesbian, bisexual, straight, transgender, or a combination of these. The clinician should inform these youths that such uncertainty is normal and that over time they will have a clearer understanding of who they are. The clinician may also provide brochures to youths facing issues of gender identity or refer them to supportive Web sites.[70]

Youths of an ethnic or another minority who are transgender may have an especially difficult time. The clinician should discuss these issues with their patients openly and connect them to appropriate supportive resources within their communities and online.

Safety. Because gender variant and transgender youths endure higher rates of physical and sexual assault, harassment, discrimination, and social rejection, clinicians should ask these youths about their safety in their homes, schools, neighborhoods, and broader community. If harassment or other harmful treatment is acknowledged, the clinician should work with the youth and family to identify and implement appropriate strategies to end the violence. Many of these youths are afraid to advocate for their own safety or uncertain how to go about doing so. They may feel shameful and think they deserve the harm inflicted on them, or they may simply accept that this is the way the world is, since in their daily lives they have never seen evidence to the contrary. The clinician should tell these youths that they deserve to expect and demand safety and respect from everyone in their lives and in all settings. Because gender variant and transgender youths have so few advocates, the clinician should offer to join with them in approaching every venue in which they experience violence, including the home and school, to work out a plan to end violence immediately and completely. Parents, clinicians, teachers, and others should also work together to ensure that schools and other community organizations create and implement policies and practices that ensure respectful treatment and appropriate accommodations for these youths. The state of Massachusetts, among others, has developed a detailed policy statement about the responsibilities of schools to affirm and support gender variant and transgender students; this statement has served as a model for other communities and states.[71] Many school districts have also developed policies prohibiting discrimination, bullying, and harassment, including that specifically based on gender identity and expression. If necessary, the clinician should call on the state child welfare services office and advocacy organizations such as the American Civil Liberties Union to join in the effort to keep these young people safe.

One of the most serious threats to safety experienced by gender variant and transgender youths is engagement in self-harming behaviors, including substance use and suicidality. These are predictable responses for any youth who is subjected to rejection and violence and who feels alone, hopeless, and afraid. Clinicians, therefore, should routinely screen not only for externally derived threats to safety but also for those that come from within. Threats to safety, whether external or internal, can be ameliorated only if they are recognized and addressed.

Isolation. Because many gender variant and transgender youths experience profound isolation and loneliness, their physical and emotional health may be compromised. Isolation may involve little or no access to accurate and supportive information, a lack of connection to transgender peers and adult role models, and little awareness of local and national resources affirming young people like them. At the same time, isolation is amplified for transgender youths who hear only negative messages in their homes, schools, peer groups, faith communities, and the media. Clinicians can ameliorate the isolation of these youths by providing accurate information about gender expression and gender identity. They should provide supportive and affirming counseling, or they should refer these youths to colleagues who have the time, comfort, and expertise to do so. Clinicians should connect these children and youths to local community resources such as support groups, GSAs, and other gender-affirming youth programs. Youths, and families, who do not have access to local programs should be informed about national organizations and Web sites created specifically for gender nonconforming children, transgender youths, and their families. (See Box 21-1.) Clinicians can also point out positive gender variant and transgender role models in the community or nationally. In certain circumstances, it is appropriate for transgender clinicians to present themselves as role models to transgender youths and their families.

Self-disclosure, or coming out. Transgender youths often reach a point in their development at which they feel a strong urge to disclose their gender identity to others. Transgender youths often have a history of gender variant expression as children. Therefore, others may have already sensed that these youths may be transgender or assumed on the basis of stereotype that they might be lesbian or gay. Some transgender youths, however, successfully conceal their gender identity, either by adapting their gender expression to fit societal expectations consistent with their birth-assigned sex or by labeling themselves or allowing others to perceive them as gay or lesbian. The process of disclosure to family and friends is often emotional and traumatic. Transgender youths who disclose their gender identity (come out) risk condemnation and rejection by family and peers. On coming out, many have faced disapproval from their schools, faith communities, and even health care professionals. Therefore, coming out should be considered carefully, weighing the risks and benefits. It is sometimes suggested that if a youth expects a negative response from parents, the youth should wait to disclose until legally and financially independent. However, many youths think that continuing to live a lie is unbearable and harmful to their self-esteem, and they come out earlier. A clinician should never reveal a youth's gender identity to parents without permission unless imminent risk of harm exists. A clinician can play an important role in the process of disclosure by helping youths assess the pros and cons of coming out and helping them choose an appropriate time, place, and approach for disclosure. Sometimes, clinicians can participate directly by facilitating the encounter in which a youth comes out to family or friends. Clinicians who feel they do not have the skills to provide such counseling effectively should refer to or collaborate with a therapist who can guide the youth and support the family through the coming out process.

Relationships and sexual decision-making. Many transgender youths have difficulty in meeting other transgender youths to establish friendships and share mutual support. Clinicians should help connect transgender youths to local LGBT teen support groups, GSAs, and other LGBT-supportive programs in the community, if they exist. Clinicians can suggest national telephone hotlines or Web sites from which transgender youths can receive accurate information and supportive counseling and can communicate with other transgender youths. (See Box 21-1.) The clinician can also serve as a supportive and reassuring lifeline until the youth is old enough to become independent and possibly move away to attend school or work in a community more accepting of transgender people.

Transgender youths may be heterosexual, homosexual, bisexual, or asexual in their attractions and sexual behaviors. Many transgender youths are afraid to reveal their gender identity to those with whom they might be interested in establishing a relationship. Therefore, some transgender youths find that their only options for experiencing gender affirmation and exploring emotional and physical intimacy are through anonymous sexual encounters on the streets, in parks, or through Internet hookups. In addition to being potentially dangerous, these encounters may be accompanied by feelings of shame and degradation, which are harmful to a youth's sense of identity and self-worth. That many transgender youths are eager to engage in the typical courting practices of adolescence, which normally take place in safer and more affirming circumstances, is evidenced in the great popularity of LGBT youth proms and other social gatherings in more and more communities across the United States.

Transgender youths who are in relationships face many of the same questions as their nontransgender peers: "Am I in love?" "What do I want from a relationship?" "Do I really want to be in this relationship?" "How do I know if this is a good relationship?" "How do I get out of this relationship?" In addition, transgender youths face the exceedingly difficult questions of how and when to tell their potential boyfriends or girlfriends about their gender identity. A transgender-supportive clinician or therapist can help youths reflect on and find answers to these questions.

As with other youths, many transgender youths know little about sexuality and how to make healthy sexual choices. Abstinence is always the appropriate option for youths who do not feel ready for a sexual relationship. Transgender youths should understand that when they are ready for a sexual relationship, they can expect to lead healthy and fulfilling sexual lives. All youths who have decided they are ready for a sexual relationship should be advised to limit their number of sexual partners and avoid mixing sex and alcohol or drugs so as to reduce their risk for infection, trauma, and sexual assault. Transgender youths, like other youths and depending on the sexual behaviors they engage in, are at risk for unplanned pregnancy and should be counseled on contraception. Safer-sex practices related to oral, vaginal, and anal sex should be reviewed in detail. Transgender youths should also be aware that *no* always means *no* in negotiating sex, and any forced or coerced sexual experience represents sexual assault.

Understanding the choices ahead. Clinicians can play an important role in supporting transgender children and youths as they and their families navigate the important choices related to transition. Transition is the process of social, emotional, psychological, legal, and physical change that transgender individuals experience as they increasingly embrace and express their inner gender identity. Historically, this process has often been impeded by a variety of societal barriers, including those imposed by health providers. Some providers refused to care for transgender patients on the basis of a professed lack of training or outright disapproval. Others saw their role as "gatekeepers," establishing stringent transition criteria determining who could or could not move forward on the transition path. A growing body of research has demonstrated the beneficial effects of transition on both the mental health and the physical health of transgender individuals and the harm that can come from withholding needed transition care.[10,54,55,72,73] This new understanding has resulted in revision of transition care standards to make them less rigidly prescriptive and restrictive and much more flexible in recognizing and supporting the varying transition choices available to transgender children, youths, and adults.[55,56]

Table 21-2 shows several of the more common transition choices made by transgender individuals. In each area, clinicians can provide valuable information, guidance, support, and advocacy. Social transition often begins in early childhood and extends through adolescence into adulthood. It commonly involves the adoption of dress, grooming style, mannerisms, interests, activities, preferred name and pronouns, and other gendered characteristics generally considered typical of an individual's gender identity. Clinicians can help address families' possible concerns about their child's gender identity or expression and also ask the gender variant child about the child's own sense of support and safety, both inside the family and outside the family. Parents should understand the importance of affirming their child's individual expression of gender. Parents should also be prepared to

Table 21-2. Common Transition Choices

Aspect	Age	Means
Social	Early childhood into adulthood	Living openly in the world consistent with gender identity, often reflected in dress, grooming, mannerisms, interests, activities, preferred name and pronouns, and other expressions of gender
Legal	Childhood into adulthood	Legal name change; change in gender designation on birth certificate, identification cards, and other documents reflecting these changes
Pubertal suppression	Initiated at onset of puberty (SMR 2), continued until youth expresses full certainty about gender identity	Gonadotropin-releasing hormone analogs
Hormone therapy	Initiated between ages 12 years and 16 years and continued into adulthood	Gender-affirming hormones (estrogen for MTF transgender individuals and testosterone for FTM transgender individuals)
Gender-affirmation surgery	Age 18 years and older, or younger with parental consent	Surgery aligning genital and other physical characteristics with gender identity (eg, orchiectomy, vaginoplasty, and breast augmentation [MTF] and mastectomy and phalloplasty [FTM])

Abbreviations: FTM, female-to-male; MTF, male-to-female; SMR, sexual maturity rating.

provide advocacy and support for their gender variant child in all settings, ensuring safety and respectful treatment no matter what their child's gender identity or expression might be.

More and more transgender children and youths pursue gender-affirming legal options as a part of their social transition. These include obtaining a legal name change reflective of their gender identity and, in more and more states, choosing the option of a change in gender designation on their birth certificates. These legal changes often make life much less stressful in the school and other settings, where often there has been resistance to using preferred names and pronouns or permitting access to gender-specific accommodations, activities, and resources without legal documentation of name and gender.

As puberty approaches for children who have been "consistent, persistent, and insistent" in asserting their transgender identity, clinicians should provide anticipatory guidance related to pubertal suppression therapy. Pubertal suppression is achieved by the administration of a gonadotropin-releasing hormone analogue, which prevents the endogenous estrogen and testosterone surges associated with puberty. This, in turn, prevents the development of the secondary sexual characteristics and physiologic events such as menarche that are associated with great psychological distress for many transgender children. Pubertal suppression therapy is considered safe and is beneficial both mentally and physically.[10,55,56,74] In addition to preventing the distressing physical changes associated with a child's birth-assigned sex, a temporary suppression of puberty may allow youths more time to mature cognitively and achieve fuller clarity and certainty related to their gender identity. If a youth eventually decides that she or he is not transgender, pubertal suppression is ended and puberty allowed to proceed as determined by biological sex. If a youth continues to assert a transgender identity, as is usually the case, then the youth can proceed with gender-affirming hormonal therapy.

The primary agents of gender-affirming hormonal therapy include estrogen (MTF transgender) and testosterone (FTM transgender). These treatments are much more effective if initiated before significant pubertal changes have taken place and allow transgender youths to achieve a physical appearance consistent with their gender identity. The beneficial impact of hormonal therapy on transgender individuals' mental health has been well-documented.[54,55,57,72,73,75] Research has found few medical risks related to hormone therapy initiated during adolescence, whereas the health risks of denying or delaying access to therapy in compromised psychological well-being and safety are significant.[10,55,56] For these reasons, hormone therapy represents the standard of care for transgender adolescents. Published guidelines have generally recommended initiating gender-affirming hormone therapy at age 16.[55,56] However, many gender centers have protocols that permit such therapy at age 14, or even younger.[55,56,76] With the recent addition of pubertal suppression in the approach to treating transgender youths, many clinicians believe it is neither medically justifiable nor developmentally justifiable to keep a young person in a peripubertal state until age 16 while that young person's cisgender peers complete their pubertal development at a much younger age. Therefore, the standard of care presented in the most recent World Professional Association for Transgender Health guidelines allows for an individualized approach in determining the appropriate age for initiating gender-affirming hormone therapy.[55]

Gender-affirming surgery is sought by many, but not all, transgender individuals to align their physical features with their inner gender identity. This often includes genital and chest or breast reconstructive surgery. This surgery often takes place at age 18 years or older but may be done at a younger age in certain circumstances with parental consent. Research shows that most patients choosing gender-affirming surgery are satisfied with their decision and also report a marked improvement in psychological well-being.[55,77]

It is important for clinicians to recognize that transition can take many forms, all valid and to be respected. Some transgender children on the brink of puberty may feel they will be comfortable with the physical changes they are about to experience and therefore decline pubertal suppression therapy. Others may decline hormonal or surgical transition options. The important thing is that clinicians have these important discussions with their patients and inform them and their parents of the options available to them, including a consideration of the pros and cons of various transition options in light of each patient's individual experience and needs.

Optimism for the future. Clinicians should not only focus on the risks that transgender youths face but also identify specific strengths that have supported their resilience growing up in an often unaccepting, sometimes hostile world. They should also challenge the belief of many transgender youths that their future will be significantly limited by their gender identity. Although some communities are more accepting and supportive of transgender people than others, US society is changing rapidly in a positive direction and many transgender adults lead happy, healthy, and fulfilling lives. Although growing up transgender can still be very challenging, the future should be seen as hopeful and exciting.

Advocacy

Because of their expertise and position of respect, pediatric clinicians are in an advantageous position to advocate on behalf of children with gender variant behaviors, transgender youths, and their families. Such advocacy is essential in supporting these children's and youths' optimal physical, social, and psychological well-being, allowing them to grow into a happy, healthy, and productive adulthood. Clinicians should encourage parents, siblings, and extended family to accept and love these young people unconditionally. The clinician should also be willing to meet with school personnel, child and youth welfare program staff, and others to share information about gender variance and transgenderism. Because schools are a major part of a child's or youth's life, and because they are often the site where significant harassment and bullying of gender variant and transgender youths take place, it is especially important that clinicians provide advocacy at all levels of local educational systems. This includes advocacy for the adoption of anti-harassment policies specifically addressing discrimination, harassment, and bullying based on gender identity and expression as well as sexual orientation. It also includes advocating for mandated training of teachers and social service providers and the implementation of policies that ensure that transgender youths are safe and treated respectfully, such as through the use of preferred names and pronouns, designation of appropriate bathrooms and changing rooms, and allowing a student to participate in graduation ceremonies and other school activities on the basis of gender identity rather than birth-assigned sex.

For clinicians seeking to advocate for societal change, encouraging the development and implementation of policies, procedures, and programs that recognize and respect the individuality of these children and youths and address their special needs for validation and safety is essential. The clinician may also provide testimony at official meetings and hearings on proposals to add gender identity and expression to laws and school policies prohibiting discrimination, harassment, and bullying. The clinician may also advocate for the inclusion of meaningful medical school, residency training, and continuing medical education curricula on the life experience and health needs of children with gender variant expression and transgender individuals and how to address these needs in a respectful and effective manner. Finally, the clinician should encourage professional organizations to develop policy statements and clinical guidelines to support them in their work with these young people and their families.

When to Refer

Refer to a child behavioral, adolescent, or gender specialist whenever children or youths

▶ Show significant gender nonconforming behaviors, particularly if they are concerning to parents or have resulted in rejection or mistreatment by family members, peers, or others. Ideally, referral will be made before possible dysphoria arises.

▶ Show signs or symptoms of gender dysphoria, including expression of dissatisfaction or distress related to their birth-assigned gender or insistence that they are of another gender.

Refer to a child and adolescent psychiatrist or another mental health professional whenever a child or a youth

▶ Experiences persistent or recurrent depressed or anxious mood that interferes with function
▶ Has acute or recurrent suicidal ideation or self-injury
▶ Evidences isolation from peers or family members
▶ Engages in substance use or other high-risk behaviors

It should be noted that referrals for therapy to change a youth's gender identity or expression are considered unethical.[14]

AAP Policy

American Academy of Pediatrics Committee on Adolescence. Office-based care for lesbian, gay, bisexual, transgender, and questioning youth. *Pediatrics*. 2013;132(1): 198–203 (pediatrics.aappublications.org/content/132/1/198)

References

1. Peletz MG. Transgenderism and gender pluralism in Southeast Asia since early modern times. *Curr Anthropol*. 2006;47(2):309–340
2. Lang S. Lesbians, men-women, and two-spirits: homosexuality and gender in Native American cultures. In: Blackwood E, Wieringa S, eds. *Female Desires: Same-sex Relations and Transgender Practices Across Cultures*. New York, NY: Columbia University Press; 1999
3. Matzner A. *'O Au No Kea: Voices from Hawai'i's Mahu and Transgender Communities*. Philadelphia, PA: Xlibris; 2001
4. Green R. Mythological, historical, and cross-cultural aspects of transsexualism. In: Denny D, ed. *Current Concepts in Transgender Identity*. London, United Kingdom: Routledge Press; 1998
5. American Academy of Pediatrics Committee on Adolescence. Office-based care for lesbian, gay, bisexual, and questioning youth. *Pediatrics*. 2013;132(1):198–203

6. Levine DA; American Academy of Pediatrics Committee on Adolescence. Office-based care for lesbian, gay, bisexual, transgender, and questioning youth. *Pediatrics*. 2013;132(1):e297–e313

7. Society for Adolescent Health and Medicine. Recommendations for promoting the health and well-being of lesbian, gay, bisexual, and transgender adolescents: a position paper of the Society for Adolescent Health and Medicine. *J Adolesc Health*. 2013;52(4):506–510

8. Shields JP, Cohen R, Glassman JR, Whitaker K, Franks H, Bertonlini I. Estimating population size and demographic characteristics of lesbian, gay, bisexual, and transgender youth in middle school. *J Adolesc Health*. 2013;52(2):248–250

9. Meier C, Harris J. Fact sheet: gender diversity and transgender identity in children. American Psychological Association Web site. http://www.apadivisions.org/division-44/resources/advocacy/transgender-children.pdf. Accessed May 8, 2018

10. Vance SR Jr, Ehrensaft D, Rosenthal SM. Psychological and medical care of gender nonconforming youth. *Pediatrics*. 2014;134(6);1184–1192

11. Meenwijk EL, Sevelius JM. Transgender population size in the United States: a meta-regression of population-based probability samples. *Am J Public Health*. 2017;107(2):e1–e8

12. Steensma TD, van der Ende J, Verhulst FC, Cohen-Kettenis PT. Gender variance in childhood and sexual orientation in adulthood: a prospective study. *J Sex Med*. 2013;10(11):2723–2733

13. American Psychiatric Association. *Diagnostic and Statistical Manual of Mental Disorders*. 4th ed. Arlington, VA: American Psychiatric Association; 2000

14. American Psychiatric Association. *Diagnostic and Statistical Manual of Mental Disorders*. 5th ed. Arlington, VA: American Psychiatric Publishing; 2013

15. Vasey PL, Bartlett NH. What can the Samoan "fa'afine" teach us about the Western concept of gender identity disorder in children? *Perspect Biol Med*. 2007;50(4):481–490

16. Drescher J, Byne W. Gender dysphoric/gender variant (GD/GV) children and adolescents: summarizing what we know and what we have yet to learn. *J Homosex*. 2012;59(3):501–510

17. Wallien MS, Cohen-Kettenis PT. Psychosexual outcome of gender-dysphoric children. *J Am Acad Child Adolesc Psychiatry*. 2008;47(12):1413–1423

18. Zucker KJ. On the "natural history" of gender identity disorder in children. *J Am Acad Child Adolesc Psychiatry*. 2008;47(12):1361–1363

19. Bonifacio HJ, Rosenthal SM. Gender variance and dysphoria in children and adolescents. *Pediatr Clin North Am*. 2015;62(4):1001–1016

20. Rosenthal SM. Transgender youth: current concepts. *Ann Pediatr Endocrinol Metab*. 2016;21(4):185–192

21. Adelson SL; American Academy of Child and Adolescent Psychiatry Committee on Quality Issues. Practice parameter on gay, lesbian, or bisexual sexual orientation, gender nonconformity, and gender discordance in children and adolescents. *J Am Acad Child Adolesc Psychiatry*. 2012;51(9): 957–974

22. Zucker KJ. Gender identity development and issues. *Child Adolesc Psychiatr Clin North Am*. 2004;13(3):551–568

23. Zucker KJ. Gender identity disorders. In: Lewis M, ed. *Child and Adolescent Psychiatry: A Comprehensive Textbook*. Philadelphia, PA: Lippincott Williams & Wilkins; 2002

24. Pleak RR. Ethical issues in diagnosing and treating gender-dysphoric children and adolescents. In: Rottnek M, ed. *Sissies and Tomboys: Gender Nonconformity and Homosexual Childhood*. New York, NY: New York University Press; 1999

25. Stein E. Commentary on the treatment of gender variant and gender dysphoric children and adolescents: common themes and ethical reflections. *J Homosex*. 2012;59(3):480–500

26. Menvielle EJ. Gender identity disorder. *J Am Acad Child Adolesc Psychiatry*. 1998;37(3):243–245

27. Gooren L. The biology of human psychosexual differentiation. *Horm Behav*. 2006;50(4):589–601

28. Hare L, Bernard P, Sánchez FJ, et al. Androgen receptor repeat length polymorphism associated with male-to-female transsexualism. *Biol Psychiatry*. 2009;65(1):93–96

29. Bentz EK, Hefler LA, Kaufmann U, Huber JC, Kolbus A, Tempfer CB. A polymorphism of the *CYP17* gene related to sex steroid metabolism is associated with female-to-male but not male-to-female transsexualism. *Fertil Steril*. 2008;90(1):56–59

30. Coolidge FL, Thede LL, Young SE. The heritability of gender identity disorder in a child and adolescent twin sample. *Behav Genet*. 2002;32(4):251–257

31. Zhou JN, Hofman MA, Gooren LJ, Swaab DF. A sex difference in the human brain and its relation to transsexuality. *Nature*. 1995;378(6552):68–70

32. Kruijver FP, Zhou JN, Pool CW, Hofman MA, Gooren LJ, Swaab DF. Male-to-female transsexuals have female neuron numbers in a limbic nucleus. *J Clin Endocrinol Metab*. 2000;85(5):2034–2041

33. Berglund H, Lindström P, Dhejne-Helmy C, Savic I. Male-to-female transsexuals show sex-atypical hypothalamus activation when smelling odorous steroids. *Cereb Cortex*. 2008;18(8): 1900–1908

34. Mallon GP, DeCrescenzo T. Transgender children and youth: a child welfare practice perspective. *Child Welfare*. 2006;85(2):215–241

35. Connolly MD, Zervos MJ, Barone CJ II, Johnson CC, Joseph CL. The mental health of transgender youth: advances in understanding. *J Adolesc Health*. 2016;59(5):489–495

36. Aitken M, Vanderlaan DP, Wasserman L, Stojanovski S, Zucker KJ. Self-harm and suicidality in children referred for gender dysphoria. *J Am Acad Child Adolesc Psychiatry*. 2016;55(6): 513–520

37. Reisner SL, Vetters R, Leclerc M, et al. Mental health of transgender youth in care at an adolescent urban community health center: a matched retrospective cohort study. *J Adolesc Health*. 2015;56(3):274–279

38. Eisenberg ME, Gower AL, McMorris BJ, Rider GN, Shea G, Coleman E. Risk and protective factors in the lives of transgender/gender nonconforming adolescents. *J Adolesc Health*. 2017; 61(4):521–526

39. Bouris A, Everett BG, Heath RD, Elsaesser CE, Neilands TB. Effects of victimization and violence on suicidal ideation and behaviors among sexual minority and heterosexual adolescents. *LGBT Health*. 2016;3(2):153–161

40. Wilber S, Ryan C, Marksamer J. *CWLA Best Practice Guidelines for Serving LGBT Youth in Out-of-Home Care*. Washington, DC: CWLA Press; 2006

41. Ray N. *Lesbian, Gay, Bisexual, and Transgender Youth: An Epidemic of Homelessness*. New York, NY: National Gay and Lesbian Task Force Policy Institute and National Coalition for the Homeless; 2006. National LGBTQ Task Force Web site. http://www.thetaskforce.org/static_html/downloads/HomelessYouth.pdf. Accessed May 8, 2018

42. Majd K, Marksamer J, Reyes C. *Hidden Injustice: Lesbian, Gay, Bisexual, and Transgender Youth in Juvenile Courts*. Washington, DC: Legal Services for Children, National Juvenile Defender Center, and National Center for Lesbian Rights; 2009

43. Toomey RB, Ryan C, Diaz RM, Card NA, Russell ST. Gender-nonconforming lesbian, gay, bisexual, and transgender youth: school victimization and young adult psychosocial adjustment. *Dev Psychol*. 2010;46(6):1580–1589

44. Earnshaw VA, Bogart LM, Poteat VP, Reisner SL, Schuster MA. Bullying among lesbian, gay, bisexual, and transgender youth. *Pediatr Clin North Am*. 2016;63(6):999–1010

45. Greytak EA, Kosciw JG, Diaz EM. *Harsh Realities: The Experience of Transgender Youth in Our Nation's Schools: A Report From the Gay, Lesbian and Straight Education Network*. New York, NY: GLSEN; 2009. GLSEN Web site. https://www.glsen.org/sites/default/files/Harsh%20Realities.pdf. Accessed May 8, 2018

46. Hatzenbuehler ML, Pachankis JE. Stigma and minority stress as social determinants of health among lesbian, gay, bisexual, and transgender youth. *Pediatr Clin North Am*. 2016;63(6): 985–997

47. Gay and Lesbian Medical Association. *Guidelines for the Care of Lesbian, Gay, Bisexual, and Transgender Patients*. Washington, DC: Gay and Lesbian Medical Association; 2006. GLMA Web site. http://glma.org/_data/n_0001/resources/live/GLMA%20guidelines%202006%20 FINAL.pdf. Accessed May 8, 2018

48. Kaiser Permanente National Diversity Council, Kaiser Permanente National Diversity Department. *A Provider's Handbook on Culturally Competent Care: Lesbian, Gay, Bisexual, and Transgendered Population*. 2nd ed. Oakland, CA: Kaiser Permanente; 2004

49. Makadon HJ, Mayer KH, Potter J, Goldhammer H, eds. *Fenway Guide to Lesbian, Gay, Bisexual, and Transgender Health*. 2nd ed. Philadelphia, PA: American College of Physicians; 2015

50. Center of Excellence for Transgender Health, University of California, San Francisco. Center of Excellence for Transgender Health Web site. http://transhealth.ucsf.edu. Accessed May 8, 2018

51. Dean L, Meyer IH, Robinson K, et al. Lesbian, gay, bisexual, and transgender health: findings and concerns. *J Gay Lesbian Med Assoc*. 2000;4(3):101–151

52. Gridley SJ, Crouch JM, Evans Y, et al. Youth and caregiver perspectives on barriers to gender-affirming health care for transgender youth. *J Adolesc Health*. 2016;59(3):254–261

53. Stevens J, Gomez-Lobo V, Pine-Twaddell E. Insurance coverage of puberty blocker therapies for transgender youth. *Pediatrics*. 2015;136(6):1029–1031

54. Spack NP, Edwards-Leeper L, Feldman HA, et al. Children and adolescents with gender identity disorder referred to a pediatric medical center. *Pediatrics*. 2012;129(3):418–425

55. Coleman E, Bockting W, Botzer M, et al; World Professional Association for Transgender Health. Standards of care for the health of transsexual, transgender, and gender nonconforming people. *Int J Transgend*. 2011;13(4):165–232

56. Hembree WC, Cohen-Kettenis PT, Gooren L, et al. Endocrine treatment of gender-dysphoric/gender-incongruent persons: an Endocrine Society clinical practice guideline. *J Clin Endocrinol Metab*. 2017;102(11):3869–3903

57. de Vries AL, McGuire JK, Steensma TD, Wagenaar EC, Doreleijers TA, Cohen-Kettenis PT. Young adult psychological outcome after puberty suppression and gender reassignment. *Pediatrics*. 2014;134(4):696–704

58. Goldenring JM, Rosen DS. Getting into adolescents' heads: an essential update. *Contemp Pediatr*. 2004;21(64):64–90

59. Zucker KJ, Wood H, Singh D, Bradley SJ. A developmental, biopsychosocial model for the treatment of children with gender identity disorder. *J Homosex*. 2012;59(3):369–397

60. Menvielle E. A comprehensive program for children with gender variant behaviors and gender identity disorders. *J Homosex*. 2012;59(3):357–368

61. de Vries AL, Cohen-Kettenis PT. Clinical management of gender dysphoria in children and adolescents: the Dutch approach. *J Homosex*. 2012;59(3):301–320

62. Hidalgo MA, Ehrensaft D, Tishelman AC, et al. The gender affirmative model: what we know and what we aim to learn. *Hum Dev*. 2013;56(5):285–290

63. Olson KR, Durwood L, DeMeules M, McLaughlin KA. Mental health of transgender children who are supported in their identities. *Pediatrics*. 2016;137(3):e20153223

64. Ehrensaft D. From gender identity disorder to gender identity creativity: true gender self child therapy. *J Homosex*. 2012;59(3):337–356

65. Edwards-Leeper L, Spack NP. Psychological evaluation and medical treatment of transgender youth in an interdisciplinary "Gender Management Service" (GeMS) in a major pediatric center. *J Homosex*. 2012;59(3):321–336

66. Ryan C, Huebner D, Diaz RM, Sanchez J. Family rejection as a predictor of negative health outcomes in white and Latino lesbian, gay, and bisexual young adults. *Pediatrics*. 2009;123(1):346–352

67. Ryan C. Engaging families to support lesbian, gay, bisexual and transgender (LGBT) youth: The Family Acceptance Project. *Prev Res*. 2010;17(4):11–13

68. DeCrescenzo T, Mallon GP. *Serving Transgender Youth: The Role of Child Welfare Systems.* Arlington, VA: Child Welfare League of America; 2002

69. Woronoff R, Estrada R, Sommer S. *Out of the Margins: A Report on Regional Listening Forums Highlighting the Experience of Lesbian, Gay, Bisexual, Transgender, and Questioning Youth in Care.* Washington, DC: Child Welfare League of America Inc, and New York, NY: Lambda Legal Defense and Education Fund Inc; 2006

70. Advocates for Youth. *I Think I Might Be Transgender, Now What Do I Do?* Washington, DC: Advocates for Youth; 2004. Advocates for Youth Web site. http://www.advocatesforyouth.org/index.php?option=com_content&task=view&id=731&Itemid=177. Accessed May 8, 2018

71. *Guidance for Massachusetts Public Schools: Creating a Safe and Supportive School Environment.* Malden, MA: Massachusetts Department of Elementary and Secondary Education; 2013. http://www.doe.mass.edu/ssce/genderidentity.pdf. Updated June 12, 2017. Accessed May 8, 2018

72. Gorin-Lazard A, Baumstarck K, Boyer L, et al. Hormonal therapy is associated with better self-esteem, mood, and quality of life in transsexuals. *J Nerv Ment Dis.* 2013;201(11):996–1000

73. White Hughto JM, Reisner SL. A systematic review of the effects of hormone therapy on psychological functioning and quality of life in transgender individuals. *Transgend Health.* 2016;1(1):21–31

74. de Vries AL, Steensma TD, Doreleijers TA, Cohen-Kettenis PT. Puberty suppression in adolescents with gender identity disorder: a prospective follow-up study. *J Sex Med.* 2011; 8(8):2276–2283

75. Costa R, Collizzi M. The effect of cross-sex hormonal treatment on gender dysphoria individuals' mental health: a systematic review. *Neuropsychiatr Dis Treat.* 2016;12:1953–1966

76. Rosenthal SM. Approach to the patient: transgender youth: endocrine considerations. *J Clin Endocrinol Metab.* 2014;99:4379–4389

77. Murad MH, Elamin MB, Garcia MZ, et al. Hormonal therapy and sex reassignment: a systematic review and meta-analysis of quality of life and psychosocial outcomes. *Clin Endocrinol (Oxf).* 2010;72(2):214–231

Children in Gay- and Lesbian-Parented Families

Cindy Schorzman, MD, and Melanie A. Gold, DO, DMQ

"Although no data have been found to suggest that children with gay or lesbian parents are different from other children in their cognitive, psychosocial, and sexual development, these children and their families face social challenges that their pediatric clinicians can help address."

Family structures in the United States, as in much of the world, are changing. The traditional structure of a working father and a homemaker mother with one or more children no longer describes most families in the United States. Alternative family structures are diverse. Unmarried couples may live together, with or without children. Single mothers and fathers, stepparents, and blended families may be created by design, by divorce, or by death. These family structures may include men whose sexual orientation is gay and women whose sexual orientation is lesbian, with or without children.

Recent estimates of children and adolescents (collectively referred to as *children* in this chapter unless otherwise specified) in the United States with at least one gay or lesbian parent range from 1 to 10 million. According to US Census data from 2010, about 1% of all-couple households were same-sex couples, and about 19% of all same-sex couples are raising children.[1] These estimates are limited by barriers to obtaining accurate numbers, in part, because many gay and lesbian parents still fear discrimination and do not report their sexual orientations.

Specific research on issues regarding gay and lesbian parenting, including the mental health of the children in these families, has historically been driven by legal issues, particularly those concerning custody. This research has focused on assessing the development and well-being of children raised by gay or lesbian parents. (Box 22-1 contains a glossary of terms associated with gender identity and sexual orientation.)

An understanding of these issues will better help prepare pediatric clinicians (ie, primary care pediatricians, pediatric subspecialists, and family physicians, internists, nurse practitioners, and physician assistants who serve as health care providers to children and adolescents) for meeting the needs, including mental health needs, of pediatric patients within the context of their family structures.

Child Development in the Context of Gay- and Lesbian-Parented Families

No consistent differences exist in the psychological profiles of children raised by gay and lesbian parents compared with children raised by heterosexual parents. During the 1990s, research became increasingly available on children conceived in the context of gay and lesbian relationships, and such research has continued through today.

Children who have gay or lesbian parents do not differ from children who have heterosexual parents in psychological health, social relationships, or cognitive or emotional functioning.[2-5] Rather, the best predictors of child behavioral problems are higher levels of parental stress and interparental conflict.[2]

The most recent research provides further support that children adopted by lesbian and gay parents are well-adjusted, not only in early childhood but also into middle childhood. A 2010 study used census data to examine the school advancement of 3,500 children with same-sex parents, finding no significant differences between households headed by same-sex

---

Box 22-1. Glossary of Terms Associated With Gender Identity and Sexual Orientation

- **Gender identity:** Personal sense of one's integral maleness or femaleness, a blend of both, or neither.

- **Gender roles:** Behaviors within a culture commonly thought to be associated with masculinity or femininity.

- **Homophobia:** Unprovoked fear, distrust, or hatred of people who are identified as or perceived as lesbian, gay, bisexual, or transgender people.

- **Sexual orientation:** Persistent pattern of emotional attraction, romantic attraction, or sexual attraction, or any combination of those attractions, to other people. Included are homosexuality (same-sex attractions), bisexuality (attractions to members of both sexes), heterosexuality (opposite-sex attractions), and asexuality (persistent lack of attraction toward any gender).

and opposite-sex parents when controlling for family background.[6] In a longitudinal study of nearly 100 adoptive families with school-aged children as they matured from early to middle childhood, Farr noted that there were no differences among heterosexual and same-sex parent family types in longitudinal psychological child outcomes and that, regardless of parental sexual orientation, children had fewer behavioral problems over time and had higher family functioning when their parents indicated experiencing less parenting stress.[2] In another recent study, using the 2011–2012 National Survey of Children's Health data set, Bos and colleagues found no differences were observed between household types on family relationships or any child outcomes.[7]

The sexual orientation of parents has not been found to affect the gender identity of their children.[3,8] Furthermore, adolescent sexual orientation is similar among adolescents raised by gay or lesbian parents and those raised by heterosexual parents.[3,9] Children raised by lesbian mothers are more likely to explore same-sex sexual relationships, particularly if their childhood family environment is characterized by an openness and acceptance of lesbian and gay relationships. However, these children are no more likely than the children of heterosexual mothers to identify themselves as gay or lesbian.[4]

Clinicians caring for a pediatric population should be aware that the psychological experience might differ for children raised in heterosexual vs homosexual parenting environments. The greatest difference reported is bullying. Although no overall increase in stigmatization may exist, children of couples who do not define themselves as heterosexual are more likely than those of heterosexual couples to be teased and to be concerned about being harassed. Some children experience shame because of conflicts between loyalty to their parents and the perceived need to conceal their parents' sexual orientation for self-preservation.[10]

This conclusion, that research to date demonstrates few discernible differences in parenting based on parental sexual orientation, is not universally accepted. Outspoken critics of the literature have highlighted the limitations of these studies, including small sample size (these studies may be more likely to conclude that no differences exist when some differences indeed exist), lack of generalizability (participants were mostly lesbian, white, well educated, and upper-middle class), lack of randomization of study populations, and lack of appropriate comparison groups.[11]

However, no studies have been published in the peer-reviewed literature that demonstrate differences in a child's development based on the sexual orientation of the parents or show any evidence that gay and lesbian parenting causes significant deleterious effects on children. Taken together, the overwhelming number of studies (despite their limitations) demonstrates no differences in children's development based on the sexual orientation of their parent or parents.[12] Adams and Light, in their analysis of temporal patterns in citation networks, found that the literature on outcomes for children of same-sex parents is marked by scientific consensus that they experience "no differences" compared to children from other parental configurations.[3]

The American Academy of Pediatrics (commonly known as the AAP) Committee on Psychosocial Aspects of Child and Family Health reviewed the available data on children of gay and lesbian parents and published a technical report in 2002 with a policy statement supporting co- or second-parent adoption by same-sex parents. Its conclusion was that "a growing body of scientific literature demonstrates that children who grow up with 1 or 2 gay and/or lesbian parents fare as well in emotional, cognitive, social, and sexual functioning as do children whose parents are heterosexual" and that "children's optimal development seems to be influenced more by the nature of the relationships and interactions within the family unit than by the particular structural form it takes."[13] Despite some reservations based on the limitations of the studies, such as those noted previously, the committee thought that the weight of the available evidence was strong enough to demonstrate "that there is no systematic difference between gay and non-gay parents in emotional health, parenting skills, and attitudes toward parenting."[13]

Social Relationships and Disclosure

All children, especially as they reach school age, must develop a wide range of relationships outside their nuclear families. The difference between dominant cultural values in the community and the family constellation may be distressing to children and add to their social isolation and uncomfortable relationships with peers.[14] Children who have gay or lesbian parents may be assumed to be homosexual and experience stigmatization by peers when their parents' sexual orientations become known. Moreover, gay and lesbian parents often fear that school staff will treat their children differently if they disclose their sexual orientations. As a result, many parents help children learn *differential disclosure*, that is, to be open about their parents' sexual orientations to some people but not to others, so harassment and social isolation can be minimized. Parents should understand that both secrecy and disclosure represent potential burdens for their children. Also, many families parented by gay and lesbian parents, including families created by adoption, may be transracial in nature. Pediatric clinicians should note that these differences can further contribute to the stressors experienced by the child and the family.

Pediatric clinicians can act as supportive listeners for families with difficult interactions with their school systems. Some providers with long-standing school relationships may choose to act as intermediaries between the family and the school to help make the educational environment more supportive and to enhance their patients' psychological well-being. They can educate child care providers and teachers and encourage schools to include information about diverse family structures in their libraries and curricula. Clinicians can also encourage families to develop a social support network in the interest of their children. In many larger cities, an active network of gay and lesbian parents works to create an environment of peer support in which their children feel more accepted than they might in other social contexts. Parent-child discussion or playgroups, story hours, and periodic communal meals have helped some parents and children seeking mutual support.

Legal Issues

Controversy regarding securing legal parental rights for gay and lesbian parents can have an impact on the mental health of patients whose families may face uncertainty and possible adversity. Legislation constantly shifts the parameters of parental rights and responsibilities. Laws have recently changed to allow for joint adoption in all 50 states and Washington, DC. Depending on specific circumstances and where someone lives, access to joint adoption may require being in a legally recognized relationship, such as marriage, civil union, or domestic partnership. Of note, however, several states still permit state-licensed child welfare agencies to refuse to place and provide services to children and families, including lesbian, gay, bisexual, and transgender (LGBT) people and same-sex couples, if doing so conflicts with their religious beliefs.[14,15]

Recognizing and helping to address the challenges to the stability of the family constellation can potentially benefit the mental well-being of patients. In the circumstance that only one person from the same-sex couple is legally recognized as a child's parent, the clinician should clarify how responsibility for the medical decisions and consent for treatment for the child will be shared and document this information in the medical record. In the event of serious injury, illness, death, or voluntary separation of the legal parent, a prior written agreement giving the other parent power of attorney in making medical decisions for the child is necessary. Curry et al give guidelines for writing agreements that specify parental rights and responsibilities.[16]

Clinical Issues in Providing Pediatric Care

The challenge for the pediatric clinician who cares for these children, including their mental health needs, lies in addressing practical concerns faced by individual families. Meeting the needs of children of gay and lesbian parents means addressing the needs of the children themselves, as well as understanding the particular issues within the context of the child's family as a whole. Gay or lesbian parents may choose not to identify their sexual orientation to their child's provider. They may worry that latent homophobia or bias among professional or nonprofessional staff will jeopardize the care their children receive or that the provider will not honor their confidentiality, particularly if the parents are concerned about legal threats to their custody rights. The challenge for the clinician caring for these children often lies in creating an environment in which members of the family feel comfortable enough to disclose and discuss the parents' sexual orientation and the family constellation.

Health care professionals have traditionally received little or no training about homosexuality.[17,18] According to a 2011 article in the *Journal of the American Medical Association,* the median reported time dedicated to LGBT-related topics in 2009–2010 was small across US and Canadian medical schools, and the quantity, content covered, and perceived quality of instruction varied substantially.[19]

In fact, evidence suggests that gay and lesbian adults find the health care system to be unresponsive and sometimes antagonistic to their unique needs and concerns.[20,21]

Little information exists about how lesbian and gay parents view pediatric care. One study found that most gay and lesbian parents perceived that their children received pediatric care that was affirming, supportive, and satisfactory. However, many specific deficiencies were noted, such as heterosexist assumptions on office forms, exclusion of the nonbiological parent from the evaluation and treatment process, and explicit insensitivity to particular family involvements.[21] In addition, parents who had not disclosed their sexual orientation to their child's medical provider had concerns that such disclosure might compromise their child's care, result in negative judgments about their parenting, and infringe on their confidentiality.

They described a significant number of concerns regarding medical providers, such as prejudice against their children, providing disparate care, lack of communication about the child's health with the nonbiological parent, and identifying parental lifestyle as the cause of any child physical or behavioral problems.[21]

Pediatric clinicians can create a safe and inclusive environment for same-sex parents and their children. Establishing a supportive health care environment requires that medical providers first examine their own attitudes toward gay and lesbian parenting. Perrin and Kulkin assert that clinicians "who cannot reconcile their personal beliefs with their professional obligation to provide supportive, understanding, and respectful care to gay and lesbian families should recognize this limitation and refer these families to a [clinician] who can better meet their needs."[21] Once the clinician has addressed these issues personally, health care staff attitudes can be similarly addressed with interventions such as diversity training and strict guidelines regarding confidentiality.

Pediatric clinicians can convey their support of all forms of families, and the office environment can reflect a supportive, safe environment for children of diverse families. Hospital and office policies regarding the use of gender-neutral language and the inclusion of nonbiological parents during the child's office visits can be discussed and enforced. Box 22-2 illustrates examples of questions to clarify family constellation in ways that can be

Box 22-2. Questions to Clarify the Family Constellation

- Is there anything about your family that would be helpful for me to know?
- Who are the adults who make up your family?
- Who are the important people in your child's life?
- Who lives at home? What is your relationship with each child caregiver?
- By what name does your child call each family member?
- Who are the other important members of your family or support system who help care for your child?
- Do you share parenting responsibilities with anyone else?
- Who helps you with parenting?
- Does anyone else participate in parenting?
- Does the biological parent or do both biological parents, if not part of the current constellation, have any involvement in child care?
- Which of your child's caregivers can give legal consent for medical care?
- Do any of your child's biological relatives have any medical conditions?

applied to any family system, including blended and adoptive families. In their work, Perrin and Kulkin identified several changes in the office or hospital environment that demonstrate support for diversity of family structures.[21] These efforts include displaying posters, magazines, books, and pamphlets that portray a wide range of family constructs. A nondiscrimination policy, prominently displayed in the waiting area, can do much to assure members of a diverse array of family structures, including, but not limited to, gay and lesbian parents and their adolescents, that the office is a safe environment for disclosure of sensitive issues (Box 22-3). Standard office forms can be modified to include gender-neutral terms, such as *parent, caregiver,* and *family member.*[18,22] Resources can be made available in the office, such as books about gay and lesbian parenting (Box 22-4), information regarding community and national support groups (Box 22-5), and standard medical forms such as medical power of attorney designation.

As the child grows and develops, in addition to standard anticipatory guidance issues, particular concerns related to mental health tend to surface at different developmental stages. In the preschool period, common concerns include how to explain the composition of one's own family and the methods of reproduction.[23] Gold and colleagues suggest that early childhood "is a good time to initiate explanations to the child about his own origin and to introduce concepts of the variety of loving relationships."[20] Pediatric clinicians can help parents empower their children to deal with these issues by encouraging them to allow the child to control the information she discloses to friends or teachers; parents should simultaneously help their children prepare for the possible negative consequences of disclosure.[19]

Parents should be encouraged to help their children come up with their own creative ways to describe their family in positive terms.[21] A gay or lesbian couple might celebrate their essential roles as 2 loving supportive parents while additionally recognizing the other important adult role models and caregivers who compose the child's extended family. For example, in the context of a lesbian couple with children, one approach to Father's Day might be to redefine it as a celebration of the child's male role models, such as writing cards to an uncle or a close male family friend.

Box 22-3. Example of Nondiscrimination Policy for the Pediatric Office

Office Nondiscrimination Policy

This office appreciates diversity and does not discriminate on the basis of race, national origin, age, religion, ability, sexual orientation, or perceived gender.

Box 22-4. Selected Books and Resources for Diverse Families

Stories of Lesbian, Gay, Bisexual, and Transgender Families

- Drucker J. *Families of Value*. New York, NY: Plenum Press; 1998. A collection of stories depicting LGBT parents and their children.

- Gillespie P, ed. Kaeser G, photog. *Love Makes a Family: Portraits of Lesbian, Gay, Bisexual, and Transgender Parents and Their Families*. Amherst, MA: University of Massachusetts Press; 1999. Combines interviews and photographs to document the experiences of LGBT parents and their children.

- Herrera D, Seyda B, photog. *Women in Love: Portraits of Lesbian Mothers and Their Families*. Boston, MA: Bulfinch Press; 1998. A collection of photographs and stories of lesbian mothers and their families.

- Rizzo C, Schneiderman J, Schweig L, et al, eds. *All the Ways Home*. Norwich, VT: New Victoria Publishers; 1995. A collection of stories written for and by lesbian and gay parents exploring what it means to be a parent in the LGBT community.

- Strah D, Margolis S. *Gay Dads: A Celebration of Fatherhood*. Putnam, MA: JP Tarcher; 2003. The stories of 24 families, including family-building resources for gay men.

Discussing Gender Identity and Sexual Identity

- Mardell A. *The ABC's of LGBT*. Coral Gables, FL: Mango Media Inc; 2016. Advice for questioning teens, teachers, and parents, or anyone who wants to learn how to talk about gender identity and sexual identity.

Legal Issues

- American Civil Liberties Union. A national organization with state-by-state reference information regarding legislation affecting LGBT families (www.aclu.org/resources-lgbt-equality).

- Doskow E, Stewart M. *The Legal Answer Book for Families*. 2nd ed. Berkeley, CA: Nolo Press; 2014. A resource for lesbian and gay couples with and without children; includes information on custody and parental rights.

- Lambda Legal. A national organization focusing on full recognition of the civil rights of LGBT people, including legal resources such as examples of hospital visitation documentation for LGBT family members (www.lambdalegal.org).

Parenting Resources

- Davis L, Keyser J. *Becoming the Parent You Want to Be: A Sourcebook of Strategies for the First Five Years*. New York, NY: Broadway Books; 1997. A guide to parenting that addresses a broad range of issues, including toilet training, punishment, parenting with a partner, and gender roles.

- Clunis DM, Green GD. *The Lesbian Parenting Book: A Guide to Creating Families and Raising Children*. Washington, DC: Seal Press; 2003. Detailed, chapter-by-chapter information on each stage of parenthood and child development.

- Rosswood E. *Journey to Same-sex Parenthood: Firsthand Advice, Tips and Stories From Lesbian and Gay Couples*. Far Hills, NJ: New Horizon Press; 2016. A guide for prospective LGBT parents to explore adoption, foster care, assisted reproduction, surrogacy, and co-parenting.

Box 22-4. Selected Books and Resources for Diverse Families (*continued*)

Books for Children

- Aldrich AR, Motz M. *How My Family Came to Be: Daddy, Papa and Me*. Oakland, CA: New Family Press; 2003. For ages 4–8 years. Loving story of how 2 men and a baby came together to make a family.

- de Haan L, Nijland S. *King and King*. Berkeley, CA: Tricycle Press; 2000. For ages 4–8 years. A prince "who has never cared much for princesses" finds true love with another prince.

- Newman L. *Heather Has Two Mommies*. 10th ed. Los Angeles, CA: Alyson Publications; 2000. For ages 2–6 years. Originally self-published in 1989, the story of a little girl named Heather and her 2 lesbian mothers.

- Newman L, Thompson C. *Daddy, Papa, and Me*. Berkeley, CA: Tricycle Press; 2009. For ages 2–6 years. Board book shows a toddler spending the day with its daddies.

- Newman L, Thompson C. *Mommy, Mama, and Me*. Berkeley, CA: Tricycle Press; 2009. For ages 2–6 years. Board book shows a toddler spending the day with its mommies.

- Parnell P, Richardson J. *And Tango Makes Three*. New York, NY: Simon & Schuster Children's Publishing; 2005. For ages 4–8 years. This tale is based on a true story about Roy and Silo, 2 male penguins living in New York City's Central Park Zoo who raise a penguin daughter.

- Parr T. *The Family Book*. New York, NY: Little Brown and Company; 2003. For ages 2–5 years. This book celebrates all kinds of families and shows how each is special in its own way.

Abbreviation: LGBT, lesbian, gay, bisexual, and transgender.

The transition to school years also poses particular challenges for children from a nontraditional family background.[21] For parents and children alike, this transition involves deciding whether to disclose their nontraditional family status to teachers and the families of the child's friends. During the early school years, peer acceptance and teasing often become concerns. In the National Lesbian Families Study, 18% of children had experienced some form of discrimination by age 5 years, and 43% had experienced homophobia by age 10 years.[23,24] Empathetic listening, role-playing about how to respond to teasing, and providing information to parents and their children through support groups can assist both parents and children in coping with stigma and discrimination.[20,22]

During adolescence, issues of sexuality tend to come to the forefront regardless of family structure; teenagers in households with lesbian and gay parents are certainly no exception, and they may have their own unique challenges. Early adolescents may feel marginalized and stigmatized by being seen as part of a nontraditional family.[20] Teenagers may feel guilty, torn between loyalty to their families and pride in their family structures

Box 22-5. Selected Web Sites of Resource Groups for Diverse Families

- COLAGE: Children of Lesbians and Gays Everywhere (www.colage.org)
- Family Equality Council (formerly Family Pride Coalition) (www.familyequality.org)
- GLSEN (formerly known as Gay, Lesbian and Straight Education Network) (www.glsen.org)
- Human Rights Campaign (www.hrc.org)
- PFLAG (formerly Parents, Families and Friends of Lesbians and Gays) (www.pflag.org)

and an intense desire to form and maintain relationships and fit in with their peers. Clinicians can help adolescents and their parents by listening in a nonjudgmental fashion and by offering resources (eg, the handout *Gay, Lesbian or Bisexual Parents: Information for Children and Parents,* available at https://patiented.solutions.aap.org) and support groups.[20] Although individual situations vary, some evidence supports encouraging adolescents to disclose their nontraditional family status to their friends. Gershon and colleagues found that adolescents who disclosed their parents' lesbian orientation to their friends reported closer friendships and higher self-esteem than those who did not.[25]

To meet the ever-changing needs of patients and their families, pediatric clinicians should have available a list of local and national support groups and community resources. They might also consider taking a proactive approach in their patients' lives by not only providing a safe, nurturing office environment but also taking steps in the community to help counteract the generalized homophobia that children of gay and lesbian parents continually face.

Advocacy

Although no evidence has been found that children raised by gay or lesbian parents will develop abnormally or be less well-adjusted than other children, these children may be faced with criticism and isolation, which may affect their self-esteems. Pediatric clinicians who care for these children should be informed about community resources and may choose to be available as consultants to schools and to gay and lesbian support groups, as there may be an opportunity to help change social attitudes and restrictive legal codes that are damaging to their patients with gay and lesbian parents. They can learn which community and national programs are supportive of gay and lesbian parents and provide guidance to those families regarding child care and school selection. Clinicians can also provide a bibliography of books for children and parents (Box 22-4) and a list of local and national resource groups (Box 22-5). Above all, pediatric clinicians have the opportunity and the responsibility to support and advise all families in achieving their maximal nurturing potentials.

Conclusion

Children will flourish in various family environments as long as these settings include adequate nurturance and guidance for optimal development. Although no data have been found to suggest that children with gay or lesbian parents are different from other children in their cognitive, psychosocial, and sexual development, these children and their families face social challenges to optimal mental health that their pediatric clinicians can help address. These challenges are best met within the context of the child's life as a whole, and the routine medical care of children and adolescents should not be overshadowed by their nontraditional family status. The diversity of the family structures of the gay and lesbian community should be recognized, and anticipatory guidance and care should be tailored to individual needs.

Acknowledgments: The authors gratefully acknowledge the expert contributions of Debra L. Bogen, MD, and Mark S. Friedman, PhD.

AAP Policy

American Academy of Pediatrics Committee on Psychosocial Aspects of Child and Family Health. Promoting the well-being of children whose parents are gay or lesbian. *Pediatrics.* 2013;131(4):827–830 (pediatrics.aappublications.org/content/131/4/827)

Perrin EC, Siegel BS; American Academy of Pediatrics Committee on Psychosocial Aspects of Child and Family Health. Technical report—promoting the well-being of children whose parents are gay or lesbian. *Pediatrics.* 2013;131(4):e1374–e1383 (pediatrics.aappublications.org/content/131/4/e1374)

References

1. Lofquist D. Same-sex couple households. *Am Community Survey Briefs.* 2011:1–4. https://www.census.gov/prod/2011pubs/acsbr10-03.pdf. Published September 2011. Accessed January 27, 2018
2. Farr RH. Does parental sexual orientation matter? A longitudinal follow-up of adoptive families with school-age children. *Dev Psychol.* 2017;53(2):252–264
3. Adams J, Light R. Scientific consensus, the law, and same sex parenting outcomes. *Soc Sci Res.* 2015;53:300–310

4. Golombok S, Tasker F, Murray C. Children raised in fatherless families from infancy: family relationships and the socioemotional development of children of lesbian and single heterosexual mothers. *J Child Psychol Psychiatry.* 1997;38(7):783–791

5. Flaks D, Ficher I, Masterpasqua F, et al. Lesbians choosing motherhood: a comparative study of lesbian and heterosexual parents and their children. *Dev Psychol.* 1995;31(1):105–114

6. Rosenfeld MJ. Nontraditional families and childhood progress through school. *Demography.* 2010;47(3):755–775

7. Bos HM, Knox JR, van Rijn-van Gelderen L, Gartrell NK. Same-sex and different-sex parent households and child health outcomes: findings from the National Survey of Children's Health. *J Dev Behav Pediatr.* 2016;37(3):179–187

8. Brewaeys A, Ponjaert I, Van Hall EV, Golombok S. Donor insemination: child development and family functioning in lesbian mother families. *Hum Reprod.* 1997;12(6):1349–1359

9. Bailey JM, Bobrow D, Wolfe M, Mikach S. Sexual orientation of adult sons of gay fathers. *Dev Psychol.* 1995;31(1):124–129

10. O'Connell A. Voices from the heart: the developmental impact of a mother's lesbianism on her adolescent children. *Smith Coll Stud Soc Work.* 1993;63(3):281–299

11. Cameron P, Cameron K, Landess T. Errors by the American Psychiatric Association, the American Psychological Association, and the National Educational Association in representing homosexuality in amicus briefs about Amendment 2 to the U.S. Supreme Court. *Psychol Rep.* 1996;79(2):383–404

12. Golombok S. Adoption by lesbian couples. *BMJ.* 2002;324(7351):1407–1408

13. Perrin EC; American Academy of Pediatrics Committee on Psychosocial Aspects of Child and Family Health. Coparent or second-parent adoption by same-sex parents. *Pediatrics.* 2002;109(2):341–344

14. Casper V, Schultz S, Wickens E. Breaking the silences: lesbian and gay parents and the schools. *Teach Coll Rec.* 1992;94(1):109–137

15. Family Equality Council. Joint adoption laws. Family Equality Council Web site. https://www.familyequality.org/get_informed/resources/equality_maps/joint_adoption_laws. Accessed January 27, 2018

16. Curry H, Clifford D, Hertz F, Daily FW. *A Legal Guide for Lesbian and Gay Couples.* 13th ed. Berkeley, CA: Nolo Press; 2005

17. Kelley TF, Langsang D. Pediatric residency training and the needs of gay, lesbian, and bisexual youth. *J Gay Lesbian Med Assoc.* 1996;3(1):5–9

18. Perrin EC. *Sexual Orientation in Child and Adolescent Health Care.* New York, NY: Kluwer/Plenum Publishers; 2002

19. Obedin-Maliver J, Goldsmith ES, Stewart L, et al. Lesbian, gay, bisexual, and transgender-related content in undergraduate medical education. *JAMA.* 2011;306(9):971–977

20. Gold MA, Perrin EC, Futterman D, Friedman SB. Children of gay or lesbian parents. *Pediatr Rev.* 1994;15(9):354–358

21. Perrin EC, Kulkin H. Pediatric care for children whose parents are gay or lesbian. *Pediatrics.* 1996;97(5):629–635

22. Ahmann E. Working with families having parents who are gay or lesbian. *Pediatr Nurs.* 1999;25(5):531–535

23. Gartrell N, Banks A, Reed N, Hamilton J, Rodas C, Deck A. The National Lesbian Family Study: 3. Interviews with mothers of five-year-olds. *Am J Orthopsychiatry.* 2000;70(4):542–548

24. Gartrell N, Deck A, Rodas C, Peyser H, Banks A. The National Lesbian Family Study: 4. Interviews with the 10-year-old children. *Am J Orthopsychiatry.* 2005;75(4):518–524

25. Gershon TD, Tschann JM, Jemerin JM. Stigmatization, self-esteem, and coping among the adolescent children of lesbian mothers. *J Adolesc Health.* 1999;24(6):437–445

Children in Self-care

Robert D. Needlman, MD

"Pediatric primary care clinicians can...help connect parents with community resources such as high-quality after-school programs, latchkey training programs, and telephone 'warm-lines' that provide safe human contact and support to children alone after school."

With most US parents employed outside the home, the after-school hours pose a challenge to families and communities. The demand for quality after-school programs continues to outpace the supply, leaving many children and adolescents (collectively referred to as *children* in this chapter unless otherwise specified) subject to informal and often shifting arrangements, including caring for themselves. While some "latchkey" children thrive, as a group these children are at risk for physical and mental health problems, including inactivity, obesity, boredom, loneliness, fear, anger, aggressive behaviors, school underperformance, risky sex, and harmful substance use.[1] Pediatric primary care clinicians (PCCs) (ie, pediatricians, family physicians, internists, nurse practitioners, and physician assistants at the front line of pediatrics), aware of these dangers, can help parents find acceptable solutions and can advocate for policies that increase high-quality after school options.

The Spectrum of Self-care

More than 50% of parents are at work when school lets out (Figure 23-1). According to the Afterschoool Alliance (www.afterschoolalliance.org), 19.4 million children were in need of after-school care in 2014, up from 15.3 million in 2004.[2] Younger children are more likely to be in programs; older ones, on their own (Figure 23-2). The true prevalence of unsupervised care is difficult to estimate. Fearing stigma or legal action, parents may underreport self-care, even to their child's PCC.

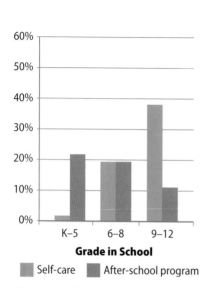

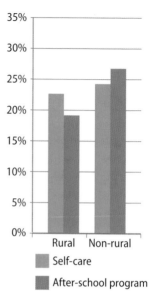

Figure 23-1. After-school care, by grade. All numbers are based on findings from the 2014 *America After 3PM survey*.

Reprinted with permission from Afterschool Alliance (2014). http://www.afterschoolalliance.org.

Figure 23-2. After-school care, both parents in workforce, by location. All numbers are based on findings from the 2014 *America After 3PM survey*.

Reprinted with permission from Afterschool Alliance (2014). http://www.afterschoolalliance.org.

Self-care comprises a spectrum. A child may be home alone, may be in the care of an older sibling, or may be caring for a younger sibling. Parents may phone home every hour, may be reachable by phone at any time, may be reachable only in emergencies, or may not be reachable at all. Sometimes grandparents help.[3] Libraries may provide formal after-school programs, informal guidance, or minimal supervision. Some children go to friends' homes (with or without the parents). Others meet at the mall, in parks, or elsewhere. Arrangements often vary from day to day and over time.[4]

Effects of Self-care: School-aged Children

Many parents and professionals believe that self-care is harmful. Children may be harmed in 4 ways: they feel bad (emotional effects), act badly (high-risk behaviors), develop badly (academic deficits), and are treated badly (risk of physical abuse or intentional injury).[5] The research, however, is mixed. Studies are divided on the question of whether children are frightened when they stay at home alone.[1,6] Not surprisingly, children who live in the relatively safe suburbs are less fearful than children in violent urban neighborhoods.[4] Increased time in self-care has been associated with poorer classroom adjustment, but it has not always been associated with poorer grades.[6–9] Measures of child self-esteem, locus of control, peer relationships, and classroom conduct do not vary significantly between self-care and parent care,[8,10,11] and some parents report that self-care builds self-confidence.[1] Generalizations are problematic. Among children of Mexican origin, for example, unsupervised self-care was associated with lying, stealing, and bullying, but only among boys.[12] In another sample, self-care was associated with increased aggression and decreased school performance, but only for children from high crime areas.[13]

The diversity of outcomes reflects differences among the groups of children studied and the details of the care they experience. Multiple factors go into determining whether a child might be exposed to self-care, and some salient factors are hard to quantify, such as a parent's judgment of her child's maturity or the strength of a parent's anxiety about leaving his child alone. There are no randomized studies to provide definitive answers. For children with special health care needs, issues of mobility, communication, and judgment, as well as potential need for administration of medication, also come into play.[14]

Effects of Self-care: Teens

One area in which there is strong agreement concerns the association of lower adult supervision with increased substance use and sex among teens.[15,16] Adolescents unsupervised at friends' homes are more at risk of succumbing to negative peer pressure than those who stay in their own homes. Those who hang out with friends without a set location are at greatest risk.[16,17] Nonpermissive parenting, family rules prohibiting substance use, and increased parental monitoring (eg, through required telephone calls) lower the risk associated with self-care, including the risk of such consequences as eating disorders.[18–20]

Early adolescents may be particularly vulnerable to the stresses and temptations of self-care. Compared with parent-supervised eighth graders, those in self-care for 11 or more hours per week reported 1.5 to 2.0 times higher levels of risk-taking, anger, family conflict, peer influence, attendance at parties, and substance use.[1] Moreover, earlier initiation of self-care was associated with increased rates of these negative behaviors. For example, 11% of eighth graders in parental care reported heavy alcohol use compared with 19.5% in self-care since junior high school and 25.5% in self-care since elementary school. While some adolescents report feeling increased self-reliance and responsibility, others experience loneliness and sadness.[21]

After-school Programs

Alternatives to self-care include care provided by relatives or hired sitters or structured after-school programs. The Afterschool Alliance has compiled numerous studies linking participation in after-school programs with higher academic achievement and less deviant and risky behavior. One critical review of the data, however, was less enthusiastic.[22] Programs aimed at obesity prevention are increasingly common, and the evidence for beneficial effects on activity level, physical fitness, and levels of lipids is growing.[23] Benefits may also extend beyond the children. High-quality after-school programming makes it easier for parents to remain in the workforce. Conversely, parents often cite inadequate after-school arrangements as a significant source of stress.[24]

The number of after-school programs has grown rapidly in the past decade. Expansion of services in low-income areas, in particular, has been financed by the US Department of Education's 21st Century Community Learning Centers (commonly known as 21CCLC) program. However, while participation in after-school programs is higher among children of ethnic minorities than in the population as a whole, the need for additional programs in low-income areas is also greater. Safety, transportation, and access to information about programs are also barriers for underserved groups. Children and youths with special health care needs (CYSHCN) may have special difficulty accessing after-school programs, which may not be equipped to accommodate their medical, developmental, or behavioral needs. Information on program accessibility is not readily available, nor is it tracked nationally. Nonetheless, CYSHCN participate in a wide range of community activities, dictated more by their personal characteristics than by their respective categories of special need.[25]

As with self-care arrangements, there is great diversity among after-school programs. Cost and quality vary widely. Among indices of program quality, warm interpersonal relationships between staff members and child participants seem to be especially important, supporting academic and personal-social outcomes.[26] The goal for all children is not merely attendance at after-school programs but rather fully engaged participation.

Decisions About After-school Care

Parents' decisions about after-school care can be relatively straightforward, or they can be fraught with guilt and worry.[1] Self-care can be a positive experience, assuming the child is mature enough; the neighborhood, safe enough; and the hours, short enough. Box 23-1 presents a commonsense checklist to help parents decide whether self-care is right for their children. Many states have adopted guidelines that attempt to help draw the line between acceptable unsupervised care and neglect, although the wording of these documents is sometimes vague; actual laws on the subject exist in only a few states. In many communities, service agencies offer "survival training" to prepare children to cope with self-care. The efficacy of such classes has been questioned, however.[5]

The Primary Care Clinician's Role

Parents are hungry for information about after-school care. Among parents using a family help desk at an urban clinic, the most frequent need (29% of visits) was information about after-school programs.[27] Primary care clinicians can ask about child care arrangements at health supervision visits for children of all ages. These discussions may be particularly important with respect to children with special health care needs. Parents of school-aged children and adolescents may have questions about out-of-school care but

---

Box 23-1. Signs of Readiness for Self-care

- **Age:** A sensible 8-year-old should be fine for a half hour or so once in a while, but most children will not be mature enough to manage being alone regularly until they are 10 or 11 years of age.

- **Interests:** The child is able to keep busy reading, drawing, making music, doing homework, and playing with toys, among other things (not just watching TV or playing video games).

- **Memory:** The child remembers commonsense safety rules, such as not opening the door and not telling telephone callers that he or she is alone.

- **Common sense:** The child can relate how to respond to a fire, a gas leak, or other emergencies.

- **Caution:** The child generally shows caution, thinking before acting. This trait is particularly important for young teens, who are tempted to engage in sexual experimentation and other experimentations.

- **Comfort:** The child seems to be truly OK with the idea of being home alone.

Abbreviation: TV, television.

be hesitant to ask. Parents need to understand that the effect of self-care varies depending on the child and the specific circumstances. Awareness of the increased rates of substance use and other risk-taking among unsupervised adolescents may lead parents to reconsider self-care for their teenagers. To date, the efficacy of pediatric guidance about out-of-school care has not been demonstrated empirically.

Primary care clinicians can provide parents with materials such as the handout *Choosing Quality Child Care: What's Best for Your Family?*, available at https://patiented.solutions.aap.org, and help connect parents with community resources such as high-quality after-school programs, latchkey training programs, and telephone "warm-lines" that provide safe human contact and support to children alone after school. Locally, service agencies such as the YMCA and Boys & Girls Clubs of America are likely to be good resources, as are public libraries. Guidance and referrals can be found through the Child Care Resource and Referral Programs in most states, easily located through a national toll-free number (800/424-2246). Primary care clinicians can advise parents to learn about the Federal Child and Dependent Care tax credit, which applies to all children younger than 13 years and to older children who have special health care needs and which can substantially lower the cost of after-school care (go to www.irs.gov and search "Child and Dependent Care").

Primary care clinicians may also play an important role in advocating for more high-quality out-of-school programs. Children's mental and physical health depends on access to intellectually stimulating, physically engaging, emotionally supportive, and, above all, safe environments. Children who face adversity in other aspects of their lives are especially dependent on such programs; in turn, these programs depend crucially on public support. Federal financing for quality after-school programs has grown steadily over the past decade, but there are constant threats to cut or eliminate this funding.[28]

AAP Policy

Donoghue EA; American Academy of Pediatrics Council on Early Childhood. Quality early education and child care from birth to kindergarten. *Pediatrics.* 2017;140(2):e20171488 (pediatrics.aappublications.org/content/140/2/e20171488)

References

1. Dwyer KM, Richardson JL, Danley KL, et al. Characteristics of eighth-grade students who initiate self-care in elementary and junior high school. *Pediatrics.* 1990;86(3):448–454

2. Afterschool Alliance. *America After 3PM: Afterschool Programs in Demand.* Washington, DC: Afterschool Alliance; 2014. http://www.afterschoolalliance.org/researchReports.cfm. Accessed January 27, 2018

3. Glaser M. "Grandma, please"! *J Long Term Care Adm.* 1994;22(1):4–6

4. Padilla ML, Landreth GL. Latchkey children: a review of the literature. *Child Welfare.* 1989; 68(4):445–454

5. Long T, Long L. *Latchkey Children: The Child's View of Self-care.* Urbana, IL: ERIC Clearinghouse on Elementary and Early Childhood Education; 1981

6. Posner JK, Vandell DL. Low-income children's after-school care: are there beneficial effects of after-school programs? *Child Dev.* 1994;65(2, spec no.):440–456

7. Pettit GS, Laird RD. Patterns of after-school care in middle childhood: risk factors and developmental outcomes. *Merrill-Palmer Q.* 1997;43:515–538

8. Vandell DL, Corasaniti MA. The relation between third graders' after-school care and social, academic, and emotional functioning. *Child Dev.* 1988;59(4):868–875

9. Galambos NL, Garbarino J. Identifying the missing links in the study of latchkey children. *Child Today.* 1983;12(4):2–4, 40–41

10. Belle D. *The After-school Lives of Children: Alone and With Others While Parents Work.* Mahwah, NJ: Erlbaum; 1999

11. Rodman H, Pratto DJ, Nelson RS. Child care arrangements and children's functioning: a comparison of self-care and adult-care children. *Dev Psychol.* 1985;21(3):413–418

12. Atherton OE, Schofield TJ, Sitka A, Conger RD, Robins RW. Unsupervised self-care predicts conduct problems: the moderating roles of hostile aggression and gender. *J Adolesc.* 2016;48:1–10

13. Lord H, Mahoney JL. Neighborhood crime and self-care: risks for aggression and lower academic performance. *Dev Psychol.* 2007;43(6):1321–1333

14. Holaday B, Turner-Henson A, Harkins A, Swan J. Chronically ill children in self-care: issues for pediatric nurses. *J Pediatr Health Care.* 1993;7(6):256–263

15. Cohen DA, Farley TA, Taylor SN, Martin DH, Schuster MA. When and where do youths have sex? The potential role of adult supervision. *Pediatrics.* 2002;110(6):e66

16. Mott JA, Crowe PA, Richardson J, Flay B. After-school supervision and adolescent cigarette smoking: contributions of the setting and intensity of after-school self-care. *J Behav Med.* 1999;22(1):35–58

17. Steinberg L. Latchkey children and susceptibility to peer pressure: an ecological analysis. *Dev Psychol.* 1986;22(4):433–439

18. Steinberg L, Fletcher A, Darling N. Parental monitoring and peer influences on adolescent substance use. *Pediatrics.* 1994;93(6, pt 2):1060–1064

19. Laird RD, Criss MM, Pettit GS, Dodge KA, Bates JE. Parents' monitoring knowledge attenuates the link between antisocial friends and adolescent delinquent behavior. *J Abnorm Child Psychol.* 2008;36(3):299–310

20. Martinson LE, Esposito-Smythers C, Blalock DV. The effect of parental monitoring on trajectories of disordered eating attitudes and behaviors among adolescents: an individual growth curve analysis. *Appetite.* 2016;107:180–187

21. Ruiz-Casares M. "When it's just me at home, it hits me that I'm completely alone": an online survey of adolescents in self-care. *J Psychol.* 2012;146(1–2):135–153

22. Apsler R. After-school programs for adolescents: a review of evaluation research. *Adolescence.* 2009;44(173):1–19

23. Beets MW, Beighle A, Erwin HE, Huberty JL. After-school program impact on physical activity and fitness: a meta-analysis. *Am J Prev Med.* 2009;36(6):527–537

24. Durlak JA, Mahoney JL, Bohnert AM, Parente ME. Developing and improving after-school programs to enhance youth's personal growth and adjustment: a special issue of AJCP. *Am J Community Psychol.* 2010;45(3–4):285–293

25. King G, Petrenchik T, Dewit D, McDougall J, Hurley P, Law M. Out-of-school time activity participation profiles of children with physical disabilities: a cluster analysis. *Child Care Health Dev.* 2010;36(5):726–741

26. Pierce KM, Bolt DM, Vandell DL. Specific features of after-school program quality: associations with children's functioning in middle childhood. *Am J Community Psychol.* 2010;45(3–4):381–393

27. Garg A, Sarkar S, Marino M, Onie R, Solomon BS. Linking urban families to community resources in the context of pediatric primary care. *Patient Educ Couns.* 2010;79(2):251–254

28. Mahoney JL, Parente ME, Zigler EF. Afterschool programs in America: origins, growth, popularity, and politics. *J Youth Dev.* 2009;4(3):23–42

Homeless Children

Patricia McQuilkin, MD, and Jason Rafferty, MD, MPH, EdM

> "It is important to keep in mind that many homeless families demonstrate an enormous amount of strength and resilience under adverse conditions and respond positively to the resources found in a medical home."

Although homelessness brings to mind the stereotype of a man panhandling on a street corner, in fact, single women and their children comprise a significant proportion of people who are homeless. Pediatric primary care clinicians (PCCs) (ie, pediatricians, family physicians, internists, nurse practitioners, and physician assistants who provide health care at the front lines of pediatrics) will likely encounter children in their practices who are experiencing or have experienced homelessness. With the passage of the McKinney Act in 1987, the US Department of Housing and Urban Development (HUD) defined a homeless individual as one "who lacks a fixed, regular, and adequate nighttime residence."[1]

This definition has been criticized for not acknowledging the dynamic nature of homelessness, particularly because it tends to exclude families and *youths* (defined in this chapter as individuals between birth and 24 years of age). To avoid the risks of living on the streets, homeless families and youths are more likely to be in and out of shelters, residing in vehicles or motels, or couch surfing with friends and relatives. Consequently, by adding the education subtitle to the renamed McKinney-Vento Act, the US Department of Education included youths living in motels and those who share temporary housing to this definition.[2] In 2011, HUD released the Final Rule Defining Homelessness, which incorporates families who are in unstable housing situations, are fleeing domestic violence, or may face homelessness in the next 14 days.[3]

In some cases, the family unit as a whole experiences homelessness. In others, an "unaccompanied youth" may not be in the custody of his or her family and may be physically disconnected from them. Youths may leave their families, either voluntarily ("runaway") or because one or more family members force them out ("thrown-away"), because they have no legal right to where they are staying ("doubling up"), or because they have no access to shelter at all ("street youth[s]").[4]

Knowledge of a child's past and present housing status is important to assessing the child's emotional and mental health. Up to a quarter of preschool children who experience homelessness have a mental health problem that would require evaluation, and by school age, the risk is 2 to 4 times greater than that among sheltered poor children of the same age.[5] Over a quarter of homeless children witness violence, and they are more than twice as likely to have problems in school, including repeating a grade or dropping out.[6] Ultimately, homelessness often contributes to high levels of toxic stress, which adversely affects the health, psychological, and developmental well-being of a child.

Numbers of Homeless

Using HUD's narrow definition of *homelessness,* it is estimated that between 2.5 and 3.5 million Americans slept in shelters, transitional housing, and public places not meant for human habitation during the course of the past year.[7] HUD conducts a point-in-time analysis annually through which in 2016 a total of nearly 550,000 people were counted as homeless. Single adults, some of whom are chronically homeless, constitute 2 in every 3 people counted (65%). Homeless families with children comprise the remaining 35% of the population.[8] In an analysis of major cities in the Unites States, homeless families make up a slightly larger fraction, at 40%, and their mayors assert that as the gap between income and affordable housing widens, the number of families without homes is increasing.[9]

According to HUD point-in-time data, on any given night, approximately 170,000 youths will have no place to stay. About 80% of these youths are living with their homeless families. The remaining 20% are "unaccompanied youth[s]."[8] It should be noted that this point-in-time count used the original, narrow HUD definition of homelessness, so these are likely underestimates that do not take into account doubling up and other unstable housing situations. This underestimation leaves hundreds of thousands of homeless children invisible to policy makers and the public.[8] In 2014, one estimate suggested an additional 7 million people lost their own homes and were "doubled-up" with others out of economic necessity.[10]

The US Department of Education is also mandated to keep a count of homeless children enrolled in US public schools, and, in the 2014–2015 academic year, nearly 1.3 million homeless children and adolescents were identified (about 95,000 were identified as unaccompanied homeless).[11] According to this count, it has been approximated that the total population of children and adolescents who experienced homelessness (enrolled and not enrolled in school) that year was 2.5 million. This number represents approximately 1 in every 30 US children on the basis of census data.[6] Despite the use of a broader definition, this figure is also likely an underestimate, given that such children may not be consistently enrolled in school and there is an incentive against disclosure because it might affect a child's school district assignment.

Homeless Families

Who are these homeless families? A typical sheltered homeless family consists of a single mother in her late 20s with 2 children and limited education.[12] Nearly 80% of these families are headed by women.[13] Among children in homeless families, 49% are younger than 6 years.[12,14] Nearly all mothers experiencing homelessness have a history of interpersonal violence, and as a result, they have severe depression (prevalence: 50%), post-traumatic stress disorder (PTSD) (prevalence: 36%), a substance use disorder (prevalence: 41%), or any combination of those conditions.[15,16]

It is estimated that 75% of homeless children and families may be doubling up with friends or relatives or living in cars or motels. These families often have a strong incentive not to disclose their living situations because it may lead to eviction or complications with their children's school districts.[11]

Unaccompanied Youths

Homeless or unaccompanied youths comprise approximately 7% of the total homeless population and 27% of all homeless youths, according to HUD point-in-time counts.[8] Among programs that count homeless youths, the US Department of Justice (DOJ) Office of Juvenile Justice and Delinquency Prevention data are most often cited. These data are often cited because they include aggregates of diverse and relevant sources for children and adolescents 10 through 18 years of age, including surveys of households, juvenile residential facilities (eg, detention centers, group homes), and law enforcement agencies. They define *homeless* as being away from home without permission for more than 1 night if the child or adolescent is younger than 15 years or 2 nights if the adolescent is older. Their most recent study, the National Incidence Studies of Missing, Abducted, Runaway, and

Thrownaway Children (NISMART) 2, showed an estimated 1,682,900 unaccompanied homeless and runaway adolescents in 1999.[17] This number is equivalent to estimates by the Research Triangle Institute based on responses to the Centers for Disease Control and Prevention's Youth Risk Behavior Survey published in 1998.[18]

In 2013, NISMART 3 was conducted, but the methods were more focused on identifying the subset of unaccompanied homeless children and adolescents who were considered missing by parental and law enforcement reports. Rates of those missing to their caregivers decreased by 32% between 1999 and 2013 from 9.2 to 6.3 per 1,000 children and adolescents. Rates of those missing to police decreased by 52% between 1999 and 2013 from 6.5 to 3.1 per 1,000 children and adolescents. The overall estimate of missing unaccompanied homeless was 238,300 to 491,000.[19]

According to the 1999 DOJ data, unaccompanied homeless adolescents include equal numbers of boys and girls, with most of them being 15 to 17 years of age. Thirty-eight percent stayed within 16 km (10 mi) of home and 83% remained within their own states of residency. Seventy-one percent of these adolescents were categorized as being in immediate danger because of factors such as a substance use disorder, sexual or physical abuse, living in an area of criminal activity, or young age (≤13 years). They are much more likely to experience and be injured by physically and sexually violent crimes.[17] Across studies, between 20% and 40% of homeless youths identified themselves as lesbian, gay, bisexual, or transgender (LGBT).[20]

In 2013, 9 sites across the country were selected as part of a federal interagency initiative, Youth Count, to pilot new methods to improve counting of unaccompanied homeless youths, particularly through increased engagement with LGBT services.[4] The Voices of Youth Count national survey has initially estimated that approximately 1 in 10 young adults (18–25 years of age) and 1 in 30 adolescents endorses an episode of unaccompanied homelessness in the last year. They found increased risk of homelessness among LGBT (120% increased risk) and unmarried parenting youths (200%).[21]

Racial Minorities

Minorities are substantially overrepresented among homeless families when compared with their representation among the US population (Table 24-1).

Of unaccompanied youths, black children in the United States have disproportionately higher rates of homelessness compared with white, non-Hispanic and Hispanic and Latino children. Youth Count estimates that black youths (13–25 years of age) have an 83% increased risk of unaccompanied homelessness.[21] Black children younger than 5 years are

Table 24-1. Race and Ethnicity Among Individuals in Homeless Families Compared With the General US Population

Demographic	Proportion of Individuals in Homeless Families[8,14]	Proportion of US Population as Reported in 2010 US Census
Black	48.0%	12.0%
Hispanic/Latino	22.0%	16.0%
American Indian/Alaskan Native/ Native Hawaiian	4.0%	0.9%
Multiple races reported	6.5%	1.9%
White, non-Hispanic	23.0%	64.0%

Derived from Henry M, Watt R, Rosenthal L, Shivji A. *The 2016 Annual Homeless Assessment Report (AHAR) to Congress. Part 1: Point-in-Time Estimates of Homelessness.* Washington, DC: Office of Community Planning and Development, US Dept of Housing and Urban Development; 2016. http://www.hudexchange.info/resources/documents/2016-AHAR-Part-1.pdf. Accessed January 27, 2018; and Child Trends. DataBank: homeless children and youth. Child Trends Web site. http://www.childtrends.org/indicators/homeless-children-and-youth. Updated October 2015. Accessed January 27, 2018.

29 times more likely to be in an emergency shelter than their white peers.[6] Furthermore, although national studies find no racial or ethnic differences in new homelessness,[18] local studies tend to suggest that such minorities are overrepresented. This discrepancy may be the result of a sampling bias, reflecting the fact that black and Native American youths are more likely to be on the streets because of low shelter access.[22]

The racial demography of homelessness has received little attention from researchers, policy makers, and advocacy groups.[6,23] The US Interagency Council on Homelessness develops a comprehensive strategic plan to prevent and end homelessness, but none of its objectives, targets, or updates have addressed the influence of racial dynamics.[24] Reports by leading nongovernmental organizations also tend not to address the role of race and ethnicity in homelessness.[10,23]

Causes of Homelessness

Family homelessness is caused by a combination of factors, including poverty, low-paying jobs, unemployment, lack of affordable housing, and interpersonal violence.[25] Vulnerable families with little social support can become homeless when seemingly minor triggers result in major catastrophe. A 2005 study by the Vera Institute of Justice showed that families who entered the New York City shelter system experienced remarkably high rates of disruption in their lives in the 5 years before becoming homeless. Sixty-nine percent had a job loss, 43% had physical health problems, 39% had emotional health problems, and 21% were exposed to interpersonal or domestic violence.[26] The economic recession during the period 2007 to 2010 caused one of the deepest downturns in the labor market in postwar history. This downturn resulted in a record high number of housing foreclosures, which compounded the problem of homelessness even further. As a result, the number of homeless children increased by 38% during this period, to include many who were previously in the middle class.[6,27]

Only 1 in 5 unaccompanied youths is reported missing; of these, 48% ran away or were asked or told to leave home by a parent or another adult.[17] Most unaccompanied youths leave home to escape dysfunctional or abusive family situations, because they feel unwanted, or they are coerced into leaving by adults at home.[28,29] There is a strong relationship between abuse and subsequent homelessness, with estimates of 17% to 35% of such youths reporting sexual abuse and 40% to 60% reporting physical abuse.[22] Other family-related factors include neglect, parental substance use, and conflict over sexual orientation, sexual activity, or pregnancy.[28] Residential instability is another contributing factor, with the majority of unaccompanied youths having a history of out-of-home placement; specifically, 70% of homeless unaccompanied youths have spent time in a foster family, group home, or other residential facility.[29] Nearly half of children in foster care report a history of running away, and 14% to 50% experience homelessness.[30]

Poverty

A clear and direct correlation exists between poverty and homelessness. Most homelessness in the United States is caused by the gap between income and the cost of housing. In 2016, 12.7% of all American families and 26.6% of all single female parent families lived below the federal poverty line.[31] According to HUD, families with the following characteristics are in the category of worst-case housing needs: those who rent, those who have incomes less than 50% of the median family income in their respective communities, and those who do not receive federal housing assistance. Further, 2 factors can lead a family to develop worst-case housing needs: paying more than one-half of their income for housing or having serious problems related to heating, plumbing, or electrical systems. Families facing such challenges are at the highest risk for becoming homeless. Worst-case housing needs are a national problem and they have expanded dramatically over the past decade, exacerbated by the impact of the economic recession on the housing market. Even with public assistance, 6 of 10 extremely low-income renters (0%–30% local mean family income) and 3 of 10 very low-income renters (30%–50% local mean family income) do not have access to affordable and available housing. Children reside in 36% of households with worst-case housing needs.[32]

Full-time employment is not a guarantee against homelessness. Of families with worst-case housing needs, 32% have at least 1 full-time worker making at least minimum wage.[32] Approximately one-fifth of all jobs in the United States do not keep a family of 4 out of poverty.[32] More and more individuals are employed by service industries, such as hotels and restaurants, which pay minimum wage and often provide only part-time work, with few or no benefits. This circumstance puts housing out of reach for many families. Fair market rent is calculated by HUD as "the amount that would be needed to pay the gross rent (rent plus utilities) of privately owned, decent, and safe housing of a modest (nonluxury) nature with suitable amenities."[33] The National Low Income Housing Coalition defines housing wage as the "…estimated full-time hourly wage a household must earn to afford a decent rental home at HUD's Fair Market Rent while spending no more than 30% of their income on housing costs."[34] Nationally, the housing wage for a 2-bedroom apartment in 2017 was $21.21 and for a 1-bedroom apartment was $17.14. The national housing wage is more than double the minimum federal wage of $7.25 per hour.[34]

Housing Shortage

A serious gap continues between the number of units needed to house low-income families and the amount of affordable housing. The National Low Income Housing Coalition concluded that the United States is experiencing a significant and prolonged shortage of affordable housing.[34] At least 1.7 million housing units are needed to fill this gap. Between the mid-1990s and 2010, about 200,000 public housing units were demolished and replaced with only 50,000 new units (57,000 families that qualify for public housing were provided vouchers instead of actual housing units, which has increased demand for the limited low-income housing supply).[6,30] This situation has been exacerbated by the federal government's decreased role in providing low-income housing over the past 30 years. HUD's budget has fallen about 56% between 1978 and 2011, leading to the loss of approximately 10,000 units of federally subsidized low-income housing annually.[23] Because of the limited supply of affordable housing, only 30% of persons who are eligible for the subsidy are able to receive it.[6,7] The median wait time for affordable housing is about 2 years,[6] and for other government housing-related resources the wait is typically 5 years and many wait lists are closed.[23]

Interpersonal Violence

Domestic violence is a leading cause of homelessness nationally, especially for women with children.[25] A study in Minnesota showed that 30% or more of mothers revealed domestic violence to be a major cause of their families' homeless situation.[35] These families are often headed by women who are fleeing a violent situation at home and have little in the way of social or financial support. They are often unable to obtain credit or child support. They may have difficulty accessing resources because they are afraid of being discovered by their abusers. The clinician needs to be aware that interpersonal violence is an important cause of homelessness for families.

Interpersonal violence is also a major cause of homelessness for youths. An important subgroup, unaccompanied youths, consists of people who are asked to leave home or are not allowed back home by a parent or guardian.[7] Family conflict and violence are the primary causes of their homelessness,[21] with 70% of youths citing relationship problems with parents as the reason for the homelessness.[36] There are also very high rates of physical abuse, sexual abuse, and neglect prior to homelessness.[21,36]

Effects of Homelessness on Children's Health

Minority Children

Minority homeless children have poorer health outcomes compared with their white counterparts, even when family income and health insurance coverage are controlled.[6] For example, black homeless children are 49% more likely to have asthma and 21% more likely to have activity limitations compared with white homeless children. Racial disparities in health outcomes persist until family income falls below 200% of the poverty line.[37]

Many mechanisms underlie the relationship between race and poor health among homeless children. Interpersonal and institutionalized discrimination contribute to differential access to medical services, dental care, and shelters. In fact, Hispanic homeless children have been found to have the poorest overall access to primary and preventive care.[37]

Ultimately, internalized discrimination, secondary to a child's witnessing firsthand the devastating effects of personal and institutional inequalities, is believed to cause physiologic stress, which has a negative influence on chronic disease. In older children, such stress reinforces feelings of injustice, powerlessness, and victimization that lead to violent behaviors and mental illness.[38] See also Chapter 25, Children Affected by Racism.

Mental Health

Children who experience homelessness have 3 times the rate of emotional and behavioral problems as their housed peers.[39] This difference is largely caused by the amount of stress and trauma that these children experience and witness.

Twenty percent of homeless preschoolers have emotional problems requiring intervention. One-third of homeless school-aged children have a major mental disorder that interferes with daily activity compared with 19% in the general population. Forty-seven percent have anxiety and depression compared with 18% in the general population, and 36% are aggressive compared with 17% in the general population. Fewer than one-third of those who might benefit from treatment are receiving assistance.[39]

Evidence that homeless children and adolescents may disproportionately have behavioral and psychological problems is persuasive. Estimates are that 23% to 67% of homeless children and adolescents meet criteria for a mental health diagnosis, including drug- and alcohol-related conditions, with the increase in prevalence occurring once a child becomes homeless. Trauma is a common experience among homeless families, with 90% of homeless adult women reporting physical or sexual assault and 80% of children in homeless families having been exposed to a serious violent event by 12 years of age.[40] The risk of sexual and physical victimization is increased among homeless adolescents, leading to further increased risk of PTSD.[41] Eighty-three percent of homeless adolescents experience physical and/or sexual assault after leaving home.[36] Homeless adolescents are 6 times more likely to meet criteria for conduct disorder, major depressive disorder, PTSD, or substance use disorders.[42] After homelessness, involvement in criminal activity is common.[43]

Attachment describes the emotional connection between a child and caregiver, particularly the desire for closeness and security in the face of stress and separation. Therefore, the health and emotional well-being of a child is closely linked to the emotional well-being of his or her parent. Increased levels of depression in homeless parents adversely affect their ability to provide supportive caregiving (including breastfeeding of newborns and infants[44]), consistent social interaction, and engagement in enriching activities. This lack of support leads to an increased stress response in the child, which contributes to poorer cognitive, emotional, and developmental outcomes.[45] Unaccompanied homeless girls have much higher rates of teenage pregnancy than their peers do,[30] which is especially concerning given that homeless adolescents are at elevated risk for mood disorders with little access to resources and supports. Unaccompanied youths are at particularly high risk for victimization, traumatic stress, and poor mental health outcomes, topics discussed later in the Unaccompanied Youths section of this chapter.

Development and Education

Developmental, educational, and psychological outcomes in homeless children are equally worrisome. Compared with other children, homeless children are 4 times as likely to have developmental delays, twice as likely to have learning disabilities, and twice as likely to repeat a grade because of frequent absences and school changes. The majority of both homeless mothers and their preschool children exhibit delays in at least one of the following areas: auditory comprehension, verbal expression, reading, and writing.[46]

Children experiencing homelessness face huge barriers to obtaining education. These children experience significant educational disruption because of multiple relocations and school changes. It takes a child 4 to 6 months to recover academically from a school transfer and 6 to 18 months to regain a sense of equilibrium, security, and control. Such educational disruptions cause significant reductions in academic achievement.[47] Multiple studies have shown that homeless children have lower performance scores and slower rates of skill acquisition in reading and math compared with housed peers who are living in either poverty or middle class.[48] Homeless children and adolescents are also at increased risk of grade retention and high school drop-out.[47,48]

In comparing the school experiences and academic achievements of adolescents in families who experienced homelessness with permanently housed adolescents whose families received public assistance, formerly homeless students had more school mobility, were more likely to repeat a grade, and had worse school experiences by maternal report and lower plans for postsecondary education by self-report. Homelessness was associated with declines in achievement during the period of maximal residential disruption. Days absent from school were hypothesized as the mediating link between homelessness and academic achievement.[47,48]

In an effort to improve the educational opportunities of homeless children, the McKinney-Vento Homeless Assistance Act of 2001 was created. It requires that school-aged youths experiencing homelessness are immediately enrolled in school and have educational opportunities equal to those of their non-homeless peers. The statute requires every public school district and charter holder to designate a *homeless liaison* to ensure that homeless students are identified and that their needs are met.[47]

Physical Health

Homeless children have significantly higher rates of acute and chronic illness compared with housed children.[27] Several factors are responsible for this disparity.

Homelessness can cause illness and aggravate existing health conditions. Living conditions in shelters are often crowded; children are more likely to be exposed to contagious diseases, and they often have poor access to health care. Families in shelters are living under stressful conditions, which can exacerbate illness. Homelessness contributes to toxic stress, which has adverse effects on child health and development. (See Chapter 13, Children Exposed to Adverse Childhood Experiences.)

Lack of access to primary and preventive care is a major issue for homeless families. Nearly 1 in 10 homeless children reports that he or she has not seen a physician in the past year.[49] Lapses in care can lead to lapses in treatment of chronic illness and decreased vaccination rates. Many homeless families use the emergency department as their primary source of health care. The lack of preventive care leaves various medical problems untreated, which leads to more use of the emergency department.

Lack of medical insurance coverage is another barrier to homeless children's obtaining primary and preventive care. One study showed that 58% of homeless children lacked health insurance compared with 15% of housed children.[49]

Rates of Illness

Health risks related to homelessness begin during the prenatal period. Statistics show increased morbidity and mortality rates related to lack of prenatal care, poor nutrition, stress, and exposure to violence, as well as increased rates of substance use. One study revealed that 20% of infants born to homeless mothers were preterm. The risk of a homeless woman giving birth to a newborn weighing less than 2 kg was 6 to 7 times that of the control group.[50] Severity of homelessness predicts low birth weight and preterm births beyond its correlation with delayed prenatal care and other risk factors.[51] Among pregnant homeless adolescents, a frequent history of severe sexual abuse and early intravenous drug use correlates with poor health outcomes in the newborn.[52]

Homeless children have 4 times as many acute illnesses as housed children. They have twice as many ear infections, 4 times as many respiratory tract infections, and 5 times more stomach problems.[27] Because homeless families live in crowded conditions, the risk of acquiring upper respiratory tract infections, diarrhea, and otitis media is increased. One study revealed that homeless children had a 50% increased rate of otitis media compared with the national average (27% vs 18%). This increase was probably the result of greater exposure to upper respiratory tract infections and second-hand smoke. Because of a lack of consistent medical care among the homeless population, otitis media is often undiagnosed and untreated, leading to possible hearing loss.[53]

Homeless children also have increased rates of chronic illness, exacerbated by their living conditions. Asthma, the most common chronic illness during childhood, is aggravated by the difficult living conditions in shelters, such as crowded conditions, increased exposure to respiratory tract infections, stress, and poor access to health care. The prevalence of asthma among a random sample of homeless children in New York City was found to be 39.8%, more than 6 times the rate for other children. Asthma in homeless children was more likely to be severe and undertreated.[54]

Other conditions that are more prevalent in homeless children include poor dentition and obesity.[55] The risk of homeless children acquiring ecto-parasitic infections such as pediculosis and scabies is higher than for housed children.[56] Homeless children are also at increased risk for elevated blood lead levels.[57]

Oral Health

The most common unmet health need among all children and adolescents is adequate dental care.[55] According to the National Health Care for the Homeless Council, the rates of poor dentition and dental caries are approximately 10 times greater among homeless children than among the general population.[57] This is particularly true among homeless children who are at high risk for tooth decay (5 times more common than asthma in the homeless population). One in 3 homeless children has not had dental care in the past year compared with 1 in 5 among housed children. Major contributing factors include the limited number of dentists who participate in public insurance, a general shortage of the dental workforce, long wait times after scheduling an appointment, and an uneven geographic distribution that neglects low-income areas.[6]

Nutrition

Children and families who are homeless are especially vulnerable to food insecurity and hunger. One episode of homelessness in the past year is the strongest predictor of hunger. Residential instability contributes to inconsistent access to community supports and entitlement programs (eg, food stamps). Families with limited financial and food storage resources often have to rely on soup kitchens, convenient stores, and fast-food restaurants, which do not offer selections with high nutritional content. In one study, more than one-third of homeless children attributed their hunger to being forced to skip meals, nearly 30% did not have enough to eat, and 15% had nothing at all.[58] It is well established that lack of good nutrition can affect a child's behavior, school performance, and cognitive development.[39,58]

Homeless children are 3 times more likely to experience iron-deficiency anemia caused by poor nutrition.[59] One study reported a 52% rate of obesity, 45% rate of anemia, and 36% rate of failure to thrive among homeless children.[58] Given the importance of adequate nutrition for development in the newborn, infant, and young child and the risk factors associated with obesity in later life, these findings are disturbing.

Increased Health Risks for Homeless Adolescents

Regardless of whether homeless adolescents are with their families or unaccompanied, they represent a particularly high-risk population. Adolescence is a challenging time in any circumstance, as teenagers learn to navigate new independence and identity alongside rapid physical change. In addition, decision-making and problem-solving skills are still developing. The lack of economic, social, and emotional resources (including supportive adult relationships) faced by homeless adolescents can interfere with their developmental trajectory, leading to dangerous consequences and high risk–taking behavior.[28] Adolescents and young adults are overrepresented among unaccompanied youths, are at an extremely high risk for victimization, and are least likely to be connected to service agencies.[8] This combination can lead to very concerning physical and mental health outcomes. (See Unaccompanied Youths section later in this chapter.)

In general, among homeless adolescents, the incidence and prevalence of HIV infection, chlamydial infection, herpes, and hepatitis B and C are increased. Increases may be caused by lack of access to educational and prevention programs, lack of condom use, multiple partners, increased drug use, and sexual victimization.[60] Homeless youths are at high risk of substance use disorders, mental illness, and blood-borne infections.[61] Mortality rate among homeless youths is approximately 11 times the expected rate based on age and sex and is mainly caused by suicide and drug overdose.[62]

Sexual Minorities

Sexual minorities are overrepresented among homeless adolescents, especially unaccompanied homeless youths. It is estimated that 2% to 40% of homeless youths identify as LGBT and their voluntary or involuntary coming out was the most common reason for becoming homeless, specifically a "throwaway."[20] The LGBT homeless youth population is at much greater risk for violence and negative health outcomes than their heterosexual peers are. In particular, they are at risk for early onset of sexual activity, involvement in prostitution or survival sex, multiple partners, and other risky behaviors leading to elevated HIV rates, substance use, mental health problems, and physical and sexual victimization.[20,63]

Unaccompanied Youths

Violence is the top reason why youths leave home and disconnect from their families. The DOJ study focusing on unaccompanied homeless youths found that 21% were physically or sexually abused in the year before leaving home.[17] A study in Seattle, WA, found that among homeless and runaway adolescents, 82% reported experiencing physical abuse; 43%, family neglect; and 26%, sexual abuse.[64]

In addition to being exposed to or experiencing violence before leaving home, adolescents are at high risk for being re-traumatized in shelters and especially on the streets.[41] A study in Los Angeles, CA, found that 1 in 4 homeless adolescents had been shot at (7% wounded); 1 in 5, had been stabbed; and 1 in 6, sexually abused.[63] In general, 62.1% of homeless youths report being beaten up; 35%, being assaulted with a weapon; 21%, being sexually assaulted[65]; and 57%, carrying a weapon for protection (several preferring guns).[66] For adult men, the greatest risk factor for engaging in aggressive behaviors is having been physically, sexually, and emotionally victimized at an earlier age.[67]

Unaccompanied adolescent and young adult women and sexual minorities are particularly susceptible to sexual victimization. As many as 43% of homeless adolescents in Los Angeles, CA, reported having engaged in survival sex, which is the exchange of sexual acts for necessary resources. Risk factors for survival sex include a history of physical or sexual abuse, depression, the need to obtain income (often for medical care), and drug or resource sharing.[68,69] Lesbian, gay, bisexual, and transgender homeless youths are 3 times more likely to engage in survival sex than their heterosexual peers are.[20] Sexual assault is a particular concern, with rates reported to be as high as 42% among female runaways[70] and 59% among LGBT homeless youths (compared with 33% among their heterosexual peers in that particular study).[71] Such behaviors have contributed to alarmingly high rates of sexually transmitted infections (estimated prevalence: 50%–70%).[72] Homeless and runaway adolescents are at 2 to 10 times greater risk for HIV infection.[73] The longer they are homeless, the less motivated they are for HIV prevention; they may report the belief that they would be better off contracting HIV because it would make them eligible for housing funds, specifically for HIV-positive people in need.[20,74]

Unaccompanied youths experience almost constant fear of victimization, which is accompanied by the stressors of living in a shelter or on the streets, obtaining necessary resources to survive, and the loss of routine and predictability in their lives. Such experiences can lead to mental health problems (depression, anxiety, and stress disorders), substance use, and reduced resiliency, and they may interfere with the individual's ability to identify and develop positive relationships.[41,43] Most unaccompanied adolescents meet criteria for mood disorders, especially major depressive disorder, and more than one-third meet PTSD criteria during their lifetimes.[30] Attempted suicide rates (18%–48% across studies) are consistently higher for unaccompanied homeless youths than for their normative peers,[22] with nearly half of heterosexual homeless youths describing suicidal ideation. Among LGBT homeless youths, that rate is as high as 75%.[71]

Homeless youths may use substances to help withstand the severe hardships they face both at home and on the streets. The prevalence of substance use across studies ranges from 70% to 90%.[75] Rates of marijuana use disorder are 6 times higher than those for housed peers, and rates of cocaine use disorder are 35 times higher.[27] Substance use is especially high among street youths, with 1 study stating that 94.0% used tobacco and alcohol, 97.0% used marijuana, 73.4% used amphetamines, 55.5% used cocaine, and 39.5% used heroin in the past year.[76]

Long-term Effects

Whether the experience of homelessness, in itself, has long-term effects on the health of a child is unknown. Although differences have been identified in the psychological and developmental characteristics of homeless children compared with housed poor children, it is not clear whether this difference is the result of events that occurred before or during homelessness. Nevertheless, it is reasonable to assume that providing needed educational, medical, and psychological services may mitigate toxic stress and limit the potential damaging effects of homelessness on the child.

Recommendations for the Care of Homeless Children and Families

It is important to keep in mind that many homeless families demonstrate an enormous amount of strength and resilience under adverse conditions and respond positively to the resources found in a medical home. In addition to identifying problems, clinicians can reinforce the strengths of the child and family, because they are crucial to helping them get through the crisis of being homeless.

Homeless Families

Families may not identify themselves as homeless. The children may actually be attending school, yet go undetected. It is important to ask questions about housing to identify homeless families. Such questions can be a part of universal previsit screening, using a tool such as Kemper's Family Psychosocial Screen. (See Appendix 2, Mental Health Tools for Pediatrics.)

Once a family is identified as homeless, the most important issue is ascertaining that any newborns, infants, children, or adolescents are living in a safe environment. If not, the family should be assisted with making contacts with a local family homeless shelter system, welfare agency, or charitable institution that can provide temporary housing. Resources that may be helpful in assisting homeless families include the toolbox of the National Association of County and City Health Officials, available at www.naccho.org/resources/toolbox; handouts from the Community Health Online Resource Center, available at www.cdc.gov/nccdphp/dch/online-resource/index.htm; "Important Resources for Families and Child Care Providers" of Child Care Aware of America, available at http://childcareaware.org/parents-and-guardians/resources; the "Rental Assistance" Web page of the US Department of HUD at www.hud.gov/topics/rental_assistance; and the Web site of the Social Security Administration at www.ssa.gov.

It should be noted that family shelters may not allow adolescent boys or adult fathers to stay, a policy that breaks apart families and forces males to leave female family members to find shelter elsewhere.[77,78] Two-thirds of cities polled in a 1995 survey reported that they do break up families because of such regulations.[79] These families also need assistance in applying for health, nutrition, and social services and, if the child is uninsured, Medicaid.

Newborns, infants, children, and adolescents need to undergo a thorough medical, developmental, and psychological history and a physical examination to identify medical conditions associated with homelessness, the factors that led to homelessness, and needs for medical care. Particular attention should be paid to preventive care and health maintenance, including immunizations, lead testing, routine oral hygiene, nutrition counseling, and psychosocial assessment. Early diagnosis and treatment of chronic medical conditions is also essential. Clinic care that is offered to children while they are homeless should be comprehensive, meeting the criteria of a medical home. In addition to primary pediatric care, clinic care should include 24-hour telephone access, referral to subspecialty care, developmental and psychological evaluation and treatment, dental care, medication and medical devices, and case management.[54]

Asthma is overrepresented among homeless children. Children often require aggressive treatment, and parents may need comprehensive education to avoid hospitalization, excessive emergency department use, and school absenteeism for their children. A child who is not sleeping at night or is keeping other family members awake because of coughing can exacerbate the stress of being homeless.

Children of families living in shelters may have frequent acute illnesses as a result of living in close quarters with other families. In treating upper respiratory tract infection, gastroenteritis, otitis media, and tinea, pediatric PCCs and other health care professionals can instruct parents about infection control measures, in addition to applying standard treatment regimens. Outbreaks of certain illnesses, such as varicella or hepatitis, may require contacting shelter personnel or the local Department of Health to initiate infection-control measures.

When a parent brings in a child who has a minor acute illness, it is important to use the visit as an opportunity to perform a thorough medical and psychosocial assessment and initiate any needed treatment and referral. Follow-up can be problematic for homeless families, and any delay in initiating a comprehensive treatment plan may impede needed health care.

Homeless children face constant traumatic stress and uncertainty (lack of routine) as well as high rates of mental health concerns and parental depression. These have all been shown to adversely affect cognitive, emotional, and social developmental trajectories. Therefore, routine behavioral and developmental screening is essential with a validated age-appropriate tool, such the Pediatric Symptom Checklist for school-aged children and adolescents. (See Appendix 2, Mental Health Tools for Pediatrics, for other examples.) A licensed mental health specialist who has experience working with homeless families should be identified for follow-up referrals, if necessary.

In addition to referrals for children with developmental assessment or psychological problems, referring parents for counseling may also be necessary. Some families are homeless because of severe parental mental health problems or substance use. A parent may become depressed as a result of being homeless. Mental health concerns and stressors of caregivers should always be addressed so as to optimize the environment needed for a child's well-being.

One of the most common reasons for a woman and her children becoming homeless is interpersonal violence. Women must be queried about this issue. (See Chapter 13, Children Exposed to Adverse Childhood Experiences.) Pediatric PCCs and other health care professionals should be aware of local resources for those exposed to or injured by interpersonal violence so that any necessary referrals can be made. Moving a family into a shelter may be necessary if the batterer is a threat.

Chronic medical and mental conditions are often not treated properly because homeless families frequently move, resulting in multiple clinicians and discontinuity of care. This circumstance may lead to under-referral, over-referral, and undertreatment. For example, a child may be referred multiple times to specialists for the same problem, the diagnostic workup may be restarted with each referral, and the specialist may never reach the point of implementing an adequate treatment plan. While the child is homeless, a more practical approach may be to initiate the workup in the primary care setting and arrange for specialty referral once the family enters permanent housing.

When a family is moving out of a shelter into permanent housing, family members will often need assistance in locating health care in their new community. This involves helping to identify a new medical home and transferring medical records to the new PCC.

Unaccompanied Youths

Distrust of adults is very common among homeless (especially victimized) youths, which limits initial contact with health care professionals, even when they are readily accessible. In addition to being based on victimization by adult figures, distrust may also be based on prior experience or fear of being forced into placement (foster care, hospitals, or detention centers) instead of having their needs met.[28] Therefore, outreach is critical because youths are unlikely to present to a traditional outpatient clinic.

In 1989, the US General Accounting Office (GAO) found that health services were not a reported priority among programs providing outreach and shelter to homeless youths. However, nearly one-quarter of unaccompanied youths reported that they receive medical care directly or through referrals from such programs.[80] In 2012, the US GAO released an updated report describing increased grant funding for programs that incorporate health care for homeless children and adolescents who are at severely high risk for morbidity and mortality. However, they continue to note challenges with limited funds, targeted resources, and redundancies and fragmentation among various services agencies.[81] Despite the lack of attention to health care, homeless youths use and depend on such services being readily available. Studies show that if such programs are available, they are used. Homeless youths appear to access care most often for pregnancy, mental health issues, trauma, sexually transmitted infections, substance use disorders, chronic conditions, and dental problems.[75]

Homeless youths also report a reluctance to seek care for reasons such as difficulty navigating the health care system, limited clinic sites, lack of coordination among PCCs and other pediatric health care professionals, specific hours for homeless youths, and long wait lists. They also report embarrassment, denial of any medical problems, and fear of a clinician's implicit and explicit biases.[75]

Unaccompanied youths have various needs, including housing, education, vocational training, preventive health care, mental health care, screening for infectious diseases, and substance use services. Services that target this population rarely address all of them. The concept and principles of the medical home are essential to overcome such challenges, but this infrastructure is difficult to support in an outreach or emergency setting, where such youths often present.

Once an unaccompanied youth is identified, the priority is to ensure that he or she is living in a safe environment. The youth should be assisted in making contacts that will enable access to safe housing. Resources specific for unaccompanied youths may not be available in all areas, but pediatric PCCs need to be familiar with local service agencies, what they offer, and how to refer patients. Adolescent girls need to be able to access women's or domestic violence shelters (or family shelters if they are pregnant or have a child). Finding shelter for adolescent boys may be especially challenging because they are often turned away from family shelters and usually cannot stay in an adult shelter until they turn 18 years of age.[79]

Whenever possible, unaccompanied youths should have access to routine preventive care, dentistry, nutrition, and social services and, if uninsured, Medicaid. The youth will also need a thorough medical, developmental, and psychological history with a comprehensive physical examination. Particular attention must be paid to signs of abuse or trauma. The youth should be counseled on sexual health, offered screening for pregnancy and sexually transmitted infections, and provided with appropriate contraception (including access to levonorgestrel-only emergency contraception, "Plan B"). Open-ended questions should be used to avoid assumptions about gender identity, sexual orientation, or sexual behaviors. Mental health screening is essential, including assessment for mood disorders, PTSD, suicidality, and substance use disorders. (See Appendix 2, Mental Health Tools for Pediatrics.)

A safety plan should be developed for instances in which the safety of the youth is threatened, and a 24-hour emergency service should be identified. Case management, referrals for subspecialty care, psychological evaluation, and treatment should be available. If the youth resides in a shelter, the precautions described earlier for infectious diseases control should be taken. All visits to the clinic, even for a minor acute illness, are an opportunity to assess safety and high-risk behaviors and to perform a thorough health assessment. Continuity of care is a particular challenge among a transient population, but it is essential for effectiveness in the face of distrust and complex presenting problems. In an attempt to develop quality outcome measures through direct interviews with homeless youths, it was found that most of them identified continuity of care as important. They desired "…rapport with 1 clinician, and 'not [having] to start all over again with repeating my story to someone else.'"[73] In addition, they stated that respect was important to "…inform me, talk to me like a regular person instead of telling me what to do."[82]

Having a caring adult figure is developmentally protective for adolescents against hopelessness and emotional distress. Homeless adolescents often lack social connectedness, particularly to adults, because of histories of violence.[73] Therefore, it is essential for PCCs and other health care professionals to create a confidential, nonjudgmental safe space that consistently promotes autonomy and respect. Over time, this space can foster resilience and trust around disclosing sensitive issues, such as sexuality, gender identity concerns, or trauma.

AAP Policy

American Academy of Pediatrics Committee on Psychosocial Aspects of Child and Family Health. The pediatricians' role in the prevention of missing children. *Pediatrics.* 2004;114(4):1100–1105. Reaffirmed January 2015 (pediatrics.aappublications.org/content/114/4/1100)

American Academy of Pediatrics Council on Community Pediatrics. Providing care for children and adolescents facing homelessness and housing insecurity. *Pediatrics.* 2013;131(6):1206–1210. Reaffirmed October 2016 (pediatrics.aappublications.org/content/131/6/1206)

American Academy of Pediatrics Council on Community Pediatrics. Providing care for immigrant, migrant, and border children. *Pediatrics.* 2013;131(6):e2028–e2034 (pediatrics.aappublications.org/content/131/6/e2028)

References

1. McKinney-Vento Act, 42 USC 11435(2), §725(2) (2002)
2. McKinney-Vento Act, Subtitle B: Education for Homeless Children and Youths, 42 USC 11435(2), §725(2) (2002)
3. Homeless emergency assistance and rapid transition to housing: defining "homeless." *Fed Regist.* 2011;76(233):75994–76019. To be codified at 24 CFR parts 91, 582, and 583. http://www.hudexchange.info/resources/documents/HEARTH_HomelessDefinition_FinalRule.pdf. Accessed January 27, 2018
4. Pergamit M, Cunningham M, Burt M, Lee P, Howell B, Bertumen K. *Youth Count! Process Study.* Washington, DC: Urban Institute; 2013
5. Bassuk EL, Richard MK, Tsertsvadze A. The prevalence of mental illness in homeless children: a systematic review and meta-analysis. *J Am Acad Child Adolesc Psychiatry.* 2015;54(2):86–96
6. Bassuk EL, DeCandia CJ, Beach CA, Berman F. *America's Youngest Outcasts: A Report Card on Child Homelessness.* Waltham, MA: National Center on Family Homelessness; 2014. http://www.air.org/sites/default/files/downloads/report/Americas-Youngest-Outcasts-Child-Homelessness-Nov2014.pdf. Accessed January 27, 2018
7. National Law Center on Homelessness and Poverty. *Homelessness in America: Overview of Data and Causes.* Washington, DC: National Law Center on Homelessness and Poverty; 2015
8. Henry M, Watt R, Rosenthal L, Shivji A. *The 2016 Annual Homeless Assessment Report (AHAR) to Congress. Part 1: Point-in-Time Estimates of Homelessness.* Washington, DC: Office of Community Planning and Development, US Dept of Housing and Urban Development; 2016. http://www.hudexchange.info/resources/documents/2016-AHAR-Part-1.pdf. Accessed January 27, 2018
9. The United States Conference of Mayors, National Alliance to End Homelessness. *Hunger and Homelessness Survey: A Status Report on Hunger and Homelessness in America's Cities.* Washington, DC: US Conference of Mayors; 2016. https://endhomelessness.atavist.com/mayorsreport2016. Accessed January 27, 2018
10. National Alliance to End Homelessness. *The State of Homelessness in America.* Washington, DC: National Alliance to End Homelessness; 2016. https://endhomelessness.org/homelessness-in-america/homelessness-statistics/state-of-homelessness-report. Accessed January 27, 2018
11. National Center for Homeless Education. *Federal Data Summary: School Years 2012-13 to 2014-15.* Browns Summit, NC: National Center for Homeless Education; 2016. https://nche.ed.gov/downloads/data-comp-1213-1415.pdf. Accessed January 27, 2018
12. Rog DJ, Holupka CS, Patton LC. *Characteristics and Dynamics of Homeless Families With Children.* Washington, DC: Office of the Assistant Secretary for Planning and Evaluation, Office of Human Services Policy, US Dept of Health and Human Services; 2007. https://aspe.hhs.gov/report/characteristics-and-dynamics-homeless-families-children. Accessed January 27, 2018
13. Solari CD, Morris S, Shivji A, de Souza T. *The 2015 Annual Homeless Assessment Report (AHAR) to Congress. Part 2: Estimates of Homelessness in the United States.* Washington, DC: Office of Community Planning and Development, US Dept of Housing and Urban Development; 2016. http://www.hudexchange.info/onecpd/assets/File/2015-AHAR-Part-2.pdf. Accessed January 27, 2018
14. Child Trends. DataBank: homeless children and youth. Child Trends Web site. http://www.childtrends.org/indicators/homeless-children-and-youth. Updated October 2015. Accessed January 27, 2018
15. Bassuk EL, Beardslee WR. Depression in homeless mothers: addressing an unrecognized public health issue. *Am J Orthopsychiatry.* 2014;84(1):73–81

16. Substance Abuse and Mental Health Services Administration. *Current Statistics on the Prevalence and Characteristics of People Experiencing Homelessness in the United States.* Rockville, MD: Substance Abuse and Mental Health Services Administration; 2011. https://www.samhsa.gov/sites/default/files/programs_campaigns/homelessness_programs_resources/hrc-factsheet-current-statistics-prevalence-characteristics-homelessness.pdf. Accessed January 27, 2018

17. Hammer H, Finkelhor D, Sedlak A. *Runaway/Thrownaway Children: National Estimates and Characteristics.* Washington, DC: Office of Juvenile Justice and Delinquency Prevention, US Dept of Justice; 2002. https://www.ncjrs.gov/html/ojjdp/nismart/04/index.html. Accessed January 27, 2018

18. Ringwalt CL, Greene JM, Robertson M, McPheeters M. The prevalence of homelessness among adolescents in the United States. *Am J Public Health.* 1998;88(9):1325–1329

19. Sedlak AJ, Finkelhor D, Brick JM. National estimates of missing children: updated findings from a survey of parents and other primary caretakers. *Juv Justice Bull.* 2017:1–17. https://www.ojjdp.gov/pubs/250089.pdf. Published June 2017. Accessed January 27, 2018

20. Ray N. *Lesbian, Gay, Bisexual, and Transgender Youth: An Epidemic of Homelessness.* New York, NY: National Gay and Lesbian Task Force Policy Institute; 2006

21. Morton MH, Dworsky A, Samuels GM. *Missed Opportunities: Youth Homelessness in America. National Estimates.* Chicago, IL: Chapin Hall at the University of Chicago; 2017

22. Robertson MJ, Toro PA. Homeless youth: research, intervention, and policy. In: Fosburg LB, Dennis DL, eds. *Practical Lessons: The 1998 National Symposium on Homeless Research.* Washington, DC: US Dept of Housing and Urban Development; 1999

23. Jones MM. Does race matter in addressing homelessness? A review of the literature. *World Med Health Policy.* 2016;8(2):139–156

24. US Interagency Council on Homelessness. *Opening Doors: Federal Strategic Plan to Prevent and End Homelessness.* Washington, DC: US Interagency Council on Homelessness; 2015. http://www.usich.gov/resources/uploads/asset_library/USICH_OpeningDoors_Amendment2015_FINAL.pdf. Accessed January 27, 2018

25. National Law Center on Homelessness and Poverty. *"Simply Unacceptable": Homelessness and the Human Right to Housing in the United States 2011.* Washington, DC: National Law Center on Homelessness and Poverty; 2011. https://www.nlchp.org/documents/Simply_Unacceptable. Accessed January 27, 2018

26. Smith N, Flores ZD, Lin J, Markovic J. *Understanding Family Homelessness in New York City: An In-depth Story of Families' Experiences Before and After Shelter.* New York, NY: Vera Institute of Justice; 2005. https://www.vera.org/publications/understanding-family-homelessness-in-new-york-city-an-in-depth-study-of-families-experiences-before-and-after-shelter. Accessed January 27, 2018

27. National Center on Family Homelessness. *Homeless Families With Children.* Washington, DC: National Center on Family Homelessness; 2009. http://www.nationalhomeless.org/factsheets/families.html. Accessed January 27, 2018

28. Moore J. *Unaccompanied and Homeless Youth: Review of Literature (1995–2005).* Greensboro, NC: National Center for Homeless Education; 2005

29. Woods JB. Unaccompanied youth and private-public order failure. *Iowa Law Rev.* 2018;103. In press

30. Aratani Y. *Homeless Children and Youth Causes and Consequences.* New York, NY: National Center for Children in Poverty, Mailman School of Public Health, Columbia University; 2009

31. Semega JL, Fontenot KR, Kollar MA. *Income and Poverty in the United States: 2016.* Washington, DC: US Census Bureau; 2017. P60-259. https://www.census.gov/library/publications/2017/demo/p60-259.html. Accessed January 27, 2018

32. Steffen BL, Carter GR, Martin M, Pelletiere D, Vandenbroucke DA, Yao YD. *Worst Case Housing Needs: 2015 Report to Congress.* Washington, DC: Office of Policy Development and Research, US Dept of Housing and Urban Development; 2015. http://www.huduser.gov/portal/Publications/pdf/WorstCaseNeeds_2015.pdf. Accessed January 27, 2018

33. Office of the Assistant Secretary for Policy Development and Research. *Fair Market Rents for the Housing Choice Voucher Program, Moderate Rehabilitation Single Room Occupancy Program, and Other Programs Fiscal Year 2018 and Adoption of Methodology Changes for Estimating Fair Market Rents*. Washington, DC: US Department of Housing and Urban Development; 2017. https://www.federalregister.gov/documents/2017/09/01/2017-18431/fair-market-rents-for-the-housing-choice-voucher-program-moderate-rehabilitation-single-room. Accessed January 27, 2018

34. Aurand A, Emmanuel D, Yentel D, Errico E, Pang M. *Out of Reach 2017: The High Cost of Housing*. Washington, DC: National Low Income Housing Coalition; 2017. http://nlihc.org/sites/default/files/oor/OOR_2017.pdf. Accessed January 27, 2018

35. Gerrard M, Shelton E, Pittman B, Owen G. *2012 Minnesota Homeless Study: Fact Sheet*. St Paul, MN: Wilder Research; 2013. https://www.wilder.org/Wilder-Research/Publications/Studies/Homelessness%20in%20Minnesota%202012%20Study/Initial%20Findings-Characteristics%20and%20Trends,%20People%20Experiencing%20Homelessness%20in%20Minnesota.pdf. Accessed January 27, 2018

36. Sznajder-Murray B, Jang JB, Slesnick N, Snyder A. Longitudinal predictors of homelessness: findings from the National Longitudinal Survey of Youth-97. *J Youth Stud*. 2015;18(8):1015–1034

37. Children's Defense Fund. *Improving Children's Health: Understanding Children's Health Disparities and Promising Approaches to Address Them*. Washington, DC: Children's Defense Fund; 2006

38. Sanders-Phillips K, Settles-Reaves B, Walker D, Brownlow J. Social inequality and racial discrimination: risk factors for health disparities in children of color. *Pediatrics*. 2009; 124(suppl 3):S176–S186

39. Buckner JC, Beardslee WR, Bassuk EL. Exposure to violence and low-income children's mental health: direct, moderated, and mediated relations. *Am J Orthopsychiatry*. 2004; 74(4):413–423

40. Biel MG, Gilhuly DK, Wilcox NA, Jacobstein D. Family homelessness: a deepening crisis in urban communities. *J Am Acad Child Adolesc Psychiatry*. 2014;53(12):1247–1250

41. Stewart AJ, Steiman M, Cauce AM, Cochran BN, Whitbeck LB, Hoyt DR. Victimization and posttraumatic stress disorder among homeless adolescents. *J Am Acad Child Adolesc Psychiatry*. 2004;43(3):325–331

42. Whitbeck LB, Johnson KD, Hoyt DR, Cauce AM. Mental disorder and comorbidity among runaway and homeless adolescents. *J Adolesc Health*. 2004;35(2):132–140

43. Martijn C, Sharpe L. Pathways to youth homelessness. *Soc Sci Med*. 2006;62(1):1–12

44. Dennis CL, McQueen K. Does maternal postpartum depressive symptomology influence infant feeding outcomes? *Acta Paediatr*. 2007;96(4):590–594

45. Milgrom J, Westley DT, Gemmill AW. The mediating role of maternal responsiveness in some longer term effects of postnatal depression on infant development. *Infant Behav Dev*. 2004; 27(4):443–454

46. Oneil-Pirozzi TM. Language functioning of residents in family homeless shelters. *Am J Speech Lang Pathol*. 2003;12(2):229–242

47. National Law Center on Homelessness and Poverty. *No Barriers: A Legal Advocate's Guide to Ensuring Compliance With the Education Program of the McKinney-Vento Act*. 2nd ed. Washington, DC: National Law Center on Homelessness and Poverty; 2016. https://www.nlchp.org/documents/NoBarriers. Accessed January 27, 2018

48. Ausikaitis AE, Wynne ME, Persaud S, et al. Staying in school: the efficacy of the McKinney–Vento Act for homeless youth. *Youth Soc*. 2015;47(5):707–726

49. Berti LC, Zylbert S, Rolnitzky L. Comparison of health status of children using a school-based health center for comprehensive care. *J Pediatr Health Care*. 2001;15(5):244–250

50. Little M, Shah R, Vermeulen MJ, et al. Adverse perinatal outcomes associated with homelessness and substance use in pregnancy. *CMAJ*. 2005;173(6):615–618

51. Stein JA, Lu MC, Gelberg L. Severity of homelessness and adverse birth outcomes. *Health Psychol.* 2000;19(6):524–534

52. Haley N, Roy E, Leclerc P, Boudreau JF, Boivin JF. Characteristics of adolescent street youth with a history of pregnancy. *J Pediatr Adolesc Gynecol.* 2004;17(5):313–320

53. Bonin E. *Adapting Your Practice: Treatment and Recommendations for Homeless Children With Otitis Media.* Nashville, TN: National Health Care for the Homeless Council Inc; 2003

54. McLean DE, Bowen S, Drezner K, et al. Asthma among homeless children: undercounting and undertreating the underserved. *Arch Pediatr Adolesc Med.* 2004;158(3):244–249

55. Chiu SH, DiMarco MA, Prokop JL. Childhood obesity and dental caries in homeless children. *J Pediatr Health Care.* 2013;27(4):278–283

56. Estrada B. Ectoparasitic infestations in homeless children. *Semin Pediatr Infect Dis.* 2003; 14(1):20–24

57. Karr C, Kline S. Homeless children: what every clinician should know. *Pediatr Rev.* 2004; 25(7):235–241

58. Kourgialis N, Wendell J, Darby P, et al. *Improving the Nutrition Status of Homeless Children: Guidelines for Homeless Family Shelters—A Report From the Children's Health Fund.* New York, NY: Children's Health Fund; 2001

59. Eicher-Miller HA, Mason AC, Weaver CM, McCabe GP, Boushey CJ. Food insecurity is associated with iron deficiency anemia in US adolescents. *Am J Clin Nutr.* 2009;90(5): 1358–1371

60. Beech BM, Myers L, Beech DJ, et al. Human immunodeficiency syndrome and hepatitis B and C infections among homeless adolescents. *Semin Pediatr Infect Dis.* 2003;14(1):12–19

61. Nyamathi AM, Christiani A, Windokun F, et al. Hepatitis C virus infection, substance use and mental illness among homeless youth: a review. *AIDS.* 2005;19(suppl 3):S34–S40

62. Boivin JF, Roy E, Haley N, Galbaud du Fort G. The health of street youth: a Canadian perspective. *Can J Public Health.* 2005;96(6):432–437

63. Zerger S, Strehlow AJ, Gundlapalli AV. Homeless young adults and behavioral health: an overview. *Am Behav Sci.* 2008;51(6):824–841

64. Tyler KA, Cauce AM, Whitbeck L. Family risk factors and prevalence of dissociative symptoms among homeless and runaway youth. *Child Abuse Negl.* 2004;28(3):355–366

65. Tyler KA, Hoyt DR, Whitbeck LB, Cauce AM. The impact of childhood sexual abuse on later sexual victimization among runaway youth. *J Res Adolesc.* 2001;11(2):151–176

66. Bender K, Thompson S, Ferguson K, Yoder J, DePrince A. Risk detection and self-protection among homeless youth. *J Res Adolesc.* 2015;25(2):352–365

67. Abbey A, Jacques-Tiura AJ, LeBreton JM. Risk factors for sexual aggression in young men: an expansion of the confluence model. *Aggress Behav.* 2011;37(5):450–464

68. Whitbeck L, Hoyt D, Yoder K, Cauce A, Paradise M. Deviant behavior and victimization among homeless and runaway adolescents. *J Interpers Violence.* 2001;16(11):1175–2104

69. Heerde JA, Hemphill SA. Sexual risk behaviors, sexual offenses, and sexual victimization among homeless youth: a systematic review of associations with substance use. *Trauma Violence Abuse.* 2016;17(5):468–489

70. Whitbeck LB, Hoyt DR, Johnson KD, Chen X. Victimization and posttraumatic stress disorder among runaway and homeless adolescents. *Violence Vict.* 2007;22(6):721–734

71. Whitbeck LB, Chen X, Hoyt DR, Tyler KA, Johnson KD. Mental disorder, subsistence strategies, and victimization among gay, lesbian, and bisexual homeless and runaway adolescents. *J Sex Res.* 2004;41(4):329–342

72. Weinstock H, Berman S, Cates W. Sexually transmitted diseases among American youth: incidence and prevalence estimates, 2000. *Perspect Sex Reprod Health.* 2004;36(1):6–10

73. Young SD, Rice E. Online social networking technologies, HIV knowledge, and sexual risk and testing behaviors among homeless youth. *AIDS Behav.* 2011;15(2):253–260

74. Collins J, Slesnick N. Factors associated with motivation to change HIV risk and substance use behaviors among homeless youth. *J Soc Work Pract Addict.* 2011;11(2):163–180

75. Edidin JP, Ganim Z, Hunter SJ, Karnik NS. The mental and physical health of homeless youth: a literature review. *Child Psychiatry Hum Dev.* 2012;43(3):354–375

76. Ginzler JA, Garrett SB, Baer JS, Peterson PL. Measurement of negative consequences of substance use in street youth: an expanded use of the Rutgers Alcohol Problem Index. *Addict Behav.* 2007;32(7):1519–1525

77. Perlman S, Sheller S, Hudson KM, Wilson CL. Parenting in the face of homelessness. In: Haskett ME, Perlman S, Cowan BA, eds. *Supporting Families Experiencing Homelessness: Current Practices and Future Directions.* New York, NY: Springer; 2014:57–78

78. Shinn M, Brown SR, Gubits D. Can housing and service interventions reduce family separations for families who experience homelessness? *Am J Comm Psychol.* 2017;60(1–2): 79–90

79. Weinreb L, Rossi PH. The American homeless family shelter "system." *Soc Serv Rev.* 1995;61(1):86–107

80. US General Accounting Office. *Report to the Honorable Paul Simon, U.S. Senate: Homelessness; Homeless and Runaway Youth Receiving Services at Federally Funded Shelters.* Washington, DC: US General Accounting Office; 1989. GAO/HRD-90–45. https://ncfy.acf.hhs.gov/library/1989/homelessness-homeless-and-runaway-youth-receiving-services-federally-funded-shelters. Accessed January 27, 2018

81. US General Accounting Office. *Homelessness: Fragmentation and Overlap in Programs Highlight the Need to Identify, Assess, and Reduce Inefficiencies.* Washington, DC: US General Accounting Office; 2012. GAO-12-491. https://www.gao.gov/products/GAO-12-491. Accessed January 27, 2018

82. Rew L. Caring for and connecting with homeless adolescents. *Fam Community Health.* 2008;31(suppl 1):S42–S51

Children Affected by Racism

Danielle Laraque-Arena, MD, and Virginia P. Young, MLS

"While it has been argued that we are in a post-racial period, the persistence of health disparities and disparities in the societal treatment of individuals decries this hopeful assertion."

Introduction and Definitions

An analysis of the effects of racism on the mental health of children can begin with an examination of generally accepted and accessible definitions of racism and race. *Racism* has 3 distinct definitions in the Webster dictionary, each covering a different aspect of the phenomenon. These are (1) the belief that "race is the primary determinant of human traits and capacities and that racial differences produce an inherent superiority of a particular race"; (2) the doctrine, political program, or political or social system founded on that belief; and (3) the act of prejudice or discrimination itself.[1] The word *race* contained in the definition of racism can be defined as "a family, tribe, people, or nation belonging to the same stock"; or "a class or kind of people unified by shared interests, habits, or characteristics"; or "an actually or potentially interbreeding group within a species"; or "a taxonomic category (as a subspecies), representing such a group."[2] In contrast with these common definitions, race is described in the sciences as a social construct, and the overlap of race, ethnicity, culture, and religion are recognized as "categories within popular and academic discourse" rather than race as an "essentialist biological category"; however, none would deny the impact, good or bad, of this social construct on certain social interactions and child well-being.[3] As noted by Williams and Mohammed, "racism often leads to the development of negative attitudes…and differential treatment (discrimination)…by both individuals and social institutions."[4]

The origins of the use of the term *race* to separate humans emerged in the late 1700s, when Swedish taxonomist Carl von Linné (Linnaeus) identified 4 main racial groups, which could be identified geographically: Europeans, Americans, Asiatics, and Africans. In the late 18th century, German anthropologist Johann Blumenbach classified 5 races: Caucasian, Mongolian, Ethiopian, American, and Malay.[5] From the first adoption of the term *race,* these divisions of variously defined "races" have been used to explain many physical and behavioral characteristics, as if the classifications derive from scientific evidence. Throughout American history, the division by race served purposes of social and class stratification, as it was used to justify slavery, unfair labor practices, and treatment of some races as less than human.[6] Racial categories and racial discrimination became part of the socioeconomic fabric of the United States.[7]

It is also useful to define the term *well-being* when examining the impact of racism on children. In 1988, the United Nations Children's Fund (UNICEF) established the Office of Research to aid in understanding issues that affect the lives of children, especially focusing on children's rights. The UNICEF Office of Research issues an annual *Innocenti Report Card* to assess child well-being in industrialized countries. The *Innocenti Report Card 7* was released in 2007, and it is organized into 3 areas: first, detailing child well-being in 29 countries as measured by 6 dimensions: (1) material well-being, (2) health and safety, (3) educational well-being, (4) family and peer relationships, (5) behaviors and risks, (6) subjective well-being; second, what children say themselves about their own life satisfaction; and third, trends in child well-being during the first decade of the 21st century.[8] A notable change in the dimensions of child well-being occurred with the release of the *Innocenti Report Card 11* in 2013. The 6 dimensions were reduced to 5, and a new dimension of "Housing and environment" replaced "Family and peer relationships" and "Subjective well-being."[9] The 5 dimensions of well-being noted in the 2013 report are helpful in evaluating the impact of racism on the well-being of children; they include material well-being, health and safety, education, behaviors and risks, and housing and environment (Table 25-1), as well as the average for all 5 dimensions, which is identified as "Overall child well-being." It is important for practitioners to recognize that well-being encompasses these domains that speak broadly to the World Health Organization (WHO) definition of health as being "a state of physical, mental, intellectual, social and emotional well-being and not merely the absence of disease or infirmity."[10] The WHO recognizes that "[h]ealthy children live in families, environments and communities that provide them with the opportunity to reach their fullest

Table 25-1. How Child Well-being Is Measured

Dimensions	Components	Indicators
Dimension 1 **Material well-being**	Monetary deprivation	Relative child poverty rate
		Relative child poverty gap
	Material deprivation	Child deprivation rate
		Low family affluence rate
Dimension 2 **Health and safety**	Health at birth	Infant mortality rate
		Low birthweight rate
	Preventive health services	Overall immunization rate
	Childhood mortality	Child death rate, age 1-19
Dimension 3 **Education**	Participation	Participation rate: early childhood education
		Participation rate: further education, age 15-19
		NEET rate (% age 15-19 not in education, employment, or training)
	Achievement	Average PISA scores in reading, math, and science
Dimension 4 **Behaviors and risks**	Health behaviors	Being overweight
		Eating breakfast
		Eating fruit
		Taking exercise
	Risk behaviors	Teenage fertility rate
		Smoking
		Alcohol
		Cannabis
	Exposure to violence	Fighting
		Being bullied
Dimension 5 **Housing and environment**	Housing	Rooms per person
		Multiple housing problems
	Environmental safety	Homicide rate
		Air pollution

From UNICEF. *Child Well-being in Rich Countries: A Comparative Overview. Innocenti Report Card 11.* Florence, Italy: UNICEF Office of Research; 2013:5. Reproduced with permission.

developmental potential."[11] From a practical and policy perspective, this framework of well-being is essential to the analysis of the impact of racism on children.

It is notable that the United States did not rank first in any measure of well-being in the *Innocenti Report Card 11*. Its rankings in the 5 dimensions of health were 26, 25, 27, 23, and 23, respectively—with an overall ranking of 26 when compared with the other 29 OECD (Organization of Economic Cooperation and Development) countries (Table 25-2). Of note, there does not appear to be a strong relationship between per-capita gross domestic product (GDP) and overall well-being.

Importantly, while the report does not claim to cover all aspects of child well-being (and, in fact, the word *racism* does not appear in its text), it does point out that the failure to protect and promote the well-being of children and adolescents is associated with increased risk for a wide range of adverse outcomes later in life. (See Table 25-1) In the literature, links between racial discrimination and violence as well as a correlation among structural racism, residential segregation, and violent crime have been documented, supporting the use of UNICEF measures of "exposure to violence" and "environmental safety" as proxy measures for racism's inverse effect on children's well-being.[12,13] The literature also notes that a "Eurocentric" examination of the social determinants of health (including the 2013 UNICEF well-being dimensions 1, 2, 3, and 5 in Table 25-1) has not considered the inequalities of broader cultural and geographic contexts—for example, the considerations of children from indigenous and minority racial and ethnic groups.[3]

The growth of research on children's perception of a stressor such as racism is important and exemplified by UNICEF's reporting on "what children say." As noted previously, the UNICEF 2007 *Innocenti Report Card* of child well-being included a sixth dimension called "Subjective well-being," which was measured in terms of children's rating of their own health, how well they liked school, and their personal well-being.[8] In that report, the United States was not among the countries reporting on this measure. By 2013, children's "Subjective well-being" had been omitted from the dimensions of well-being, to be included as a separate measure in its own right. Figure 25-1 displays the children's life satisfaction league table (2009/2010). As noted, the chart shows the proportion of children aged 11, 13, and 15 who answered 6 or more on a scale of 1 to 10 in rating their overall satisfaction with life, with 0 = "the worst possible life for me" and 10 = "the best possible life for me." In this rating of 29 countries, the United States ranks 23rd in life satisfaction.[9]

Table 25-2. A League Table of Child Well-being

		Overall Well-being	Dimension 1	Dimension 2	Dimension 3	Dimension 4	Dimension 5
		Average Rank (All 5 Dimensions)	Material Well-being (Rank)	Health and Safety (Rank)	Education (Rank)	Behaviors and Risks (Rank)	Housing and Environment (Rank)
1	Netherlands	2.4	1	5	1	1	4
2	Norway	4.6	3	7	6	4	3
3	Iceland	5	4	1	10	3	7
4	Finland	5.4	2	3	4	12	6
5	Sweden	6.2	5	2	11	5	8
6	Germany	9	11	12	3	6	13
7	Luxembourg	9.2	6	4	22	9	5
8	Switzerland	9.6	9	11	16	11	1
9	Belgium	11.2	13	13	2	14	14
10	Ireland	11.6	17	15	17	7	2
11	Denmark	11.8	12	23	7	2	15
12	Slovenia	12	8	6	5	21	20
13	France	12.8	10	10	15	13	16
14	Czech Republic	15.2	16	8	12	22	18
15	Portugal	15.6	21	14	18	8	17
16	United Kingdom	15.8	14	16	24	15	10
17	Canada	16.6	15	27	14	15	11
18	Austria	17	7	26	23	17	12

Table 25-2. A League Table of Child Well-being (continued)

		Overall Well-being	Dimension 1	Dimension 2	Dimension 3	Dimension 4	Dimension 5
		Average Rank (All 5 Dimensions)	Material Well-being (Rank)	Health and Safety (Rank)	Education (Rank)	Behaviors and Risks (Rank)	Housing and Environment (Rank)
19	Spain	17.6	24	9	26	20	9
20	Hungary	18.4	18	20	8	24	22
21	Poland	18.8	22	18	9	19	26
22	Italy	19.2	23	17	25	10	21
23	Estonia	20.8	19	22	13	26	24
24	Slovakia	20.8	25	21	21	18	19
25	Greece	23.4	20	19	28	25	25
26	United States	24.8	26	25	27	23	23
27	Lithuania	25.2	27	24	19	29	27
28	Latvia	26.4	28	28	20	28	28
29	Romania	28.6	29	29	29	27	29

Twenty-nine developed countries are ranked according to the overall well-being of their children. Each country's overall rank is based on its average ranking for the 5 dimensions of child well-being. Lack of data on a number of indicators means that the following countries, although OECD and/or EU members, could not be included in the league table of child well-being: Australia, Bulgaria, Chile, Cyprus, Israel, Japan, Malta, Mexico, New Zealand, the Republic of Korea, and Turkey. A light lavender background indicates a place in the top third of the table, mid lavender denotes the middle third, and dark lavender the bottom third.
From UNICEF. Child Well-being in Rich Countries: A Comparative Overview. Innocenti Report Card 11. Florence, Italy: UNICEF Office of Research; 2013:2. Reproduced with permission.

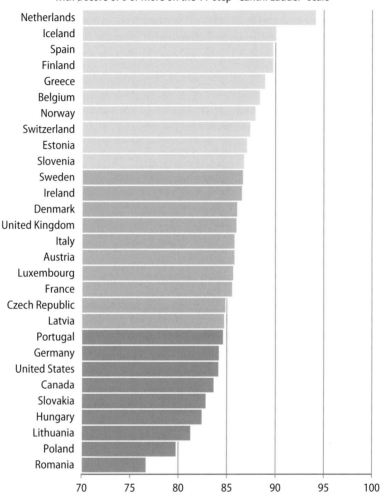

Percent of children aged 11, 13, and 15 who rate their life satisfaction
with a score of 6 or more on the 11-step "Cantril Ladder" scale

Figure 25-1. The children's life satisfaction league table (2009/2010).

From UNICEF. *Child Well-being in Rich Countries: A Comparative Overview. Innocenti Report Card 11.*
Florence, Italy: UNICEF Office of Research; 2013:39. Reproduced with permission.

The current chapter focuses on racism as a social determinant of child
well-being—a term that incorporates concepts of health, fulfillment, and
happiness. It reviews select key articles that emerged from our literature
review in the areas of definitions and characteristics of racism, relationship
of reported racism to child health and well-being, and individual and societal paths toward resolution of racism. We acknowledge that our review is

not comprehensive but meant to raise awareness and to begin the conversation, that surely others will add greatly to that ongoing conversation, and that a more robust research agenda will be needed to guide effective interventions; however, on the basis of the current state of the field, we propose some concrete actions pediatric primary care clinicians (PCCs) (ie, pediatricians, family physicians, internists, nurse practitioners, and physician assistants at the front lines of pediatrics) may consider in their practice to care effectively for children and adolescents (collectively called *children* in this chapter unless otherwise specified) who are affected by racism.

Epidemiology

Describing the incidence and prevalence of racism—the extent of racism nationally and globally—is a difficult process, complicated by the lack of uniformity in the definition of racism and the lack of agreed-upon measures or perceptions of racism. Additionally, studies have reported on the direct experiences of racism, vicarious racial discrimination, caregivers' reports of their child's racism experiences, and children's own reports of experiences and perceptions of racism. Given these caveats, a brief review of the literature is instructive. Search terms for the key words *epidemiology of racism* in PubMed yields 1,103 results (April 10, 2017). Review of these articles shows a diversity of topic areas related to racism. They include, for example, police encounters, housing/housing practices, segregation, crime and punishment, juvenile justice, depression, post-traumatic stress disorder, mental illness, health disparities, epigenetics, intergenerational experiences, nursing care, health and labor-power, paranoia, scientific racism, prevention, policy, medical teaching, public health, research, medical mistrust, sexism, gender, poverty, survival, violence, sexual assault, abuse, bad outcomes, a variety of health conditions and outcomes (eg, diabetes, hypertension, obesity, cardiovascular, HIV/AIDS, asthma, perinatal, birth, lead poisoning, sickle cell, substance use, cancer, palliative care, pregnancy outcomes, infant mortality), protective factors, life course, adoption, school, working conditions, socioeconomics, social identity, profiling, inequality, homophobia, resilience, cultural competence, acculturation, Tuskegee, apartheid, implicit bias, microaggressions, and refugee status. When the key word *children* is added to the search for *epidemiology of racism,* PubMed yields 141 (April 10, 2017) articles. Topics of smoking, preschool, social-emotional development, and life course are highlighted, in addition to those noted previously.

Despite the number of studies identified in the literature review noted previously, few studies examine the prevalence of the experience of racial discrimination in populations of children. In one study, a convenience sample of 277 children was recruited with the demographics of 31% African American, 38% Latino, 7% West Indian/Caribbean, 19% multiracial, 4% European American, and 2% other.[14] These children were administered a questionnaire that described settings or contexts (school and community) where they might have experienced reported discrimination; 88% of the children had at least one experience of racial discrimination, and 11.6% had these experiences in at least half of the 23 situations described in the questionnaire. These experiences included incidents between children and individuals of both similar and different racial/ethnic identities; incidents, both blatant and subtle; and some, ambiguous in nature. The result of this exploratory study speaks to the almost universal experience of racial discrimination in this diverse group of children. This finding supports the need to further explore this phenomenon and its impact on the life satisfaction of children.

The report of the peer-reviewed literature is only one source of information on the epidemiology of racial discrimination and children. The incidence and prevalence of racially based violence is an important area of study and would necessitate the review of many additional sources: national and state-level government databases, such as the Centers for Disease Control and Prevention "Leading Causes of Death Reports"[15]; the non–peer-reviewed literature, such as conference proceedings, government and nonprofit organization reports—either originating on the organization Web site or published in documents like the "Grey Literature Report"[16]; and news media resources. The difficulty in locating data and conducting research on gun violence has been documented as an example of access limitations.[17]

Racism, Health, and Well-being in Children and Adolescents

As noted previously, in the *Innocenti Report Card 11* health and safety are but subsets of overall well-being. A systematic review of 121 studies examining the relationship between reported racism and health and well-being for children is instructive in some key principles.[3] The authors of this review chose the following health outcomes in their review of the impact of reported racism: negative mental health, positive mental health, physical health, general health, negative general health, positive general health, well-being/life satisfaction/quality of life (QoL), negative pregnancy/birth, positive pregnancy/birth, and behavioral problems/delinquent behavior. This categorization did not include some broader determinants of health and well-being, such as material and educational well-being. Nonetheless, it is helpful to review their results and the measures used to assess reported (subjective) racism and its relationship to the selected outcomes.

Priest et al[3] note the use of different instruments as exposure measures in the studies reviewed. These include, for example, the Everyday Discrimination Scale (EDS)[18] and the Experiences of Discrimination (EOD).[19,20] The majority of the 121 studies reported interpersonal racial discrimination, and a minority reported on systemic racism. Internalized racism was also examined. Reports were from children or their caregivers. Health outcomes were reported, with mental health being the most commonly reported outcome. From the analysis, 46% of reported outcomes were negatively associated with racial discrimination, 18% were positively associated, and 3% were conditionally associated. Anxiety, depression, and negative self-esteem were the most commonly reported negative health outcomes related to racial discrimination. Importantly, there was a negative association between racial discrimination and favorable health outcomes such as resilience, self-esteem or self-worth, positive adjustment, and social and psychological adaptation. There was a positive association between racial discrimination and externalizing conditions, such as aggression and conduct problems, and between racial discrimination and internalizing problems. There was also a positive association between racial discrimination and health-related behaviors, such as drug use and cigarette smoking. Notably, a weaker relationship was reported between racial discrimination and physical health outcomes, although this may reflect delayed onset of those physical ailments such as hypertension, obesity, and other chronic diseases. The use of biomarkers that measure allostatic load and chronic diseases (eg, salivary cortisol) was suggested by this and other studies.

While well-being, life satisfaction, and QoL outcomes were negatively associated with racial discrimination in the Priest et al review,[3] other studies showed no significant associations. There is an evident need for longitudinal studies in better understanding the direction of the relationships reported.

While there have been consistent patterns of association between racial discrimination and health outcomes reported in a number of studies and in the systematic review by Priest et al,[3] a number of mediators deserve mention. These include emotions such as anger and perceived threat as well as individual factors such as identity, cultural orientation, and self-esteem. These findings suggest that much more study is needed to understand factors that can either aggravate or mitigate exposure to racism. Other obvious areas of needed study are positive parenting and socialization, social support, and ethnic identity.

In one study, the protective role of ethnic identity is examined.[21] The authors point to the role of cultural values and identity in supporting psychological well-being and resilience, for example, coping with the adverse conditions of urban poverty, where a disproportionate number of black and Latino adolescents reside. Citing the "identity-focused cultural-ecological model,"[22] they discuss the balance between risk contributors and protective factors. They cite this model in better understanding the variable response of youth to stressful situations; factors include, for example, youth's perceptions of the experience, their adaptations to stresses, the resources available to them, and micro-system as well as macro-system influences (eg, neighborhoods, social policies, government systems). The role of culture is argued to be pivotal and a strong moderator of the experience of racial discrimination—and in their treatise, resultant antisocial behavior. The contribution of cultural assets and a strengths-based approach in support of adolescents has been a useful framework for positive development.[23,24] The findings of the study by Williams et al confirmed, in a group of minority youth, that youth's cultural heritage and pride in that heritage helped youth to cope with the negative effects of racial/ethnic discrimination.[21] Ethnic identity was also protective in relation to family-related stressors and economic hardship. However, not surprisingly, the authors also found that youth engaged in actively exploring the meaning of their racial/ethnic group memberships were vulnerable to the negative effects of discrimination. This latter effect may be caused by increased sensitivity and awareness of subtle or implicit biases and microaggressions, as well as overt, violent, and often repeated encounters. In general, the findings speak to the need for more research and more nuanced or complex interpretations of the role of racial identity, the role of racial discrimination, and the interventions that might effectively buffer adolescents from negative outcomes.

As noted, there is not uniformity in how we measure exposure to racial discrimination. In that respect, the importance in understanding the child's perception of exposure to racism is informed by the work of Pachter et al.[25] In this report, the development and testing of a new self-report instrument, the Perceptions of Racism in Children and Youth (PRaCY) is described. Theoretically driven instruments are few, as are examinations of how children perceive the world. The PRaCY is based on stress theory[26] and seeks to examine not only the frequency of occurrences of racist events but the valid and reliable measurement of perceptions of racism in a multidimensional way, reflecting both the emotional response and the adaptation or coping mechanisms in the face of these occurrences. The authors developed two

10-item questionnaires for children aged 8 to 13 and adolescents 14 to 18—the first such instruments for use in children this young and ethnically diverse, including African American, Latino, West Indian/Caribbean, and multicultural/multiracial populations.[25] While this sampling is diverse, it is acknowledged that it is not all-inclusive; for example, Asian and Southeast Asian children were not included in validation studies. Interestingly, this tool provides additive scores, as well as sub-scores reflecting perceptions of racism that relate to skin color, ethnicity, language, accent, and emotional and coping responses. The authors indicate that more research is needed to examine other variables associated with perceptions of racism and to examine the possible impact of these perceptions on outcomes across a range of domains (eg, clinical, public health).

While we have reviewed selected studies in this chapter, a literature review of this research area yields a relative lack of studies recommending evidence-based interventions that mitigate the impact of racism on health outcomes and child well-being. In addition, as noted, there are a variety of instruments used in singular studies making reasonable comparisons difficult. There is recognition that understanding the experience of racism from the child's and adolescent's perceptions may give additional clues to effective interventions. Societal efforts toward primary prevention are clearly needed and are discussed in the next sections.

Individual Responses to Racism: Case Examples of Social Activism, Resilience, Socialization, and Coping

There are countless examples of individual responses to systemic and personal racism.[27] In this section, we thought it instructive to cite a few case examples of individuals who have dealt with the reality of racism and with the evident inequities resulting from such exposure.

In her publication of *"Outstanding Services to Negro Health": Dr Dorothy Boulding Ferebee, Dr Virginia M. Alexander, and Black Women Physicians' Public Health Activism,*[28] noted author Vanessa Northington Gamble, MD, PhD, describes the lives of 2 black women from very different backgrounds; one (Ferebee, born 1898) from an elite black family and the other (Alexander, born 1899) from a racially diverse poor and working class background. Both women entered medical school—one at Tufts and the other at Women's Medical College of Pennsylvania—where they encountered both racism and sexism. The evidence of that discrimination included being subjected to, for example, "insulting" stories, preferential treatment of other students, and lack of selection for internships despite academic excellence. Dr Ferebee's experiences as a leader in black women's organizations provided the pathway for her activism. She was pivotal in the operation of the first black sorority Alpha Kappa Alpha (AKA) and led the AKA-sponsored Mississippi Health Project, which was focused on improving the health of low-income rural families. Dr Ferebee served as the president of the National Council of Negro Women from 1949–1953. Dr Alexander's approach began on a much smaller scale, with the opening of a practice in her home called the Aspiranto Health Home, providing care without the racism she observed in Philadelphia hospitals. Her Quaker beliefs provided the foundation and funding (through the Quaker Friends' Race Relations Committee) for her expansion to research on health disparities in north Philadelphia. Dr Alexander was the first black woman to earn a master's degree in Public Health at Yale.[28] Both of these women chose to integrate medicine, public health, and social activism in order to make right the inequities that they suffered and saw rampant in their communities.

Another notable example of resilience and social activism is David Satcher, MD, PhD, the founder of the *Journal of Health Care for the Poor and Underserved* and the director of the Satcher Health Leadership Institute. Dr Satcher was raised in poverty and rose to the rank of the 16th US Surgeon General. An inspirational leader with whom this author (Laraque-Arena) has had an opportunity to have long conversations, Satcher's economic circumstances did not dictate what he would achieve. Born and raised in Anniston, AL, 1 of 10 children of a farmer with only elementary school–level education, Satcher stated, "I may have come from a poor family economically, but they were not poor in spirit."[29] Satcher told the *Los Angeles Times:* "We had a rich environment from the spirit of my parents, both of whom had a vision for their children. They didn't keep us out of school working in the fields. They made it clear that school came first, and that teachers were heroes."[29] Another noted asset in Satcher's life was his parents' deep religious beliefs, which in the literature is often cited as a buffer to the potential negative consequences of poverty and racism.[30]

The circumstances that allow individuals such as those described previously to overcome adversity related to racism have been studied. One such study[31] defines social capital as "the ability to secure benefits through membership in networks or other social structures"—specifically 6 types of associations (home-country friends meetings, civil society organizations, school-parent meetings, community associations, labor unions, and political parties). The authors report possible mitigating effects of social capital on racial discrimination. The previously described examples of Drs Ferebee (sorority membership and National Council of

Negro Women) and Alexander (Quaker Friends participation) clearly demonstrate the essential role social capital played in the ability of these individuals to succeed.

In a commentary by Harrell et al, the authors examine racism in the context of social neurosciences and discuss the array of cognitive and self-controlling behaviors that can mitigate the effects of racism.[32] The authors propose models in which psychological processes and physiologic pathways link 4 forms of racism to health-related physiologic changes. (See Figure 25-2 and also the conceptual model from Sanders-Phillips et al.[33]) Harrell et al[32] and others[34] discuss interventions addressing the various forms of racism, based on the described models of racism. Individualized approaches discussed include mindful meditation and progressive relaxation to counter the physiologic responses to racism. Other stress management techniques involve cognitive behavioral therapy, restructuring the response to racism as a stressor. What is most notable in the discussion by Harrell et al[32] is the recognition of this stressor—racism—as precipitating the physiologic responses of other types of trauma, validating and creating awareness in the clinical arena of the impact of racism on the health of individuals, hence the recognition that treatment is merited and available. This awareness contrasts with the response often experienced by those exposed to racism that their reactions are exaggerated or not at all justified.

Also deserving of mention is the socialization of children: direct and indirect, intentional or more implicit, messages given to them in response to anticipated or actual exposure to racism. "Racial socialization" colloquially refers to the steps that parents take in raising their children's awareness of the racial context of their lives and preparing them to meet those challenges and/or to solidify their racial identity. More strict definition of racial social-ization refers to "the process in which individuals are taught certain cultural values and beliefs that pertain to their racial group membership."[35] Relevant to the discussion of racial socialization are the variables of *racial identity* and *ethnic identity*. While these 2 terms are often collapsed, one refers to belonging to a racial group and the other, belonging to an ethnic group with shared cultural values and beliefs. All 3 variables are postulated to buffer the mental health effects of racial discrimination, hence leading to the belief that socialization regarding racial identity and ethnic identity is an inter-vention that is protective against the negative impact of racial discrimina-tion. The literature does support the notion that the 3 concepts—racial socialization, racial identity, and ethnic identity—are distinct constructs.[36]

In one study of 106 African American adolescents, boys reported having been given more "cultural alertness" to messages of discrimination,

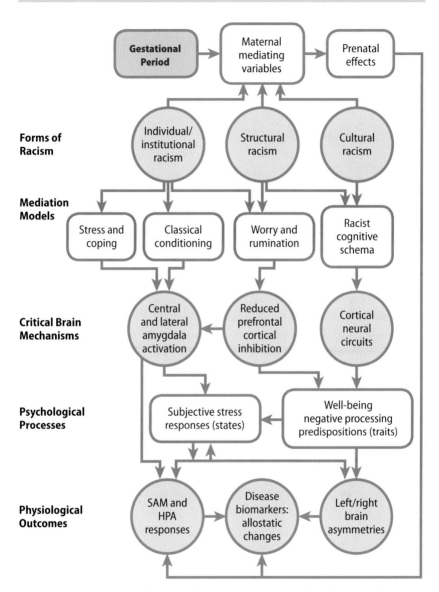

Figure 25-2. Proposed models, psychological processes, and physiological pathways that link four forms of racism to health-related physiological changes.

From Harrell CJP, Burford TI, Cage BN, et al. Multiple pathways linking racism to health outcomes. *Du Bois Rev.* 2011;8(1):152. Reproduced with permission.

as well as ways to cope with these experiences.[37] The authors concluded that such racial socialization is important in teaching teens strategies for managing racial discrimination. However, it remained unclear whether preparation for such racial bias was supportive of the mental health of these teens. The authors reported an association between this type of preparation and depressive symptoms among the teens; however, the authors also reported that context matters: messages delivered in the context of "democratic/involved parenting" yielded more positive outcomes (eg, school engagement) than those delivered by less democratic and involved parenting. The authors' definition of democratic or involved parenting, while not entirely clear, is generally understood to indicate an approach that is more authoritative, rather than authoritarian, and engages the teen in discussion and problem-solving. This finding certainly would call upon the pediatric community to understand the impact of racism, the necessary discussions with parents of ethnically diverse children at greater risk of experiencing racism, support for activities that build resilience in children, and support for the positive aspects of racial and ethnic identity.

One last area deserves mention. In easing conversations regarding race and in leading individuals and ultimately society to be more reflective about the impact of prejudice, it is useful to look at the worlds of entertainment and the arts. Many performers and artists have stimulated direct, confrontational dialogue on racism in ways often avoided in other settings. These include rap artists; creative youth organizations (eg, Urban Word NYC); comedians (eg, Sasheer Zamata[38]); and writers (eg, Dick Gregory). *Narrative medicine* (defined as "medicine practiced with the narrative competence to recognize, interpret and be moved to action by the predicaments of others") has provided a framework for self-expression in the context of professional development.[39] Using media such as these to communicate may enable individuals to express their views more freely, provide emotional depth to difficult conversations, and potentially lead to better understanding of the impact of issues such as racial discrimination on health.

While this chapter cannot review in depth the full variety of individual coping and recovery responses to the experience of racism, the narrative of those who have succeeded personally and professionally in the face of such trauma, the corresponding neuroscience research linking physiologic responses to effective therapeutic interventions, and the important role of parents and the broader society in alleviating the distress of children facing racism all provide hope that the health care professional community will react and support individuals and communities oppressed by racism.

Societal Responses to Racism: Laws, Regulations, and Social Networks

Societal responses to racism run the gamut from laws and regulations to social networks. The legacy of slavery, racial segregation, and apartheid is well-known to most. Following the abolition of slavery with the Thirteenth Amendment to the US Constitution in 1865, repeated attempts to remedy racial discrimination have been enacted by legislation and judicial decree. The 14th and 15th constitutional amendments granted equal protection of laws (14th) and the right to vote (15th) to US citizens, excluding women, who were not guaranteed the right to vote until the passage of the Nineteenth Amendment to the US Constitution ratified in 1920.[40] The US Supreme Court ruled against school segregation in *Brown v Board of Education* (347 US 483) in 1954.[41] The Civil Rights Act of 1964, the Voting Rights Act of 1965, and the Fair Housing Act of 1968 were signed in efforts to eliminate racial barriers to access to public places and services; participation in elections; and the sale, rental, and financing of housing.[42] In 1965, President Lyndon B. Johnson endorsed a plan for affirmative action in the United States, articulated in the following statement: "You do not take a person who for years has been hobbled by chains and liberate him, bring him up to the starting line of a race and then say, 'You are free to compete with all the others' and believe that you have been fair."[43] In 1967, the US Supreme Court ruled in *Loving v Virginia* (388 US 1) that prohibition of interracial marriage was a violation of the US Constitution.[44] The legislation and judicial decisions included herein are a selection of notable efforts to address discrimination in the United States and are provided as an overview.

The national discussion of the needed societal response to past and current racially biased policies and opportunities continues today.[45,46] The recent national debates around the Black Lives Matter movement, in response to a number of police shootings of unarmed black individuals—including children and adolescents—underscores the continuing importance of our attention to the impact of racism and underprivilege.[47,48] In addition, the increasing diversity of the population of the United States demands that discussions of equity and fair treatment extend to all individuals and populations—beyond those traditionally the focus of policies (eg, African Americans/blacks, Native Americans, Mexican Americans, and mainland Puerto Ricans)—to all those who are discriminated against, for whatever reasons, including race, ethnicity, color, religion, gender, sexual orientation, disability, veterans, and immigration status. The resolution of discrimination demands a system and the rule of law to reaffirm the inherent rights of infants, children, adolescents, young adults, adults, and elders to be treated civilly and to have access to all opportunities such as good health, education, economic advancement, and legal representation. While it has been argued that we are in a post-racial period, the persistence of health disparities and disparities in the societal treatment of individuals decries this hopeful assertion. Aja and Bustillo review the conceptual model of affirmative action as a set of positive antidiscrimination policies aimed at the inclusion of stigmatized groups in "preferred positions in society, with aims to promote institutional desegregation."[46]

Lastly, beyond laws and regulation—critically important to drive forward change—is the continued quest of civil societies to have their individual members engage respectfully in open exchange of ideas. The pediatric community, in its exceptional role in the care of children and adolescents, can support progressive laws and policies to advance this kind of equitable treatment.

The Primary Care Clinician's Role in Caring for Children Affected by Racism

While recognizing that there is much to learn about buffering children against the negative effects of racism, including the possible vicarious effects of racial discrimination experienced by individuals close to children such as family members or friends, pediatric PCCs have the opportunity to develop a trusting relationship with families and children that provides the opening for honest conversations on a whole host of experiences, both positive and negative, that impact the lives of all children.[49,50] No assumptions can be made by the PCC regarding the perception of families. Race, ethnic, and language concordance, among other attributes, may mediate the comfort level that families feel in engaging their PCC in conversations regarding their perceptions of racism and the impact of racism on their lives. There is no cookbook approach to these conversations. Asking permission to engage, reflecting an openness to discuss, and perhaps offering use of a validated scale such as the PRaCY[25] are among the options that PCCs consider in support of families and youth. Other tools and published works are also available to guide these discussion as aides to PCCs and parents.[51] However, there is currently little evidence in the literature to support the value of routine screening, and further research is needed. The usual steps of assessing social determinants such as food security, economic security, and housing; asking about the school environment and bullying; and identifying adverse childhood experiences are important components of health supervision. Most important is the strength-based assessment of the myriad potential child, family, and neighborhood assets. *Bright Futures: Guidelines for Health Supervision of Infants, Children, and Adolescents,* 4th Edition, recommends psychosocial/behavioral assessment (ie, history, surveillance) at every visit and formal psychosocial screening for maternal depression during infancy and depression and substance use during adolescence.[52]

When discussions emerge identifying racism as a stressor in a child and family's life, the following anticipatory guidance may be useful:

▶ Teach self-regulation techniques (mindful meditation and progressive relaxation) to deal with anger, anxiety, and depression.

▶ Engage in conversation with parents on their views regarding the role of ethnic, cultural, and religious identity.

▶ Ask about supportive social structures, eliciting the parent's and child's views.

▶ When appropriate, discuss with parents that it is unclear whether preparation for racial bias is supportive of the mental health of children and that the context of those discussions is highly personal and specific to their family's view of the world.

▶ Offer parenting and child resources such as "Racism and Violence: Using Your Power as a Parent to Support Children Aged Two to Five" (article), Zero to Three (www.zerotothree.org/resources/1598-racism-and-violence-using-your-power-as-a-parent-to-support-children-aged-two-to-five).

▶ Consider mentorship programs that build resilience in children experiencing the negative consequences of racism.

Conclusion

The experience of racial discrimination is prevalent in the lives of children. Understanding of the ways to support children effectively is in a nascent stage; however, the willingness of PCCs to indicate their openness to discussion of racism may be supportive of those parents and children who are open to such guidance or acknowledgment. Strong advocacy to correct continued social injustices is clearly in the domain of pediatric health care professionals. The well-being of children, in all its dimensions, will be determined by the maturation of our societal norms to recognize the inherent uniqueness and wonder of every individual.

AAP Policy

Flores G; American Academy of Pediatrics Committee on Pediatric Research. Racial and ethnic disparities in the health and health care of children. *Pediatrics*. 2010; 125(4):e979–e1020. Reaffirmed May 2013 (pediatrics.aappublications.org/content/125/4/e979)

References

1. Racism. Merriam-Webster Web site. https://www.merriam-webster.com/dictionary/racism. Accessed January 27, 2018
2. Race [No. 3 noun]. Merriam-Webster Web site. https://www.merriam-webster.com/dictionary/race#h3. Accessed January 27, 2018
3. Priest N, Paradies Y, Trenerry B, Truong M, Karlsen S, Kelly Y. A systematic review of studies examining the relationship between reported racism and health and wellbeing for children and young people. *Soc Sci Med*. 2013;95:115–127
4. Williams DR, Mohammed SA. Racism and health I: pathways and scientific evidence. *Am Behav Sci*. 2013;57(8)
5. Witzig R. The medicalization of race: scientific legitimization of a flawed social construct. *Ann Intern Med*. 1996;125(8):675–679
6. Smedley A, Smedley BD. Race as biology is fiction, racism as a social problem is real: anthropological and historical perspectives on the social construction of race. *Am Psychol*. 2005(1):16–26
7. Bailey ZD, Krieger N, Agénor M, Graves J, Linos N, Bassett MT. Structural racism and health inequities in the USA: evidence and interventions. *Lancet*. 2017;389(10077):1453–1463
8. UNICEF. *Child Poverty in Perspective: An Overview of Child Well-being in Rich Countries*. *Innocenti Report Card 7*. Florence, Italy: UNICEF Office of Research; 2007
9. UNICEF. *Child Well-being in Rich Countries: A Comparative Overview. Innocenti Report Card 11*. Florence, Italy: UNICEF Office of Research; 2013
10. World Health Organization (WHO). Constitution of WHO: principles. WHO Web site. http://www.who.int/about/mission/en. Accessed January 27, 2018
11. Bruner C. *Health Equity and Young Children: Improving Healthy Development, Closing Health Disparities, and Ensuring School Readiness*. Des Moines, IA: Child and Family Policy Center; 2014
12. Krivo LJ, Peterson RD, Kuhl DC. Segregation, racial structure, and neighborhood violent crime. *AJS*. 2009;114(6):1765–1802
13. Sanders-Phillips K. Racial discrimination: a continuum of violence exposure for children of color. *Clin Child Fam Psychol Rev*. 2009;12(2):174–195
14. Pachter LM, Bernstein BA, Szalacha LA, Garcia Coll C. Perceived racism and discrimination in children and youths: an exploratory study. *Health Soc Work*. 2010;35(1):61–69
15. National Center for Injury Prevention and Control, Centers for Disease Control and Prevention. *Leading Causes of Death Reports, 1981-2015*. Atlanta, GA: Centers for Disease Control and Prevention; 2017. https://webappa.cdc.gov/sasweb/ncipc/leadcause.html. Accessed January 27, 2018
16. New York Academy of Medicine. Grey Literature Report Web site. http://www.greylit.org. Accessed January 27, 2018
17. Kellermann AL, Rivara FP. Silencing the science on gun research. *JAMA*. 2013;309(6):549–550
18. Clark R, Coleman AP, Novak JD. Brief report: initial psychometric properties of the everyday discrimination scale in black adolescents. *J Adolesc*. 2004;27(3):363–368
19. Krieger N. Racial and gender discrimination: risk factors for high blood pressure? *Soc Sci Med*. 1990;30(12):1273–1281

20. Krieger N, Smith K, Naishadham D, Hartman C, Barbeau EM. Experiences of discrimination: validity and reliability of a self-report measure for population health research on racism and health. *Soc Sci Med.* 2005;61(7):1576–1596

21. Williams JL, Aiyer SM, Durkee MI, Tolan PH. The protective role of ethnic identity for urban adolescent males facing multiple stressors. *J Youth Adolesc.* 2014;43(10):1728–1741

22. Swanson DP, Spencer MB, Dell'Angelo T, Harpalani V, Spencer TR. Identity processes and the positive youth development of African Americans: an explanatory framework. *New Dir Youth Dev.* 2002;(95):73–99

23. Duncan PM, Garcia AC, Frankowski BL, et al. Inspiring healthy adolescent choices: a rationale for and guide to strength promotion in primary care. *J Adolesc Health.* 2007; 41(6):525–535

24. Frankowski BL, Leader IC, Duncan PM. Strength-based interviewing. *Adolesc Med: State Art Rev.* 2009;20(1):22–40

25. Pachter LM, Szalacha LA, Bernstein BA, Coll CG. Perceptions of Racism in Children and Youth (PRaCY): properties of a self-report instrument for research on children's health and development. *Ethn Health.* 2010;15(1):33–46. https://www.ncbi.nlm.nih.gov/pmc/articles/PMC2891186/. Accessed June 7, 2018

26. Lazarus RS, Folkman S. *Stress, Appraisal, and Coping.* New York, NY: Springer Publishing Co Inc; 1984

27. deShazo RD, Smith R, Skipworth LB. Black physicians and the struggle for civil rights: lessons from the Mississippi experience; part 2: their lives and experiences. *Am J Med.* 2014;127(11):1033–1040

28. Gamble VN. "Outstanding Services to Negro Health": Dr. Dorothy Boulding Ferebee, Dr. Virginia M. Alexander, and Black Women Physicians' Public Health Activism. *Am J Public Health.* 2016;106(8):1397–1404

29. Cimons M. To heal a nation: as head of CDC, Dr. David Satcher takes a holistic view. Although healthy minds in fit bodies are important, he knows firsthand that we must also cure social ills—including violence. *Los Angeles Times.* March 1, 1994. http://articles.latimes.com/1994-03-01/news/vw-28674_1_david-satcher. Accessed January 27, 2018

30. Satcher, David. In: *Contemporary Black Biography.* Detroit, MI: Thomson Gale; 2007. http://www.encyclopedia.com/people/history/us-history-biographies/david-satcher. Accessed January 27, 2018

31. Kim C-O, Cho B-H. Can geographic bridging social capital improve the health of people who live in deprived urban neighborhoods? *Int J Health Serv.* 2016;46(4):767–789

32. Harrell CJP, Burford TI, Cage BN, et al. Multiple pathways linking racism to health outcomes. *Du Bois Rev.* 2011;8(1):143–157

33. Sanders-Phillips K, Settles-Reaves B, Walker D, Brownlow J. Social inequality and racial discrimination: risk factors for health disparities in children of color. *Pediatrics.* 2009; 124(suppl 3):S176–S186

34. Paradies Y, Priest N, Ben J, et al. Racism as a determinant of health: a protocol for conducting a systematic review and meta-analysis. *Syst Rev.* 2013;2:85

35. Berkel C, Murry VM, Hurt TR, et al. It takes a village: protecting rural African American youth in the context of racism. *J Youth Adolesc.* 2009;38(2):175–188

36. Lee DL, Ahn S. The relation of racial identity, ethnic identity, and racial socialization to discrimination-distress: a meta-analysis of Black Americans. *J Couns Psychol.* 2013;60(1):1–14

37. Lambert SF, Roche KM, Saleem FT, Henry JS. Mother-adolescent relationship quality as a moderator of associations between racial socialization and adolescent psychological adjustment. *Am J Orthopsychiatry.* 2015;85(5):409–420

38. To get to "SNL," comic Sasheer Zamata "followed the fun." *Fresh Air.* April 13, 2017. http://www.npr.org/programs/fresh-air/2017/04/13/523717679/fresh-air-for-april-13-2017. Accessed January 27, 2018

39. Charon R. Narrative medicine: form, function, and ethics. *Ann Intern Med.* 2001;134(1):83–87

40. U.S. Constitution. Cornell Law School Web site. https://www.law.cornell.edu/constitution. Accessed January 27, 2018

41. *Brown v Board of Education,* 347 US 483 (1954). https://www.law.cornell.edu/supremecourt/text/347/483. Accessed January 27, 2018

42. US House of Representatives. Constitutional amendments and major Civil Rights Acts of Congress referenced in *Black Americans in Congress.* History, Art and Archives Web site. http://history.house.gov/Exhibitions-and-Publications/BAIC/Historical-Data/Constitutional-Amendments-and-Legislation/. Accessed January 27, 2018

43. Johnson LB. Commencement address at Howard University: "To Fulfill These Rights." The American Presidency Project Web site. http://www.presidency.ucsb.edu/ws/index.php?pid=27021. Accessed January 27, 2018

44. *Loving v Virginia,* 338 US 1 (1967). https://www.law.cornell.edu/supremecourt/text/388/1. Accessed January 27, 2018

45. Friedman RA, ed. Affirmative action in education. *Georgetown J Gender Law.* 2007;8(2):395–415

46. Aja AA, Bustillo D. Judicial histories and racial disparities: affirmative action and the myth of the "post racial." *Hamline J Public Law Policy.* 2015;36(1):26–53

47. Charles D, Himmelstein K, Keenan W, Barcelo N; White Coats for Black Lives National Working Group. White Coats for Black Lives: medical students responding to racism and police brutality. *J Urban Health.* 2015;92(6):1007–1010

48. Bassett MT. #BlackLivesMatter—a challenge to the medical and public health communities. *N Engl J Med.* 2015;372(12):1085–1087

49. Laraque D. Health promotion: core concepts in building successful clinical encounters. *Pediatr Ann.* 2008;37(4):225–231

50. Heard-Garris NJ, Cale M, Camaj L, Hamati MC, Dominguez TP. Transmitting trauma: a systematic review of vicarious racism and child health [published online April 26, 2017]. *Soc Sci Med.* doi:10.1016/j.socscimed.2017.04.018

51. Zero to Three. Racism and violence: using your power as a parent to support children aged two to five. Zero to Three Web site. https://www.zerotothree.org/resources/1598-racism-and-violence-using-your-power-as-a-parent-to-support-children-aged-two-to-five. Published August 21, 2017. Accessed January 27, 2018

52. Promoting mental health. In: Hagan JF Jr, Shaw JS, Duncan PM, eds. *Bright Futures: Guidelines for Health Supervision of Infants, Children, and Adolescents.* Elk Grove Village, IL: American Academy of Pediatrics; 2017:115–150

Children With Chronic Medical Conditions

Ruth E. K. Stein, MD

"Regardless of the nature of a child's condition,
the primary goal of care is to contain or
minimize its effect and to provide maximal
opportunity for the child to function and
develop physically, socially, cognitively,
and emotionally."

Introduction

All children experience mental health issues regardless of their physical
health status, but these issues are even more integral to the care of children
and adolescents with ongoing health conditions. Some mental health issues
are transient; others, long-lasting and may themselves qualify as chronic
conditions. Children and adolescents who have chronic mental or physical
health conditions may be referred to, collectively, as *children with special
health care needs* (commonly known as CSHCN). This chapter, however, is
devoted to a discussion of how having a health condition of an ongoing
nature affects the delivery of primary care and the ways that the delivery of
integrated physical and mental health care can help ameliorate the effects of
these conditions on the mental health of the child and family. For the most
part, this discussion focuses on children who have primarily physical health
conditions, a situation in which it is frequently a little easier to separate the
physical and mental health components, but much of the discussion applies
to the presence of a primary ongoing mental health condition as well.

The first part of this chapter is devoted to issues of definition, prevalence, and general effects on the child and family of a significant ongoing
health condition and to important considerations in the general management of these conditions. The second part focuses on mental health issues at
different phases of the life cycle and care of children during these phases.

Definition and Audience

While all children experience minor illnesses and injuries, most do not experience ongoing consequences from these episodes. Some children, however, have more serious or recurrent impairments or disruptions of their health for prolonged periods. Some authorities have referred to them as *having chronic illness,* but some are not ill. Other authors have referred to them as *having disabilities* or *handicaps,* but many do not exhibit these characteristics. *Children and youths with special health care needs* (CYSHCN) has now become the preferred term. In addition, the subgroup of children who are more severely affected, that is, whose conditions involve more than one body system and either functional limitation or technology dependence (or both), has been referred to as *children with medical complexity.*

The term *children with special health care needs* was originally introduced as a euphemism for the other terms used earlier to describe these children with ongoing conditions.[1] More recently, the Maternal and Child Health Bureau has used *CYSHCN* to include children who do not currently have any condition or impairment but who are *at risk* for one, such as foster children, adopted children, or those living in poverty.[2] Because no agreement exists on which children to include in the at-risk category, CYSHCN are referred to in this chapter as *children who have ongoing or chronic conditions.* When the term *youth* is used in this chapter, it refers to children and adolescents aged 6 through 18 years.

Ongoing or *chronic conditions* also requires a definition. In fact, many current definitions are similar. One useful definition has 3 key components: the presence of a condition, a duration or expected duration of at least 1 year, and at least 1 of 3 consequences for the child or adolescent.[3] These consequences are having a functional limitation (something that prevents the child or adolescent (collectively called simply *child* or *children* in this chapter) from participating in age-appropriate activities), increased use of health care services beyond those used by age-mates, and reliance on compensatory mechanisms (medication, special treatments, assistive devices, or personal assistance) to function.

The definition adopted by the Maternal and Child Health Bureau combines the final 2 categories of consequences and considers *at-risk* children as well: "Those children who have or are at increased risk for a chronic physical, developmental, behavioral, or emotional condition and who also require health and related services of a type or amount beyond that required by children generally."[2] Because no validated method currently exists for fully operationalizing the Maternal and Child Health Bureau definition that includes those at risk, and because the concept of compensatory mechanisms is conceptually and critically distinct from receipt of services, the definition with 3 key components is used in this chapter. Compensatory mechanisms are especially important as medical care experts find new ways to minimize functional limitations and therefore allow children to carry on with their normal activities and to function as healthy children do, because of those treatments, often without other consequences of the underlying condition. Unless these special aspects of care are considered, children whose compensatory mechanisms are successful may be counted as healthy; thus, the success of treatments and the need to sustain them will be underappreciated, undercounted, and underfunded.

The use of an umbrella definition that includes children regardless of their diagnoses is important because the epidemiology of ongoing conditions in children and adolescents includes a few common conditions, congenital malformations and inborn errors of metabolism, malignancies, and a wide range of acquired injuries and illnesses. Thinking of CYSHCN as sharing some common characteristics of duration and consequences without necessarily naming any conditions is far more convenient for many purposes other than biomedical treatment and especially for understanding the emotional stresses experienced by the developing child and family. This approach, which had been referred to as "generic" or "non-categorical" is useful on many levels, but it should not obscure the need for disease-specific biomedical treatments of the condition.

The primary audience for this chapter is pediatric primary care clinicians (PCCs)—that is, pediatricians, family physicians, internists, nurse practitioners, and physician assistants who provide frontline, longitudinal health care to children.

Prevalence

Estimates suggest that between 15% and 20% of children have some impairment or underlying condition that qualifies them as CYSHCN, depending on how the definition is applied, but other studies have cited far greater percentages. Some experience only minor, if any, difficulties from their conditions, but some are severely affected.[4] Between one-half and two-thirds of the children who meet the definition experience a functional limitation, either with or without other types of consequences. Approximately 10% of all children who have ongoing conditions experience consequences in all 3 categories (functional limitations, increased use of services, and need for compensatory mechanisms), and these are often the children with the most severe conditions.[5] Children with technology dependence comprise a unique group among CYSHCN. These are children who require both a medical device or procedure to compensate for the loss of a vital bodily function and substantial, ongoing care to prevent further disability or death. It is estimated that between 0.1% to 0.25% of children in the United States have technology dependence.

Three factors will likely lead to increased identification of children with ongoing conditions. The first factor is improvements in early detection and diagnosis as a result of advances in molecular genetics and the appreciation of familial risk. Second is the use of preventive interventions that postpone the full onset of manifestations of some conditions to which children are genetically vulnerable, thus increasing the number of children receiving care for conditions that are not yet fully manifested. Finally, medical advances increase the number of children who survive their conditions, sometimes with prolonged need for treatments and dependence on medical interventions and technology.

Effects of the Condition

Ongoing conditions vary in severity from very mild, requiring little health care, to extremely debilitating, affecting every aspect of life and requiring intensive health care services. However, all ongoing conditions have some implications for children's long-range health and service needs and in many cases for children's longevity as well. Additionally, all conditions affect how families view their children and their children's vulnerabilities. Research has demonstrated that there is not always a correlation between the pediatric clinician's sense of the severity of the condition and the family's perception of its effect or influence on their lives. Even children with conditions that the medical community views as minor or inconsequential may create a sense of vulnerability or concerns that make this child seem "special" in the eyes of the family members. Moreover, families differ in the way that they may perceive the impact of the same condition or similar conditions. For example, one family may view asthma as normative because many other family members have it, while another may think that it is a catastrophic condition.

Children with functional limitations tend to experience fewer of the usual activities and opportunities for socialization that are important for normal development. Depending on the age of the child and the level of functional limitations, these effects vary considerably. Motor or sensory impairments may limit exploratory opportunities to varying degrees and therefore the child's exposure to experiences in the environment that can influence the child's developmental trajectory. Even children who do not have limitations are sometimes restricted by their parents, resulting in limitations of opportunity for developing important social skills and psychological well-being. When these restrictions of opportunities and experiences are not based on the demands of the condition itself, we consider them to be overprotection. Many families fall into this pattern because of concerns for the child's potential health vulnerability. This tendency has been described even when there is absolutely no basis in medical fact for the overprotection, such as when there is a functional cardiac murmur. This excessive worry and overprotection is referred to as *the vulnerable child syndrome.* While it occurs in children with typical health and development, it is extremely common to see some level of overprotection and concern among parents of children who have an ongoing health condition.

Another common pattern is to see parents spoiling or giving in to their child's wishes because of, for example, a desire to make up for some of the unpleasant medical procedures that the child is undergoing. This behavior can vary from providing the child with an extra treat after a blood drawing, to allowing the child to be exempted from chores, to indulging the child excessively. While the parental intentions may be good, children, especially young ones, are often more worried, rather than reassured, by these deviations from normal family rules. It is important for the pediatric clinician and his or her team to help the family understand this fact before the behavior becomes a real problem. A return to "normal" family behavior is reassuring for the child.

Effects on Delivery of Care

Developing and Promoting Partnerships With Families

Unlike with acute conditions, after which life quickly returns to normal, the disruption caused by ongoing conditions continues or ameliorates slowly. In the long term, families bear the brunt of the care responsibilities, and they need to be full partners with other members of the health care team in the care of the child.

The traditional medical approach poses some barriers to the formation of partnerships with families. First, medicine tends to be paternalistic and hierarchical, characteristics often associated with entirely prescriptive decision-making that discourages the sharing of decision-making with family members. Effective management of a chronic condition or impairment requires the clinician to understand that the parents are the experts in rearing their child, and they assume most of the day-to-day care. Within a short time, some parents will know more, especially about rare conditions, than the average PCC does, and their expertise should be valued and respected. Even at the beginning, the importance of the parents' role with and knowledge about their own child necessitates active involvement and sharing of responsibility that may run counter to the traditional hierarchical paternalism of the health care system. This shared decision-making process leads to better health outcomes for the child.[6]

The second barrier is emphasis on the deficit model, which focuses entirely on what is *wrong* with the patient, rather than seeing the child's strengths and assets. Primary care clinicians are trained to focus on the problem and fix it. For the most part, chronic conditions cannot be cured entirely, and the challenge for both the family and the clinician is to live with this reality and to minimize disruption in the child's life as much as possible, while still maximizing the child's longer-term future health and potential. Accomplishing this task requires focusing on the whole child: on both assets and impairments and helping the family to rear the child with as few limitations as possible.

When communication and mutual respect are established among health care professionals and family members, a care plan can be developed that includes the priorities of all parties, is medically and culturally acceptable, and has a far better chance of being implemented and being successful than a plan that does not recognize the parents' critical role.

Goals of Care

Regardless of the nature of a child's condition, the primary goal of care is to contain or minimize its effect and to provide maximal opportunity for the child to function and develop physically, socially, cognitively, and emotionally. This process involves providing optimal biomedical treatment of the condition and helping the family *normalize* the entire family's life experiences as much as possible. To accomplish this, clinicians should place as few restrictions on the child's activities as possible, limiting only activities that are absolutely necessary to avoid. Additionally, the care plan should be implemented in a way that minimizes the burden on the family as much as possible. Achieving an understanding of the family's burden may require gathering information about the child and family that is sometimes beyond the usual inquiry. As a result, clinicians may be perceived by families as intrusive; however, most families are able to understand this exploration of their family life once it is explained to them. For example, information about the family's routines and preferences may help in suggesting minor modifications in the type or timing of medication administration or procedures that will make the child's care less disruptive. Family members may not know on their own whether they can safely modify schedules. Tailoring care to the individual family also requires a longitudinal and developmental framework in which the management strategies and responsibilities shift over time as the parents become increasingly comfortable with the management of the condition and with the child's developmental progress.

Coordination of Care

Families of CYSHCN often depend on services from multiple parts of the health care system, as well as services from other sectors. Dealing with multiple sectors, each of which has its own requirements and regulations, can be daunting, and families need assistance in learning how to use these services. Responsibility for this assistance often falls to members of the primary care team.

The deliberate organization of patient care activities between 2 or more participants is referred to as *coordination of care* (www.ahrq.gov/ professionals/prevention-chronic-care/improve/coordination/atlas2014/ chapter2.html). In addition to coordinating care within the health care sector, the care team may need to coordinate and integrate health care services with services of other community agencies and resources in the educational, recreational, and human services sectors. Family coalitions that range from disease-specific organizations to more general groups of parents of children with ongoing conditions, such as Family Voices (www. familyvoices.org) and the Federation for Children with Special Health Care Needs (www.fcsn.org), may provide critical advice and networking. Other families in the practice who have struggled with and ultimately succeeded in finding resources may be willing to partner with parents of a child with the same or another condition. These arrangements vary from informal networking to formal parent-to-parent programs. In some instances, opportunities for care coordination can be found through private agencies, insurance companies, or Title V programs. However, for these care coordination efforts to be most successful they need to be family centered. Familiarity with these programs and resources can be extremely helpful.

Family-Centered Care

Family-centered care is based on *mutual, beneficial partnerships between families and health care professionals,* a philosophy first articulated by Shelton et al.[7] It recognizes each family's strengths, regardless of the family's circumstances, and how these strengths can add positively to the family's health care experiences. The core concepts of family-centered care are listed in Box 26-1.[8,9] Communication principles central to family-centered care are the subject of Chapter 2, Family-Centered Care: Applying Behavior Change Science.

Periodic Reassessment

At each stage in the care of a child with an ongoing condition, it is important to ensure that the family (including all the primary caregivers, whenever possible, and patients with the developmental capacity to participate), the PCC, and other health care team members, including subspecialists, agree on the priorities and on the plan. Many programs use a written plan that outlines the next phase of care and builds on the mutual priorities. Although this step may be time-consuming initially, it saves time in the long run. An agreed-on plan may encourage adherence to therapy better than presumptive decisions that are made quickly and unilaterally. It is also important to remember that circumstances change over time and the plan will need to be revised as the goals and priorities for care evolve.

Mental Health Considerations

Children with ongoing conditions and their family members often experience more stress and difficulty in adjusting to the demands of their lives than other families do. As a result, families with children with ongoing

---

Box 26-1. Core Concepts of Patient- and Family-Centered Care

- **Dignity and Respect.** Health care practitioners listen to and honor patient and family perspectives and choices. Patient and family knowledge, values, beliefs and cultural backgrounds are incorporated into the planning and delivery of care.

- **Information Sharing.** Health care practitioners communicate and share complete and unbiased information with patients and families in ways that are affirming and useful. Patients and families receive timely, complete and accurate information in order to effectively participate in care and decision-making.

- **Participation.** Patients and families are encouraged and supported in participating in care and decision-making at the level they choose.

- **Collaboration.** Patients, families, health care practitioners, and health care leaders collaborate in policy and program development, implementation and evaluation; in research; in facility design; and in professional education, as well as in the delivery of care.

From Patient- and family-centered care. Institute for Patient- and Family-Centered Care Web site. http://www.ipfcc.org/about/pfcc.html. Accessed March 8, 2018. Reproduced with permission.

conditions are more likely than others in a PCC's practice to need social-emotional support and assistance from mental health services. Having a keen appreciation of their emotional challenges enables the pediatric staff to provide anticipatory counseling and to recognize when more-intensive services are needed. The chance of success in addressing these extra mental health stresses is greatly enhanced by an integrated approach to care of the physical and mental health components. An integrated approach is one through which the general and mental health care are provided in a coordinated fashion, whether in a primary care or specialty setting. This approach can be accomplished by the PCC, who comprehensively manages the physical and the mental health conditions, or by a team of social workers, psychologists, and others, who collaborate with the PCC to provide anticipatory guidance and support throughout the stages of care.

Parenting is challenging even when there are no special issues, but having a child with a special health care need makes this role even more difficult. Despite this difficulty, most families rise to the challenge effectively. Rearing a child who is diagnosed as having a special health care need results in a great deal of physical, emotional, and financial strain, and in many cases the entire family experiences significant social isolation, placing considerable burdens and demands on family members. Some studies suggest that parents who assume major caregiving responsibilities for children with severe conditions are at increased risk for physical and mental health problems and divorce, while others contest these findings. However, it is clear that parenting a child with special health care needs is something that was not in the family's plan and provides the family with extra challenges to overcome. When they successfully overcome these challenges, many families state that it adds to their cohesion and sense of accomplishment; others are not able to rise to the challenges without substantial personal costs.

Siblings and the children themselves are often stigmatized when conditions are visible, either because of the condition itself or its treatment, which may alter the child's appearance. In addition, many siblings are left to function more independently than usual because parental attention may be focused on the child with a condition. They may feel jealous, abandoned, and sad, or they may assume increased adult responsibilities and become "adultified," missing out on some childhood experiences. Sometimes these children become caregivers for the sibling with an ongoing condition or take on the care of younger, healthy siblings. For siblings with fewer personal strengths, the effects of these changes in family dynamics can exact a significant emotional toll. Others seem to rise to the demands and become superachievers, and many go on to caregiving roles in their adult lives.

Conditions that are not obvious can be particularly challenging emotionally, because children and families face issues regarding whether to disclose a condition (and, if so, when) and must navigate between the world of the well and the world of the condition. The lack of visibility creates uncertainty. Parents and children also seem to have great difficulty with conditions that fluctuate in severity, even when most of the time the children are relatively well: when there is no stable level of greater dysfunction, children and families do not know what to expect and cannot begin to deal with a condition and accommodate to it.

Families describe the emotional toll of unpredictability and uncertainty as particularly challenging, and research has confirmed that any type of uncertainty is particularly challenging for people to deal with from an emotional perspective.[10]

Transition times are especially stressful. Transition times include stages and events such as becoming ambulatory, entering school or child care, moving from one school or community to another, and moving into latency, adolescence, or adulthood. When healthy age-mates move from one major stage to another, the family of a child with an ongoing condition is often confronted with the ways in which its own child is different or with the need to make special accommodations to ensure that medical safety or special needs are managed appropriately. Clinicians can anticipate that these are times when families may need extra help and support and also prepare families for the issues that they may face at the time of the transition.

Throughout this discussion, it is important to recognize that many parents and siblings find it helpful to know that their reactions are similar to the reactions of others and to be linked with other families that have faced comparable struggles. Especially when there are extra tasks or ambivalent feelings, knowing that their feelings are not unusual can relieve some stress. Additionally, providing an opportunity for parents and siblings to talk about their challenges and find respite when needed may help prevent serious mental health problems in family members.

Next we outline some of the important stages of illness and diagnosis and some of the common emotional reactions.

Emotional Reactions to the Diagnosis

The detection and confirmation of a condition herald the first stage of management. No matter the age of a child when a diagnosis is made, discovery that the child has a significant ongoing health condition sets off a fairly predictable set of emotional reactions, although intensity and duration of the reactions of individuals may vary. Parents normally go through a series of reactions at the time of diagnosis. These reactions may include shock, denial, anger, sadness, and anxiety. Well described by Drotar et al (in their discussion of adaptation to the birth of a child with a congenital malformation, but applicable to all new diagnoses) (Figure 26-1), the initial reaction is usually shock, which is often accompanied by numbness and may prevent the parents or youth from absorbing any additional information. This reaction is usually fairly brief and is one of the reason why it is either best if both parents can be informed at the same time (so they know they have been told the same thing) or helpful if a single parent can bring someone else along for support.

Denial is a problem when it interferes with obtaining needed treatments and services, but it can serve as an effective part of many individuals' coping mechanisms when it does not. Dealing with denial or with sadness and anger can be challenging even for a clinician skilled in caring for children with complex or serious conditions, especially when the anger is directed at the clinician. Anger is often directed at others, and navigating a family's anger can be especially hard for the staff treating the patient, because it is

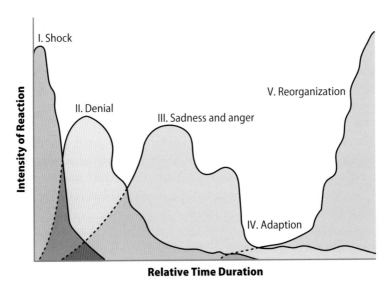

Figure 26-1. Hypothetical model of a normal sequence of parental reactions to the birth of a malformed infant.

From Drotar D, Baskiewicz A, Irvin N, Kennell J, Klaus M. The adaptation of parents to the birth of an infant with a congenital malformation: a hypothetical model. *Pediatrics*. 1975;56(5):710–717.

most often focused on some minor act of omission or commission; staff are likely to take the anger personally, especially when they do not directly understand or when they forget what the family is experiencing. Care should be taken to recognize the displaced anger and to avoid letting it negatively affect the clinician-patient relationship.

These reactions to confirmation of a diagnosis, that is, part of the grief that results from loss of the idealized perfect child, are to be expected. Ultimately, the family moves into a period of acceptance or equilibrium during which they can resume their lives, activities, and personal development in the context of the new normal. This reorganization (a restoration of general emotional well-being) is an important accomplishment and a necessary phase for child development to progress.

It is important to remember that different members of the family may go through these stages at different rates. When they do, the differences can complicate their communication with and relationship with one another and with members of the health care team. Sometimes, one of the parents remains in one phase of reaction; if this stasis occurs in the denial phase, it may interfere with adherence to recommended care. Other times, one parent remains in or easily reverts to the phase of anger or becomes very depressed. When parents are angry, or if one of them is having trouble adapting, the physician should avoid overreacting to parents' behavior. Demonstrating this patience may be especially difficult if the anger is displaced onto the medical team. Nevertheless, it is important to recognize that anger is part of the family's (mal)adaptation to the condition and to make sure that all members of the team maintain a professional relationship. Recognizing this fact may help the clinician focus on the common goal of improving the child's care and avoid getting into a pattern of deteriorating communication.

The chain of reactions described by Drotar et al[11] is reactivated by many factors, such as revisits to the clinician, exacerbations, complications, and readmissions. But other factors also precipitate a cascade of emotions, such as milestones that are not achieved on time, important events that are missed, and transitions to new experiences that are more complicated or require special adjustment for a child with special health care needs. Usually, the cascade of emotions that is precipitated by these events is shorter than at the time of the original diagnosis, but that is not always the case.

One factor that the Drotar model does not include is that of *guilt*, which we have found to be a universal feature of the emotional disappointment that results from having a child who faces health challenges. Addressing this guilt is important. Parents often fantasize about the characteristics and opportunities that their child will have in life, and seeing that in reality their child may be constrained by physical or mental health concerns makes parents worry about what they might have done differently to prevent this outcome. These guilty feelings may or may not be based on factual issues, but the concerns are real to the person who is feeling guilty and the PCC should be prepared to listen and respond appropriately. A highly effective technique for identifying these concerns and reassuring the parent or child is to universalize the concern by stating that most people worry about something they might have thought or done, or that had happened, that might have led to a different outcome or prevented the child's condition. Allowing a few moments of silence thereafter usually produces useful information, and it can serve as the basis of discussion. When parents are encouraged to share their worries, they often can be reassured that the source of their guilty feelings is often unrelated to the child's condition. Reassuring parents that these kinds of worries are not unusual can relieve angst.

Reassuring a family is more challenging when a condition has a known genetic component or if a family member was involved in a traumatic event that led to the health condition. However, even then it can be useful to point out that we all carry harmful genes and none of us chooses to receive them or to pass them on intentionally to our children or that unintentional injuries can occur to anyone. Even in the case of intentional trauma, most parents did not intend to inflict long-term damage on their child, and in most cases the parent himself or herself has been traumatized by a family that did not parent effectively. While discussing guilt may not remove it, normalizing the feeling helps the family focus on what it and the care team can do now and in the future to help the child thrive as much as possible.

Ongoing Care

It is important to recognize that the mental and physical health care provided to CYSHCN are not entirely separable. How we provide care in a sensitive and integrated manner is key to long-term success and to minimizing the mental health stress that family members experience. Therefore, it is important to review some of the best guidance for how care should be provided.

The care team includes the child's medical subspecialists or surgical subspecialists (or both), the PCC, and other primary care team members; it also includes any involved mental health specialists, whether inside the practice or linked through traditional community referral, telemedicine, or telephonic consultation, or as part of the subspecialty group providing care. Many aspects of management, goals of treatment, and family challenges are similar across the full range of physical, developmental, and behavioral conditions. Ideally, the child will receive family-centered care that is accessible, compassionate, comprehensive, continuous, and coordinated within a medical home. While family-centered care may be a goal for all children, it is an essential component of the care of CYSHCN: their care differs from the care of those with acute conditions in the degree to which the family needs to be involved actively in care decisions to ensure adherence to ongoing treatment. Also, ongoing care requires more care decisions and adherence over long periods of time; therefore, incorporating family concerns and needs is critically important. Moreover, many CYSHCN need long-term treatments that require the clinicians and the parents to figure out how these treatments can best be implemented in the home. Making choices that fit as well as possible into the family's routines and preferences has been shown to enhance adherence and reduce stress.

The treatment plan should be developed in partnership with the family and the PCC and, when appropriate, the mental health specialist or specialists and relevant medical or surgical subspecialists. While the clinical care responsibilities may be shared with a subspecialist or the staff of a referral hospital, the team in the medical home needs to work out a pattern of communication through which the various responsibilities of each of the parties are delineated. The primary care team needs to determine regular mechanisms for communication, ascertain key issues that need to be monitored, and determine how these responsibilities are to be divided amongst all providers. In the case of children with rare conditions, especially when the medical expert is far from the patient's home, the PCC should make sure that the delegated responsibilities are clearly understood and that the subspecialist with expertise in the child's rare condition has reviewed the special issues to monitor and the indications for further consultation to ensure the best possible care.

It is important to remember that, because of the usual shock reaction, confirming a diagnosis and discussing its implications with parents and their child are ongoing processes that are never accomplished in a single conference. Moreover, different issues become relevant as the condition and its treatments progress and as the child ages. Parents should be encouraged to ask questions regularly, because they are usually unable to absorb a great deal of information at the time of confirmation of the diagnosis. Members of the medical team should suggest that parents write down their questions and concerns and other people's questions and advice and discuss them at each subsequent visit. This mechanism provides a socially acceptable way to ask naive or awkward questions and can enable family members to address issues they may find embarrassing or difficult to bring up. In cases in which the condition is life-threatening, it may be appropriate to involve a palliative care specialist to talk about quality of life issues early in the care of the child and family. Reducing unnecessary worries helps the family's emotional health.

Some clinicians are uncomfortable sharing uncertainty about answers to questions posed by family members. In most instances, the key questions that the parents want answered are related to what will happen to their child. Even the most expert clinicians cannot answer such questions except in a probabilistic way. When talking about the prognosis of a single child, statistics are not very helpful, because any event or outcome is either 100% or 0%, and even the most experienced practitioner cannot make absolute predictions. Parents repeatedly state that a cornerstone to working well with clinicians over time is honesty, including sharing uncertainty or seeking additional information when the clinician does not have ready answers.

When the information provided is especially distressing, many parents want to seek a second opinion. This desire can be awkward if the family is thinking about it and the PCC is not aware of their thoughts. In these situations, it can be helpful if the clinician raises the possibility and offers that if, at any time, the family would like a second opinion, she or he would be happy to recommend places where this consultation can be accomplished responsibly; she or he can also offer to make study results available so the child will not need additional testing. For some families, the offer of opening the results to scrutiny is reassuring by itself. For others, who wish to follow through on the offer, the offer prevents the need for repeated tests and the awkwardness of the family's worrying about raising the issue with the clinician or finding a way to discuss and reconcile conflicting recommendations.

Health Care Supervision

Because many children with ongoing conditions have more contact with the health care system than other children do, their parents often assume that they are receiving a full package of services, but often this assumption is not true. The actual number of visits that focuses on issues of health care supervision for children with ongoing conditions is much lower than for the general population. Many subspecialists assume that these services are being provided elsewhere. However, studies show that many children with ongoing conditions do not receive all the recommended immunizations and routine screenings. Unless there is a contraindication, CYSHCN should receive all immunizations and screenings. In addition, many children with ongoing conditions may need screening for specific vulnerabilities caused by their primary diseases or by the medications that they take.

The usual anticipatory guidance should also be provided, although in the case of children with developmental impairments, the guidance should be adjusted to the appropriate developmental stage. This process may be complex, because children with ongoing conditions may develop normally or even be precocious in some areas while lagging in others.

Systematically identifying adverse childhood experiences and social risk factors in both the child and the parents is important to CYSHCN, as it is to all children. Psychosocial surveillance is an important activity for all children, but it is especially important for CYSHCN because their rates of mental health conditions, especially anxiety and depression, are increased compared with those of the general population. In addition to the surveillance offered to all children at routine health supervision visits, the existence of a chronic health condition justifies routine, periodic psychosocial screening of the child for mental health symptoms and functional impairment, using validated measures. (See Chapter 1, Healthy Child Development.) Assessment of the impact on the child's caregivers, using a tool such as the Caregiver Strain Index, Parenting Stress Index, or a screening for parental depression, may also be useful. This assessment is particularly key because of the strong evidence that mental health problems and psychosocial tensions can alter adherence of the children and their parents to the therapeutic plan that has been developed. Poor adherence can lead to poorer prognosis and quality of life and can be life-threatening in the presence of a serious ongoing condition. When there are problems with adherence or periods of poor control of symptoms, further exploration of psychosocial issues is needed, because these are often the key reasons underlying the change in adherence. It is especially important to involve the mental health specialists of the care team when these issues arise. When sharing responsibility for the care of CYSHCN with subspecialists, the PCC should determine who is providing the routine screening, immunizations, anticipatory guidance, mental health screening, and support and who is monitoring these special risks to prevent failures, duplications, or omissions of care. If a division of services exists, the family should know this and the reasons that they need to make regular visits to multiple providers.

Many models set up how this coordination can be accomplished. In some cases, either the PCC or the subspecialists have embedded mental health staff such as psychologists, social workers, or psychiatrists who work in a colocated or integrated fashion with physical health specialists. This setup is preferable, because it does not impose yet another "problem" and set of providers on a family that is often already overburdened with appointments. In other cases, it may be necessary to refer the child or family for specialized and separate mental health services. When this referral is necessary, it is helpful if the family receives the message that rearing a child or an adolescent with a chronic condition is challenging, and most families need extra support in doing so. This communication minimizes their chance of seeing the referral as yet another form of pathology and reduces the stigma of having to have extra help.

Of note, too, is the increasing evidence that some medical conditions and medications are associated with specific types of learning problems, so a full assessment of the child's success in school is important. School learning problems often present as behavioral problems, as the child tries to compensate for learning difficulties. Also, children who are absent from school more than usual may have social difficulties or be bullied (or both), especially if they are stigmatized in any way. Helping the child and family deal with these issues in a proactive way is important to their long-term outcomes.

Emotional Impact of Acute Illness, Injury, or Exacerbation

Children with ongoing conditions experience the same minor illnesses that affect others in the community. However, every evaluation of a seemingly minor primary concern requires the treating clinician to consider whether the symptoms are complications of the underlying disease process, undesirable or harmful side effects related to medication taken to treat the condition, or a typical intercurrent event. Even when the child has a minor illness or injury, clinicians should also consider whether the condition or its treatment requires the child to receive any special care or medication adjustment or any additional emotional support.

In evaluating a patient and a management plan for an acute minor illness, the clinician should check with the parents and the patient, if he or she is an older child, about whether they have any special concerns or questions. This responsibility is most essential in an encounter in which the treating clinician does not know the family, given that the family is often able to distinguish between the child's current and baseline condition in ways that may not be immediately obvious to someone who does not know the patient well. In many instances, the patient or parents will raise practical issues in daily management that may not have occurred to the clinician. This circumstance is particularly true when they have experienced similar circumstances in the past. Box 26-2 lists some of the questions to consider in the management of acute illness or injury. In addition to remembering the medical complexity of evaluating children with acute conditions who

Box 26-2. Assessing Acute Conditions in Children With Ongoing Health Conditions

- Can the primary concern and associated symptoms be explained by the child's underlying condition?

- Can the primary concern and associated symptoms be explained by the current or recent medications or other treatments?

- Might the primary concern and associated symptoms represent a complication of the child's underlying condition or a special vulnerability caused by the underlying condition? If so, what special evaluations should be performed?

- How do the child's current physical and laboratory findings differ from the child's baseline findings?

- Has the child skipped, vomited, or failed to absorb recent medications, and might this circumstance be causing a problem?

- What features of the child's condition are of most concern to the family or patient? What do they think the problem is? Can these features be explained by the presumptive diagnosis of the acute condition?

- What events or circumstances worry the family or patient most? Is this worry a realistic concern, and can something be done to reassure the family?

- In light of the acute diagnosis, does the child need a modification of usual care or medication? Can this modification be handled at home? If the situation can be handled at home, what is the plan for follow-up, and should it be modified in light of the child's underlying condition?

have underlying chronic health conditions, one should also remember that having an acute illness may bring back the full set of emotional reactions outlined in the discussion of diagnosis earlier in this chapter. The acute care visit may be a good opportunity to conduct a brief mental health update (Appendix 2, Brief MH Update) and, in some instances, a psychosocial screening.

Involving and Preparing the Child

The care team should provide developmentally appropriate information to the child about his or her treatment. The child should also be involved in the timing, nature of, and assent for special procedures, especially when real choices exist. As the child matures, it is important to communicate directly with the child, rather than exclusively through the parents, and to assess the child's responses to reasonable choices. Explanations that may have been given to a young child require expansion and revision as the child matures. As the child matures and acquires better understanding of the condition and its implications, he or she may need some extra emotional support and clinicians should be sensitive to that. Daily care routines are optimally shifted to the child as early as possible, and well before adolescence, to prepare the child to become independent and responsible for self-care and self-management. This shift helps move care of the condition out of the domain of rebellion against parental involvement that is a normal part of adolescent individuation. This emphasis on the child also promotes individualized goal-setting processes and ensures the child's inclusion.

Just as with other responsibilities, special care for the condition starts out as the parents' duty and must become the child's responsibility to the fullest extent possible. As the child ages, the care team also starts preparing adolescents with ongoing health conditions for transitioning their care to clinicians trained to care for adults. To do this, the primary communication about symptoms and concerns needs to be owned by the youth to the fullest extent possible. Otherwise, the youth will not have the necessary skills to communicate with adult health care professionals.

An important emotional consideration is assessing the child's understanding of the condition and the treatments of it. Many children experience elements of their treatments as related to punishment for real or imaginary misbehaviors. Identifying this magical thinking and acknowledging that other children often wonder about things that have happened and the reasons for them may help normalize their fantasies and enable discussion of their unnecessary guilt.

Rehospitalization

Hospitalization is traumatic for anyone, but it may be especially so for CYSHCN, for whom it may stir up memories of previous traumatic events. With hospitalization, as with other aspects of managing ongoing conditions, communication at an age-appropriate level with the child is helpful, and providing choices ("Should I try the IV injection on the left or the right first?") helps the child deal with the loss of control.

Regardless of the reason for the hospitalization, it is important to do some anticipatory counseling regarding discharge. Children will often have had special attention and privileges during the hospitalization and may also have regressed in their behaviors. So they may try to continue those patterns when they go home. Many parents do not realize that returning to their normal routines as much as possible is the best thing they can do for their child's mental health: children feel safest in the presence of their normative rules and routines, while being given in to makes them worry about their conditions and health issues being more serious than they are. Giving this anticipatory advice takes only a minute, but it can help avert problems in behavior later on and help reduce the child's anxiety on discharge.

It is important also to note that children and adolescents who have "frequent" readmissions are at particular risk of having primary or secondary mental health issues, and the more quickly these are recognized and addressed, the better the chance of reversing the maladaptive pattern of care. When these issues exist, it is critical that there be adequate communication between the hospital staff and the patients' medical home team, so the mental health services can continue after discharge.

The Role of Home Health Care

Medical advances in treatments and technologies permit children with complex medical conditions to be cared for at home, where their social and developmental needs are met more effectively than in institutional settings. Children who benefit from home health care vary widely in their needs for assistive technology and in the intensity and duration of their health care needs. Variability in illness trajectory and the inability to identify a definitive prognosis present additional challenges. In addition to facing the increasing complexity of the child's illness, parents find themselves increasingly in the role of care providers in the home and community.[12] To care for their child at home, parents must develop specialized skills and knowledge to manage the child's condition and the technology on which their child depends. High-acuity care in the home may include tracheostomy care, long-term ventilation, enteral and parenteral feeding, and the use of intravenous drugs (the latter via central lines). Thus, the child's care requirements can significantly affect daily family functioning, leaving parents and caregivers physically and emotionally exhausted and isolated, often with little personal time and limited financial resources.

These more-intensive services, often accompanied by the need to have home visiting personnel or nursing personnel (or both) in the home place extra burdens on the social-emotional health of all the family members and on their privacy. The care team should be especially alert to their needs for emotional help and support.

Transition to Adult Care

Transitions from pediatric to adult-centered health care involve changes in providers and activities across all areas of an adolescent's life. This transition should be carefully planned. For adolescents with a chronic condition, this planning is complicated and time-consuming; fortunately, guidelines and algorithms are available to assist the care team.[13,14] However, it is worth noting in this context that teens with uneven development (social or mental immaturity) or with intermittent problems in functioning caused by physical illness or mental health problems are particularly vulnerable in these transitions: although the need for guardianship is apparent in those who are chronically unable to function at an age-appropriate level, it may be less so in those with intermittent or inconsistent needs, who are often assumed able to be independent when they reach the age of majority. In most places, once they reach the age of majority their parents or adult siblings will be excluded from information and be unable to act on their behalves without advanced planning and the documentation of appropriate permission to act on their behalves, partially or completely. Thus, anticipating and raising the questions about planning for transition may be especially important for this subgroup.

Facing the End of Life

While most CYSHCN lead full and long lives, a subgroup of individuals do not survive into adulthood. Many of these children and their families are highly resilient and inspiring to us all, but they also need and deserve our help and special attention. In most instances, the end of life is the end of a long journey and there has been a solid partnership with the family for a while. Sometimes, it is a matter of helping make the final days take place where the child and family want them. Other times, just being there to listen to them and to anticipate their needs, provide support, and share the experience may be a great comfort to them. At times, the child is ready to let go before the parents are, and helping give permission for that to happen on the child's terms can be a gift. Alternatively, the child may continue to fight for life when the parents are ready to give up; allowing parents to voice their inevitable ambivalence about wanting the suffering to end, but not wanting the child to die, can help ease their guilt.

Regardless of how the final days are played out, there is an important role for the care team in following up with the family, staying in touch, and providing mental health support. Special attention should be paid to the siblings and their understanding of what has transpired, assuring them that the death of their sibling is not their fault and addressing their concerns about their own vulnerabilities. They may also have a hard time with their grieving parents, who may initially lack the energy to be fully involved with their other children's lives. This lack of energy may give rise to questions about their parents' love for them or even to acting-out behaviors. It may be important for the care team to help them and their parents strengthen bonds at this time of great pain.

Summary of Overarching Principles

There are some key principles in the delivery of social-emotional care to CYSHCN and their families. First and foremost, families have told us the key to an integrated approach is trust and honest communication. Both require the family and the members of the care team to be willing to share some vulnerabilities. A second principle is being supportive of the fact that rearing and caring for a child with an ongoing condition is hard work and, for the most part, parents are doing the best that they can. Acknowledging what they are doing well and the assets of their children (not just their problems) goes a long way. Third, it is important to inquire how you can help. Sometimes, there are simple things that you can do; at other times, there may not be. But you can always listen without judging them. Sometimes that is all it takes to be helpful, as allowing them to vent may be the best help. Finally, a method that has been extremely helpful is universalizing feelings and concerns: helping family members feel that they are not alone in having thoughts that are ambivalent or negative and expressing your understanding of their predicament.

In sum, using an integrated approach to the physical and mental health of CYSHCN and their families is the pinnacle of pediatric care and requires the best of all you have learned over the years of practice; it is also far and away the most rewarding as well as challenging practice a pediatric clinician can have.

AAP Policy

American Academy of Pediatrics, American Academy of Family Physicians, American College of Physicians Transitions Clinical Report Authoring Group. Supporting the health care transition from adolescence to adulthood in the medical home. *Pediatrics.* 2011;128(1):182–200. Reaffirmed August 2015 (pediatrics.aappublications.org/content/128/1/182)

American Academy of Pediatrics Committee on Pediatric Emergency Medicine and Council on Clinical Information Technology, American College of Emergency Physicians Pediatric Emergency Medicine Committee. Emergency information forms and emergency preparedness for children with special health care needs. *Pediatrics.* 2010;125(4):829–837. Reaffirmed October 2014 (pediatrics.aappublications.org/content/125/4/829)

American Academy of Pediatrics Council on Children With Disabilities. Supplemental Security Income (SSI) for children and youth with disabilities. *Pediatrics.* 2009; 124(6):1702–1708. Reaffirmed February 2015 (pediatrics.aappublications.org/content/124/6/1702)

American Academy of Pediatrics Council on Children With Disabilities and Medical Home Implementation Project Advisory Committee. Patient- and family-centered care coordination: a framework for integrating care for children and youth across multiple systems. *Pediatrics*. 2014;133(5):e1451–e1460 (pediatrics.aappublications.org/content/133/5/e1451)

American Academy of Pediatrics Medical Home Initiatives for Children With Special Needs Project Advisory Committee. The medical home. *Pediatrics*. 2002;110(1):184–186. Reaffirmed May 2008 (pediatrics.aappublications.org/content/110/1/184)

References

1. Nelson R, Stein REK. Children with special needs: recommendations and rationale. In: Klerman L, ed. *Research Priorities in Maternal and Child Health*. Washington, DC: Office for Maternal and Child Health, Health Services Administration, Public Health Service, US Dept of Health and Human Services; 1982

2. McPherson M, Arango P, Fox H, et al. A new definition of children with special health care needs. *Pediatrics*. 1998;102(1, pt 1):137–140

3. Stein REK, Bauman LJ, Westbrook LE, Coupey SM, Ireys HT. Framework for identifying children who have chronic conditions: the case for a new definition. *J Pediatr*. 1993;122(3):342–347

4. Bethell C, Blumberg SJ, Stein REK, Strickland B, Robertson J, Newacheck PN. Taking stock of the CSHCN screener: a review of common questions and current reflections. *Acad Pediatr*. 2015;15(2):165–176

5. Stein REK, Sliver EJ. Operationalizing a conceptually based noncategorical definition: a first look at US children with chronic conditions. *Arch Pediatr Adolesc Med*. 1999;153(1):68–74

6. Sobo EJ, Kurtin PS, eds. *Optimizing Care for Young Children With Special Health Care Needs: Knowledge and Strategies for Navigating the System*. Baltimore, MD; Paul H. Brookes Publishing Co; 2007

7. Shelton TL, Jeppson ES, Johnson BH. *Family-Centered Care for Children With Special Health Care Needs*. Washington, DC: Association for the Care of Children's Health; 1987

8. Johnson BH, Schlucter J. Family-centered home health care. In: Libby RC, Imaizumi SO, eds. *Guidelines for Pediatric Home Health Care*. 2nd ed. Elk Grove Village, IL: American Academy of Pediatrics; 2008

9. Ahmann E. *Home Care for the High-risk Infant: A Family-Centered Approach*. Gaithersburg, MD: Aspen Publishers Inc; 1996

10. Jessop DJ, Stein REK. Uncertainty and its relation to the psychological and social correlates of chronic illness in children. *Soc Sci Med*. 1985;20(10):993–997

11. Drotar D, Baskiewicz A, Irvin N, Kennell J, Klaus M. The adaptation of parents to the birth of an infant with a congenital malformation: a hypothetical model. *Pediatrics*. 1975;56(5):710–717

12. Ward C, Glass N, Ford R. Care in the home for seriously ill children with complex needs: a narrative literature review. *J Child Health Care*. 2015;19(4):524–531

13. American Academy of Pediatrics, American Academy of Family Physicians, American College of Physicians-American Society of Internal Medicine. A consensus statement on health care transitions for young adults with special health care needs. *Pediatrics*. 2002;110(6, pt 2):1304–1306

14. American Academy of Pediatrics, American Academy of Family Physicians, American College of Physicians Transitions Clinical Report Authoring Group. Supporting the health care transition from adolescence to adulthood in the medical home. *Pediatrics*. 2011;128(1):182–200

Adolescents Who Are Pregnant or Parenting

Julie M. Linton, MD; Keli Beck, MD; and Daniel P. Krowchuk, MD

> "Pediatric primary care clinicians...can build
> on effective strategies to support pregnant
> and parenting teens as they endeavor to
> become loving parents and continue
> their journey to adulthood."

Background

Despite declining rates of teen pregnancy in the United States, teen pregnancy continues to be associated with societal, economic, and educational disadvantages for mothers and their children. Only 38% of teen girls who become pregnant prior to age 18 will get a high school diploma. Pregnant and parenting teens are known to have higher risks of depression, substance use disorders, intimate partner violence, and poverty. Their children often experience consequences as well, including a risk of preterm birth, abuse and neglect, lower standardized test scores, and higher chance of becoming teen parents themselves.[1] Likelihood of teen pregnancy is influenced by many factors: individual goals, societal pressure, family values, pubertal timing, age at first intercourse, risk-taking behaviors, and knowledge of contraceptive choices, among others.[2]

Although the United States has higher rates of births to teen mothers than most other industrialized nations do, these rates have steadily declined since the 1970s, when data were initially collected[3–5] (Figure 27-1). From 1991 to 2015, decreases occurred in the teen birth rates of all racial and ethnic groups, with the greatest decrease for non-Hispanic black teens (73%) and Asian and Pacific Island teens (75%). Birth rates for non-Hispanic white teens dropped 63%, and rates among Hispanic teens dropped 67%.[3] Despite these declines, a significant disparity exists between white teens and other racial and ethnic groups. In 2015, the pregnancy rate (per 1,000 girls) among non-Hispanic white teens (16.0) was approximately half of that of

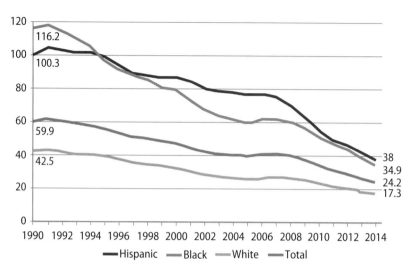

Figure 27-1. Birth rates per 1,000 females ages 15-19, by race/ethnicity, 1990-2014.
From Martin JA, Hamilton BE, Ventura SJ. *Births: Final Data for 2014.* Hyattsville, MD: National Center for Health Statistics; 2015.

non-Hispanic black teens (31.8) and Hispanic teens (34.9). Declines in teen birth rates have been accompanied by decreases in rates of pregnancy and elective termination.[3,4] Wide differences in birth and abortion rates are also prevalent among various ethnicities. The rate of teen fatherhood declined 54% between 1991 and 2014; this decline was far more substantial among black teens than among white teens (67% vs 47%).[6,7] While these trends are encouraging, much work remains to mitigate disparities and enhance support for pregnant and parenting teens.

While birth, pregnancy, and abortion rates have declined, the proportion of teens who report having sex has not. Recent data suggest that improved utilization rates and effectiveness of contraceptive methods are solely responsible for the declines noted earlier.[4] Rates of contraception use with first sexual encounter have increased from 48% in 1982 to 79% in 2013. Today, approximately 86% of female teens and 93% of male teens report using contraception during their most recent sexual encounter.[7]

Contraceptive options have expanded as well to include long-acting reversible contraceptives (LARCs). These methods eliminate the need to remember to take something daily or with each sexual encounter. The percentage of women at risk for unintended pregnancy who are using a LARC has increased from 1.1% to 11.1% between 2006 and 2013.[8] Because of their efficacy and the practical application in the life of a busy teen, both the

American Academy of Pediatrics (AAP) and the American Congress of Obstetricians and Gynecologists (ACOG) have recommended LARCs as the preferred contraceptive choice among teens.[9,10]

Pregnant and Parenting Teens: A Public Health Perspective

Social Determinants of Health

Teen pregnancy may have social, educational, legal, emotional, and financial consequences not only for the mother but for the father, grandparents, and others. These factors represent social determinants of health, defined as the social, economic, and environmental factors that shape the health of individuals and communities.[11] A 3-generation approach[12] to issues affecting pregnant and parenting teens incorporates the impact of teen pregnancy on the next generation, that is, the future offspring of the teen's child.

Risk factors for teen pregnancy are numerous and include demographic, social, and environmental components. As discussed earlier, pregnancy and birth rates are higher among black and Hispanic teens compared with non-Hispanic white teens.[4] Teen birth rates in rural counties are nearly one-third higher compared with the rest of the country.[13] Factors contributing to higher birth rates among rural teens include higher poverty rates, less access to health services, loss of population in the region, and lower rates of college enrollment.[13] Females with low cognitive ability are at increased risk for early initiation of sexual activity and early pregnancy,[14] and those with intellectual disability seem to be at particularly high risk for pregnancy.[14,15] Academically, teens that are behind their peers are often the ones who become pregnant. Even a pregnant teen's decision about her pregnancy may be affected by socioeconomic factors. Teenagers who choose pregnancy termination tend to come from higher socioeconomic backgrounds and have mothers with higher educational levels. These girls have higher educational aspirations, greater feelings of control over life, and higher levels of subsequent educational achievement than those who continue a pregnancy.[16]

Although depression rates among adolescents who are not pregnant and those who are do not appear to differ,[17] stress symptoms, particularly in the setting of comorbid depression, are associated with increased incidence of unintended pregnancy.[17,18] Conversely, unintended pregnancy may place adolescents at risk for depression.[19] Amidst the conventional dichotomy of unintended and intended pregnancy are teens with mixed, contradictory, or not fully established intentions about pregnancy.[20] Pregnancy ambivalence is associated with mild depression, which may begin to illuminate the complex interplay between mental health and increased risk for adolescent pregnancy.[20] Among teens with mild depression, symptoms such as lack of motivation and anhedonia may manifest as ambivalence about active prevention of pregnancy and pregnancy itself, in the event that a pregnancy occurs.

Other psychosocial risk factors associated with adolescent parenthood include daily cigarette smoking, age of first antisocial personality disorder or conduct disorder symptoms,[21] homelessness,[22] and running away.[23,24] Among youths who live in urban communities, dual substance use with marijuana and alcohol has a particularly high association with becoming pregnant or getting someone else pregnant.[25] Reports suggest that youths of a sexual minority are more likely to become pregnant than students who identify as heterosexual or report only opposite-gender sexual partners.[26]

Last, adolescent pregnancy has a strong association with adverse childhood experiences (ACEs), including child abuse and neglect, exposure to domestic violence, having a household member with substance use disorder, mental illness, criminal behavior, and divorced or separated parents.[24,27] In fact, teens who have been maltreated are more than twice as likely as their peers who have not been maltreated to experience teen childbirth,[28] and teen girls who are in foster care are nearly twice as likely to become pregnant as those not in foster care.[29] Immigrant teens fleeing violence in countries of origin and seeking safe haven in the United States often face risks of sexual exploitation or human trafficking that can increase risk of pregnancy.

Once pregnant, teens seem to be at increased risk for experiencing family or intimate partner violence.[15,30–33] Outside the home, community violence, which may be particularly high among urban minority adolescent mothers, can threaten mental health and school performance.[32,34] The experience of violence may not only predispose teens to risk for pregnancy but also adversely affect health and well-being during and after the pregnancy.

Repeat Teen Pregnancy

Repeat teen pregnancy can amplify adverse outcomes for both teen parents and their children. Depression, earlier initiation of sexual activity, and greater number of lifetime sexual partners are all associated with an increased risk of multiple adolescent pregnancies.[18,19,21] The more health risk behaviors reported by adolescents, the greater likelihood of experiencing or causing multiple adolescent pregnancies.[21]

Mothers who live with the father of their child, those who do not return to school within 6 months, or those who receive significant child care assistance from the child's grandmother are most likely to have a repeat pregnancy soon after the first.[15,35] The second pregnancy is more likely to end in elective termination than the first. If the second pregnancy is carried, the mother frequently enters into prenatal care later than with her first baby. Statistically, the second baby is at greater risk for low birth weight and greater risk for death by homicide.[36]

Teen Fathers

Teen fathers are a crucial and often neglected population in conversations surrounding pregnant and parenting teens. Data regarding teen fathers can be difficult to quantify because information on age and race and ethnicity of the father is often missing on birth certificates of children born to females younger than 25 or to unmarried females.[3] As an example, in 2015 the age of the father was not reported for 12% of all births, 31% of births to all females younger than 20, and 28% of all extramarital births.[3] Teen fatherhood rates vary considerably by race. In 2014, the rate among black males aged 15 to 19 was almost twice that of their white counterparts.[6] Earlier data suggest that, in most instances, male sexual partners are approximately 3 years older than their female partners. The age difference between fathers and their teen partners may be greater than average in some racial and ethnic groups.[37,38]

Fathers, in the setting of teen pregnancy, may be just as likely as the mothers to have been exposed to ACEs such as domestic violence, parental separation, or parental divorce, or any combination of those experiences.[39] Other predictors of adolescent fatherhood include delinquency, lower maternal education, early adolescent dating, non-Hispanic black or Hispanic race and ethnicity, and having a teen father themselves.[40] Enhanced attention to the risks and opportunities for potential teen fathers before pregnancy occurs, during pregnancy, and in the postpartum period is critical to improving outcomes for these teens and their children.

Consequences of Teen Pregnancy

Risks for Teen Mothers

Adolescents who become pregnant predominantly have good physical outcomes. In fact, many studies have shown that adolescents are more likely to have a successful vaginal delivery compared with their older counterparts.[41] Reported risks to the pregnant adolescent include anemia, preeclampsia, preterm delivery, low birth weight newborns, and small for gestational age newborns.[41–43] Some of these can be attributed to late entry to prenatal care,[42,44] and controversy exists as to whether these outcomes are confounded by socioeconomic factors. However, when studies control for socioeconomic disparities, teen pregnancies are associated with higher rates of preterm delivery and low birth weight or small for gestational age newborns, indicating the importance of maternal age.

Most teens facing unintended pregnancy experience a range of normal emotional reactions, including regret, mild depression, and anxiety.[16] However, pregnant and parenting teens face greater risk for experiencing depressive symptoms than pregnant and parenting adult women do.[17] Psychosocial factors associated with perinatal depression include perceived lack of social support, ACEs, self-efficacy, social isolation, body dissatisfaction, and low socioeconomic status.[17] Among adolescents, depression in the perinatal period is a risk factor for substance and alcohol use and for a harsher parenting style.[17] Some evidence suggests that the association between teen pregnancy and depression is attributable to ACEs.[27]

Early motherhood increases risk for educational underachievement and poorer economic circumstances.[45] Although most women who become pregnant as teenagers eventually complete their high school education, women who were teen parents continue to remain educationally behind their age-matched peers. Only 38% of teen girls who have a child before age 18 earn a high school diploma by age 22. Sixty-six percent of teen mothers receive either their GEDs or their high school diplomas by age 22, compared with 94% of those who did not give birth as teens.[46] Thirty percent of teen girls who have dropped out of high school cite pregnancy or parenthood as a reason. Finally, 61% of women who have children after enrolling in community college do not finish their education.[47]

Risks for Newborns

Newborns born to teen mothers are at risk of being born preterm, having a low birth weight, and being small for gestational age.[41–43] These outcomes increase the risks for neonatal intensive care unit admissions, difficulty feeding, and multiple other medical complications. Some studies have shown an almost 2-fold increase in nonchromosomal congenital anomalies in newborns of teen mothers. Most experts believe these anomalies to be caused by nutritional deficiencies and a lack of folic acid supplementation in teens.[1] While initial data suggest an increased risk of postneonatal death for babies of teen parents, that risk seems to disappear once socioeconomic factors are controlled for.[18] The most consistently repeated risks to newborns are those of preterm birth and low birth weight.[41,43]

Years later, the children of prior teen mothers continue to face increased risk for poverty, death, poor educational outcomes, and involvement with state-sponsored family services programs.[48] Among children of adolescent mothers, risk factors for adverse behavioral outcomes include black or Hispanic/Latino race/ethnicity and housing insecurity.[49] The children of teen parents are twice as likely to be placed in foster care as children born to older parents.[29] Among adolescents with a history of maltreatment, adolescent parenthood is strongly associated with risk of subsequent maltreatment in their children.[50] Prenatal violence places teens at risk for preterm birth, delivery of low birth weight preterm infants, and alcohol use.[30] Summative ACEs of mothers are associated with delivery of newborns with lower birth weight and reduced gestational age.[51] In fact, higher ACE scores, rather than teen pregnancy itself, have been associated with higher rates of fetal death.[27]

Although adolescent mothers may face risks such as lower self-esteem, more parenting stress, and lower quality of home environment, there is no difference in how children of these adolescent mothers and those of non-adolescent mothers develop attachment.[52] Nevertheless, the higher than normal rate of postpartum depression in teen mothers, when compared with adults, may influence maternal-child bonding and the amount of energy that the developmentally immature mother is able to put into guiding and teaching her child.[15] Depression during pregnancy, the strongest risk factor for postpartum depression, is associated with harsher parenting style, attachment difficulties, children's behavioral changes, and maternal suicide.[17] Postpartum depressive symptoms in adolescent mothers are associated with poorer academic achievement and problem behavior for their children, beginning in toddlerhood and extending through adolescence.[17]

Supporting Pregnant and Parenting Teens

Initial Engagement With the Health Care System

Pregnant teenagers may not seek care for the classic symptoms of pregnancy and instead may seek care for unrelated physical concerns. Primary care clinicians (PCCs) (ie, pediatricians, family physicians, internists, nurse practitioners, and physician assistants who care for young women of childbearing age) must always consider pregnancy, regardless of the symptoms the teen exhibits. For this reason, the most recent menstrual period should be a routine vital sign for all teen girls and recorded at every office visit. The validity of the stated most recent menstrual period should be questioned if any clinical concern for pregnancy exists, and a urine or serum pregnancy test should be performed. Pregnancy should always be considered in a young woman who has secondary amenorrhea. Other symptoms that suggest pregnancy are fatigue, nausea, dizziness or syncope, urinary frequency, weight gain, breast tenderness or enlargement, and abdominal tenderness or enlargement. For anyone with these symptoms, a pregnancy test should be performed; if results are positive, referral to an obstetrician or a family physician practicing obstetrics should be made. Often it is safe to defer pelvic and breast examinations at this initial encounter unless otherwise clinically indicated.

Should the patient have any symptoms suggestive of a sexually transmitted infection (STI), appropriate testing should be performed at this initial visit. The population at risk for pregnancy is often at higher risk for STIs; thus, any PCC should have a high index of suspicion to test and treat when results are positive.

Pregnancy Options and Early Support

Once a teen pregnancy has been confirmed, several issues must be addressed. Many teens are unprepared for being pregnant or becoming parents. During the visits, it is important to support the teen while sharing the diagnosis. Hopefully, the PCC will be familiar with appropriate community resources, accessible for questions, and supportive in the setting of crisis.[17,19,53]

The PCC should privately inform the teen of the pregnancy. Her reaction will depend on several factors: whether the pregnancy was suspected or not, wanted or unwanted, and intended or unintended. If desired by the adolescent, the PCC can offer assistance informing parents or family members of the pregnancy or provide resources for problem pregnancy counseling. Pregnancy options should be discussed in a nonjudgmental fashion. Some teens will decide that they are not ready to parent, and they may want to terminate the pregnancy (if legally able to do so) or to make a plan for adoption. Primary care clinicians who have moral or religious objections to discussing pregnancy options are encouraged to refer patients to another health care professional (eg, pediatrician, family practitioner, internist, obstetrician/gynecologist, or midwife) or to a family planning center that is able to do so. Regardless of the decision reached, the teen will need ongoing support from her PCC and possibly from a counselor or mental health specialist. Primary care clinicians should be familiar with state laws governing the ability of minors to consent for various health care services, including abortion.[54]

If the decision is made to continue the pregnancy, prenatal care may be provided by a teen-friendly PCC who is able to offer support and offer referrals to appropriate community resources. Many teens will need educational, social, and financial assistance during the pregnancy and while parenting. A number of tools are available to conduct screening for social determinants of health and help identify barriers to care.[11,55–58] Referral to community resources may enhance receipt of other community resources for families[55] and ultimately enhance access to care. Box 27-1 lists the ways a PCC can help the pregnant teenager.

Enhancing Support During and After Pregnancy

Addressing Mental Health Issues for Pregnant and Parenting Teens

Several barriers can impede access to mental health services for pregnant and parenting teens. These include inadequate or insufficient availability of mental health services; lack of insurance, lack of time availability, or lack of transportation, or any combination of those issues; and concerns about confidentiality.[53,59] Mental health services may be exceptionally limited in rural communities, particularly for minority teens.[59,60] Among minority youths, particular barriers may include language differences, community stigma, and cultural mistrust. Given the extensive barriers for pregnant and parenting teens in accessing mental health services, gateway agencies, including the Department of Public Health, schools, churches, and juvenile justice agencies, may allow access to and encourage use of mental health care.[53]

The PCC provides a pivotal role in facilitating access to mental health services for pregnant and parenting teens. Consistent use of brief but effective screening tools provides a means to identify symptoms and to elicit dialogue regarding parental stressors, symptoms of depression, history of trauma, and parenting experiences.[53] (See Appendix 2, Mental Health Tools for Pediatrics.) When treatment is needed, integrated mental health care offers an optimal strategy to engage teen mothers in behavioral health services.[53] Innovative programs offer models to incorporate mental health for teen parents within primary care medical homes or obstetric medical

---

Box 27-1. How a Primary Care Clinician Can Support a Pregnant Teenager

- Help the teenager think through her options for the pregnancy.
- Screen for depression, substance use, suicidality, risk of homelessness, and other urgent social determinants of health.
- Facilitate an appointment for prenatal care or immediate evaluation if indicated.
- Offer to help the teen inform her immediate family or create a plan to do so.
- Facilitate the teen's return to school.
- Link the teen to evidence-based support programs in the community for pregnancy and parenting.

homes or both.[19,61,62] Group prenatal care through CenteringPregnancy programs is associated with improved perinatal outcomes[63,64] and may also offer particular benefit for teens, including a referral base and enhanced social support.

Key to supporting mental health of pregnant and parenting teens is helping them to build positive relationships with their children. Evidence-based programs in the medical setting and the community can offer support services that meet the unique needs of pregnant and parenting teens. For instance, home visiting programs can benefit families through supporting positive parenting practices, enriching the child's home environment, and supporting the child's development.[65,66] These programs may be particularly effective for low-income, first-time adolescent mothers.[65,67] Targeted interventions for adolescent parents can also effectively include fathers, which can improve experiences for children and families.[68] Box 27-2 offers suggestions for enhanced support of parenting teens and their children.

Prevention

Prevention of unintended teen pregnancy must include multilevel approaches that integrate access to contraception, evidence-based counseling regarding options, and community-based approaches to support positive youth development. Contraception in today's world includes a diversity of options regarding route of administration, drug content, and duration. Primary care clinicians and other health care professionals caring for adolescents should be skilled in counseling regarding options available and recognize that LARCs are considered the contraceptive method of choice by

---

Box 27-2. How a Primary Care Clinician Can Help Teen Parents and Their Children

- Help the teen mother engage in positive parenting techniques.
- Screen early and often for postpartum depression.
- Encourage use of LARCs to prevent repeat teen pregnancy.
- Actively engage the father to feel welcome at baby health supervision visits.
- Teach the infant's grandparents modern child-rearing concepts.
- Encourage the young mother to continue her education.
- Refer the family to evidence-based support services as needed.
- Watch for behavioral and school problems in the child.

Abbreviation: LARC, long-acting reversible contraceptive.

both the AAP[10] and the ACOG.[9] Primary care clinicians can be trained in LARC insertion and thus can offer LARCs at the time of the adolescent's presentation for contraception.

Contraceptive use by adolescents is contingent upon access and effective counseling. Health care professionals can facilitate pregnancy prevention by routinely offering education about risks and prevention methods. Web resources, such as those of the Centers for Disease Control and Prevention, may be helpful (eg, "Contraception" at www.cdc.gov/reproductivehealth/ UnintendedPregnancy/Contraception.htm). Many teens who become pregnant seem not to have understood their actual risk at the time of conception.[69] Recent evidence has revealed strategies to improve use of effective contraception among adolescents. Specifically, the CHOICE project studied 9,000 females, including those aged 14 to 19 years. They found that approximately 70% of adolescents, when counseled consistently, chose a LARC and that those who did so had greater continuation rates than those who chose other methods. As a result, there was a significant reduction in teen pregnancy, birth, and abortion rates compared with the national average (decreases of 78%, 79%, and 77%, respectively).[70]

From a public health perspective, population-based approaches that target particular groups of adolescents may be particularly promising. For instance, most male adolescents believe that they should be responsible for pregnancy prevention.[71] Clear, consistent messages for male adolescents, their parents, and schools are a critical part of teen pregnancy prevention.[71] College students may also benefit from targeted interventions.[47] Given notably high rates of teen pregnancy in particularly vulnerable groups, including those in foster care,[29] teens facing homelessness,[22] and sexual minority youths,[26] innovative population-based strategies are critical to mitigate risk and build resilience. Barriers to successful program implementation for populations at greatest risk may include difficulty with recruitment and retention.[72]

Given the persistently high rates of teen pregnancy among minority adolescents, interventions must emphasize unique needs among this population without stereotyping the adolescents served.[73] For Hispanic adolescents, unique considerations include language barriers, lack of access to health insurance for undocumented teens, cultural barriers, and immigration-related fears. Opportunities include parental engagement and efforts to work with partners to address unequal power dynamics.[73] Several effective programs specifically for Hispanic youths have been developed for HIV prevention and have been successful.[74] Incorporating some of these strategies into culturally relevant reproductive life planning should be considered.

For teens who are already parents, programs to reduce repeat births (secondary pregnancy prevention) are particularly crucial and need a different emphasis than the programs for primary prevention (preventing the first birth). Successful secondary prevention programs require effective personnel who maintain close, sustained relationships with teen mothers with an emphasis on school completion and family planning.[75] Regardless of the type of program developed for secondary prevention, PCCs should always remember that the pregnant teenager is an adolescent who happens to be pregnant, not a pregnant woman who happens to be an adolescent.

Community-based approaches that incorporate reproductive life planning into community culture may ultimately help all adolescents reach their educational and social potentials. In schools, evidence-based approaches are critical, and abstinence-only education is not as effective as comprehensive sex education.[76] Schools can also incorporate efforts to provide condoms,[77] emphasize males in contraceptive education,[78] and incorporate efforts to prevent repeat teen pregnancy.[78] Positive youth development programs, based in schools, public health departments, or other community-based organizations, may offer opportunities to promote these skills. Early communication with partners about sexual topics, particularly among girls in steady relationships, is associated with consistency in hormonal contraceptive use.[79] Accordingly, adolescents may benefit from strategies that improve communication skills. Given the clear association between teen pregnancy, mental health symptoms,[18] and ACEs,[24] prevention efforts must incorporate strategies that mitigate stress and build resilience among teens with these risk factors.

Conclusion

Much work remains to prevent unintended teen pregnancy and to enhance support for pregnant and parenting teens. In particular, social determinants of health and mental health are critical considerations. Innovative strategies that incorporate evidence-based interventions to address the needs of populations and include cross-sector support are particularly promising. Pediatric PCCs and other health care professionals can build on effective strategies to support pregnant and parenting teens as they endeavor to become loving parents and continue their journey to adulthood.

Acknowledgments: The authors would like to acknowledge that this chapter is a revised version of one published in the *American Academy of Pediatrics Textbook of Pediatric Care,* 2nd Edition, Chapter 122, Adolescent Pregnancy and Parenthood, coauthored by Dianne S. Elfenbein, MD, and Marianne E. Felice, MD.

AAP Policy

American Academy of Pediatrics Committee on Adolescence. Addendum—adolescent pregnancy: current trends and issues. *Pediatrics.* 2014;133(5):954–957 (pediatrics. aappublications.org/content/133/5/954)

American Academy of Pediatrics Committee on Adolescence. Condom use by adolescents. *Pediatrics.* 2013;132(5):973–981 (pediatrics.aappublications.org/content/132/5/973)

American Academy of Pediatrics Committee on Adolescence. Contraception for adolescents. *Pediatrics.* 2014;134(4):e1244–e1256 (pediatrics.aappublications.org/content/134/4/e1244)

American Academy of Pediatrics Committee on Adolescence. Emergency contraception. *Pediatrics.* 2012;130(6):1174–1182 (pediatrics.aappublications.org/content/130/6/1174)

American Academy of Pediatrics Committee on Adolescence. The adolescent's right to confidential care when considering abortion. *Pediatrics.* 2017;139(2):e20163861 (pediatrics.aappublications.org/content/139/2/e20163861)

Marcell AV, Wibbelsman C, Seigel WM; American Academy of Pediatrics Committee on Adolescence. Male adolescent sexual and reproductive health care. *Pediatrics.* 2011;128(6):e1658–e1676. Reaffirmed May 2015 (pediatrics.aappublications.org/content/128/6/e1658)

Pinzon JL, Jones VF; American Academy of Pediatrics Committee on Adolescence and Committee on Early Childhood. Care of adolescent parents and their children. *Pediatrics.* 2012;130(6):e1743–e1756. Reaffirmed July 2016 (pediatrics.aappublications.org/content/130/6/e1743)

References

1. Ruedinger E, Cox JE. Adolescent childbearing: consequences and interventions. *Curr Opin Pediatr.* 2012;24(4):446–452
2. Santelli JS, Melnikas AJ. Teen fertility in transition: recent and historic trends in the United States. *Annu Rev Public Health.* 2010;31:371–383
3. Martin J, Hamilton B, Osterman M, Driscoll A, Mathews T. Births: final data for 2015. *Natl Vital Stat Rep.* 2017;66(1):1–68
4. Kost K, Maddow-Zimet I. *U.S. Teenage Pregnancies, Births and Abortions, 2011: National Trends by Age, Race and Ethnicity.* New York, NY: Guttmacher Institute; 2016. http://www.guttmacher.org/report/us-teen-pregnancy-trends-2011. Accessed March 8, 2018
5. Guttmacher Institute. US teen pregnancy, birth and abortion rates reach the lowest levels in almost four decades. https://www.guttmacher.org/news-release/2016/us-teen-pregnancy-birth-and-abortion-rates-reach-lowest-levels-almost-four-decades. Published April 5, 2016. Accessed March 8, 2018
6. Martin J, Hamilton B, Osterman M, Curtin S, Matthews T. Births: final data for 2014. *Natl Vital Stat Rep.* 2015;64(12):1–64
7. Guttmacher Institute. Adolescent sexual and reproductive health in the United States. https://www.guttmacher.org/fact-sheet/american-teens-sexual-and-reproductive-health. Published September 2016. Updated September 2017. Accessed March 8, 2018

8. Pazol K, Daniels K, Romero L, Warner L, Barfield W. Trends in long-acting reversible contraception use in adolescents and young adults: new estimates accounting for sexual experience. *J Adolesc Health*. 2016;59(4):438–442

9. Committee on Gynecologic Practice Long-Acting Reversible Contraception Working Group. Increasing access to contraceptive implants and intrauterine devices to reduce unintended pregnancy. *Obstet Gynecol*. 2015;126(4):e44–e48

10. American Academy of Pediatrics Committee on Adolescence. Contraception for adolescents. *Pediatrics*. 2014;134(4):e1244–e1256

11. Gorski P, Kuo A; American Academy of Pediatrics Council on Community Pediatrics. Community pediatrics: navigating the intersection of medicine, public health, and social determinants of children's health. *Pediatrics*. 2013;131(3):623–628

12. Cheng T, Johnson S, Goodman E. Breaking the intergenerational cycle of disadvantage: the three generation approach. *Pediatrics*. 2016;137(6):e20152467

13. Ng A, Kaye K. *Sex in the (Non) City: Teen Childbearing in Rural America*. Washington, DC: The National Campaign to Prevent Teen and Unplanned Pregnancy; 2015

14. Shearer DL, Mulvihill BA, Klerman LV, Wallander JL, Hovinga ME, Redden DT. Association of early childbearing and low cognitive ability. *Perspect Sex Reprod Health*. 2002;34(5): 236–243

15. American Academy of Pediatrics Committee on Adolescence and Committee on Early Childhood, Adoption, and Dependent Care. Care of adolescent parents and their children. *Pediatrics*. 2001;107(2):429–434

16. American Academy of Pediatrics Committee on Adolescence. The adolescent's right to confidential care when considering abortion. *Pediatrics*. 2017;139(2):e20163861

17. Siegel R, Brandon A. Adolescents, pregnancy, and mental health. *J Pediatr Adolesc Gynecol*. 2014;27(3):138–150

18. Hall K, Kusunoki Y, Gatny H, Barber J. The risk of unintended pregnancy among young women with mental health symptoms. *Soc Sci Med*. 2014;100:62–71

19. Bhat A, Reed SD, Unützer J. The obstetrician-gynecologist's role in detecting, preventing and treating depression. *Obstet Gynecol*. 2017;129(1):157–163

20. Francis J, Malbon K, Braun-Courville D, Lourdes L, Santelli J. Ambivalence about pregnancy and its association with symptoms of depression in adolescent females initiating contraception. *J Adolesc Health*. 2015;56(1):44–51

21. Cavazos-Rehg PA, Spitznagel EL, Krauss MJ, et al. Understanding adolescent parenthood from a multisystemic perspective. *J Adolesc Health*. 2010;46(6):525–531

22. Begun S. The paradox of homeless youth pregnancy: a review of challenges and opportunities. *Soc Work Health Care*. 2015;54(5):444–460

23. Thrane LE, Chen X. Impact of running away on girls' pregnancy. *J Adolesc*. 2012;35(2): 443–449

24. Garwood SK, Gerassi L, Jonson-Reid M, Plax K, Drake B. More than poverty: the effect of child abuse and neglect on teen pregnancy risk. *J Adolesc Health*. 2015;57(2):164–168

25. Green KM, Musci RJ, Matson PA, Johnson RM, Reboussin BA, Ialongo NS. Developmental patterns of adolescent marijuana and alcohol use and their joint association with sexual risk behavior and outcomes in young adulthood. *J Urban Health*. 2017;94(1):115–124

26. Lindley LL, Walsemann KM. Sexual orientation and risk of pregnancy among New York City high-school students. *Am J Public Health*. 2015;105(7):1379–1386

27. Hillis SD, Anda RF, Dube SR, Felitti VJ, Marchbanks PA, Marks JS. The association between adverse childhood experiences and adolescent pregnancy, long-term psychosocial consequences, and fetal death. *Pediatrics*. 2004;113(2):320–327

28. Noll JG, Shenk CE. Teen birth rates in sexually abused and neglected females. *Pediatrics*. 2013;131(4):e1181–e1187

29. Ng A, Kaye K. *Why It Matters: Teen Childbearing and Child Welfare*. Washington, DC: The National Campaign to Prevent Teen and Unplanned Pregnancy; 2013

30. Covington DL, Justason BJ, Wright LN. Severity, manifestations, and consequences of violence among pregnant adolescents. *J Adolesc Health.* 2001;28(1):55–61

31. Wiemann CM, Agurcia CA, Berenson AB, Volk RJ, Rickert VI. Pregnant adolescents: experiences and behaviors associated with physical assault by an intimate partner. *Matern Chil Health J.* 2000;4(2):93–101

32. Kennedy AC, Bennett L. Urban adolescent mothers exposed to community, family, and partner violence: is cumulative violence exposure a barrier to school performance and participation? *J Interpers Violence.* 2006;21(6):750–773

33. Gessner B, Perham-Hester K. Experience of violence among teenage mothers in Alaska. *J Adolesc Health.* 1998;22(5):383–388

34. Lewin A, Horn I, Valentine D, Sanders-Phillips K, Joseph J. How does violence exposure affect the psychological health and parenting of young African American mothers? *Soc Sci Med.* 2010;70(4):526–533

35. East P, Felice M. *Adolescent Pregnancy and Parenting: Findings From a Racially Diverse Sample.* Mahwah, NJ: Lawrence Erlbaum Associates; 1996

36. Overpeck MD, Brenner RA, Trumble AC, Trifiletti LB, Berendes HW. Risk factors for infant homicide in the United States. *N Engl J Med.* 1998;339(17):1211–1216

37. Taylor D, Chavez G, Chabra A, Boggess J. Risk factors for adult paternity in births to adolescents. *Obstet Gynecol.* 1997;89(2):199–205

38. Lindberg LD, Sonenstein FL, Ku L, Martinez G. Age differences between minors who give birth and their adult partners. *Fam Plann Perspect.* 1997;29(2):61–66

39. Tan LH, Quinlivan JA. Domestic violence, single parenthood, and fathers in the setting of teenage pregnancy. *J Adolesc Health.* 2006;38(3):201–207

40. Sipsma H, Biello KB, Cole-Lewis H, Kershaw T. Like father, like son: the intergenerational cycle of adolescent fatherhood. *Am J Public Health.* 2010;100(3):517–524

41. Kawakita T, Wilson K, Grantz KL, Landy HJ, Huang CC, Gomez-Lobo V. Adverse maternal and neonatal outcomes in adolescent pregnancy. *J Pediatr Adolesc Gynecol.* 2016;29(2): 130–136

42. Beers L, Hollo R. Approaching the adolescent-headed family: a review of teen parenting. *Curr Probl Pediatr Adolesc Health Care.* 2009;39(9):216–233

43. Kirbas A, Gulerman HC, Dagler K. Pregnancy in adolescence: is it an obstetrical risk? *J Pediatr Adolesc Gynecol.* 2016;29(4):367–371

44. Shrim A, Ates S, Mallozzi A, et al. Is young maternal age really a risk factor for adverse pregnancy outcome in a Canadian tertiary referral hospital? *J Pediatr Adolesc Gynecol.* 2011; 24(4):218–222

45. Boden JM, Fergusson DM, John Horwood L. Early motherhood and subsequent life outcomes. *J Child Psychol Psychiatry.* 2008;49(2):151–160

46. Perper K, Peterson K, Manlove J. *Child Trends Fact Sheet: Diploma Attainment Among Teen Mothers.* Washington, DC: Child Trends; 2010. Publication #2010-01

47. Antonishak J, Connolly C. *Preventing Unplanned Pregnancy and Completing College: An Evaluation of Online Lessons.* 2nd ed. Washington, DC: The National Campaign to Prevent Teen and Unplanned Pregnancy; 2014

48. Jutte D, Roos N, Brownell M, Briggs G, MacWilliam L, Roos L. The ripples of adolescent motherhood: social, educational, and medical outcomes for children of teen and prior teen mothers. *Acad Pediatr.* 2010;10(5):293–301

49. Hoffman L, Bann C, Higgins R, Vohr B; Eunice Kennedy Shrive National Institute of Child Health and Human Development Neonatal Research Network. Developmental outcomes of extremely preterm infants born to adolescent mothers. *Pediatrics.* 2015;135(6):1082–1092

50. Putnam-Hornstein E, Cederbaum JA, King B, Eastman AL, Trickett PK. A population-level and longitudinal study of adolescent mothers and intergenerational maltreatment. *Am J Epidemiol.* 2015;181(7):496–503

51. Smith M, Gotman N, Yonkers K. Early childhood adversity and pregnancy outcomes. *Matern Child Health J.* 2016;20(4):790–798

52. Andreozzi L, Flanagan P, Seifer R, Brunner S, Lester B. Attachment classifications among 18-month-old children of adolescent mothers. *Arch Pediatr Adolesc Med.* 2002;156(1):20–26

53. Hodgkinson S, Beers L, Southammakosane C, Lewin A. Addressing the mental health needs of pregnant and parenting adolescents. *Pediatrics.* 2014;133(1):114–122

54. Guttmacher Institute. An overview of minors' consent law. https://www.guttmacher.org/state-policy/explore/overview-minors-consent-law. Published 2017. Updated March 1, 2018. Accessed March 8, 2018

55. Garg A, Toy S, Tripodis Y, Silverstein M, Freeman E. Addressing social determinants of health at well child care visits: a cluster RCT. *Pediatrics.* 2015;135(2):e296–e304

56. Fazalullasha F, Taras J, Morinis J, et al. From office tools to community supports: the needs for infrastructure to address the social determinants of health in paediatric practice. *Paediatr Child Health.* 2014;19(4):195–199

57. Garg A, Butz AM, Dworkin PH, Lewis RA, Thompson RE, Serwint JR. Improving the management of family psychosocial problems at low-income children's well-child care visits: the WE CARE Project. *Pediatrics.* 2007;120(3):547–558

58. Kenyon C, Sandel M, Silverstein M, Shakir A, Zuckerman B. Revisiting the social history for child health. *Pediatrics.* 2007;120(3):e734–e738

59. Murry VM, Heflinger CA, Suiter SV, Brody GH. Examining perceptions about mental health care and help-seeking among rural African American families of adolescents. *J Youth Adolesc.* 2011;40(9):1118–1131

60. Foy JM; American Academy of Pediatrics Task Force on Mental Health. Enhancing pediatric mental health care: report from the American Academy of Pediatrics Task Force on Mental Health. Introduction. *Pediatrics.* 2010;125(suppl 3):S69–S74

61. Leplatte D, Rosenblum KL, Stanton E, Miller N, Muzik M. Mental health in primary care for adolescent parents. *Ment Health Fam Med.* 2012;9(1):39–45

62. Ashby B, Ranadive N, Alaniz V, St John-Larkin C, Scott S. Implications of comprehensive mental health services embedded in an adolescent obstetric medical home. *Matern Child Health J.* 2016;20(6):1258–1265

63. Ickovics J, Kershaw T, Westdahl C, et al. Group prenatal care and perinatal outcomes: a randomized controlled trial. *Obstet Gynecol.* 2007;110(2, pt 1):330–339

64. Ickovics JR, Earnshaw V, Lewis JB, et al. Cluster randomized controlled trial of group prenatal care: perinatal outcomes among adolescents in New York City health centers. *Am J Public Health.* 2016;106(2):359–365

65. Howard KS, Brooks-Gunn J. The role of home-visiting programs in preventing child abuse and neglect. *Future Child.* 2009;19(2):119–146

66. Sama-Miller E, Akers L, Mraz-Esposito A, et al. *Home Visiting Evidence of Effectiveness Review: Executive Summary.* Washington, DC: Office of Planning, Research and Evaluation; Administration for Children and Families; US Dept of Health and Human Services; 2016. http://homvee.acf.hhs.gov/About-Us/5/Executive-Summary/20/2. Accessed March 8, 2018

67. Olds D. The nurse-family partnership: an evidence-based preventive intervention. *Infant Ment Health J.* 2006;27(1):5–25

68. Florsheim P, Burrow-Sanchez JJ, Minami T, McArthur L, Heavin S, Hudak C. Young parenthood program: supporting positive paternal engagement through coparenting counseling. *Am J Public Health.* 2012;102(10):1886–1892

69. Centers for Disease Control and Prevention. Prepregnancy contraceptive use among teens with unintended pregnancies resulting in live births—Pregnancy Risk Assessment Monitoring System (PRAMS), 2004–2008. *MMWR Morb Mortal Wkly Rep.* 2012;61(2):25–29

70. Birgisson NE, Zhao Q, Secura GM, Madden T, Peipert JF. Preventing unintended pregnancy: the Contraceptive CHOICE project in review. *J Womens Health (Larchmt).* 2015;24(5):349–353

71. Marcell AV, Wibbelsman C, Seigel WM; American Academy of Pediatrics Committee on Adolescence. Male adolescent sexual and reproductive health care. *Pediatrics.* 2011;128(6):e1658–e1676

72. Mezey G, Meyer D, Robinson F, et al. Developing and piloting a peer mentoring intervention to reduce teenage pregnancy in looked-after children and care leavers: an exploratory randomised controlled trial. *Health Technol Assess.* 2015;19(85):1–509

73. Scott M, Berger A, Caal S, Hickman S, Moore K. *Preventing Teen Pregnancy Among Latinos: Recommendations From Research, Evaluation, and Practitioner Experience.* Bethesda, MD: Child Trends; 2014

74. Villarruel AM, Jemmott JB III, Jemmott LS. A randomized controlled trial testing an HIV prevention intervention for Latino youth. *Arch Pediatr Adolesc Med.* 2006;160(8):772–777

75. Klerman LV. *Another Chance: Preventing Additional Births to Teen Mothers.* Washington, DC: The National Campaign to Prevent Teen Pregnancy; 2004. http://www.healthyteennetwork. org/wp-content/uploads/2014/05/Another-Chance-Preventing-Additional-Births-to-Teen-Mothers.pdf. Accessed March 20, 2018

76. Kohler P, Manhart L, Lafferty W. Abstinence-only and comprehensive sex education and the initiation of sexual activity and teen pregnancy. *J Adolesc Health.* 2008;42(4):344–351

77. American Academy of Pediatrics Committee on Adolescence. Condom use by adolescents. *Pediatrics.* 2013;132(5):973–981

78. Key JD, Gebregziabher MG, Marsh LD, O'Rourke KM. Effectiveness of an intensive, school-based intervention for teen mothers. *J Adolesc Health.* 2008;42(4):394–400

79. Johnson AZ, Sieving RE, Pettingell SL, McRee AL. The roles of partner communication and relationship status in adolescent contraceptive use. *J Pediatr Health Care.* 2015;29(1):61–69

Children in the Juvenile Justice System

Robert E. Morris, MD, and Evalyn Horowitz, MD

"Primary care clinicians who understand the juvenile justice system in their geographic location are prepared to assist delinquent youths and their families before, during, and after incarceration."

History of the Juvenile Justice System

Policies and regulations for juvenile detention and rehabilitation in the United States have been refined, then redirected toward newer philosophies, and then returned to older ways. Today's methods for directing behavior and those of 1910 are not unalike.[1] A review of this history provides insights into the opportunities and challenges pediatric health care professionals and other child advocates experience today in preventing juvenile delinquency and in interacting with the juvenile justice system.

Under English law, parental control was primary. In 1797, the first New York penitentiary opened. Because the state presumed its potential was to provide rehabilitation, juveniles were brought to criminal court. Community groups began lobbying for children to be handled separately from adults, and, in 1824, the first House of Refuge for children with juvenile delinquency was founded in New York. Shortly before the Civil War, in 1851, the Children's Aid Society built the New York Juvenile Asylum to house children younger than 12 years.[2]

Throughout this chapter, the term *youth* or *youths* refers to individuals who, based on age, are subject to the juvenile justice system in the jurisdiction in which they live.

The Civil War brought immigrants, poverty, violence, and chaos to the United States. Parents worked long hours, and children and adolescents ran the streets, causing passage of disorderly conduct laws and more incarceration of youths. Children older than 7 years and adolescents were housed with adults in jails and prisons. In 1875, the Society for the Prevention of Cruelty to Children was formed, defining child neglect and holding parents responsible. By 1892, a separate juvenile court system was founded.

With the Progressive Era of US history (1900–1918) came women's suffrage, child labor laws, and the 8-hour workday. Journalism and political satiric cartoons became a tool for public persuasion, and psychological theories for treating children flourished. These forces helped shape the rights of juveniles who had been incarcerated, and society began to feel responsible to reform youthful offenders before their criminal activity was entrenched or strengthened through incarceration.[3,4]

Over the next 75 years, juvenile justice law was honed. Girls who had been incarcerated were separated from boys, and their housing was improved. In most cases, juvenile hearings were conducted apart from adult courts, and proceedings were considered civil rather than judicial cases.

In the late 1960s, in *Kent v United States,* it was decided that the informal process of determining whether a juvenile should be tried in juvenile or adult court failed to provide sufficient due process protection for children.[5] A year later, an Arizona juvenile court placed a sentry adolescent, the Mr Gault case, at 15 years of age, in detention until age 21 years for a status offense.[3] (A status offense is behavior that is unique to the juvenile status, such as truancy or running away.) On appeal, the US Supreme Court held, according to Article 5 of the Bill of Rights (ratified in 1791) and the 14th Amendment (ratified in 1868) regarding due process, that children had a right to receive fair treatment under the law, including the following rights:

- ▶ To receive notice of charges
- ▶ To obtain legal counsel
- ▶ To confront and cross-examine their accusers
- ▶ To avoid self-incrimination
- ▶ To receive a transcript of the proceedings
- ▶ To appeal[6]

The 1970s brought several new developments. The 1970 case *In re Winship* held that when a juvenile is held responsible for criminal behavior, the previous standard of a *preponderance of evidence* (ie, the facts indicate the juvenile's behavior was "likely" to be true) now rose to a standard of *beyond a reasonable doubt* (ie, the evidence must be proved beyond any other logical explanation, similar to adult law). The 1971 case *McKeiver v Pennsylvania* found that juveniles charged with a criminal law violation and adjudicated in juvenile court are not entitled to a jury trial. The 1968 Juvenile Delinquency

Prevention and Control Act was reauthorized as the Juvenile Justice and Delinquency Prevention Act in 1974 and again reauthorized in 2002, providing federal funding to states with community programs to discourage juvenile delinquency.[3] The law created the following programs:

▶ The Office of Juvenile Justice and Delinquency Prevention
▶ The Runaway Youth Program
▶ The National Institute for Juvenile Justice and Delinquency Prevention[1,3,6]

The law required separation of "young and impressionable" juvenile delinquents from convicted adults. Part of the rationale behind the separation of juvenile and adult offenders was the evidence that youths learned to behave as more skillful criminals.[7]

By the late 1980s, violent crime rose, peaking in 1994. Highly publicized shootings and shocking crimes by juveniles led citizens to fear that, for some juveniles, violence was a way of life. Retrospectively, it seems media claims greatly exaggerated the role of juveniles in perpetrating crime. In response to this perception of a crime wave, legislation swung back to "get tough on crime," and the Juvenile Justice Act was amended, allowing states to try younger juveniles as adults for certain violent crimes with resulting lengthy prison sentences. The juvenile justice system became increasingly similar to the adult criminal justice system, reflecting the sentiment that youths who commit serious crimes must be held accountable and punished for their crimes, not just "reformed."[4]

Today, throughout the 50 states, correctional facilities for youths, much like those for adults, have vastly different infrastructure and focus. Beyond simply corralling youths with aberrant behavior, their management points toward different goals, from simple containment, to punishment, to attempts to model nurturing and rehabilitation.[8] Some systems are centralized and run by the state, including both preadjudication facilities and postadjudication facilities. Other states have decentralized systems, allowing counties or other jurisdictions to presort and house juveniles during preadjudication, as determined appropriate by the local courts. In nearly all states, depending on age, a youth may be remanded to adult court for certain serious crimes.[4]

Mental Health Care in Juvenile Justice Facilities

In the 1970s, congressional attempts at health care reform called for standards of care throughout the health care system, leading the American Medical Association (AMA) to investigate health care standards in correctional institutions. The AMA found a lack of standards, and this finding resulted in the development of correctional health care standards by various national organizations.[9] By the 1990s, medical, dental, and mental health standards became formalized for correctional institutions of all sizes and in all jurisdictions. However, accreditation and adherence to the standards is voluntary. Often, compliance with standards is forced on states or jails through lawsuits brought by federal authorities or prisoner rights organizations.

The facility health care workers may be on-site for a portion or the entirety of the day, depending on the size and population of the facility. It is well-known that one poor outcome will cause years of financial and political upheaval for the facility; thus, the correctional administration generally facilitates access to health care, enabling the individuals who have been incarcerated to receive appropriate health benefits. However, in some institutions, because of budget, culture, and lack of oversight, health care may be doled out. Federal Medicaid rules currently prohibit payment for all incarcerated people inside correctional facilities, and many private insurance companies also decline to cover care of incarcerated people; thus, health care costs can strain the budgets of the governmental jurisdiction responsible for the facility. More assistance, although not uniformly, is offered for hospitalizations but not for urgent care or emergency visits. Difficulties in providing care often occur because of insufficient internal staffing during lean funding years and when outside specialty services are needed. Specialty health care outside the facility is expensive, even though fees are often discounted: inmates may be seen as threatening to the outside physicians' other patients, and payment to providers can be slow. For these reasons, some private specialty physicians refuse to see prisoners in their practices. University or public facilities often become the default care providers. In the absence of mandatory national adherence to accreditation standards, variability in quality of care for small, decentralized, and state-run juvenile detention centers persists.

Processing Youths Through the Juvenile Justice System

The arresting officers are the first "judges" of what is best for the youth and community, dealing with nonviolent crime on the basis of their best judgment. The officer may issue a warning and accompany the youth home to discuss with the parents, usually maintaining a record of the contact. Or, the officer may take the youth to the police station and ask the parent to come there to discuss the situation.[10]

In cases in which the youth does not have a parent or guardian or anyone else who can or will parent the youth, or resides in a house that is not fit to live in, is abused or neglected, or is threatening people or property, then the youth may be placed in a community shelter or foster care. For more serious crimes or for a re-offense, the youth may be sent to a juvenile hall that generally holds preadjudicated youths; the hall may also be used for short-term incarceration as a punishment or deterrent to further offending or for placement when other release settings have failed.[4,5,8]

If the youth's offense leads to more than an officer's warning, variable legal processes occur, usually culminating in a juvenile court hearing. Youths may not be incarcerated for status offenses. More serious offenses that are irrelevant to age can range from minor offenses such as petty theft or property destruction to more serious crimes involving violence, bodily harm, sexual offenses, and other felonies.

Before disposition, referred to as the hearing, an evaluation of the youth is usually performed by a social worker or probation officer who recommends to the judge the appropriate disposition of the case.[4,10,11] This evaluation may include structured assessment tools such as the Youth Assessment and Screening Instrument (Orbis Partners, Ottawa, Ontario, Canada), a review of family and school history, mental or physical health records, past criminal history, and statements from parents, friends, teachers, faith leaders, or the victim of the youth's crime, plus the youth's own statement. At this point, it is important for the youth's primary care clinician (PCC) (ie, the pediatrician, family physician, internist, nurse practitioner, or physician assistant who has provided longitudinal health care) to provide records, to support and encourage the parents and youth, and to make suggestions about actions parents or community members may take to advocate for the youth and to provide support and control of the youth after release.

At the disposition hearing, the sentence depends on the offense, the state in which the crime occurred, and, sadly, the race and ethnicity of the offender.[6,12] The youth may be released to the parent or guardian, community service may be required, and there may be ongoing supervision by a probation officer, social workers, or others who work with youths,[10,13] or Multisystemic Therapy (MST) (see Interventions for Young Offenders section later in this chapter). A youth on probation in the community may be required to attend a special segregated school. Courts often order individual, group, or family counseling, structured after-school programs, or weekend or other short-term detention in a county restricted, locked facility. If there is a splintered or an unsupportive family situation, the youth can be made a ward of the court, allowing the judge to control the care in an out-of-home or locked setting, assisting with the treatment and guidance of the minor and limiting or ending parental control.

Youths who reoffend, in some cases, those who are involved in gang activity or who have little or no family support, may then be placed in a community juvenile "jail" or "ranch." As noted previously, these facilities can be centralized (regional or even state run) or community centered and may involve schooling. Depending on the offense, detention may vary in duration, with eventual release to family or foster care on probation.[13]

States have developed increasingly more severe programs for youths with violent or recalcitrant behavior (eg, high-discipline or boot camps). These military-like work camps seek to provide a highly structured environment with the aim of instilling responsibility and self-discipline. Such programs have failed uniformly, sometimes with tragic consequences. One such example was the death resulting from staff neglect of a 14-year-old boy sent to a Florida boot camp for trespassing at a school, that is, a probation and parole violation related to a previous charge, but itself a relatively minor offense. After this 2006 episode, the Florida boot camps were closed.[14]

There are far fewer resources and less discretion in adult courts, whose primary goal is to punish offenders and protect society. If a youth is remanded directly to adult criminal court because of repeated crimes or a serious crime and convicted in a jury trial, the youth will receive an adult sentence, including possibly life without parole in a case of murder. This sentencing practice is currently being challenged in a number of jurisdictions.[15]

Interventions for Young Offenders

Currently, rather than being referred initially to social services systems to prevent the stigma of justice system involvement, youths who have recently begun to offend against laws are more likely to be referred to the juvenile justice system, which will largely determine both sanctions and mandated rehabilitation programs. Some programs include outpatient therapy. For example, MST, an evidence-based treatment program addressing antisocial behavior in children and adolescents, is variably available in the United States. The treatment uses trained case managers and their supervisors to evaluate the challenges facing the child or adolescent and the family. Plans are developed in conjunction with the family, instituted, and evaluated, usually over a 3- to 5-month period. The program is action oriented, with a solution for each problem. For example, if a teenager is not getting to school, a person such as a relative, coach, or neighbor is identified to be responsible for getting the teenager to school. Curfew problems could be addressed by engaging the teenager in appropriate evening activities. Individual cognitive behavioral therapy (CBT), drug counseling, and effective parenting training are often part of the program. The case manager should be available by phone 24 hours a day for crises. A team of several case managers and their supervisors meets weekly to address successes and failures. Family meetings with the case manager are conducted at a time convenient for the family.[16] Under some circumstances, the child's or adolescent's PCC may be asked to participate; for example, there could be a health condition that affects the youth and requires optimal medical management so that the youth can regularly attend school. It should be noted that MST can be utilized outside the justice system, thus preventing criminal stigma that can follow the youth into adulthood.

A number of states and local jurisdictions have programs aimed at young offenders 10 to 12 years of age. All programs involve case managers and provide integrated services (Box 28-1). Several other evidence-based outpatient programs are therapeutic foster care,[17] dialectical behavioral therapy, functional family therapy, and motivational enhancement therapy; these are available for children and adolescents with certain mental health diagnoses or who have committed certain types of crimes. These therapies are sometimes used while youths are incarcerated.

Box 28-1. Typical Services Offered by Intensive Outpatient Rehabilitation Programs to Young Offenders

- Crisis management services
- Comprehensive assessment of all aspects of the child: physical health, mental health, substance abuse, school functioning, family economic problems or strengths, vocational needs, family and social functioning
- Skills training for youth and family
- Cognitive problem solving
- Self-control methods
- Behavior cognitive training
- Family training
- Tutoring
- School involvement
- Adult role models

From Burns BJ, Howell JC, Wiig JK, et al. *Treatment, Services, and Intervention Programs for Child Delinquents.* Washington, DC: Office of Juvenile Justice and Delinquency Prevention, Office of Justice Programs, US Dept of Justice; 2003. Child Delinquency Bulletin Series NCJ 193410. https://www.ncjrs.gov/html/ojjdp/193410/contents.html. Accessed March 8, 2018.

Interventions for Incarcerated Youths

For delinquents who are incarcerated, rehabilitation becomes part of the therapeutic milieu. Generally, smaller institutions with only 25 to 30 youths have better outcomes and less violence, as demonstrated by the Missouri State System and others.[18]

A variety of theoretical frameworks support programs for incarcerated youths. A widely accepted set of principles that guide rehabilitation programs for incarcerated youths involves attention to the criminogenic risks of each youth (Box 28-2). Evidence shows that the criminogenic risks are the most important issues to address during rehabilitation, while excluding other factors often found in delinquent youths that research shows are not relevant to reducing recidivism. When addressing criminogenic risks, counselors must consider the degree of risk to reoffend (ie, youths at high risk to reoffend, defined as those with more criminogenic risk factors in their histories, require more-intensive services). Also important during rehabilitation are the principles of responsivity (ie, interactions are tailored to learning styles and abilities) and professional override (ie, trained professional staff make decisions based on the current situation).[19] A logical inference of this theoretical framework supports the notion that youths at low risk require little or no services because they are unlikely to reoffend.

Despite the enthusiasm for using this criminogenic risk evaluation during incarceration, Lipsey recently reported on a meta-analytic overview designed to assess the factors that make up effective rehabilitation interventions. He found that the criminogenic risk principles were important first steps but that programs were most effective if done in the child's community as opposed to during incarceration. The data showed that the best interventions included CBT, mentoring, and group counseling. Not surprisingly,

---

Box 28-2. Criminogenic Risks for Youths to Reoffend

- History of antisocial behavior or low self-control
- Personal attitudes, values, or beliefs supportive of crime
- Procriminal associates and isolation from anticriminal peers and role models
- Current dysfunctional family features
- Callous personality factors
- Substance use

Derived from Andrews DA, Bonita J, Hoge RD. Classification for effective rehabilitation: rediscovering psychology. *Crim Justice Behav.* 1990;17(1):19–52.

high-quality programs worked best for high-risk offenders, and these programs were usually research or demonstration programs.[19] Evaluations of routine practices generally had about half the effect of high-quality programs because they were not conducted with fidelity to the original program.[20]

Aggression is a significant issue for many incarcerated youths. Aggression replacement training uses several short problems that illustrate issues in moral reasoning, anger control, or prosocial skill building. Small groups of youths are guided through these exercises by trained staff over about a 10-week period.[21]

Recently, a series of initiatives has taken juvenile detention into the "case management" realm in many parts of the United States. Behavioral therapy is provided pre-detention and continued post-detention, and it is also provided when youths are placed into group homes, work camps, and locked schools, because these facilities are often utilized by the juvenile justice system.[22] Therapeutic interventions, such as CBT, MST, functional family therapy, and dialectical behavioral therapy, attempt to redirect erring youths to a more productive lifestyle.[23] In the past decade, attempts were made to classify these programs by effectiveness, with some recent decreases in overall juvenile incarceration.[24] The states have various levels of commitment. One example is the IMPACT (Integrated Managed Partnership for Adolescent and Child Community Treatment) program in Boulder, CO, which uses evidence-based motivational and behavioral intervention skills to engage clients in treatment to stabilize their mental health and substance use disorders.[25] Other states have no apparent interventional involvement beyond physical incarceration, although this is changing as requirements for programing are increasingly mandated. Community development of youth programs involving local mental health, recreational, and social service workers have the potential to be plausible rehabilitation programs.

The concept of *restorative justice* involves reciprocal relationships between the offended community and the youth offender, who is required to engage in activities to restore the community to its pre-offense status. In return, the community takes some responsibility for rehabilitation and care of the youth.

A complete discussion of various rehabilitation strategies in use throughout the United States is beyond the scope of this chapter. However, many child advocates believe that all effective interventions must, at a minimum, address the intrinsic and extrinsic factors known as criminogenic risks to effectively reduce the risk for reoffending.

In 2014, the Models for Change Resource Center Partnership and the National Center for Mental Health and Juvenile Justice published a white paper documenting system improvements undertaken in states and communities over the past decade and outlining new models, publications, toolkits, and training curricula that provide guidance to other sites interested in tackling similar reforms.[26] See Box 28-3.

Pediatric PCCs are unlikely to be extensively involved in the lives of youths who are incarcerated. However, the parents may turn to their son's or daughter's PCC for advice. Alternatively, the youths may form an attachment to PCCs or therapists after repeated or extended incarcerations, especially if these health care professionals also work outside the juvenile detention facility in the community. Because many youths (≥50%) have co-occurring mental and substance use disorders,[27] the National Commission on Correctional Health Care *Standards for Health Services in Juvenile Detention and Confinement Facilities* mandates that youths with these co-occurring disorders should be assessed and treated by appropriate clinicians while in detention.[9]

Anoshiravani and colleagues reported on the causes of hospitalizations in California's detained youths and found that mental illness, often with comorbid substance use disorders, required long inpatient stays and represented the major cause for hospitalization of detained youths.[28] This finding highlights the substantial need for mental health services for detained youths.

Box 28-3. Significant State Innovations Related to Mental Health of Adjudicated Youths

- New school, probation and police-based diversion models for youth with mental health needs

- New mental health training resources for juvenile justice staff and police

- Resources to support family involvement within the juvenile justice system

- Advanced protocols and processes for screening and assessment to identify mental health needs and risk among juveniles

- New resources for implementing evidence-based practices for justice-involved youth

- New guidelines for juvenile competency

From Mental Health and Juvenile Justice Collaborative for Change: A Training, Technical Assistance and Education Center and a Member of the Models for Change Resource Center Partnership. *Better Solutions for Youth With Mental Health Needs in the Juvenile Justice System.* Delmar, NY: National Center for Mental Health and Juvenile Justice; 2014. https://www.ncmhjj.com/resources/better-solutions-youth-mental-health-needs-juvenile-justice-system. Accessed March 8, 2018. Reproduced with permission.

The parents should be urged to advocate for treatment of these disorders while their son or daughter is incarcerated and prepare to continue treatment for the youth after release. Parents, even if they are geographically far removed from their son or daughter, should work to maintain contact with both their child and the staff at the correctional facility. When a youth with a substance use disorder is released, the court will often mandate that the youth attend a substance use disorder treatment program that the court or jurisdiction will reimburse. Generally, it is the probation or parole officer who is responsible for ensuring that the youth attends any mandated treatment programs after release.

Failure to ensure continuing care after release remains a major problem for incarcerated youths. When PCCs become aware that their patients will soon be released, they should contact the facility's medical department to plan for a smooth transition back to community care. The youth's probation or parole officer can be a useful ally in working to keep the youth in care. Most correctional facilities provide the medical and mental health records to the child's community PCC if the youth and parents consent. If the youth is released on psychotropic medication, the PCC may play an important role in helping the patient remain on medication until psychiatric evaluation.

Advocating for the Health Care of Youths in the Juvenile Justice System

The American Academy of Pediatrics (AAP) Committee on Adolescence published a comprehensive policy statement in 2011 that advocates for involvement of the youth's community PCC during and after incarceration so that medical and behavioral health is optimized. Therefore, the institution should refer the youth back to the PCC in the community. When the youth does not have an existing community PCC, the institutional staff should work with the family (or foster family), parole agents, local public health agencies, and community PCCs to develop a plan to coordinate care after release. The institutional staff, in planning for the youth's release, should help the youth and family apply for appropriate health insurance. In some jurisdictions, youths in the correctional system remain in the foster care system. If this is the case, the youth may be eligible for Medicaid insurance beyond the usual cutoff age. The AAP policy statement also discusses the need for adequate funding of medical and behavioral health and education in juvenile facilities and suggests that pediatric health care professionals advocate for a reversal of federal law to allow Medicaid and other insurance funding of incarcerated juveniles.

Preventing Juvenile Delinquency

Primary care clinicians caring for children and families and advocating through their organizations can also undertake "upstream" activities to prevent juvenile delinquency and decrease the number of incarcerated youths.[29]

Surveillance, Screening, and Anticipatory Guidance

Many factors may contribute to later delinquency. In early life, these may include fetal complications, fetal exposure to substances such as alcohol, brain injury, toxic exposures to chemicals, experiences of violence in the environment, physical or mental abuse, difficult temperament, and hyperactivity. In addition, a wide variety of pathological family structures and functions may contribute to future delinquency. Toddlers and older children who exhibit aggression, repeated lying, risk-taking, lack of empathy, or animal cruelty and those whose parents practice harsh, erratic discipline are at risk for later delinquency. Substance use disorder; depression; victimization as a result of crime, abuse (physical, sexual, or emotional abuse), bullying, or other factors; and exposure to violence are often proximal to overt delinquency. Problems at school, peer rejection, association with deviant peers, unemployment, school drop-out, and residence in neighborhoods with gang warfare, high rates of violence and crime, prostitution, or visible illegal substance or alcohol use compound the risk for delinquency. When youths are carrying weapons, dealing drugs, or involved in gangs, their behavior becomes obviously delinquent.[30,31] The PCC who is alert to risk factors can make early referrals to programs that work to prevent later delinquency.

Additional information for assessing youths at risk for delinquency can be found in the AAP publication *Addressing Mental Health Concerns in Primary Care: A Clinician's Toolkit*.[32] The Juvenile Justice Fact Sheet in the toolkit provides suggestions for working with youths involved in the juvenile justice system. In this book, Chapter 1, Healthy Child Development, discusses promotion of mental health; surveillance of children and families for mental health problems; psychosocial screening of children, adolescents, and their families; primary care intervention when concerns are identified; and referral to mental health specialty care when needed. Children and adolescents also benefit from evaluation and appropriate treatment of traumatic stress, which may contribute to aggressive behavior and, in turn, juvenile delinquency.

Early Intervention

Because there is evidence that very early childhood experiences have profound and long-lasting effects on an individual's behavior throughout life,[33] programs early in life, even during the prenatal period, may be the most effective interventions to provide protection from developing delinquency. Olds and others developed a model program of home visits by trained public health nurses; these visits begin during the prenatal period and continue until the child is 18 months of age. Follow-up conducted years after the program, in some cases 20 years later, has shown multiple benefits for these children, including significantly reduced delinquency and improved school outcomes compared with control groups.[34,35]

A Chicago-based program that provided an enhanced grade school experience and comprehensive family services from kindergarten through third grade resulted in higher rates of school completion, more college attendance, and fewer felony arrests compared with the control group. This intervention began later in life and had fewer positive effects compared with the early childhood nurse visitors.[36] The Rand Corporation has published information about a number of effective preschool programs.[37]

Primary care clinicians faced with disruptive children who are living in dysfunctional families with overly punitive parents or families experiencing major disruptions may benefit from referral to a parenting program. These have a number of titles, including New Beginnings, Positive Parenting, and Parent Training programs.[38-41]

Several programs are available for children with fetal alcohol spectrum disorder. Box 28-4 gives examples of successful programs for children at risk for future behaviors likely to bring them into contact with police and the juvenile justice system.

Delinquent youths rarely begin to offend without an early history of maladaptive behavior, often beginning before age 12 years. Behavioral problems are often present for at least 5 years before coming to the attention of juvenile courts; in one study, one-third of offenders were diagnosed as having disruptive behavior by age 13 years. Specific professional help is rarely provided to these young children.[42] Appendix 2, Mental Health Tools for Pediatrics, lists tools that can be used to assist in the timely identification of children experiencing maladaptive behavior and emotional disturbance.

A recent article by Assink and his colleagues,[43] identifying factors for persistent delinquent behavior among juveniles, provides useful guidance to PCCs in identifying youths in their practice who are at heightened risk for life-course persistent delinquent behaviors compared with adolescent-limited offending. The authors suggest that risk for persistent offending is

Box 28-4. Behavioral Interventions for Youths With Fetal Alcohol Spectrum Disorder

- **Good Buddies:** A children's friendship training to teach appropriate social skills to individuals with FASD.

  Children with FASD often have difficulty learning subtle social skills from their own experiences; those kinds of skills are typically "learned by osmosis" on the playground, such as how to slip into a group, appropriate sharing, or dealing with teasing. This intervention uses a group format to teach age-appropriate social skills over 12 weekly sessions for parent and child. Sessions are organized around and toward each child by hosting a playdate with a classmate or peer.

- **Families Moving Forward:** A program to provide support for families who deal with challenging FASD behaviors.

  This intervention, based in part on positive behavior support techniques, is most appropriate for children with severe, clinically significant behavioral problems. It is a feasible, low-intensity, sustained model of supportive consultation with a parent or caregiver (rather than directly with the child). The intervention lasts 9–11 mo, with at least 16 every-other-week sessions, typically lasting 90 min each. Services are carried out by mental health specialists with specialized training.

- **Parents and Children Together:** Parents and Children Together is a group program designed to improve behavior regulation skills, executive functioning, and parent effectiveness.

  Parents and Children Together is a prevention/early intervention program that provides in-home counseling, skill building, and support. The program is based on the HOMEBUILDERS model of family preservation using a neurocognitive habilitation program to improve self-regulation and executive function.

Abbreviation: FASD, fetal alcohol spectrum disorder.

related to quantitative rather than qualitative risks (eg, the more risks, the higher the likelihood for ongoing delinquency). Primary care clinicians are encouraged to inquire into the many risk factors for delinquency, as listed in Box 28-5. Early referral to multifaceted interventions targeting problems in multiple domains is warranted when there are many risk factors.[43]

Gender-Specific Interventions

Gender-responsive or gender-specific principles aim to meet girls' individual developmental needs, personal characteristics, and life circumstances. The principles include safety and safe spaces, attention to relationships, and a collaborative approach with power shared across systems (including power sharing with the girl).

Safety and safe spaces involves both physical safety and emotional and intellectual safety. Many girls who offend have been the subject of male violence involving both physical abuse and sexual abuse. Use of same-gender staff helps create safer living environments in correctional programs.

Box 28-5. Domains Associated With Risk of Persistent Offending According to a Meta-analytic Review

Domains With Higher Risk
- Criminal history
- Aggressive behavior
- Alcohol/drug use
- Sexual behavior
- Social relationships (especially with antisocial peers)
- Emotional and behavioral problems
- School/employment difficulties

Domains With Smaller Effect on Risk
- Family risk issues (Fathers, siblings, and family systems appear to be more important, while mother relationships are less important.)

Domains With Higher Risk for Females and Suggesting Gender-Specific Interventions
- Aggression
- Neurocognition/physiology (genetic factors regarding brain function)

Domains With Moderating Effects on Risk
- Gender: For example, boys and girls tend to have different life experiences, such as greater exposure to physical and sexual violence in girls (see the section Gender-Specific Interventions).
- Age: For example, older youths may have higher risks of persistent offending.
- Cultural minorities: Interventions should be culturally matched to the juvenile (see the section Ethnic and Other Minority Interventions).

Derived from Assink M, van der Put CE, Hoeve M, de Vries SL, Stams GJ, Oort FJ. Risk factors for persistent delinquent behavior among juveniles: a meta-analytic review. *Clin Psychol Rev*. 2015;42:47–61.

Emotional and intellectual safety involves allowing girls to feel comfortable in expressing their emotions, beliefs, goals, and fears. This therapeutic milieu helps girls engage in individual growth.

Research devoted to girls' relationships stresses the importance of relationships in molding girls toward socialization and caregiving roles. Rehabilitation programs can focus on the centrality of relationships in girls' lives by developing opportunities for girls to connect with adult individuals and enhancing their connection to their community.

When girls are encouraged to collaborate in developing program design and taking leadership roles, they are empowered to actively participate in their rehabilitation. Programs that focus on strengths rather than deficits give girls that have often experienced negative effects from trauma renewed control over their lives. Because girls may be simultaneously involved in multiple care and rehabilitation systems, it is important for the organizations to use the same principles when working with girls. This consistency can be accomplished by forming collaborative partnerships among programs that provide services to girls.[44]

Ethnic and Other Minority Interventions

Until recently, concerns regarding justice-involved youths of ethnic minority or other minorities focused on disproportionate arrests, confinement, and sentencing of minority youths. In response to the excessive involvement of minority youths in correctional facilities, several programs were developed in individual cities. These programs were generally not financed by governmental agencies and were often unsuccessful in reducing disproportion because of inadequate funding.

G. Roger Jarjoura reviewed the effective strategies for mentoring African American boys and listed 10 effective programs operating in cities in the United States. Although the programs were focused on African American boys, the concepts can be applied to other ethnic groups.

The following principles inform these interventions:

1. "Begin with a big vision for the ultimate outcome: productively engaged adult citizens." (The mentoring relationships are based on mutuality, trust, and empathy that are more likely to result in positive youth outcomes by contributing to social-emotional development, cognitive development, and identity development.)

2. "Effective mentoring is all about relationships, but context is also important." (The cultural competency of mentors allows youths to develop a healthy ethnic identity that can counter the negative messages that many of these boys receive in school and society.)

3. "Trauma experiences and exposure to violence complicate adolescent development and must be addressed." (African American youths are likely to be raised with violence all around them. Some of the youths have learning disorders, difficulties with problem-solving, and difficulties with decision-making. Strengths-based mentoring can build skills in these areas. Structured group experiences are designed to build emotional intelligence in the context of interpersonal relationships. The programs also use trauma-informed care to allow healing and growth.)

4. "Model mentoring programs for African American boys tend not to be traditional one-on-one mentoring programs." (These programs work

with youths in groups led by one or several adults, often connected with schools, to enhance educational success and career development.)

5. "A hallmark of effective mentoring programs for African American boys is advocacy." (It is especially important that there is strong advocacy for boys involved in the justice system.)

6. "Access to model programs is complicated." (Many of these programs are designed and led by visionary founders and they struggle to maintain a secure level of funding. Therefore, each program tends to thrive in only one setting and is unlikely to be available on a large scale.)

7. "When you are inclined to look for role models among relatives, youth in the child welfare system are at a particular disadvantage." (Minority youths are less likely to have a natural mentor compared with white youths, although when they have natural mentors, they are relatives that come from the extended family. When youths are caught up in the child welfare system, it is important to connect them with culturally competent African American mentors and role models.)

8. "To have hope for the future, it helps to see how it will turn out." (A challenge for these youths is that their future appears to be one in which they are more likely to go to prison rather than college. When mentoring is done well, youths are exposed to inspiring adult role models who give hope for the future. Once youths believe there is hope, they are more likely to do what is asked of them in the program.)[45]

Diagnosis and Treatment of Mental Disorders Associated With Offending

Specific mental health diagnoses can be precursors to criminal behaviors, according to the fifth edition of the *Diagnostic and Statistical Manual of Mental Disorders (DSM-5)*.[46]

Oppositional defiant disorder (ODD) is characterized by an angry and irritable mood along with argumentative and defiant behavior. These youths also display spiteful or vindictive behavior at a minimum of 2 times in the past 6 months. This behavior causes distress in the individual and others and is not the result of another mental health diagnosis such as psychosis or substance use disorder.[46]

Conduct disorder (CD) involves a repetitive and persistent pattern of behavior that violates the basic rights of others or major age-appropriate norms or rules. Criteria include exhibiting aggression to people or animals. Destruction of property, deceitfulness, theft, and serious violation of rules are also criteria. There is clinically significant impairment of social, academic, or occupational functioning with onset before 18 years of age.[46] Youths with CD often have contact with the juvenile justice system. An intervention using an evidence-based parenting program in the United Kingdom reduced the likelihood of their progressing to contact with the juvenile justice system.[47] Other community-based and institutional interventions are described earlier in this chapter in the Interventions for Incarcerated Youths section.

The *DSM-5* includes a new diagnosis: disruptive mood dysregulation disorder (DMDD), defined as severe recurrent temper outbursts grossly out of proportion in intensity or duration to the situation or provocation. The outbursts are inconsistent with the child's developmental level and happen 3 or more times per week, with irritable or angry mood between outbursts. The disorder occurs between 6 and 18 years of age.[18] Children with DMDD meet criteria for another mental health diagnosis 92.8% of the time. For example, in a recent review, nearly all youths with DMDD were also diagnosed as having ODD, and 61% of youths with CD and 58% of youths with ODD met DMDD criteria.[48]

Treatments for these 3 overlapping diagnoses are similar, including psychotherapeutic interventions, such as parental intervention and MST, and, in some cases, pharmacological agents, that is, psychostimulants and selective serotonin reuptake inhibitors.[48,49] Typically, PCCs involve mental health specialists, that is, therapists and psychiatrists, to co-treat children and adolescents with these conditions.

Conclusion

Primary care clinicians can help prevent delinquency by providing parenting support to at-risk families and referring young children with disruptive behavior to treatment. After a youth becomes involved with the juvenile justice system, PCCs can provide support and counseling for the youth's parents as the youth traverses the system from arrest to adjudication, sanctions, and rehabilitation. Primary care clinicians who understand the juvenile justice system in their geographic location are prepared to assist delinquent youths and their families before, during, and after incarceration. Juvenile correctional facilities generally welcome the involvement of the youth's community PCC if the parents and youth consent.

As Barnert et al point out in their publication aimed at academic pediatricians: "Opportunities exist in clinical care, research, medical education, policy, and advocacy for pediatricians to lead change and improve the health status of youth involved in the juvenile justice system."[50]

AAP Policy

American Academy of Pediatrics Committee on Adolescence. Health care for youth in the juvenile justice system. *Pediatrics*. 2011;128(6):1219–1235 (pediatrics. aappublications.org/content/128/6/1219)

References

1. Laub JH. A century of delinquency research and delinquency theory. In: Rosenhein MK, Zimring FE, Tanenhaus DS, Dohn B, eds. *A Century of Juvenile Justice*. Chicago, IL: University of Chicago Press; 2002:179–205
2. Grossberg M. Changing conceptions of child welfare in the United States, 1820–1935. In: Rosenhein MK, Zimring FE, Tanenhaus DS, Dohn B, eds. *A Century of Juvenile Justice*. Chicago, IL: University of Chicago Press; 2002:3–41
3. Government Affairs Office, Division for Public Education, American Bar Association. Juvenile Justice and Delinquency Prevention Act. American Bar Association Web site. https://www.americanbar.org/advocacy/governmental_legislative_work/priorities_policy/criminal_justice_system_improvements/juvenile_justice_delinquency_prevention_act.html. Updated June 2016. Accessed March 8, 2018
4. King M. *Guide to the State Juvenile Justice Profiles*. Pittsburgh, PA: National Center for Juvenile Justice; 2006
5. Scott ES, Steinberg L. Adolescent development and the regulation of youth crime. *Future Child*. 2008;18(2):15–33
6. Snyder HN, Sickmund M. *Juvenile Offenders and Victims: 2006 National Report*. Washington, DC: US Dept of Juvenile Justice and Delinquency Prevention; 2006
7. MacArthur Foundation. Report finds no benefit to sending juvenile offenders to expensive institutional placements [press release]. Chicago, IL: MacArthur Foundation; December 9, 2009. https://www.macfound.org/press/press-releases/report-finds-no-benefit-to-sending-juvenile-offenders-to-expensive-institutional-placements. Accessed March 8, 2018
8. National Juvenile Justice Network. *Advances in Juvenile Justice Reform, 2007-2008*. Washington, DC: National Juvenile Justice Network. http://www.njjn.org/uploads/digital-library/NJJN-Advances_2007-2008.pdf. Accessed March 8, 2018
9. National Commission on Correctional Health Care. *Standards for Health Services in Juvenile Detention and Confinement Facilities*. Chicago, IL: National Commission on Correctional Health Care; 2004
10. Juvenile Division. Superior Court of California, County of Santa Clara, Web site. http://www.scscourt.org/court_divisions/juvenile/juvenile_home.shtml. Accessed March 8, 2018
11. Cocozza JJ, Shufelt JL. *Juvenile Mental Health Courts: An Emerging Strategy*. Delmar, NY: National Center for Mental Health and Juvenile Justice; 2006. https://www.ncmhjj.com/resources/juvenile-mental-health-courts-emerging-strategy. Accessed March 8, 2018
12. Males M, Macallair D. *The Color of Justice*. San Francisco, CA: Center on Juvenile and Criminal Justice; 2000. http://www.cjcj.org/uploads/cjcj/documents/coj.pdf. Accessed March 8, 2018
13. Petteruti A, Velázquez T, Walsh N; Justice Policy Institute. *The Costs of Confinement: Why Good Juvenile Justice Policies Make Good Fiscal Sense*. Washington, DC: Justice Policy Institute; 2009. http://www.justicepolicy.org/research/78. Accessed March 8, 2018
14. Merzer M. U.S.: no charges in Florida boot camp death. NBCNews.com Web site. http://www.nbcnews.com/id/36599286/ns/us_news-crime_and_courts/t/us-no-charges-florida-boot-camp-death/#.WrFgppch2Hs. Published April 16, 2010. Accessed March 20, 2018
15. Brown SA. *Trends in Juvenile Justice State Legislation 2001 – 2011*. Washington, DC: National Conference of State Legislatures; 2012. http://www.ncsl.org/documents/cj/trendsinjuvenilejustice.pdf. Accessed March 8, 2018

16. Henggeler SW, Schoenwald SK, Borduin CM, Rowland MD, Cunningham PC, eds. *Multisystemic Treatment of Antisocial Behavior in Children and Adolescents.* 2nd ed. New York, NY: Guilford Press; 2009

17. Hahn RA, Lowy J, Bilukha O, et al. Therapeutic foster care for the prevention of violence: a report on recommendations of the Task Force on Community Preventive Services. *MMWR Recomm Rep.* 2004;53(RR-10):1–8

18. Abrams DE. *A Very Special Place in Life: The History of Juvenile Justice in Missouri.* Jefferson City, MI: Missouri Juvenile Justice Association; 2003

19. Andrews DA, Bonita J, Hoge RD. Classification for effective rehabilitation: rediscovering psychology. *Crim Justice Behav.* 1990;17(1):19–52

20. Lipsey MW. The primary factors that characterize effective interventions with juvenile offenders: a meta-analytic overview. *Vict Offender.* 2009;4(2):124–147

21. Goldstein AP, Nensén R, Daleflod B, Kalt M, eds. *New Perspectives on Aggression Replacement Training: Practice, Research and Application.* Chichester, West Sussex, England: John Wiley & Sons Ltd; 2004

22. Redding RE. The effects of adjudicating and sentencing juveniles as adults: research and policy implications. *Youth Violence Juv Justice.* 2003;1(2):128–155

23. Lipsey MW, Wilson DB. Effective intervention for serious juvenile offenders: synthesis of research. In: Loeber R, Farrington DP, eds. *Serious and Violent Juvenile Offenders: Risk Factors and Successful Interventions.* Thousand Oaks, CA: Sage; 1998:313–345

24. Lipsey MW, Wilson DB, Cothern L. Effective interventions for serious juvenile offenders. *Juv Justice Bull.* 2000. https://www.ncjrs.gov/pdffiles1/ojjdp/181201.pdf. Published April 2000. Accessed March 8, 2018

25. Boulder County IMPACT. Colorado Implementation Collaborative Web site. http://www.coloradoimplementation.com/boulder-county-impact.html. Accessed March 8, 2018

26. Mental Health and Juvenile Justice Collaborative for Change: A Training, Technical Assistance and Education Center and a Member of the Models for Change Resource Center Partnership. *Better Solutions for Youth With Mental Health Needs in the Juvenile Justice System.* Delmar, NY: National Center for Mental Health and Juvenile Justice; 2014. https://www.ncmhjj.com/resources/better-solutions-youth-mental-health-needs-juvenile-justice-system. Accessed March 8, 2018

27. Grisso T, Underwood L. Screening and assessing mental health and substance use disorders among youth in the juvenile justice system. National Center for Mental Health and Juvenile Justice Web site. https://www.ncmhjj.com/resources/screening-assessing-mental-health-substance-use-disorders-among-youth-juvenile-justice-system. Published January 2003. Accessed March 8, 2018

28. Anoshiravani A, Saynina O, Chamberlain L, et al. Mental illness drives hospitalizations for detained California youth. *J Adolesc Health.* 2015;57(5):455–461

29. American Academy of Pediatrics Committee on Adolescence. Health care for youth in the juvenile justice system. *Pediatrics.* 2011;128(6):1219–1235

30. Loeber R, Farrington DP. Never too early, never too late: risk factors and successful intervention for serious and violent juvenile offenders. *Stud Crime Crime Prev.* 1998;7(1):7–30

31. Loeber R, Farrington DP, Petechuk D. *Child Delinquency: Early Intervention and Prevention.* Washington, DC: Office of Juvenile Justice and Delinquency Prevention, Office of Justice Programs, US Dept of Justice; 2003. Child Delinquency Bulletin Series NCJ 186162

32. Juvenile justice fact sheet. In: *Addressing Mental Health Concerns in Primary Care: A Clinician's Toolkit.* Elk Grove Village, IL: American Academy of Pediatrics; 2010

33. Shonkoff JP, Boyce WT, McEwen BS. Neuroscience, molecular biology, and the childhood roots of health disparities: building a new framework for health promotion and disease prevention. *JAMA.* 2009;301(21):2252–2259

34. Donelan-McCall N, Eckenrode J, Olds DL. Home visiting for the prevention of child maltreatment: lessons learned during the past 20 years. *Pediatr Clin North Am.* 2009;56(2):389–403

35. Olds DL, Kitzman H, Hanks C, et al. Effects of nurse home visiting on maternal and child functioning: age-9 follow-up of a randomized trial. *Pediatrics*. 2007;120(4):e832–e845

36. Reynolds AJ, Temple JA, Ou SR, et al. Effects of a school-based, early childhood intervention on adult health and well-being: a 19-year follow-up of low-income families. *Arch Pediatr Adolesc Med*. 2007;161(8):730–739

37. Karoly LA, Kilburn MR, Cannon JS. *Early Childhood Interventions: Proven Results, Future Promise*. Santa Monica, CA: Rand Corp; 2005

38. Forgatch MS, Beldavs ZG, Patterson GR, DeGarmo DS. From coercion to positive parenting: putting divorced mothers in charge of change. In: Kerr M, Stattin H, Engels R, eds. *What Can Parents Do? New Insights Into the Role of Parents in Adolescent Behavior*. Chichester, West Sussex, England: John Wiley & Sons Ltd; 2008:191–209

39. Zhou Q, Sandler IN, Millsap RE, Wolchik SA, Dawson-McClure SR. Mother-child relationship quality and effective discipline as mediators of the 6-year effects of the New Beginnings Program for children from divorced families. *J Consult Clin Psychol*. 2008; 76(4):579–594

40. DeGarmo DS, Patterson GR, Forgatch MS. How do outcomes in a specified parent training intervention maintain or wane over time? *Prev Sci*. 2004;5(2):73–89

41. Webster-Stratton C, Hammond M. Treating children with early-onset conduct problems: a comparison of child and parent training interventions. *J Consult Clin Psychol*. 1997;65(1): 93–109

42. Stouthamer-Loeber M, Loeber R. Lost opportunities for intervention: undetected markers for the development of serious juvenile delinquency. *Crim Behav Ment Health*. 2002;12(1):69–82

43. Assink M, van der Put CE, Hoeve M, de Vries SL, Stams GJ, Oort FJ. Risk factors for persistent delinquent behavior among juveniles: a meta-analytic review. *Clin Psychol Rev*. 2015;42:47–61

44. Sherman FT, Greenstone JH. The role of gender in youth systems: Grace's story. In: Sherman FT, Jacobs FH, eds. *Juvenile Justice: Advancing Research, Policy, and Practice*. Hoboken, NJ: John Wiley & Sons Inc; 2011:131–155

45. Jarjoura GR. *Effective Strategies for Mentoring African American Boys*. Washington, DC: American Institutes for Research; 2013. http://www.air.org/resource/effective-strategies-mentoring-african-american-boys. Accessed March 8, 2018

46. Disruptive impulse-control, and conduct disorder. In: American Psychiatric Association. *Diagnostic and Statistical Manual of Mental Disorders*. 5th ed. Washington, DC: American Psychiatric Association; 2013:462–463

47. Bonin EM, Stevens M, Beecham J, Byford S, Parsonage M. Costs and longer-term savings of parenting programmes for the prevention of persistent conduct disorder: a modelling study. *BMC Public Health*. 2011;11:803

48. Baweja R, Mayes SD, Hameed U, Waxmonsky JG. Disruptive mood dysregulation disorder: current insights. *Neuropsychiatr Dis Treat*. 2016;12:2115–2124

49. Benarous X, Consoli A, Guilé JM, Garny de La Rivière S, Cohen D, Olliac B. Evidence-based treatments for youths with severely dysregulated mood: a qualitative systematic review of trials for SMD and DMDD. *Eur Child Adolesc Psychiatry*. 2017;26(1):5–23

50. Barnert ES, Perry R, Morris RE. Perspectives: juvenile incarceration and health. *Acad Pediatr*. 2016;16(2):99–109

Promoting Mental Health Beyond the Medical Home

Promoting the Mental Health of Young Children

David P. Steffen, DrPH, MSN; Jill Kerr, DNP, MPH; and Jonathan Kotch, MD, MPH

"We, as a society, cannot tolerate the great loss that would result from failure to implement relatively simple interventions early in life that have been shown to boost resilience and protect young children from adverse experiences."

Introduction: What Today's Young Children Face

Demographics

The demographics of young children (aged 0–4) in the United States have changed dramatically during the past 15 years. According to the Pew Research Center,[1] the US Census Bureau estimates from July 1, 2015, indicated for the first time that a majority, 50.2%, of all births, were to women of racial or ethnic minority, many of whom had immigrated to the United States. Most of this growth was from Hispanic births; however, there has been a dramatic decline in births and birth rates since the Great Recession of 2007. Although Hispanics represent the largest population of minority infants, followed by African Americans and Asians, the birth rates declined most for Hispanic women and immigrant women.

The US minority population is younger than its white population and has a large proportion of 20- to 34-year-old women who are at the height of their childbearing years. The "Annual Summary of Vital Statistics,"[2] however, indicates that in 2013 birth rates among 20- to 29-year-olds declined, while birth rates for women 30 to 39 increased. Overall, the birth rate declined to 62.5 births per 1,000 women per year, the lowest rate ever reported.

This demographic change to mostly minority births in the United States is important to child health trends because a large proportion of young children of racial or ethnic minority live in a family with low incomes. More than 20 years of research makes it undeniably clear that poverty can impede development and health. In 2014, more than 44% of children lived in households with incomes of less than twice the federal poverty level (FPL).[3] (See Chapter 17, Children in Poverty.)

Poverty and Toxic Stress

Toxic stressors may include child abuse or neglect, parental substance use disorder, maternal depression, witness to domestic violence, or separation from loved ones. Many children exposed to these stressors go on to develop physical and mental health problems, even into adulthood. Some will be counted among the 11% to 20% of children in the United States who have a behavioral or emotional disorder. Emergency department (ED) visits increased by more than 20% for children 1 to 4 years of age between 2006 and 2011. This increase was likely related to an almost 61% increase in ED use for behavioral disorders, accounting for more than 75% of the patient visit increases for 1- to 4-year-olds.[4]

Toxic stress is strongly associated with income level. Nearly 67% of children with family incomes less than 100% of the FPL have experienced an adverse childhood experience (ACE), as opposed to 27% of children with family incomes above 400% of the FPL.[5]

According to the National Center for Children in Poverty, there are 7 risk factors associated with poverty that contribute most to young children's adversity.

▶ Being born to a teen mother
▶ Being born to a single parent
▶ Being born to a parent with low education
▶ Living in a large family
▶ Experiencing residential mobility
▶ Living in a household without an employed parent
▶ Living in a household without English speakers

Of the 37 million infants and children younger than 6 years, 39% do not have any of the risk factors, 41% have 1 or 2, and 20% have 3 or more.[6] Nearly all children have at least one adverse childhood experience (commonly known as an ACE) during their lifetimes (national average is

3.6). Adverse childhood experiences during early childhood are associated with poor early childhood mental health and social development.[5] See Chapter 13, Children Exposed to Adverse Childhood Experiences, for further discussion.

The Annie E. Casey Foundation annual *Kids Count Data Book* provides a longitudinal tracking of a total of 16 child health indicators with 4 sub-indicators in each of 4 categories: economic well-being, education, health, and family and community. Trends in these categories were highlighted with the release of the 2016 data book.[3] Between 2012 and 2015, there were several encouraging trends: the teen birth rates hit historical lows, the number of families with at least one person with a high school diploma increased slightly, and health insurance coverage increased slightly. However, there were discouraging trends as well: the proportion of children in single-parent homes increased, as did the proportion of children living in high poverty areas. The percentage of young children not in preschool increased to 53%. Individual state data reports show significant variation among states.

Rationale for Intervention During Early Childhood

Events in the early months of life lay a foundation and a future trajectory for every young child's health and development. A strong rationale exists for the very earliest of interventions in the development and growth of children, the proverbial "first 1,000 days," as the marginal effect on child health of therapeutic interventions diminishes over time. The loss aversion argument is also compelling: namely, we, as a society, cannot tolerate the great loss that would result from failure to implement relatively simple interventions early in life that have been shown to boost resilience and protect young children from adverse experiences.

This chapter focuses on several community-level strategies: early home visiting and medical home–visitation programs, medical-legal partnerships, initiatives to improve children's mental health in out-of-home care, Early Intervention (EI) services, and Head Start. It also outlines the role of pediatricians (primary care clinicians [PCCs] and, in some instances, pediatric subspecialists, collectively referred to as *pediatric clinicians*) and other pediatric health care professionals (family physicians, nurse practitioners, physician assistants, and other members of the pediatric medical home team) in advocating for key mental health services that address needs of young children and their families.

Visitation Programs to Enhance Children's Development and Mental Health

Maternal, Infant, and Early Childhood Home Visiting Program

As evidence of the critical importance of intervening early in vulnerable children's lives has mounted, so has interest in early home visiting programs. These programs were initially funded predominantly by small private and public sources, but early home visiting that meets certain outcome criteria has gained Affordable Care Act (ACA) support and other public and private financing, indicative of the confidence that funders have in family-focused health interventions. The Maternal, Infant, and Early Childhood Home Visiting Program (MIECHV), administered by the Health Resources and Services Administration and the Administration for Children and Families, funds states, territories, and tribal entities to develop and implement evidence-based home visiting programs. These programs use models proven to improve maternal and child health and produce other positive outcomes, such as fewer incidents of child abuse and neglect; fewer injuries; better speech development and readiness for school; reductions in behavioral problems, depression, and substance use disorder; and, for mothers, fewer incidents of substance use disorder, increased participation in the labor market, better spacing of births, and decreased necessity of public support.[7]

Programmatic goals, target populations, and interventions may vary, but all programs are delivered in homes by staff trained to improve knowledge, beliefs, and behaviors.[8] By seeing the young child interacting in the home environment with family and developing a caring, trusting relationship, the home visitor can better assess and respond to real needs, develop tailored strategies, and coordinate services for individual families. This format is far superior to standardized one-size-fits-all institutional treatment and appointment scheduling. One major opportunity within home visiting is education regarding online health promotion–related messages and Web sites, including those of the American Academy of Pediatrics (AAP). Many adolescents are used to communicating by cell phone, and the home visitor can introduce the many apps that give opportunities for health-related reminders and information, such as Text4baby, Zero to Three, Bright Futures, The Incredible Years, Triple P – Positive Parenting Program, Familias Unidas, Autism Navigator, and many other information sheets and resources developed by the AAP and the Centers for Disease Control and Prevention.[7,9]

Variations in Programs

The implementation of home visiting programs varies widely. Some programs begin during pregnancy, such as the Nurse-Family Partnership (NFP) and Early Head Start programs, whereas others begin at birth or even later. The length of most programs is 2 to 4 years, which ensures there will be adequate time to develop a strong relationship between parents, child, and home visitor. The background for home visitors' educational preparation ranges from professionals with a bachelor's or master's degree in nursing to paraprofessionals who live in the communities being served, many of whom possess language and cultural skills that match those of the clients.[10] Paraprofessionals have not been proven to be as effective as professional nurses in general home visiting. However, home visitation by community health workers has recently been shown to be cost-effective in some specialized areas of intervention, such as reducing asthma-related hospital care of children.[11]

The varying structure of programs is based on disparate levels of resources and differing goals. Some programs, such as Healthy Families America, have a specific outcome in mind, for example, attempting to prevent child abuse and neglect, while working on generally recognized core activities, such as improving parenting skills and promoting healthy child development.[12] Other programs focus on improving mothers' lives by supporting their efforts to return to school, to postpone subsequent pregnancies, and to earn a living.[13] Programs emphasizing the personal relationship between parents and home visitors, such as Parents as Teachers, Home Instruction of Parents of Preschool Youngsters, and Parent-Child Home Program, can bridge the isolation between families and their communities. By providing social support, empathic relationships, practical assistance, and shared responsibility, home visitors attempt to stimulate and nurture changes in parents' attitudes, knowledge, and behavior.[12]

Home Visiting Program Examples and Results

In 2005, the federal government reauthorized MIECHV funding for 17 home-visitation models that they deemed *evidence-based* and to be meeting certain process and outcome criteria. A variety of home visiting programs were judged to be effective and were therefore reauthorized as part of the ACA in 2010. The federal home visiting program invested close to $2 billion in grants to states to augment and rigorously research home visiting programs. These programs were designed to ameliorate poverty by promoting parental skills and motivation and by linking the community health and social service system to families.[14] Their preliminary findings indicate that home visiting will be most effective in breaking the cycle of poverty when implemented as an integral piece of childhood care systems, which in turn represent a broad commitment to increasing community and caregiver capabilities.

One of the most rigorously evaluated and widely replicated of these programs is the Colorado-based nonprofit NFP model of home visitation. This model is constantly being refined and reevaluated under the guidance of early childhood researcher David Olds, PhD. It supports Eckenrode and colleagues'[15] argument that altering a mother's life course has important implications for her children. A mother's ability to assume responsibilities associated with a steady job and postpone a second pregnancy may make it possible for her to emerge from poverty and focus her efforts on her child. A 19-year follow-up of a randomized trial showed that girls born to high-risk mothers (unmarried and low-income) who had prenatal and infancy home visitation based on the NFP model had significantly less involvement with the criminal justice system, had fewer children, and were less likely to have received Medicaid than were high-risk girls in the comparison group.

Involvement of Fathers

Until recently, the primary focus of home visiting had been almost exclusively on the mother-child relationship. During the past decade, however, there has been outreach to fathers and other family members. The NFP found that nurse home visitation had significantly more fathers in attendance than did paraprofessional home visitation.[8] Recently, Holmberg and Olds[16] reported that father attendance in home visiting was associated with factors such as the number of completed maternal home visits, maternal cohabitation with the partner, being married, and white, non-Hispanic race.

Because the presence of the father is a positive influence on the child's and mother's life (except when he is abusive),[17] it is important to engage him in the family parenting and family functioning process. Paternal presence has generally been low, between 2% and 32% of visits, in the NFP. Reports indicate that some success in engaging men has come from having more "male" types of activities, such as sporting events, outdoor events such as cookouts and picnics, coaching, and martial arts; fathers have been drawn in and then integrated into healthy parenting topics and principles of successful fatherhood.[7]

In their study of the differences in fathers' frequency of attendance, Holmberg and Olds reported that more of the difference was attributable to intangible clinic and nurse visitor characteristics, most likely the skill of the home visitor.[16] This finding brings attention to the vital importance of the quality of interaction between visitor and family, particularly the visitor's ability to bring in, involve, and engage in a conversational relationship with the father. Holmberg and Olds conclude that "the ability to remain interpersonally available to the mother and father in the same visit, attitudes about the role of fathers in the program, skill in advocating for father involvement, [and] comfort in working with fathers will be important next steps for research in this area."

Panter-Brick et al[18] performed a systematic review of the literature regarding father engagement in young families. They found that father or couple effects were rarely considered. They pointed out 7 important disincentives for father engagement in parenting programs: cultural, institutional, professional, operational, content, resource, and policy biases. Their conclusion was that to engage fathers more, there must be significant, conscious efforts to modify parenting programs to reverse the existing, almost unconscious, gender biases.

Attaining Other Outcomes

Results from a variety of programs' evaluations document some change in parents' attitudes as a result of the home visiting programs, and often in their behaviors.[13] Despite promoting the importance of prenatal care and the use of preventive health visits, none of the 6 evaluation studies showed improvements in immunization rates or number of health supervision visits. Results of assessments of children's development and behavior similarly suggested only modest improvement.

All home visiting programs depend on changes in parents' behavior to nurture children's health and development. However, the complexity and variety of the family situations affect the consistency with which a home visiting program can be implemented. To expand and develop home visitation, improved methods are needed to evaluate programs. This evaluation includes examining context, service intensity and units, family engagement, and training and characteristics of home visitors. There needs to be an accurate understanding and measurement of risk. Assessment of the involvement of family members, in addition to that of the mother and child, requires further exploration. Strengthening home visiting programs to produce better outcomes for the children and families requires ensuring that the programs are an integrated component of a system of support rather than a separate intervention model.[9] Results from evaluations of home visiting programs to date suggest that expectations for home visiting without clear standards of technical fidelity and clear, faithful commitment to clients can be only modest and, most important, that home visiting cannot be the only strategy for serving families with young children at risk for poor mental health and development.

Further research is needed on father participation and "organizational, team, and nurse factors.... [P]romising targets of intervention [are] increasing safe, nurturing father involvement in home visits." Dr Olds is increasing efforts to retain nurses: continuity of personnel enhances technical implementation of the program and strengthens the relationship of the nurse with parents. Mothers are reportedly 7 to 8 times more likely to drop out if they lose their current nurse visitor.

Another area of future research in home visitation will be to determine whether models can be generated that maintain the proven effectiveness of nurse visitation while reducing costs and perhaps increasing cultural competence of visitors through pairing community health workers or local parents with a nurse visitor. A recent study[19] showed that a universal prevention model delivered by a nurse–parent educator team reduced unnecessary and after-hours health care use.

Universal Home Visiting

Buoyed by the predominantly positive findings and the experiences of other countries, some advocates in the United States have proposed universal nurse home visiting of families with newborns.[20] The main reason for this proposal is that even the most experienced and educated parents have difficulty with and questions regarding parenting their children, each of whom may have a different temperament. Universal home visiting has the potential to remove the stigma of being high-risk, provide a common experience for all mothers in the region, and foster open dialogue about parenting and the care of children. Universal home-visitation models are more likely to be viewed favorably in cultures that share a communitarian ethic, which is not as widely held a view in the United States.[21]

Medical Home–Visitation Model

An example of a medical home–visitation model is HealthySteps, an early childhood program of Zero to Three, a private nonprofit founded by national and international pediatric leaders, including Shonkoff and Brazleton among others. The program fosters relationships among the key influencers of overall health from birth to age 3: PCCs, parents and families, and comprehensive support services. HealthySteps is an evidence-based, interdisciplinary program that facilitates healthy social-emotional and behavioral development. There are more than 100 pediatric and family practice HealthySteps sites in 15 states in which at-risk young children are required to be "visited" in their pediatric medical "home" by a specifically designated additional staff person, the HealthySteps specialist. This specialist has advanced training in one or more pediatric fields and ensures that children receive appropriate developmental screening and other services, including home visiting when indicated, designed to ensure general child health, focusing particularly on emotional and mental health.[22]

Medical-Legal Partnerships

Legal problems greatly affect health issues. Medical-legal partnerships have been developing since 1993. According to the National Center for Medical-Legal Partnership, there are currently 294 health institutions in 41 states in the United States that have adopted the medical-legal partnership model.[23] O'Toole and colleagues[24] demonstrated that pediatric residents who worked in clinics with social and legal resources had confidence to screen for social determinants of health. These partnerships will become more important with changes in immigration laws, Medicaid, and the ACA.

Partnerships are being formed between PCCs and legal aid, law school students, and pro bono lawyers in the community. Some partnerships are colocated in the clinical setting.[25] They may provide direct legal aid or align strategies with health care services. This model can help improve young children's health and mental health by dealing with legal needs that affect well-being. Some examples of legal needs that affect health are government entitlements, housing (including mitigation of lead exposure), immigration status, domestic violence, and expulsion from child care.

Custody issues are something medical-legal partnerships have traditionally helped with. With the current opioid use crisis, however, more young children are being deprived by death of one or both parents at alarming rates and subsequently raised by grandparents or put into foster care. As of this writing, there have been no studies on the long-term effects on young children's mental health after exposure to the adverse life events associated with this epidemic.

Out-of-Home Child Care

Non-parental child care comes in various types, and any given child may participate in more than one type of non-parental care. In most states, non-parental care of 3 or more unrelated children for 4 or more hours per day at least once a week is considered to be the kind of child care falling under state regulatory authority. A facility providing group care for fewer than 6 babies and children 0 to 5 years of age would be considered a child care home, whereas a facility providing group care for 6 or more such babies and children constitutes a child care center, regardless of the shape of the building in which the care is given. It is important, however, to recognize that these definitions may vary by state. Community-based child health professionals should be aware of the number, location, and variety of early care and education programs operating in their service areas.

According to the US National Household Education Survey, approximately 60% of US babies and children 0 to 5 who are not in kindergarten are in some form of regular, non-parental care every week.[26] Therefore, early care and education programs are the best places to reach groups of such babies and children and their families, between birth and kindergarten entry. The opportunities for promoting health, safety, and psychosocial development are enormous. Primary care clinicians are urged to discuss child care as part of the AAP recommended schedule of anticipatory guidance. In addition, the community-based clinician or designee can support individual child care facilities or the early care and education community in the ways described in the Roles for Child Health Professionals section of this chapter.

Child Care Quality

All states have some way of measuring child care quality (quality rating and improvement systems, or QRIS), and, in some cases, states may attach benefits to higher quality ratings, such as higher reimbursement rates for centers serving children who are eligible for public subsidy. Child health professionals should be aware of how child care centers and homes are rated in order to be better positioned to help families choose the best child care experiences for their children. Information about the availability and quality ratings of local child care facilities can be obtained from Child Care Resource and Referral (CCR&R) agencies. (See http://childcareaware.org for your state and local CCR&R.)

Involvement in the QRIS process at the local or state level is an opportunity for pediatric health care professionals and other child advocates willing to contribute their time to improving the quality of early care and education overall. Children's health and their safety in child care are important components of quality, contributing to their physical, cognitive, and social-emotional development and readiness for school.[27,28] The child health professional can be a powerful advocate for health and safety in child care in the QRIS and state regulatory processes.

Mental Health Promotion in Early Care and Education Programs

The Institute of Medicine and the National Academy of Sciences have documented the positive effects that appropriately timed EI and health promotion services can have on lifelong health and developmental outcomes.[29] However, the quality of early childhood education (ECE) in our country varies greatly.[30] Expulsion rates from early childhood programs are extremely high.[31] Thirty-nine percent of child care providers in Massachusetts reported at least one expulsion in the prior year, for an expulsion rate more than 13 times higher than that of kindergarten through 12th grade.[32] Most of these expulsions are caused by children's challenging behaviors.

Child care can be an effective setting to address children's social, emotional, and behavioral needs. Evidence-based classroom teacher training in promoting mental health and responding to challenging behaviors is available (eg, The Incredible Years at www.incredibleyears.com and Center on the Social and Emotional Foundations for Early Learning at http://csefel.vanderbilt.edu), and the PCC or designee can encourage child care providers to avail themselves of these programs. Child care can also be a focus around which to organize parenting trainings. Finally, child care mental health consultants can work with teachers and parents in the child care setting through education, training, and coaching to address the social-emotional needs of young children to improve mental health outcomes and reduce expulsions.[33,34]

Roles for Child Health Professionals

Chapter Child Care Contact

Most states have a pediatrician member of the AAP Council on Early Childhood serving as the state chapter child care contact (CCCC). Each CCCC is supported in mobilizing efforts to improve the health and safety of children in child care and engage parents in discussions about their options for quality care. The CCCC also serves as a liaison between his or her state AAP chapter and the national AAP regarding early care and education initiatives. Pediatricians and other child health professionals are encouraged to work with their CCCC and to increase their involvement in AAP child care activities.

Child Care Health Consultants

Most states are served by child care health consultants (CCHCs), who are child health professionals with interest in and experience with children, with knowledge of resources and regulations, and who are comfortable linking health resources with facilities that provide primarily education and social services.[35] A fully trained and qualified CCHC can assess the health and safety status of child care facilities; consult collaboratively with child care providers on-site and by telephone or electronic media; help develop or update health policies and procedures; provide referral for health, mental health, and social needs; link children and families to medical and dental homes, children's health insurance programs (including Medicaid and the Children's Health Insurance Program), and services for special health care needs; consult with a child's pediatric clinician about medications as needed, in collaboration with parents or guardians; interpret standards, regulations, and accreditation requirements related to health and safety; and provide technical advice to child care providers, separate and apart from the enforcement role of a regulatory inspector. Pediatric clinicians may receive referrals from CCHCs and in turn work with CCHCs, most of whom are nurses, to facilitate the implementation of medical plans for their patients in out-of-home care. Working together, pediatric clinicians, their designees, and CCHCs can promote quality, health, and safety for child care in their communities.

In response to the need for scientific evidence of the efficacy and cost-effectiveness of the CCHC roles, initial investigations sought to measure the impact of child care health consultation on specific child outcomes, such as injury, upper respiratory tract illness,[36] and emotional health and challenging behaviors.[37,38] Although value was found in promoting specific areas and activities of child care health consultation, a synthesis of the overall impact of the service was not addressed until Alkon et al[39] examined the impact of child care health consultation on ECE program policies and practices in California. They concluded that child care health consultation can improve the written health and safety policies and may improve practices in ECE centers.

Even more recently, researchers not only have demonstrated that child care health consultation can have a favorable impact on child health outcomes[40] but also have shown that child care health consultation is associated with improved health policies and practices and increased access to health care among children in ECE programs. Finally, in a randomized controlled trial, Alkon et al[41] documented a statistically significant decrease in measures of body mass index among children 3 to 5 years of age in ECE programs receiving a nutrition and physical activity intervention delivered by CCHCs.

Early Childhood Mental Health Consultants

An early childhood mental health consultant is a professional with mental health expertise who engages one or more early childhood caregivers and/or family members in a problem-solving and capacity-building intervention implemented within a collaborative relationship that aims to improve the ability of staff, families, programs, and systems to prevent, identify, treat, and reduce the impact of mental health problems among babies and children from birth to age 6 and their families.[42]

In a systematic review of 14 rigorous studies that reported on child-level outcomes of early childhood mental health consultation services, investigators found consistent associations with reductions in teacher-reported externalizing behaviors. (The findings for teacher-reported internalizing behaviors were more mixed.) Teacher ratings of prosocial behaviors were improved in most of the studies that reported on this domain.

Collaboration

Child care health consultation and early childhood mental health consultation each have a place in a system of services to support children and families in out-of-home child care. Pediatric clinicians can work with CCHCs and early childhood mental health consultants to build the capacity of parents and early care and education professionals to enhance positive social-emotional development in all young children in their care as part of a universal approach to mental health promotion.[33]

Early Intervention Services

Pediatricians are specialists in the complex care of children with special health care needs.[43] There is enormous potential and need for the pediatrician to take a central leadership role in care coordination for young children who receive services under the Individuals with Disabilities Education Act (IDEA).

The IDEA is a federal law that dictates how states provide EI services and special education to children with special health care needs. Part C covers babies and toddlers from birth until 3 years of age. Services are outlined in an Individualized Family Service Plan (IFSP). Part B covers children after their third birthday until age 21 years with an Individualized Education Program (IEP), administered by the local education agency.

A child who demonstrates a delay in development, speech, language, gross or fine motor skills, or emotional disturbance may be referred by the pediatric clinician, parent, child care center staff, or hospital staff for evaluation.[44] If the infant or child is younger than 3 years, the public health department does the initial screening in the home or child care center. When the child is between 3 and 5 years of age, the EI team of the public school system evaluates the child, again in a child care center or in a preschool or an EI office associated with the local school system. If the child's delay was not identified until after kindergarten entry, the kindergarten through 12th grade intervention team begins the process. The evaluation is by a multidisciplinary team (not necessarily including the child's PCC). With parental permission, the child is screened and, if found to have significant delays, referred for a full evaluation.

There are different working definitions of disability, and with young children it is often difficult to differentiate between a mental health problem and a behavioral or emotional problem. A functional behavioral assessment must be used to decide whether the behavior is associated with a disability. If the child is eligible for EI or special education services, the team, in collaboration with the parent, determines which services to recommend (occupational therapy, physical therapy, speech-language therapy, special education, or a combination of those) and with what frequency.

The IFSP (for 0- to 3-year-olds) determines whether the services will be in the home or at an office. Some states provide services recommended by the IFSP free of charge; others apply fees. The IEP (3- to 5-year-olds), on the other hand, will determine whether the services will be in either a school or child care setting or an EI office. These services are free of charge. The IDEA regulations require that all services take place in the "least restrictive environment."

Many professionals and paraprofessionals are involved in developing and implementing the IFSPs and IEPs, including, but not limited to, social workers, occupational therapists, physical therapists, speech-language pathologists, nurses, psychologists, early childhood special educators, and pediatric subspecialists. Many PCCs have a low level of involvement in these processes, and some think that an established diagnosis is necessary before making an EI referral. This perception is associated with a decreased rate of referral of children with speech delay, particularly among English-language learners, despite parental concern of inappropriate development.[45]

Parents may not perceive the PCC as part of the care team; however, with PCC involvement there are often improved behavioral outcomes and parent satisfaction.[42] Without specific parental authorization in accordance with HIPAA (Health Insurance Portability and Accountability Act) or

FERPA (Family Educational Rights and Privacy Act), the PCC of an infant or a child receiving EI services may be unaware of goals and progress. However, PCCs can make significant contributions through communication (with parents, therapists, and agencies), information exchange, and service delivery coordination. The PCC has the ability to request a meeting of the EI team or to visit providers in their workplaces. The PCC can attend an IFSP or IEP meeting virtually or by phone. At a minimum, parents should be instructed to bring copies of the plans and updates to be part of the child's medical record. If the PCC is unaware of the EI system or process, the local Area Health Education Center may be available to provide training.

Head Start

Head Start is an evidence-based program of the US Department of Health and Human Services, providing comprehensive ECE, health, nutrition, and parent involvement services to low-income children and their families.[46] Head Start has personnel to ensure program fidelity: health services coordinators, parent services coordinators, and nurse health consultants, nutrition professionals, mental health consultants, oral health consultants, home visitors, and social workers as needed.

Head Start's major goal is to ensure that enrolled children enter elementary school with an educational foundation at least equivalent to that of peers in a family with more economic advantages. In the mid-1990s, in response to the emerging research about the critical importance of development in very early childhood, Early Head Start was developed to serve pregnant women, babies, and toddlers. Eligibility for services is determined by FPL, but factors such as homelessness, child disabilities, foster care, or Supplemental Security Income allow the program to accept some over-income families. Currently, 80% of enrolled children are 3- to 4-year-olds served in preschool classrooms designed to nurture their social, emotional, and behavioral development.[46]

Head Start encourages parents' involvement as classroom volunteers and requires staff to make home visits. In these ways, the program aims to preserve each family's ethnic, cultural, and linguistic heritage. Each Head Start program has a designated staff member, usually with a health-related background, serving as the Head Start health services coordinator. This person systematically evaluates enrolled children's health histories and ensures that each child receives screenings and referrals for preventive medical, dental, vision, nutrition, and mental health services; EI; and service coordination. This evaluation involves coordinating with other program staff who screen the children to ensure age-appropriate developmental, sensory, behavioral, motor, language, social, cognitive, and emotional skills. These screenings are mandated to be conducted by the 40th day of enrollment.[46] Successful follow-up of findings involves partnering with the child's medical home. If the child does not have a medical home, the coordinator links the child's family to a PCC and works to ensure that the child continues to receive comprehensive health care, even after graduating from Head Start.

During the past 50 years, Head Start has served 30 million children and their families. Head Start outcomes have been extensively evaluated, with mixed results. Lee and colleagues[47] looked at data from the Early Childhood Longitudinal Study–Birth Cohort (about 6,950 children) and examined kindergarten readiness (academic skills and social-emotional well-being) in children who had attended Head Start compared with those who had experienced other types of child care (prekindergarten, other center-based care, other non-parental care, or parental care). Head Start participants had higher early reading and math scores than did children who had not been in center-based care; however, the Head Start participants demonstrated higher levels of conduct problems than those in parental care. The benefits of Head Start were more pronounced for children who had low initial cognitive ability, children of parents with low levels of education, and children who attended Head Start for more than 20 hours per week. Puma and colleagues[48] found positive comparative health effects; however, they were not retained after the end of third grade.

Primary care clinicians can serve as referral agents for Head Start and can connect with local Head Start programs in a variety of ways.[49]

▶ Designate a staff person to be the coordinator of interactions with Head Start.

▶ Arrange a meeting early in each school year between the office coordinator and the Head Start health services coordinator.

▶ Have the designated staff member link the practice to Head Start with business cards and educational pamphlets. Consider formalizing a partnership.

▶ Become a member of the Health Services Advisory Committee, which is designed to improve services by connecting with the health community.

▶ Participate in the quarterly, mandated meeting of the Health Services Advisory Committee.

▶ Participate in the development of IFSPs or IEPs for children from the practice who are in Head Start.

▶ Consider arranging a field trip to different types of classrooms (regular education, blended, or self-contained) for pediatric residents, medical students, and office staff.

▶ Volunteer to accept Head Start patients who do not have a medical home.

The Pediatric Clinician as Mental Health Advocate

Pediatric clinicians and other child advocates can have a multilevel impact on improving child mental health by advocating for funding of the programs mentioned in the Child Care Health Consultants and Early Childhood Mental Health Consultants sections of this chapter and by involving themselves as advisers and participants in these programs. In addition, they can work at the community level to ensure that parenting programs and key early childhood mental health services are available and accessible, evidence based, family driven, and linguistically and culturally competent. The pediatric clinician can be a leader in judiciously selecting from among these evidence-based programs that, when matched to local characteristics and strengths, invested in, and run effectively, can be successful in removing road blocks to children's positive mental health and resilience. When vetted interventions are managed well, scaled correctly, and held accountable for results, health effects can be maximized.

Summary

Social determinants of health, such as poverty, and events in the early years of life may create or mitigate toxic stress and lay the foundation for every young child's health and development. A strong rationale exists for the very earliest of interventions in the development and growth of children.

Several community-based approaches have been shown to improve young children's health, education, and mental health outcomes. These approaches include maternal, infant, and early childhood home visiting programs; medical home visitation; medical-legal partnerships; initiatives to improve the quality of out-of-home child care; the EI program; and Head Start. Pediatric clinicians can improve the health and mental health of young children by ensuring that children and families who can benefit from these programs receive them and by involving themselves in advisory and advocacy efforts to improve and sustain them. In addition, child health professionals can advocate for key therapeutic services that address the mental health needs of young children and their families. These services include evidence-based parenting programs as well as psychosocial therapies specific to the young child and family.

AAP Policy

American Academy of Pediatrics Council on Community Pediatrics. Community pediatrics: navigating the intersection of medicine, public health, and social determinants of children's health. *Pediatrics.* 2013;131(3):623–628. Reaffirmed October 2016 (pediatrics.aappublications.org/content/131/3/623)

Garner AS, Shonkoff JP; American Academy of Pediatrics Committee on Psychosocial Aspects of Child and Family Health; Committee on Early Childhood, Adoption, and Dependent Care; and Section on Developmental and Behavioral Pediatrics. Early childhood adversity, toxic stress, and the role of the pediatrician: translating developmental science into lifelong health. *Pediatrics.* 2012;129(1):e224–e231. Reaffirmed July 2016 (pediatrics.aappublications.org/content/129/1/e224)

Gleason MM, Goldson E, Yogman MW; American Academy of Pediatrics Council on Early Childhood, Committee on Psychosocial Aspects of Child and Family Health, and Section on Developmental and Behavioral Pediatrics. Addressing early childhood emotional and behavioral problems. *Pediatrics.* 2016;138(6):e20163025 (pediatrics. aappublications.org/content/138/6/e20163025)

Weitzman C, Wegner L; American Academy of Pediatrics Section on Developmental and Behavioral Pediatrics, Committee on Psychosocial Aspects of Child and Family Health, and Council on Early Childhood; Society for Developmental and Behavioral Pediatrics. Promoting optimal development: screening for behavioral and emotional problems. *Pediatrics.* 2015;135(2):384–395 (pediatrics.aappublications.org/content/135/2/384)

References

1. Cohn D. It's official: minority babies are the majority among the nation's infants, but only just. Pew Research Center Web site. http://www.pewresearch.org/fact-tank/2016/06/23/its-official-minority-babies-are-the-majority-among-the-nations-infants-but-only-just. Published June 23, 2016. Accessed December 29, 2017
2. Osterman MJ, Kochanek KD, MacDorman MF, Strobino DM, Guyer B. Annual summary of vital statistics: 2012–2013. *Pediatrics.* 2015;135(6):1115–1125
3. Annie E. Casey Foundation. *2016 Kids Count Data Book.* Baltimore, MD: Annie E. Casey Foundation; 2016. http://www.aecf.org/resources/the-2016-kids-count-data-book. Accessed December 29, 2017
4. Kerker BD, Zhang J, Nadeem E, et al. Adverse childhood experiences and mental health, chronic medical conditions, and development in young children. *Acad Pediatr.* 2015;15(5):510–517
5. Halfon N, Long P, Chang DI, Hester J, Inkelas M, Rodgers A. Applying a 3.0 transformation framework to guide large-scale health system reform. *Health Aff (Millwood).* 2014;33(11):2003–2011

6. *US Federal Poverty Guidelines Used to Determine Financial Eligibility for Certain Federal Programs: 2017 Poverty Guidelines.* Washington, DC: Office of the Assistant Secretary for Planning and Evaluation; 2017. https://aspe.hhs.gov/poverty-guidelines. Accessed January 2, 2018

7. Forum on Promoting Children's Cognitive, Affective, and Behavioral Health; Board on Children, Youth, and Families; Institute of Medicine; National Research Council. *Strategies for Scaling Effective Family-Focused Preventive Interventions to Promote Children's Cognitive, Affective, and Behavioral Health: Workshop Summary.* Washington, DC: National Academies Press; 2014

8. Olds DL, Sadler L, Kitzman H. Programs for parents of infants and toddlers: recent evidence from randomized trials. *J Child Psychol Psychiatry.* 2007;48(3-4):355–391

9. Azzi-Lessing L. Home visitation programs: critical issue and future directions. *Early Child Res Q.* 2011;26(4):387–398

10. Jones Harden B, Chazan-Cohen R, Raikes H, Vogel C. Early Head Start home visitation: the role of implementation in bolstering program benefits. *J Commun Psychol.* 2012;40(4): 438–455

11. Campbell JD, Brooks M, Hosokawa P, Robinson J, Song L, Krieger J. Community health worker home visits for Medicaid-enrolled children with asthma: effects on asthma outcomes and costs. *Am J Public Health.* 2015;105(11):2366–2372

12. Donelan-McCall N, Eckenrode J, Olds DL. Home visiting for the prevention of child maltreatment: lessons learned during the past 20 years. *Pediatr Clin North Am.* 2009;56(2): 389–403

13. Fergusson DM, Boden JM, Horwood LJ. Nine-year follow-up of a home-visitation program: a randomized trial. *Pediatrics.* 2013;131(2):297–303

14. Minkovitz CS, O'Neill KM, Duggan AK. Home visiting: a service strategy to reduce poverty and mitigate its consequences. *Acad Pediatr.* 2016;16(3)(suppl):S105–S111

15. Eckenrode J, Campa M, Luckey DW, et al. Long-term effects of prenatal and infancy nurse home visitation on the life course of youths: 19-year follow-up of a randomized trial. *Arch Pediatr Adolesc Med.* 2010;164(1):9–15

16. Holmberg JR, Olds DL. Father attendance in nurse home visitation. *Infant Ment Health J.* 2015;36(1):128–139

17. Lundahl BW, Tollefson D, Risser H, Lovejoy MC. A meta-analysis of father involvement in parent training. *Res Social Work Pract.* 2008;18(2):97–106

18. Panter-Brick C, Burgess A, Eggerman M, McAllister F, Pruett K, Leckman JF. Practitioner review: engaging fathers—recommendations for a game change in parenting interventions based on a systematic review of the global evidence. *J Child Psychol Psychiatry.* 2014;55(11): 1187–1212

19. Kilburn MR, Cannon JS. Home visiting and use of infant health care: a randomized clinical trial. *Pediatrics.* 2017;139(1):e20161274

20. Dodge KA, Goodman WB, Murphy RA, O'Donnell K, Sato J, Guptill S. Implementation and randomized controlled trial evaluation of universal postnatal nurse home visiting. *Am J Public Health.* 2014;104(suppl 1):S136–S143

21. Dodge KA, Goodman WB, Murphy RA, O'Donnell K, Sato J. Randomized controlled trial of universal postnatal nurse home visiting: impact on emergency care. *Pediatrics.* 2013;132(suppl 2):S140–S146

22. What is HealthySteps? HealthySteps Web site. https://www.healthysteps.org/article/what-is-healthysteps-11. Accessed January 2, 2018

23. National Center for Medical-Legal Partnership Web site. http://medical-legalpartnership.org. Accessed January 2, 2018

24. O'Toole JK, Burkhardt MC, Solan LG, Vaughn L, Klein MD. Resident confidence addressing social history: is it influenced by availability of social and legal resources? *Clin Pediatr (Phila).* 2012;51(7):625–631

25. Sandel M, Hansen M, Kahn R, et al. Medical-legal partnerships: transforming primary care by addressing the legal needs of vulnerable populations. *Health Aff (Millwood).* 2010;29(9): 1697–1705

26. Mamedova S, Redford J. *Early Childhood Program Participation, From the National Household Education Surveys Program of 2012.* Washington, DC: National Center for Education Statistics, Institute of Education Sciences, US Dept of Education; 2015. NCES 2013-029.REV. https://nces.ed.gov/pubsearch. Published May 2015. Accessed January 2, 2018

27. Banghart P, Kreader JL. *What Can CCDF Learn From the Research on Children's Health and Safety in Child Care?* Washington, DC: Urban Institute; 2012. Brief no. 3

28. Friedman SL, Brooks-Gunn J, Vandell D, Weinraub M. Effects of child care on psychological development: issues and future directions for research. *Pediatrics.* 1994;94(6, pt 2):1069–1070

29. Shonkoff J. From neurons to neighborhoods: old and new challenges for developmental and behavioral pediatrics. *J Dev Behav Pediatr.* 2003;24(1):70–76

30. Fuller B, Kagan SL, Loeb S, Chang Y-W. Child care quality: centers and home settings that serve poor families. *Early Child Res Q.* 2004;19(4):505–527

31. Gilliam WS. *Early Childhood Expulsions and Suspensions Undermine Our Nation's Most Promising Agent of Opportunity and Social Justice.* Princeton, NJ: Robert Wood Johnson Foundation; 2016

32. Gilliam WS, Shahar G. Preschool and child care expulsion and suspension: rates and predictors in one state. *Infants Young Child.* 2006;19(3):228–245

33. Perry DF, Allen MD, Brennan EM, Bradley JR. The evidence base for mental health consultation in early childhood settings: a research synthesis addressing children's behavioral outcomes. *Early Educ Dev.* 2010;21(6):795–824

34. Raver CC, Knitzer J. *Ready to Enter: What Research Tells Policymakers About Strategies to Promote Social and Emotional School Readiness Among Three- and Four-Year-Olds.* New York, NY: National Center for Children in Poverty, Columbia University Mailman School of Public Health; 2002

35. American Academy of Pediatrics, American Public Health Association, National Resource Center for Health and Safety in Child Care and Early Education. *Caring for Our Children: National Health and Safety Performance Standards; Guidelines for Early Care and Education Programs.* Elk Grove Village, IL: American Academy of Pediatrics; 2011

36. Ulione MS. Health promotion and injury prevention in a child development center. *J Pediatr Nurs.* 1997;12(3):148–154

37. Johnson K. Inclusivity in mental health consultation to the childcare community. *Zero Three.* 2000;20(4):15–18

38. Alkon A, Ramler M, MacLennan K. Evaluation of mental health consultation in child care centers. *Early Child Educ J.* 2003;31(2):91–99

39. Alkon A, Bernzweig J, To K, Wolff M, Mackie JF. Child care health consultation improves health and safety policies and practices. *Acad Pediatr.* 2009;9(5):366–370

40. Isbell P, Kotch J, Savage E, Gunn E, Lu L, Weber D. Improvement of child care programs' health and safety policies, and practices, and children's access to health care, linked to child care health consultation. *NHSA Dialog.* 2013;16(2):34–52

41. Alkon A, Crowley A, Neelon S, et al. NAPSACC intervention in child care improves nutrition and physical activity knowledge, policies, practices, and children's BMI. *BMC Pediatr.* 2014; 14:215

42. Duran F, Hepburn K, Irvine M, et al. *What Works? A Study of Effective Early Childhood Mental Health Consultation Programs.* Washington, DC: Georgetown University Center for Child and Human Development; 2009

43. Coker TR, Moreno C, Shekelle PG, Schuster MA, Chung PJ. Well-child care clinical practice redesign for serving low-income children. *Pediatrics.* 2014;134(1):e229–e239

44. Lipkin PH, Okamoto J; American Academy of Pediatrics Council on Children With Disabilities and Council on School Health. The Individuals with Disabilities Education Act (IDEA) for children with special educational needs. *Pediatrics.* 2015;136(6):e1650–e1662

45. Silverstein M, Sand N, Glascoe FP, Gupta VB, Tonniges TP, O'Connor KG. Pediatrician practices regarding referral to early intervention services: is an established diagnosis important? *Ambul Pediatr.* 2006;6(2):105–109

46. US Department of Health and Human Services Head Start Bureau. *Head Start Program Performance Standards and Other Regulations.* Washington, DC: Administration for Children and Families, Administration on Children, Youth and Families; 2015

47. Lee R, Zhai F, Brooks-Gunn J, Han WJ, Waldfogel J. Head Start participation and school readiness: evidence from the Early Childhood Longitudinal Study–Birth Cohort. *Dev Psychol.* 2014;50(1):202–215

48. Puma M, Bell S, Cook R, et al. *Third Grade Follow-up to the Head Start Impact Study: Final Report.* Washington, DC: Administration for Children and Families; 2012. OPRE Report 2012-45

49. Bull MJ. Consider working with Head Start/Early Head Start to meet needs of vulnerable patients. *AAP News.* 2014;35(1):8

Promoting the Health of Adolescents

Breena Welch Holmes, MD, and Paula M. Duncan, MD

"Primary care clinicians and other child advocates can have a positive effect on adolescents' development by helping to create opportunities for all young people to feel connected, to learn to make good decisions, to help others, and to develop skills such as managing stress and taking responsibility for their own behaviors."

Introduction

Adolescence presents unique challenges for health promotion. The role of schools as the primary community of children and adolescents is the topic of Chapter 31, Promoting Mental Health in Schools. This chapter focuses on the role of the larger community in helping adolescents to develop autonomy and explore new behaviors. Through community-based systems of care, pediatricians, family physicians, nurse practitioners, and physician assistants (hereafter referred to as *primary care clinicians* [PCCs]) can partner with community organizations and service providers to promote healthy outcomes and deliver high-quality preventive and treatment services to adolescents.

Frameworks for Healthy Adolescent Development

Protective factors are individual or environmental characteristics, conditions, or behaviors that reduce the effects of stressful life events, increase an individual's ability to avoid risks or hazards, and promote social-emotional competence to thrive in all aspects of life now and in the future. One of these factors is resilience, the ability to cope with and adapt to change. Being resilient allows children and adolescents to overcome difficulties in their lives.

In the 1990s, researchers developed a framework of developmental assets, that is, the strengths and resources that promote positive development in adolescents as they transition from childhood. The Search Institute, a social science research group, identified 40 positive factors that promote healthy development in young people. A greater number of assets in the lives of adolescents correlate with fewer risk-taking behaviors.[1]

Primary care clinicians and other child advocates can have a positive effect on adolescents' development by helping to create opportunities for all young people to feel connected, to learn to make good decisions, to help others, and to develop skills such as managing stress and taking responsibility for their own behaviors. The components of healthy adolescent development can be characterized according to 3 prominent frameworks: Protective Factors, Strengths, and Developmental Tasks; Circle of Courage; and the 7 Cs Model of Resilience.

Protective Factors, Strengths, and Developmental Tasks

Bright Futures: Guidelines for Health Supervision of Infants, Children, and Adolescents, the 2017 preventive services guidelines, describes the individual protective factors, strengths, and developmental tasks of adolescence (Box 30-1).

Circle of Courage

Another way to describe the opportunities adolescents need to thrive is the Circle of Courage, a framework used by Brendtro and colleagues, who identified generosity, independent decision-making, mastery, and belonging as essential to a healthy adolescence.[2] Ideally, the activities adolescents pursue at the community level would provide opportunities to develop these qualities.

7 Cs Model of Resilience

Lerner and Pittman's work has identified 5 Cs (competence, confidence, connection, character, and caring) as key components of a positive youth development framework, and Lerner and colleagues tested them through their 4-H study work.[3] On the basis of his work with young people, Ginsburg has added coping and control to the original 5 Cs.[4]

In his book *Reaching Teens: Strength-Based Communication Strategies to Build Resilience and Support Healthy Adolescent Development,* Ginsburg describes a strengths-based approach and core principle. He also describes "wisdom from model" strengths-based programs that work with adolescents who are traditionally labeled "at risk."[5]

Box 30-1. Individual Protective Factors, Strengths, and Developmental Tasks of Adolescence

- Forming caring and supportive relationships with family members, other adults, and peers
- Engaging in a positive way with the life of the community
- Engaging in behaviors that optimize wellness and contribute to a healthy lifestyle
- Demonstrating physical, cognitive, emotional, social, and moral competencies (including self-regulation)
- Exhibiting compassion and empathy
- Exhibiting resiliency when confronted with life stressors
- Using independent decision-making skills
- Displaying a sense of self-confidence, hopefulness, and well-being

Derived from Hagan JF, Shaw JS, Duncan PM, eds. *Bright Futures: Guidelines for Health Supervision of Infants, Children, and Adolescents.* 4th ed. Elk Grove Village, IL: American Academy of Pediatrics; 2017.

Assessing the Adolescent Environment

Adolescents need opportunities to grow in each of the areas just outlined (eg, opportunities to help others, to practice independent decision-making, and to establish relationships with peers). Families often provide a setting for this growth and development, but by adolescence school activities, community organizations, faith-based groups, and sports teams often supply young people with development opportunities. The inventory in Box 30-2 can help PCCs assess their respective communities' programs and services for adolescents.

Box 30-2. Strengths-Based Practices Inventory

- Does the program help adolescents feel respected, valued, and treated as if they are knowledgeable and capable?
- Does the program help adolescents and families acquire knowledge, skills, and self-confidence to do things for themselves?
- Does the program focus on helping adolescents and families develop positive relationships within their own lives?

Derived from Green BL, McAllister CL, Tarte JM. The Strengths-Based Practices Inventory: a tool for measuring strengths-based service delivery in early childhood and family support programs. *Fam Soc.* 2004;85(3):326–334.

Pediatric PCCs who work toward positive adolescent development in their communities should also be familiar with the information in Table 30-1.

Sabaratnam and Klein have identified and tested an inventory tool for use by community organizations for assessment and implementation of the positive youth development approach.[6]

Kretzmann and McKnight have also developed a framework for use at the community level.[7]

Table 30-1. Features of Community-Based Positive Developmental Settings

Feature	Descriptors	Opposite Poles
Physical and psychological safety	Safe and health-promoting facilities and practices that increase safe peer group interaction and decrease unsafe or confrontational peer interactions.	Physical and health dangers; fear; feelings of insecurity; sexual and physical harassment; verbal abuse.
Appropriate structure	Limit setting; clear and consistent rules and expectations; firm enough control; continuity and predictability; clear boundaries; age-appropriate monitoring.	Chaotic; disorganized; laissez-faire; rigid; overcontrolled; autocratic.
Supportive relationships	Warmth; closeness; connectedness; good communication; caring; support; guidance; secure attachment; responsiveness.	Cold; distant; overcontrolling; ambiguous support; untrustworthy; focused on winning; inattentive; unresponsive; rejecting.
Opportunities to belong	Opportunities for meaningful inclusion, regardless of one's gender, ethnicity, sexual orientation, or disabilities; social inclusion, social engagement, and integration; opportunities for sociocultural identity formation; support for cultural and bicultural competence.	Exclusion; marginalization; intergroup conflict.
Positive social norms	Rules of behavior; expectations; injunctions; ways of doing things; values and morals; obligations for service.	Normlessness; anomie; laissez-faire practices; antisocial and amoral norms; norms that encourage violence; reckless behavior; consumerism; poor health practices; conformity.
Support for efficacy and mattering	Youth based; empowerment practices that support autonomy; making a real difference in one's community; being taken seriously. Practices that include enabling, responsibility granting, and meaningful challenge. Practices that focus on improvement rather than on relative current performance levels.	Unchallenging; overcontrolling; disempowering; disabling. Practices that undermine motivation and desire to learn, such as excessive focus on current relative performance level rather than improvement.

Table 30-1. Features of Community-Based Positive Developmental Settings (*continued*)

Feature	Descriptors	Opposite Poles
Opportunities for skill building	Opportunities to learn physical, intellectual, psychological, emotional, and social skills; exposure to intentional learning experiences; opportunities to learn cultural literacies, media literacy, communication skills, and good habits of mind; preparation for adult employment; opportunities to develop social and cultural capital.	Communities that promote bad physical habits and habits of mind; practices that undermine school and learning.
Integration of family, school, and community efforts	Concordance; coordination; synergy among family, school, and community.	Discordance; lack of communication; conflict.

Reproduced with permission from *Community Programs to Promote Youth Development*. Copyright © 2002, National Academy of Sciences. Courtesy of the National Academies Press, Washington, DC.

Positive Adolescent Development Focus

As part of their preventive services visits with each adolescent, adolescent PCCs identify individual patient strengths through developmental surveillance, give feedback about progress on the developmental tasks to the patient and (if appropriate) the patient's parents, and practice shared decision-making when a change needs to be made. As community members, they play an additional role. On the basis of their roles as board members, team physicians, volunteer coaches, community health leaders, and parents, they provide consultation about using the positive youth development approach and advocating for this approach with funders.[8] Primary care clinicians understand the importance of community partners in the lives of adolescents.[9] These partners may include state and national organizations of the American Academy of Pediatrics (AAP), state health departments, schools, faith-based organizations, and community organizations such as 4-H and Boys & Girls Clubs of America. Primary care clinicians can advocate for programs that have demonstrated effectiveness by being aware of what programs work for promoting healthy adolescent development. For example, Lerner and colleagues have reported that participants in 4-H, when compared with young people in other out-of-school programs, had better outcomes in healthy behaviors, academic competence, school engagement, and community contribution.[3] The Big Brothers Big Sisters of America mentoring programs evaluation in 2013 has shown improved social acceptance among participants compared with youths who have not yet been matched with a mentor. When followed over time, participants also showed improvement or maintenance of scholastic competence, educational expectations, attitudes toward risky behavior, and parental trust.[9,10] Opportunities for community service are also associated with risk reduction among adolescents; for this reason, the Community Preventive Services Task Force of the Centers for Disease Control and Prevention recommends youth development–focused behavioral interventions coordinated with community service.[11]

In recent years, many youth advocacy organizations have become more aware of, and focused on, positive youth development strategies.[6]

In addition, pediatric practices often have a staff person who is in charge of knowledge about and links to community resources. Among these resources are programs with a positive adolescent development focus or proven efficacy for easy referral of patients seen for preventive services and acute care visits in the medical home.

Risk Reduction Focus

Health promotion activities at the community level also focus on the prevention of the 6 risk behaviors that result in the greatest morbidity and mortality for adolescents and adults: unhealthy nutrition, inadequate physical activity, unhealthy sexual behaviors, substance use and use disorder, unintentional injury–related behaviors, and intentional injury–related behaviors.

Pediatric PCCs can provide consultation to other child advocates on risk reduction in a specific area. This consultative role can result from personal interest or expertise on the part of a clinician or in response to a critical need identified among the patient population or in the community (eg, prescription drug misuse or teen suicide), identified by community partners such as local public health or community mental health agencies.

Recent research has identified several community-based strategies for adolescent risk reduction. Safe, supervised recreational activities and physical activity promote healthy development. Neighborhoods and communities can work together with health professionals to improve the built environment. Researchers have shown that increasing the percentage of park space in a neighborhood increases the percentage of 8- to 12-year-olds without overweight.[12] Undoubtedly, there are mental health benefits as well.

Retail environments that support healthy choices are also important to an adolescent's mental health, especially the adolescent's decision-making regarding nutrition, tobacco, and alcohol. Pediatric PCCs can advocate for laws to regulate the marketing and sale of nonnutritious food, tobacco, and alcohol to adolescents.

Communities can also promote healthy attitudes about sexuality. Accepting one's changing body and exploring sexual feelings and identity are among the developmental tasks of adolescence.[13] Pediatric PCCs can advocate for medically accurate sexuality education in schools and for an emotionally and physically safe environment for young people who are gay, lesbian, bisexual, or transgender. The Centers for Disease Control and Prevention Community Preventive Services Task Force has identified competence, improved decision-making, self-determination, and improved communication skills as critical components in a recommended sexuality risk reduction program.

Community-based substance use disorder prevention is most effective when it involves programs to help individuals develop skills along with policies that support healthy behaviors. Communities must make enforcement of these policies a high priority.[14]

A physically safe environment is also critical to healthy adolescent development. School programs about bullying and Internet safety can contribute to a community-wide effort to promote a positive climate. (See Chapter 31, Promoting Mental Health in Schools.) Injury prevention at the community level might include safe driving legislation and enforcement, seat belt and bike helmet legislation, and gun violence prevention.

Pediatric PCCs are ideal advocates for wellness and mental health support for adolescents and can encourage opportunities for strength-building activities. Nutrition, exercise, sleep, sunshine, reading, music, sports, and spirituality all contribute to an adolescent's sense of well-being.[15] These factors are essential components of a strategy to promote mental health. Communities also need ongoing resource development to help adolescents in crisis, those experiencing problems in school, and those in need of mental health treatment.

Schools continue to play a vital role in adolescents' mental health. See Chapter 31, Promoting Mental Health in Schools, for an in-depth discussion of the Whole School, Whole Community, Whole Child model (www.ascd.org/programs/learning-and-health/wscc-model.aspx) and the various ways schools can promote mental health and resilience through initiatives that address bullying, promote Internet safety, prevent suicide, incorporate trauma-informed practices, address drop-out risks, and provide healthy extracurricular activities. Schools can also offer mental health screening and referral or provide on-site treatment services that are typically more accessible and less stigmatizing than community-based mental health services or do both. Pediatric advocates can partner with mental health advocates to seek school policies that create a healthy climate for students and funding for school-based mental health services.

Media can have significant effects on adolescent health behavior choices. Opportunities for education about safe, effective, and healthy media use can be promoted by families, schools, health care professionals, and community organizations.[16]

Finally, pediatric PCCs are a valuable source of support for parents and guardians, who may benefit from an understanding of strengths and positive youth development.[17,18] Building on relationships often forged when children were much younger, the medical home provides adolescents and their families a supportive extension of the community. A helpful resource for parents is the AAP publication *Building Resilience in Children and Teens: Giving Kids Roots and Wings*.

Ginsburg's book *Reaching Teens*[5] is an excellent guide to implementation of the strengths-based approach for health care professionals, social workers, educators, and all professionals who work in youth-serving organizations.

Adolescents in Special Circumstances

Pediatric PCCs should recognize the special needs of certain groups within a community and strive to create opportunities for these vulnerable young people. Adolescents with special health care needs and vulnerable families who, because of income level or geography, lack access to social, cultural, and economic resources can be supported by health care professionals, public health professionals, and community organizations. The section Care of Special Populations, in this book, addresses concerns for those exposed to adverse childhood experiences; families new to the United States; children and adolescents in foster or kinship care; youths from military families; those who are lesbian, gay, or bisexual; youths with gender expression and identity issues; those in gay- and lesbian-parented families; those in self-care; those facing homelessness; those affected by racism; adolescents who are pregnant or parenting; and adolescents in the juvenile justice system.

Conclusion

Pediatric PCCs play a vital role in ensuring that their communities support the developmental tasks of adolescence. Bright Futures provides specific guidance to assist: Box 30-3 identifies specific recommendations.

A comprehensive, coordinated approach promotes healthy outcomes among adolescents. Pediatric PCCs are an essential component of this

Box 30-3. Recommendations for Promoting Community Relationships and Resources

- Learn about the community, understand its culture, and collaborate with community partners.

- Recognize the special needs of certain groups (eg, people who have recently immigrated to the United States, families of children with special health care needs).

- Link families to needed services.

- Establish relationships and partnerships with organizations and agencies that serve as local community resources, including schools and early care and education programs.

- Encourage adoption of referral networks that have demonstrated effective partnerships with medical homes and parents of young children.

- Consult and advocate in partnership with groups and organizations that serve the community, such as schools, parks, and recreation agencies; businesses; and faith groups.

- Encourage parents to find support in family, friends, and neighborhoods.

- Encourage families and all children and adolescents, especially adolescents, to become active in community endeavors to improve the health of their communities.

- Consider colocating in the medical home mental health, care coordination, oral health, legal, social service, or parenting education professionals to address unmet needs of families.

Derived from Hagan JF, Shaw JS, Duncan PM, eds. *Bright Futures: Guidelines for Health Supervision of Infants, Children, and Adolescents.* 4th ed. Elk Grove Village, IL: American Academy of Pediatrics; 2017.

cooperative effort. Health promotion for adolescents involves the medical home, community-based organizations, schools, parents and guardians, and the adolescents themselves. By helping to develop strengths-based programs, reduce risks to health and safety, and foster the growth of developmental assets, pediatric PCCs can encourage positive adolescent development.

Acknowledgments
Additional information: Coauthor Paula M. Duncan died October 25, 2017.

AAP Policy

American Academy of Pediatrics Committee on Adolescence. Achieving quality health services for adolescents. *Pediatrics.* 2008;121(6):1263–1270. Reaffirmed March 2013 (pediatrics.aappublications.org/content/121/6/1263)

American Academy of Pediatrics Council on Communications and Media. Media use in school-aged children and adolescents. *Pediatrics.* 2016;138(5):e20162592 (pediatrics.aappublications.org/content/138/5/e20162592)

References

1. Scales PC, Leffert N. *Developmental Assets*. Minneapolis, MN: Search Institute; 1999
2. Brendtro LK, Brokenleg M, Van Bockern S. *Reclaiming Youth at Risk: Our Hope for the Future*. Bloomington, IN: Solution Tree; 2002
3. Lerner RM, Lerner JV, et al. *The Positive Development of Youth: Comprehensive Findings From the 4-H Study of Positive Youth Development*. Chevy Chase, MD: National 4-H Council; 2013. http://www.4-h.org/About-4-H/Research/PYD-Wave-9-2013.dwn. Accessed January 2, 2018
4. Ginsburg KR, Jablow MM. *Building Resilience in Children and Teens: Giving Kids Roots and Wings*. 3rd ed. Elk Grove Village, IL: American Academy of Pediatrics; 2015
5. Ginsburg KR, Kinsman SB, eds. *Reaching Teens: Strength-Based Communication Strategies to Build Resilience and Support Healthy Adolescent Development*. Elk Grove Village, IL: American Academy of Pediatrics; 2014
6. Sabaratnam P, Klein JD. Measuring youth development outcomes for community program evaluation and quality improvement: findings from Dissemination of the Rochester Evaluation of Asset Development for Youth (READY) tool. *J Public Health Manag Pract*. 2006;(suppl):S88–S94
7. Kretzmann JP, McKnight JL. *Discovering Community Power: A Guide to Mobilizing Local Assets and Your Organization's Capacity*. Chicago, IL: Asset-Based Community Development Institute, Northwestern University; 2005
8. Hagan JF, Shaw JS, Duncan PM, eds. *Bright Futures: Guidelines for Health Supervision of Infants, Children, and Adolescents*. 4th ed. Elk Grove Village, IL: American Academy of Pediatrics; 2017
9. Davis WS, Berry P, Shaw JS. Using Bright Futures to improve community child health. *Pediatr Ann*. 2008;37(4):232–237
10. Valentino S, Wheeler M. *Big Brothers Big Sisters Report to America: Positive Outcomes for a Positive Future; 2013 Youth Outcomes Report*. Tampa, FL: Big Brothers Big Sisters of America; 2013. http://bbbsnew.org/wp-content/uploads/YOS2013.pdf. Accessed January 2, 2018
11. Community Preventive Services Task Force. HIV/AIDS, other STIs, and teen pregnancy: youth development behavioral intervention to reduce sexual risk behaviors in adolescents coordinated with community service. The Community Guide Web site. https://www.thecommunityguide.org/findings/hivaids-other-stis-and-teen-pregnancy-youth-development-behavioral-interventions-reduce-2. Published October 2007. Accessed January 2, 2018
12. Roemmich JN, Epstein LH, Raja S, Yin L, Robinson J, Winiewicz D. Association of access to parks and recreational facilities with the physical activity of young children. *Prev Med*. 2006; 43(6):437–441
13. American Academy of Pediatrics Committee on Psychosocial Aspects of Child and Family Health, and Committee on Adolescence. Sexuality education for children and adolescents. *Pediatrics*. 2001;108(2):498–502
14. Practicing effective prevention. Substance Abuse and Mental Health Services Administration Web site. https://captus.samhsa.gov/prevention-practice/prevention-approaches. Updated January 11, 2016. Accessed January 2, 2018
15. American Academy of Pediatrics Adolescent Sleep Working Group, Committee on Adolescence, and Council on School Health. School start times for adolescents. *Pediatrics*. 2014;134(3):642–649
16. American Academy of Pediatrics Council on Communications and Media. Media use in school-aged children and adolescents. *Pediatrics*. 2016;138(5):e20162592
17. Frankowski BL, Leader IC, Duncan PM. Strength-based interviewing. *Adolesc Med State Art Rev*. 2009;20(1):22–40
18. Eccles J, Gootman JA, eds. *Community Programs to Promote Youth Development*. Washington, DC: National Academies Press; 2002

Promoting Mental Health in Schools

Barbara L. Frankowski, MD, MPH; Stephanie Daniel, PhD; and Howard Taras, MD

"The nature and quality of school health and mental health programs can affect pediatric clinicians' success with disease management as well as illness and injury prevention."

Introduction

Mental health problems affect about 1 in 5 school-aged children. In the United States, about 1 in every 4 to 5 adolescents and young adults aged 13 to 18 has a mental disorder with impairment in functioning during that person's lifetime. Negative impacts can be observed on children's and adolescents' abilities to function within their families, with their peers, and in the school environment. Some of the more common mental disorders that students experience include attention disorders, autism spectrum disorder, anxiety disorders, depression, oppositional defiant and conduct disorders, disordered eating, and substance use. Many of these problems are revealed for the first time as children enter the more complex social environment of school, with the added demands of formal education. In fact, some of these problems are identified in the school before the child's primary care clinician (PCC) (pediatrician, family physician, internist, nurse practitioner, or physician assistant who provides frontline, longitudinal care) becomes aware of them.

Children with mental health problems often experience lower educational achievement than their peers do.[1] Indeed, untreated mental health needs and physical health problems are substantial barriers to school learning and academic success for children and adolescents.[2] Less than 25% of children and adolescents with mental health problems, however, have received treatment within the past 6 months,[3] and only 36% have received treatment in their lifetimes.[4] Surprisingly, of the estimated 36% of children who receive treatment for their mental health issues, nearly two-thirds receive treatment only at school.[5]

Pediatric clinicians (PCCs and pediatric subspecialists, collectively) need to be aware of the context beyond the family that is supporting the child. They can be advocates for improvement of their communities. For school-aged children, the most influential community setting is the school. Because 98% of school-aged children attend public, charter, or private school,[6] it is not surprising that schools have an enormous influence, both positive and negative, on the health and well-being of our nation's children. The nature and quality of school health and mental health programs can affect pediatric clinicians' success with disease management as well as illness and injury prevention. Moreover, pediatric clinicians can influence the nature and quality of these programs. Pediatric clinicians need familiarity with how schools work, knowledge of how to work with schools on behalf of their patients, and knowledge of advocacy techniques that help improve school health programs. Armed with this knowledge, pediatric clinicians can influence the health of their own school-aged patients.

This chapter outlines the role of schools in supporting healthy mental, emotional, and behavioral development of children; how schools can help identify problems and offer initial treatment; and how pediatric clinicians, schools, and communities can work together to help meet the needs of children with more serious mental, emotional, and behavioral problems.

The Whole School, Whole Community, Whole Child Model

The Whole School, Whole Community, Whole Child (WSCC) model combines and builds on elements of the traditional coordinated school health approach and the whole-child framework (Figure 31-1). In the WSCC model, the child is the center of the model, with emphasis placed on the relationship between the healthy development and educational attainment of the child. The child is encircled by the whole-child tenets: being healthy, safe, engaged, supported, and challenged. Achieving this requires alignment, integration, and collaboration among the school, health, and community sectors, to improve each child's learning and health. Next, the 10 components that provide the full range of learning and health support systems to each child, in each school, in each community, are listed: health education; physical education and physical activity; nutrition environment and services; health services; counseling, psychological, and social services; social and emotional climate; physical environment; employee wellness; family engagement; and community involvement. Finally, community

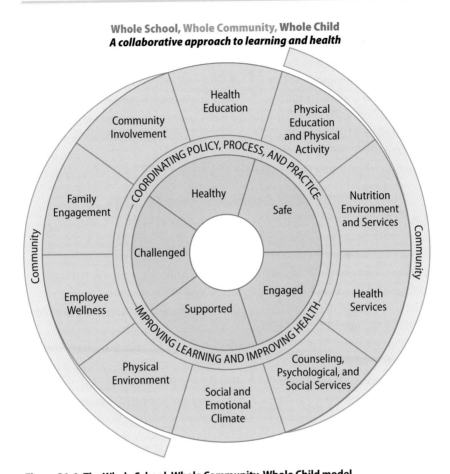

Whole School, Whole Community, Whole Child
A collaborative approach to learning and health

Figure 31-1. The Whole School, Whole Community, Whole Child model.
From Whole School, Whole Community, Whole Child. ASCD Web site. http://www.ascd.org/programs/
learning-and-health/wscc-model.aspx. Accessed January 2, 2018.

input, resources, and collaboration are needed to support students in
achieving optimal health and learning.

ASCD (Association for Supervision and Curriculum Development) and
the Centers for Disease Control and Prevention (CDC) encourage use of the
WSCC model as a framework for improving students' learning and health
in our nation's schools.

Many communities have local school health advisory council (SHAC)
or other community or school-level wellness committees that convene
throughout the year to address issues associated with the health, wellness,
and safety of their local school-aged children and adolescents. Some states

require the establishment of annual SHAC or wellness committee goals to address these issues broadly for children and teens in their communities. Pediatric clinicians may have opportunities to contribute to their local SHAC or other community or school-level wellness committee initiatives. Information about committees like these in your area can typically be obtained from your school district or from your health department. Additional information about SHACs can also be found by searching for the Department of Public Education or Board of Education for your state or by searching your state's Department of Health and Human Services Web site.

Youth Risk Behavior Survey Findings

The CDC Youth Risk Behavior Surveillance System (YRBSS)[7] uses the Youth Risk Behavior Survey (YRBS) to monitor 6 priority health-risk behaviors that contribute to the leading causes of death and disability among adolescents and adults: behaviors that contribute to unintentional injuries and violence; tobacco use; alcohol and other drug use; sexual behaviors related to unintended pregnancy and sexually transmitted infections (STIs), including HIV infection; unhealthy dietary behaviors; and physical inactivity. The YRBSS includes school-based national, state, and large urban school district YRBSs conducted among representative samples of students in grades 9 through 12. A middle school survey is also conducted in interested states and communities. The YRBS has been conducted biennially since 1991. Additional information about YRBSS is available at www.cdc.gov/healthyyouth/data/yrbs/index.htm. Individual states can add additional questions to their YRBS; the results of these state surveys are often found on state health department Web sites. Pediatric clinicians can usually obtain results for school districts and individual schools from school district superintendents or their local health departments. These data do not link to individual students; rather, they provide a valuable snapshot of some of the risky behaviors reported by students from a specific school district.

Information about behaviors affecting mental health can be helpful for pediatric clinicians working with schools. For example, YRBS (2015) data from high school students revealed that

▶ Of those students, 29.9% reported that in the past 12 months they had felt so sad or hopeless almost every day for 2 or more weeks in a row that they stopped doing some usual activities.

▶ Furthermore, 17.7% of students responding contemplated suicide, 14.6% made a plan, and 8.6% attempted suicide in the previous 12 months.

▶ In addition, 20.2% of students reported being bullied on school property in the previous 12 months.

▶ A total of 63.2% reported ever drinking alcohol, with 32.8% reporting drinking in the past 30 days.

▶ Also, 38.6% reported ever using marijuana, with 21.7% using in the past 30 days.

▶ Finally, 5.2% reported ever using cocaine; 6.4%, ever using a hallucinogen; 7.0%, ever using an inhalant; and 16.8%, ever using a prescription medication (such as stimulants meant for treating attention-deficit/hyperactivity disorder [ADHD]) that was not their own.

Students of Sexual and Gender Minorities

Students who orient or identify as lesbian, gay, bisexual, transgender, or questioning (LGBTQ) are an especially vulnerable population. In 2015, 2 questions ascertaining sexual or gender minority status were added to the national YRBS for the first time. The prevalence of all the risk behaviors listed previously are significantly higher among those orienting or identifying as LGBTQ.[8]

Another source of information about sexual and gender minority students comes from the National School Climate Survey, a biennial report that began in 1999 and includes a sample of more than 10,000 secondary students from all 50 states and the District of Columbia.[9] It is sponsored by GLSEN (Gay, Lesbian and Straight Education Network). The 2015 survey report showed that

▶ **Most LGBTQ students have experienced harassment and discrimination at school.** Eighty-five percent experienced verbal harassment, and 66% experienced LGBTQ-related discrimination at school. Because of feeling unsafe or uncomfortable, 32% of students missed at least 1 day of school in the past month, and many avoided bathrooms (39%) and locker rooms (38%).

▶ **Hostile school climates negatively affect LGBTQ students' educational outcomes and mental health.** Lesbian, gay, bisexual, transgender, and questioning students who experienced high levels of victimization were twice as likely to report they do not plan to pursue postsecondary education, had lower grade point averages, had lower self-esteem, and had higher levels of depression.

▶ **School-based supports have a positive effect on school climate.** Lesbian, gay, bisexual, transgender, and questioning students in schools with a GSA (gay-straight alliance) or a comprehensive antibullying policy experienced lower levels of victimization. Also, students with an LGBTQ-inclusive curriculum were more likely to report that their classmates were somewhat or very accepting of LGBTQ students (76% vs 42%, respectively).

▶ **School climates are slowly improving for LGBTQ students.** Lesbian, gay, bisexual, transgender, and questioning students reported a decrease in homophobic remarks. The incidence of harassment and assault related to sexual orientation was also lower than in prior years. (Changes in harassment and assault based on gender expression were similar to those for sexual orientation.)

School-Based Mental Health Services

There are numerous barriers to obtaining needed mental health services, with lack of adequate insurance coverage, nationwide and local shortages of appropriate professionals, stigma, and transportation being among the major ones. School-based mental health services are continuing to evolve as a strategy to address these concerns, by removing barriers to accessing mental health services and improving coordination of those services. School-based mental health services offer the potential for prevention efforts that positively affect school climate, as well as screening and intervention strategies. Existing school-based mental health services range from minimal support services provided by a school counselor to comprehensive, integrated programs of prevention, identification, and treatment within a school. In some schools, comprehensive mental health services are provided in an existing school-based health center (SBHC). Pediatric clinicians should become familiar with the mental health services that already exist in the schools that serve their patient populations.

In 2004, the American Academy of Pediatrics (AAP) Committee on School Health published a policy statement on school-based mental health services[10] that set out a 3-tiered model of services and needs as a way to categorize components of a school's mental health program (Table 31-1). This model still holds true today, and it is a good way for a pediatric clinician to assess the services that are currently available for patients who are students at a particular school.

Tier 1: Systems for Positive Development and Systems of Prevention

The first tier includes a variety of preventive mental health programs and services. Activities in this tier are designed to target all children in all school

Table 31-1. A Three-Tiered Model of School-Based Services

Tier	Target Population	Examples of School Resources[a]	Examples of Community Resources[a]
Tier 1: Systems for Positive Development and Systems of Prevention [primary prevention (low-end need/low cost per student programs)]	All students in all school settings	• Enrichment and education • General health education • Promotion of social-emotional development • Drug and alcohol education • Support transitions • Conflict resolution • Parent involvement	• Youth development programs • Public health and safety programs • Prenatal care • Immunizations • Recreation and enrichment • Child abuse education
Tier 2: Systems of Early Intervention [early-after-onset problems (moderate need, moderate cost per student)]	Students with identified MH needs, function well enough to engage in daily activities	• Pregnancy prevention • Violence prevention • Drop-out prevention • Learning/behavior accommodations • Work programs	• Early identification to treat health problems • Monitoring health problems • Short-term counseling • Foster placement/group homes • Family support • Shelter, food, and clothing • Job programs
Tier 3: Systems of Care [treatment of severe and chronic problems (high-end need/high cost per student)]	Students with more severe MH symptoms and diagnoses, require multiple services	• Special education for learning disabilities, emotional disturbance, and other health impairments	• Emergency/crisis treatment • Family preservation • Long-term therapy • Probation/incarceration • Disabilities programs • Hospitalization

Abbreviation: MH, mental health.
[a] Include facilities, stakeholders, programs, and services.
Adapted with permission from Adelman HS, Taylor L. Mental health in schools: moving in new directions. *Contemp School Psychol.* 2012;16(1):9–18.

settings. Preventive programs focus on decreasing risk factors and building resilience, including providing a positive, friendly, and open social environment at school, and they focus on ensuring that the school is LGBTQ friendly, culturally competent, and trauma informed. Each student should have access to community and family supports associated with healthy emotional development.

School Connectedness

A sense of student connectedness to schools has a positive effect on academic achievement and decreases risky behaviors.[11] Social-emotional well-being is important to student motivation and engagement in learning; interventions that address this well-being can foster connectedness and are likely to promote successful student academic adjustment.[12] For example, schools should provide students with varied curricular and extracurricular activities (beyond sports programs) to increase the chances that each student will experience success in some aspect of school life. Schools should strive to provide opportunities for positive individual interactions with adults at school so each student has positive adult role models and opportunities to develop a healthy relationship with an adult outside his or her family. *School connectedness*, that is, the belief held by students that adults and peers in the school care about their learning as well as about them as individuals, is an important protective factor. Research has shown that young people who feel connected to their school are less likely to engage in many risk behaviors, including early sexual initiation; alcohol, tobacco, and other drug use; and violence and gang involvement. Students who feel connected to their school are also more likely to have better academic achievement, including higher grades and test scores; to have better school attendance; and to stay in school longer. See www.cdc.gov/healthyyouth/protective/school_connectedness. htm for more information about school connectedness.

School Policies

Behavioral expectations, rules, and discipline plans should be well publicized among teachers and school staff, students, and their parents and guardians. Often these expectations are outlined in the school handbook or school district handbook (or both) and distributed to students and their families at the beginning of a school year. These materials may also be posted on the school Web site or school district Web site (or both) for easy access.

Positive Behavioral Interventions and Supports

Teachers often need assistance with behavior management and use of positive behavior incentives. One of the foremost advances in school-wide discipline is the emphasis on school-wide systems of support that include proactive strategies for defining, teaching, and supporting appropriate student behaviors to create positive school environments. Instead of using a piecemeal approach of individual behavior management plans, all school staff members implement a continuum of positive behavioral support for all students within a school in multiple areas, including the classroom and nonclassroom settings (such as hallways, buses, and restrooms). Positive Behavioral Interventions and Supports (PBIS) is a proactive approach to establishing the behavioral supports and social culture needed for all students in a school to achieve social, emotional, and academic success. Attention is focused on creating and sustaining primary (school-wide), secondary (classroom or other groups of students), and tertiary (individual) systems of support that improve lifestyle results (eg, personal, health, social, family, recreation) for all students by making targeted misbehavior less effective, efficient, and relevant and desired behavior more functional. Pediatric clinicians should determine whether the PBIS system is being implemented in area schools, and they can encourage and provide support and guidance to school staff who are working with students with identified mental health issues or challenges. Additional training and resources about PBIS are available at www.pbis.org.

Physical Activity
Pediatric clinicians can advise schools about the benefits of physical activity to health and academic success, and they can encourage schools and parents to avoid eliminating recess and other physical activities as consequences for misbehavior.[13] Physical activity and exercise can help with decreasing behavioral problems for some students.

Health Education and Sexuality Education
A major component of the WSCC model is health education, including sexuality education. Beginning in the 1970s, concerns over teen pregnancy, and later HIV/AIDS, prompted widespread public support for sex education in schools. Most states today have a policy requiring HIV education, usually in conjunction with broader sex education. As of March 1, 2016,[14]

▶ Twenty-four states and the District of Columbia require public schools to teach sex education (21 of which mandate sex education and HIV education).

▶ Thirty-three states and the District of Columbia require students to receive instruction about HIV/AIDS.

▶ Twenty states require that, if provided, sex education and HIV education must be medically, factually, or technically accurate.

The Guttmacher Institute maintains an updated list of state-level sex and HIV education requirements on its Web site (www.guttmacher.org/state-policy/explore/sex-and-hiv-education).

Beyond teaching facts about preventing STIs and about early, unintended pregnancy (which is costly to our health care and social welfare systems), sexuality education in school provides the opportunity to augment what students learn at home and elsewhere and to reinforce positive behavioral expectations around relationships. At its best, sexuality education is a lifelong process of acquiring information and forming attitudes, beliefs, and values. It encompasses sexual development, sexual and reproductive health, interpersonal relationships, affection, intimacy, body image, and gender roles, sexual orientation, and gender identity. However, what sexuality education looks like can vary widely from school to school. Pediatricians and other health care professionals are encouraged to know what is happening at their state levels as well as in local school districts. Pediatric clinicians can turn to many reliable sources when advocating for optimal sexuality education in schools. See, for example, "Sexual Risk Behaviors: HIV, STD, and Teen Pregnancy Prevention" at www.cdc.gov/healthyyouth/sexual behaviors and Sexuality Information and Education Council of the United States at www.siecus.org. Refer also to Chapter 12, Healthy Sexual Development and Sexuality, for further information.

Substance Use Prevention

Schools are appropriate settings for drug prevention programs for 3 reasons[15]: prevention must focus on children before their beliefs and expectations about psychoactive substances are established, schools offer the most systematic way of reaching young people, and schools can promote a broad spectrum of drug-related educational policies.

Many curricula designed for school use have been proven to be effective and are delivered to students in ways that are interesting, interactive, and developmentally appropriate.[16,17] Although many program approaches are available, some effective programs focus on enhancing students' problem-solving skills or aiding them to evaluate the influence of the media. Other effective programs help improve students' self-esteem, reduce stress and anxiety, or increase activities. One of the most studied programs is LifeSkills Training,[18] a universal school-based prevention approach (most often implemented among seventh graders) that teaches general personal and social skills training combined with drug-refusal skills and normative education. LifeSkills Training produces positive behavioral effects on reducing alcohol, tobacco, and illicit drug use.

Discipline

Publication of the Adverse Childhood Experiences Study has informed many professionals that stress and psychological trauma experienced by children can increase the probability of developing mental disorders that may initially manifest as behavioral problems.[19] These adverse childhood experiences range from sexual abuse, grief and loss, parental divorce or separation, exposure to violence, child abuse or neglect, and parental illicit use of drugs to natural disasters, school crises, military deployments, familial mental illness, and poverty. Schools should strive to train their faculties in trauma-informed interactions and discipline and should avoid out-of-school suspension and expulsion as first-line consequences for many behavioral problems at school.[20] Pediatric clinicians can assist schools in reframing behavioral problems as potential mental health issues and can recommend further assessment and therapy for students as an alternative to a disciplinary approach.

Trauma-Informed Schools and Restorative Justice

In recent years, school districts have begun to examine what motivates students' atypical behaviors and to identify other methods of discipline, rather than simply adopting a zero-tolerance attitude that may exclude the student from his or her educational opportunities and classmates to keep others on campus safe. *Restorative justice* is a discipline approach that brings all parties together to resolve conflict, promote academic achievement, and address school safety.[21] In some schools, these techniques are being taught to staff members as well as to student leaders as a way to deal with multiple school-related issues, ranging from bullying to disruptive behaviors in the classroom.[22]

Schools are increasingly recognizing that many students have been traumatized by abuse, neglect, and exposure to homelessness, family violence, and extreme poverty. These problems impede students' ability to focus and learn and to function respectfully. Trauma-informed care is a method for teachers that not only acknowledges these barriers to learning but also provides teachers with tools to address these issues. The basis of these tools is to make these students feel safe at school, understood, and "heard."[23,24] In some schools, mental health specialists work with teachers, school administrators, and school nurses to use evidence-based approaches such as cognitive behavioral strategies and mindfulness techniques to lower the stress levels of students and reduce the maladaptive effects of trauma on their school functioning.[25] For more information about interventions applicable to students affected by trauma, see www.samhsa.gov/nctic/trauma-interventions.

Bullying Prevention

Bullying is unwanted, aggressive behavior among school-aged children that involves a real or perceived power imbalance. The behavior is repeated, or has the potential to be repeated, over time. Both students who are bullied and students who bully others may have serious, lasting emotional and behavioral problems. Because bullying is so widespread, every school should have activities in place that address bullying prevention and clear policies that define the consequences and the action steps that take place when bullying is reported or discovered. Extensive resources for schools that include student, parent, and community involvement can be found through the CDC at www.stopbullying.gov.

Suicide Prevention

A variety of suicide prevention programs are available for schools, including some specifically developed to increase awareness among students, teachers, and parents of the warning signs and risk factors for suicidal behavior. Talk Saves Lives and More Than Sad are 2 programs developed by the American Foundation for Suicide Prevention (AFSP). Many states have local AFSP chapters that can provide trainings to schools or can provide some of these training materials to the schools within their state for free or at reduced costs. If your state does not have a local chapter, you can contact AFSP directly through their Web site (https://afsp.org).

Schools should have an effective protocol in place to respond to a local adolescent suicide in order to prevent "copycat" suicides.[26-28]

Tier 2: Systems of Early Intervention

The second tier consists of targeted mental health services that are designed to help students who have identified mental health needs but who function well enough to engage successfully in social, academic, and other daily activities. Services in this tier could include the provision of group or individual therapy to students identified with ADHD, social anxiety, mild depression, substance use, issues with bullying, and other common behavioral or mental health issues (eg, anger management, self-control, social relatedness), depending on what resources are available at the school. In an effort to enhance education outcomes for all children and adolescents, some states have piloted an approach referred to as an *interconnected systems framework*. This approach is intended to integrate PBIS with school-based mental health services. Additional information about this approach, including implementation guides, is available online (www.pbis.org/school/school-mental-health/interconnected-systems).

School-based mental health services increase protective factors and reduce risk factors among students. As reported by Albright and colleagues,[29] examples of improved outcomes include

▶ Treating depression in adolescents

▶ Increasing positive self-esteem

▶ Improving family relationships

▶ Improving academic performance

▶ Decreasing symptoms of depression and anxiety resulting from bullying

For students in special education with learning difficulties and who also have behavioral issues, this tier may consist of either the behavioral components of these students' Individualized Education Programs (commonly known as IEPs) or the individual health service plans that address these students' behavioral issues.

Staff Training in Recognition of Mental Health Problems

Mental Health First Aid (www.mentalhealthfirstaid.org) is training program available to school personnel and other community citizens (including pediatric clinicians) in many states. Mental Health First Aid is an 8-hour course that helps individuals to understand and recognize signs of mental health illness and addiction and to know how to respond appropriately.

Attention-deficit/Hyperactivity Disorder

Attention-deficit/hyperactivity disorder (with and without hyperactivity) is a chronic disorder that affects 4% to 12% of 6- to 12-year-olds, and it results in challenging personal, clinical, educational, and societal problems. Attention-deficit/hyperactivity disorder often first presents in the school environment, and the school is an important partner in the diagnosis and management. The AAP publication *ADHD: Caring for Children With ADHD; A Resource Toolkit for Clinicians,* 2nd Edition, is a recommended source of information for those treating these children, adolescents, and young adults.

Like pediatric clinicians, school personnel find ADHD both challenging and time-consuming to manage, and many educators may have little accurate knowledge about ADHD. Communication and coordination of efforts among students, families, schools, community mental health agencies, and pediatricians can be daunting. With motivation and effort, however, communities can identify ways to coordinate services for students. One such community effort in North Carolina[30] resulted in a consensus of school personnel and community PCCs on all the following shared operating procedures:

1. Ideal ADHD assessment and management principles (facilitated by the AAP guidelines for children 6–12 years of age)

2. An inventory of relevant services currently available in the community
3. A common entry point (a team) at schools for children needing assessment because of inattention and classroom behavioral problems, whether the problems present first to a medical provider, the behavioral health system, or the school
4. A protocol followed by the school system, recognizing the schools' resource limitations but meeting the needs of community health care professionals for classroom observations, psychological testing, parent and teacher behavior rating scales, and functional assessments
5. A packet of information about each child who is determined to need medical assessment
6. A contact person or team at each PCC's office to receive the packet from the school and direct it to the appropriate clinician
7. An assessment process that investigates comorbidities and applies appropriate diagnostic criteria
8. Evidence-based interventions
9. Processes for follow-up monitoring of patients after establishment of a treatment plan
10. Roles for central participants (school personnel, PCCs, school nurses, and mental health specialists) in assessment, treatment, and follow-up monitoring of students with attention problems
11. Forms for collecting and exchanging information at every step
12. Processes and key contacts for flow of communication at every step
13. A plan for educating school and health care professionals about the new processes

Substance Use Rehabilitation

Illicit drug use usually has negative consequences on students' academic, social, and behavioral performance at school.[31] Schools may offer after-school programs, incorporating life-skills training into drug education curricula, helping parents become better informed, providing counseling, identifying problem behaviors for early intervention, and promptly referring students to health care professionals for detailed assessment and intervention. School-based health centers have the capacity to counsel students who need such treatment plans or to refer students to other available evaluation and treatment resources within the community (or to do both).

Schools may be able to partner with rehabilitation programs to provide care for individual students and help successfully reintegrate them. The school's roles in such a collaborative relationship may include identifying any underlying learning disabilities that may have contributed to the problem, making special accommodations for students when necessary, providing remedial work so students can catch up with their classmates, helping reinforce expectations for students to attend school and to adhere to follow-up or monitoring as prescribed by the health care professional or rehabilitation facility, and assisting with finding after-school programs. Involved PCCs, mental health specialists, or rehabilitation programs should identify any mental health diagnoses and notify the schools of their relevance to the student's safety at school, to the student's educational program, and to school personnel or operations in general. (Check state confidentiality regulations regarding need for student consent.) Health care professionals should also provide schools with treatment plans (such as individual health plans or 504 plans) that may affect the school day while maintaining the student's confidentiality to the extent that is possible.

Learning Differences and Disorders
Learning difficulties and learning disorders make it more difficult for students to keep up with their classmates and can therefore cause behavioral and social problems, contribute to anxiety and depression, and lead to substance use as a coping mechanism. It is important to identify students struggling with learning difficulties as early as possible to offer appropriate assistance and prevent further comorbidities.

Drop-Out Prevention
While multiple factors contribute to risk for dropping out of school, adolescent mental health seems to play a role in student drop-out. Major depressive disorder, disruptive behavioral disorders, and substance use disorders have been found to be associated with school drop-out.[32,33] Stoep and colleagues[34] found that greater than 50% of US adolescents who drop out of school have a psychiatric disorder and that the disorder itself is responsible for the drop-out decision (with rates of disorder ranging anywhere from 44%–61% among adolescents with low socioeconomic status [SES] to high SES, respectively). Among children and adolescents with mental health problems, chronic absenteeism and behavioral problems in the classroom may contribute to poor academic progress and success and, in turn, increase risk for school drop-out in adolescence.[20]

Tier 3: Systems of Care
The third tier of health services targets the smallest population of students and addresses needs of those with more severe mental health symptoms and diagnoses. These students may require the services of a multidisciplinary team of professionals, usually including special education services,

individual and family therapy, pharmacotherapy, and care coordination among school, medical home, pediatric subspecialty practice if involved, and social agencies. In addition, most schools will want to have specialized emergency plans in place that would enable school personnel to respond quickly to incidents such as a suicide death, or other traumatic death, of a student in the school or a violent act or natural disaster in the community.

School-Based Mental Health Service Delivery Models

One of the realities in many communities is that, for children with limited access to mental health services, schools are often the major de facto mental health specialist, even though school personnel (social workers, guidance counselors, psychologists, and school nurses) are often tasked with many other responsibilities, including administration and supervision of testing; management and oversight of qualification for special educational services for students; responding to truancy, including spending time in truancy court; and developing care plans for students diagnosed as having chronic disease or illness. A growing number of school systems are adding school-based mental health screening, evaluation, and treatment services to address this gap.

School-based mental health services increase children's and adolescents' access to mental health services and help their families overcome many of the barriers (eg, financial or economic, transportation, cultural, geographic, other family circumstances) associated with getting more traditionally rendered mental health services.[35] Currently, several different models of school-based mental health services are provided in some schools across the United States.

Mental Health Screening and Referral

Some schools may have strong medical home or community connections that allow expedited referral for early treatment. These schools may choose to have screening procedures in place for early identification of issues such as depression or substance use. There are many benefits to screening students who are experiencing learning or behavioral problems or who are otherwise at risk for social, emotional, and academic problems (Box 31-1).

The Rapid Assessment for Adolescent Preventive Services (www.possibilitiesforchange.com/raaps) is an example of a proprietary evidence-based risk assessment tool that includes built-in educational materials for school-based health providers to use with students and their families; this tool can be incorporated into a school-based health clinic

Box 31-1. Benefits of Screening for Mental Health Problems in School

- Screening identifies students with immediate needs and those who need further mental health assessment.

- Screening helps identify mental health needs and other risk factors that may contribute to child and adolescent morbidity and mortality, and it provides opportunities for educating patients and their families about strategies for reducing risk.

- Screening allows school health or mental health providers the opportunity to connect identified students to services, potentially ameliorating conditions that are affecting learning and behavior.

- Screening provides opportunities for coordinating referral and treatment efforts across school and community health and mental health providers and agencies to prevent duplication of service efforts and to improve the continuity of care.

setting to be used as a previsit "intake questionnaire" prior to annual health care visits, prior to mental health visits, or at other times when the student needs to be evaluated for risky behaviors. This tool can also be administered repeatedly over time to monitor changes in risk behaviors for a given student. In addition, the AAP *Bright Futures Tool and Resource Kit* (https://brightfutures.aap.org/materials-and-tools/tool-and-resource-kit/Pages/default.aspx) contains previsit questionnaires for assessing risks, forms for chart documentation, and educational information appropriate for use in school-based clinic settings with students and their parents or guardians.

There are a number of evidence-based screening tools that school-based clinicians can choose to use within their practices to identify risk for mental health problems as well as other health risks. Many of these tools are public domain tools that are available for free, while others are available for purchase. (See Chapter 1, Healthy Child Development, and Appendix 2, Mental Health Tools for Pediatrics.)

If access to early treatment or prompt referral is not available, it is not advisable to institute screening in schools.

Care Coordination and Counseling

Students with emotional disabilities are at a higher risk of dropping out of school compared with students without emotional disabilities.[36] To decrease drop-out rates and increase access to mental health services, additional care coordination and counseling services are currently being integrated within many public schools. Some schools have targeted efforts to students with poor attendance records or other risk factors associated with risk for dropping out of school. For example, school staff may be designated to schedule regular meetings, both individual and group, with this high-risk group of students. The meetings develop personal connections and relationships between school staff and students by offering guidance and problem-solving to address barriers to school success and by rewarding students' accomplishments through verbal feedback, praise, and small incentives. Services may also involve collaborations with local mental health agencies, partnerships with universities, and services funded and operated by school or local mental health entities, as described in the following section.

Mental Health Services Within Comprehensive School-Based Health Centers

School-based health centers are widely recognized as a critical resource for early screening, evaluation, and treatment of mental (and physical) health problems among school-aged children and adolescents.[10,35,37] Some comprehensive SBHCs provide the full range of medical and nursing care, mental health care, and nutrition services to enrolled students. The focus in this model is treating the whole child. Comprehensive school-based care can be provided in a brick-and-mortar facility located on the campus of the school or on a mobile medical unit (providing opportunities to serve more than one school within a given school district or region). Research suggests that there is decreased stigma associated with receiving mental health services in an SBHC setting relative to community health centers and providers: students are 10 to 21 times more likely to come to an SBHC for mental health services than a community health center or another community provider.[38] When the comprehensive SBHC is not considered the primary medical home, care should be coordinated with the medical home. The care provided is intended to complement, rather than compete with, existing primary care services.

Combined Mental Health and Nursing Services

Other SBHCs operate under a wellness center model, providing nursing services and the services of a licensed mental health provider in tandem. Again, care provided under this model is ideally coordinated with the medical home and other members of the school team.

Other schools in the United States use a School-Based Child and Family Support Team model (an example of which can be found at https://childandfamilypolicy.duke.edu/project/evaluation-of-school-based-child-and-family-support-teams-initiative-100-schools-project). The purpose of this model is to identify and coordinate appropriate services and support for children at risk of school failure or out-of-home placement by addressing the physical, social, legal, emotional, and developmental factors that affect academic performance. Referrals are generated through self-referral by students or from school personnel and families. Teams composed of a clinical school social worker and a registered nurse assess and offer interventions specific to the need of the student and the student's family through direct service or referral to appropriate resources in the community.

School-Based Mental Health Treatment Without Medical or Nursing Services

Some models of school-based care focus primarily on the provision of mental health services for students, coordinating care with other health care providers and community agencies as needed. For example, in one child psychiatry consultation model in North Carolina, students can receive psychiatric consultation and care planning by a psychiatrist on-site at schools.[39] Therapy services rendered by a licensed mental health provider are also available in some models of child psychiatry consultation programs. Referrals for these services can be made by school personnel, juvenile justice personnel, or PCCs. Within this model of care, options are available for the psychiatrist to assume the care and treatment of the student's psychiatric condition or to evaluate the student, develop a care plan, and direct the student back to the referring clinician for ongoing treatment and medication management in the medical home and ongoing consultation with the psychiatrist. Other variations on this model of psychiatric consultation exist. The National Network of Child Psychiatry Access Programs (http://web.jhu.edu/pedmentalhealth/nncpap_members.html) is a resource for identifying what psychiatric consultation services might be available to you within your state.

Telepsychiatry is also being explored as an option. The University of Arizona Telemedicine Program, for example, serves patients in areas of limited accessibility. One psychiatrist provides telemental health services to adolescents and their families on the Navajo reservation using a wireless telecommunications system with direct connections into the 2 high school clinics in Tuba City, AZ. Mental health services are provided without the students' leaving their schools.[40]

Another example of mental health–only services on-site at schools involves expanding the roles of existing school support staff to provide mental health assessment and treatment services. Some school social workers or guidance counselors may be assigned to schools where they provide mental health evaluation and treatment services, in addition to fulfilling their more traditional roles and responsibilities within other assigned schools.

Other schools provide contracted mental health services for their students involving an outside organization or mental health agency that establishes a working relationship with a school system. Contracted agencies have a designated mental health professional assigned to one or more schools to provide counseling services. Universities, for example, may collaborate with local public schools to provide mental health services in the school setting. Graduate students often provide supervised counseling and care management services to students for course credit or as volunteer experience. Under these circumstances, graduate student trainees are supervised by a licensed professional from their university. Pediatric clinicians can contact their local universities to see if such a program exists or could be developed.

All these mental health–only models of school-based care provide opportunities for increasing access to mental health services for students on-site at schools, eliminating many of the barriers to accessing mental health services within the community.

With all models of care, coordination of services with the primary medical home is paramount to ensure all the child's or adolescent's needs are met and to avoid duplication of services. Partnerships with other community agencies are also important to ensure the needs of the student and family are fully met. Mental health services offered in schools are intended to complement initiatives focused on a positive school climate.

Community Connections

Pediatric clinicians can find additional information about working with schools from the AAP Council on School Health Web site (www.aap.org/en-us/about-the-aap/Committees-Councils-Sections/Council-on-School-Health/Pages/School-Health.aspx) or the School-Based Health Alliance Web site (www.sbh4all.org).

Pediatric clinicians may also find it beneficial to become familiar with the contact person(s) in the neighboring school districts who can help them navigate their school mental health system or systems. In some instances, the first contact could be the school nurse, a school social worker, or the guidance counselor. Box 31-2 lists key knowledge necessary for establishing a relationship with a local school. In addition, some states have a State School Nurse Consultant located within the Department of Health or Department of Education who may also be helpful. Check with your local AAP chapter to determine if there is a local AAP Council on School Health contact.

Box 31-2. Establishing a Relationship With Local Schools

- Identify contact person(s) at school or district level (eg, school nurse, social worker, guidance counselor).

- Learn rules around establishing communication about an individual student (confidentiality forms that may need to be signed by family, as well as HIPAA and FERPA regulations[a]).

- Determine what services are already in place.

- Identify community agencies that can assist with social determinants of health (external stressors): housing, clothing, employment, safety in neighborhoods, after-school care. Some states may have already established 211 or Help Me Grow call centers.

- Identify emergency referral sources.

- Establish community mental health referral sources.

Abbreviations: HIPPA, Health Insurance Portability and Accountability Act; FERPA, Family Educational Rights and Privacy Act.

[a] The US Department of Health and Human Services provides guidance on HIPAA and FERPA regulations as they relate to children and adolescents in schools (www.hhs.gov/hipaa/for-professionals/faq/ferpa-and-hipaa).

Summary

Ideally, schools are places where students are healthy, safe, engaged, supported, and challenged. Schools may also be places where children and adolescents receive mental health services not otherwise available or not as easily accessed in their communities. Schools have opportunities to promote students' mental health through programs that ensure a positive climate for sexual and gender minorities, school connectedness for all students, positive behavior incentives, trauma-informed discipline policies, physical activity, sexuality education, parent and family engagement, and other tier-1 preventive strategies. They can also implement tier-2 strategies to identify emerging mental health problems and facilitate or provide care and tier-3 strategies to provide multidisciplinary systems of care for students who are experiencing significant social, emotional, behavioral, or mental health problems. A number of school-based service delivery models have been developed. Effective collaboration among school personnel, pediatric clinicians, and community mental health and social service providers is a key element in the success of these school-based models and, in turn, the students served by these models.

AAP Policy

American Academy of Pediatrics Adolescent Sleep Working Group and Committee on Adolescence. School start times for adolescents. *Pediatrics*. 2014;134(3):642–649 (pediatrics.aappublications.org/content/134/3/642)

American Academy of Pediatrics Council on School Health. Out-of-school suspension and expulsion. *Pediatrics*. 2013;131(3):e1000–e1007 (pediatrics.aappublications. org/content/131/3/e1000)

American Academy of Pediatrics Council on School Health. Role of the school nurse in providing school health services. *Pediatrics*. 2016;137(6):e20160852 (pediatrics. aappublications.org/content/137/6/e20160852)

American Academy of Pediatrics Council on School Health. School-based health centers and pediatric practice. *Pediatrics*. 2012;129(2):387–393 (pediatrics. aappublications.org/content/129/2/387)

Breuner CC, Mattson; American Academy of Pediatrics Committee on Adolescence and Committee on Psychosocial Aspects of Child and Family Health. Sexuality education for children and adolescents. *Pediatrics*. 2016;138(2):e20161348 (pediatrics. aappublications.org/content/138/2/e20161348)

Levy S, Schizer M; American Academy of Pediatrics Committee on Substance Abuse. Adolescent drug testing policies in schools. *Pediatrics*. 2015;135(4):782–783 (pediatrics.aappublications.org/content/135/4/782)

Levy S, Schizer M; American Academy of Pediatrics Committee on Substance Abuse. Technical report—adolescent drug testing policies in schools. *Pediatrics*. 2015;135(4): e1107–e1112 (pediatrics.aappublications.org/content/135/4/e1107)

Schonfeld DJ, Demaria T; American Academy of Pediatrics Committee on Psychosocial Aspects of Child and Family Health and Disaster Preparedness Advisory Council. Supporting the grieving child and family. *Pediatrics*. 2016;138(3):e20162147 (pediatrics.aappublications.org/content/138/3/e20162147)

References

1. Stagman S, Cooper JL. *Children's Mental Health: What Every Policymaker Should Know*. New York, NY: National Center for Children in Poverty; 2010. http://www.nccp.org/publications/pdf/text_929.pdf. Accessed January 3, 2018
2. Brown MB, Bolen LM. The school-based health center as a resource for prevention and health promotion. *Psychol Sch*. 2008;45:28–38
3. Jensen PS, Goldman E, Offord D, et al. Overlooked and underserved: "action signs" for identifying children with unmet mental health needs. *Pediatrics*. 2011;128(5):970–979
4. Merikangas KR, He J, Burstein M, et al. Service utilization for lifetime mental disorders in U.S. adolescents: results of the National Comorbidity Survey-Adolescent Supplement (NCS-A). *J Am Acad Child Adolesc Psychiatry*. 2011;50(1):32–45
5. Center for Mental Health Services. *Identifying Mental Health and Substance Abuse Problems of Children and Adolescents: A Guide for Child-Serving Organizations*. Rockville, MD: Substance Abuse and Mental Health Services Administration; 2012. https://store.samhsa.gov/product/Identifying-Mental-Health-and-Substance-Use-Problems-of-Children-and-Adolescents-A-Guide-for-Child-Serving-Organizations/SMA12-4700. Accessed January 3, 2018

6. Noguera P. *City Schools and the American Dream: Reclaiming the Promise of Public Education.* New York, NY: Teachers College Press; 2003

7. Centers for Disease Control and Prevention. Youth Risk Behavior Surveillance System (YRBSS). Centers for Disease Control and Prevention Web site. https://www.cdc.gov/healthyyouth/data/yrbs. Accessed January 3, 2018

8. Kann L, Olsen EO, McManus T, et al. Sexual identity, sex of sexual contacts, and health-related behaviors among students in grades 9–12—United States and selected sites, 2015. *MMWR Surveill Summ.* 2016;65(9):1–202

9. Kosciw JG, Greytak EA, Giga NM, Villenas C, Danischewski DJ. *The 2015 National School Climate Survey: The Experiences of Lesbian, Gay, Bisexual, Transgender, and Queer Youth in Our Nation's Schools.* New York, NY: GLSEN; 2016

10. American Academy of Pediatrics Committee on School Health. School-based mental health services. *Pediatrics.* 2004;113(6):1839–1845

11. McNeely CA, Nonnemaker JM, Blum RW. Promoting school connectedness: evidence from the National Longitudinal Study of Adolescent Health. *J Sch Health.* 2002;72(4):138–146

12. Archambault I, Janosz M, Morizot J, Pagani L. Adolescent behavioral, affective, and cognitive engagement in school: relationship to dropout. *J Sch Health.* 2009;79(9):408–415

13. Division of Adolescent and School Health, National Center for Chronic Disease Prevention and Health Promotion. *The Association Between School-Based Physical Activity, Including Physical Education, and Academic Performance.* Atlanta, GA: Centers for Disease Control and Prevention; 2010. https://www.cdc.gov/healthyschools/health_and_academics/pdf/pa-pe_paper.pdf. Accessed January 3, 2018

14. State policies on sex education in schools. National Conference of State Legislators Web site. http://www.ncsl.org/research/health/state-policies-on-sex-education-in-schools.aspx. Published December 21, 2016. Accessed January 3, 2018

15. Faggiano F, Vigna-Taglianti FD, Versino E, Zambon A, Borraccino A, Lemma P. School-based prevention for illicit drugs' use. *Cochrane Database Syst Rev.* 2005;(2):CD003020

16. Office of Educational Research and Improvement. *Drug Prevention Curricula: A Guide to Selection and Implementation.* Washington, DC: US Dept of Education; 1988. https://babel.hathitrust.org/cgi/pt?id=umn.31951003082644n;view=1up;seq=3. Accessed January 3, 2018

17. McBride N. A systematic review of school drug education. *Health Educ Res.* 2003;18(6):729–742

18. Botvin LifeSkills Training Program [substance abuse and violence prevention curriculum]. White Plains, NY: National Health Promotion Associates; 2016

19. Division of Violence Prevention, National Center for Injury Prevention and Control. Adverse childhood experiences (ACEs). Centers for Disease Control and Prevention Web site. https://www.cdc.gov/violenceprevention/acestudy/index.html. Updated April 1, 2016. Accessed January 3, 2018

20. American Academy of Pediatrics Council on School Health. Out-of-school suspension and expulsion. *Pediatrics.* 2013;131(3):e1000–e1007

21. González T. Keeping kids in schools: restorative justice, punitive discipline, and the school to prison pipeline. *J Law Educ.* 2012;41(2):281–335

22. Davis M. Restorative justice: resources for schools. Edutopia Web site. https://www.edutopia.org/blog/restorative-justice-resources-matt-davis. Updated October 29, 2015. Accessed January 3, 2018

23. McInerney M, McKlindon A. *Unlocking the Door to Learning: Trauma-Informed Classrooms and Transformational Schools.* Pittsburgh, PA: Education Law Center; 2014. https://www.elc-pa.org/wp-content/uploads/2015/06/Trauma-Informed-in-Schools-Classrooms-FINAL-December2014-2.pdf. Accessed January 3, 2018

24. Sypniewski RL. Increasing the awareness of trauma informed care in the school setting: giving practitioners the tools to actively participate in trauma related care [doctor of nursing practice project]. University of San Francisco; 2016:72

25. Mendelson T, Tandon SD, O'Brennan L, Leaf PJ, Ialongo NS. Brief report: moving prevention into schools; the impact of a trauma-informed school-based intervention. *J Adolesc.* 2015; 43:142–147

26. Adler RS, Jellinek MS. After teen suicide: issues for pediatricians who are asked to consult to schools. *Pediatrics.* 1990;86(6):982–987

27. Schonfeld DJ, Demaria T; American Academy of Pediatrics Committee on Psychosocial Aspects of Child and Family Health and Disaster Preparedness Advisory Council. Supporting the grieving child and family. *Pediatrics.* 2016;138(3):e20162147

28. Guidelines for schools responding to a death by suicide. University of Southern California School of Social Work Web site. https://sowkweb.usc.edu/download/about/centers-affiliations/ncscb-guidelines-schools-responding-death-suicide. Accessed January 3, 2018

29. Albright A, Michael K, Massey C, Sale R, Kirk A, Egan T. An evaluation of an interdisciplinary rural school mental health programme in Appalachia. *Adv Sch Ment Health Promot.* 2013;6(3):189–202

30. Foy JM, Earls MF. A process for developing community consensus regarding the diagnosis and management of attention-deficit/hyperactivity disorder. *Pediatrics.* 2005;115(1):e97–e104

31. Sanders CE, Field TM, Diego MA. Adolescents' academic expectations and achievement. *Adolescence.* 2001;36(144):795–802

32. Bardone AM, Moffitt TE, Caspi A, Dickson N, Silva PA. Adult mental health and social outcomes of adolescent girls with depression and conduct disorder. *Dev Psychopathol.* 1996; 8(4):811–829

33. Lynskey MT, Coffey C, Degenhardt L, Carlin JB, Patton G. A longitudinal study of the effects of adolescent cannabis use on high school completion. *Addiction.* 2003;98(5):685–692

34. Stoep AV, Weiss NS, Kuo ES, Cheney D, Cohen P. What proportion of failure to complete secondary school in the US population is attributable to adolescent psychiatric disorder? *J Behav Health Serv Res.* 2003;30(1):119–124

35. Bains RM, Diallo AF. Mental health services in school-based health centers: systematic review. *J Sch Nurs.* 2016;32(1):8–19

36. Zablocki M, Krezmien MP. Drop-out predictors among students with high-incidence disabilities: a national longitudinal and transitional study 2 analysis. *J Disabil Policy Stud.* 2012;24(1):53–64

37. Kopec MT, Randel J, Naz B, et al. Using the Guidelines for Adolescent Preventive Services to estimate adolescent depressive symptoms in school-based health centers. *Fam Med.* 2010;42(3):193–201

38. Keeton V, Soleimanpour S, Brindis CD. School-based health centers in an era of health care reform: building on history. *Curr Probl Pediatr Adolesc Health Care.* 2012;42(6):132–156

39. Mental health consultation clinic. School Health Alliance for Forsyth County Web site. http://shaforsyth.com/our-programs/mental-health-consultation-clinic. Accessed January 3, 2018

40. Telemedicine. University of Arizona College of Medicine – Tucson Web site. http://psychiatry.arizona.edu/patient-care/telemedicine. Accessed January 3, 2018

Appendixes

[a] These tools are updated regularly at www.aap.org/mentalhealth.

Algorithm: A Process for Integrating Mental Health Care Into Pediatric Practice

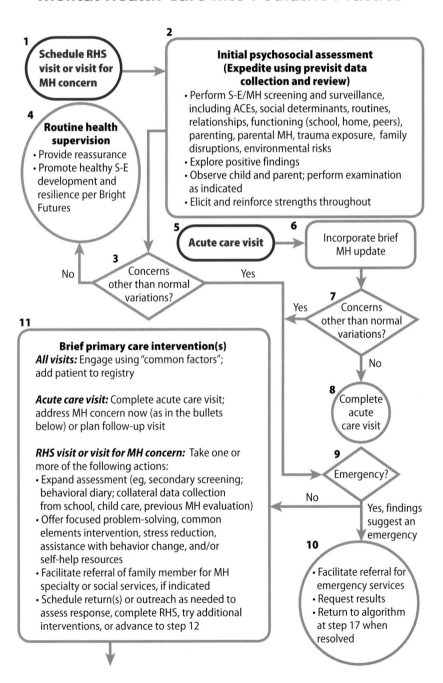

1 Schedule RHS visit or visit for MH concern

2 Initial psychosocial assessment (Expedite using previsit data collection and review)
- Perform S-E/MH screening and surveillance, including ACEs, social determinants, routines, relationships, functioning (school, home, peers), parenting, parental MH, trauma exposure, family disruptions, environmental risks
- Explore positive findings
- Observe child and parent; perform examination as indicated
- Elicit and reinforce strengths throughout

4 Routine health supervision
- Provide reassurance
- Promote healthy S-E development and resilience per Bright Futures

5 Acute care visit

6 Incorporate brief MH update

3 Concerns other than normal variations?
No / Yes

7 Concerns other than normal variations?
Yes / No

8 Complete acute care visit

9 Emergency?
No / Yes, findings suggest an emergency

11 Brief primary care intervention(s)
All visits: Engage using "common factors"; add patient to registry

Acute care visit: Complete acute care visit; address MH concern now (as in the bullets below) or plan follow-up visit

RHS visit or visit for MH concern: Take one or more of the following actions:
- Expand assessment (eg, secondary screening; behavioral diary; collateral data collection from school, child care, previous MH evaluation)
- Offer focused problem-solving, common elements intervention, stress reduction, assistance with behavior change, and/or self-help resources
- Facilitate referral of family member for MH specialty or social services, if indicated
- Schedule return(s) or outreach as needed to assess response, complete RHS, try additional interventions, or advance to step 12

10
- Facilitate referral for emergency services
- Request results
- Return to algorithm at step 17 when resolved

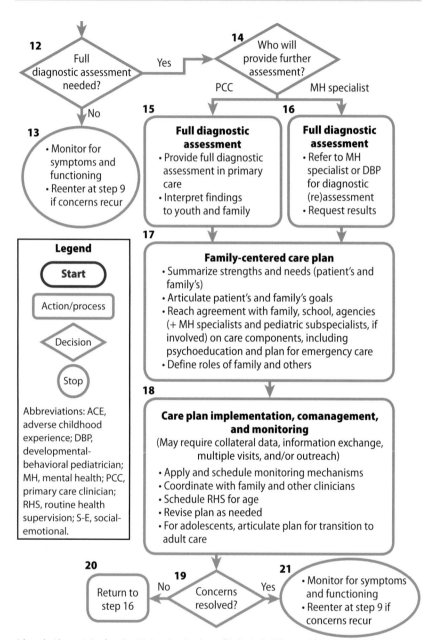

Adapted with permission from Foy JM; American Academy of Pediatrics Task Force on Mental Health. Enhancing pediatric mental health care: algorithms for primary care. *Pediatrics*. 2010;125(suppl 3):S109–S125.

2

Mental Health Tools for Pediatrics

The following table is a snapshot of a work in progress of the American Academy of Pediatrics (AAP) Mental Health Leadership Work Group (MHLWG). It is a compilation of tools that are potentially useful at each stage of a clinical process through which mental health content can be integrated into pediatric primary care. This process is depicted by algorithms in Appendix 1. A number of chapters offer, in addition, guidance in interpreting results of commonly used screening tools, including a number of those included in the following table.

Several points about the table bear noting.

▶ The sequence of tools within each section does not reflect the recommendation or preference of the AAP MHLWG for one tool over another.

▶ In a number of instances, there are options for use of a tool at more than one place in the process. In these instances, a full description accompanies the first mention. Subsequent mentions of the tool include only the tool abbreviation and any reference numbers. In addition to facilitating access to further reading, this setup will assist readers in locating the tool's full description where it appears in the table.

▶ Information about psychometric properties of each tool is available in the latest version of the tool at www.aap.org/mentalhealth.

Table A2-1. Mental Health Tools for Pediatrics

Psychosocial Measure	Tools and Description	Number of Items and Format	Age-group and Any Languages Reading Level if Specified	Administration and Scoring Time Training[a]	Source
Initial Psychosocial Assessment (Algorithm Step 2): Previsit or Intra-visit Data Collection and Screening					
Surveillance	Bright Futures surveillance questions[1]	Unlimited	0–21 y English Spanish	Variable	AAP/MCHB freely accessible Source: https://brightfutures.aap.org/materials-and-tools/tool-and-resource-kit/Pages/default.aspx
	Bright Futures previsit and supplemental questionnaires[1]	Variable	0–21 y English Spanish	Variable	AAP/MCHB freely accessible Source: https://brightfutures.aap.org/materials-and-tools/tool-and-resource-kit/Pages/default.aspx
	HEADSSS mnemonic[2] Assesses for **H**ome/environment, **E**ducation and employment, **A**ctivities, **D**rugs, **S**exuality, **S**uicide/depression, and **S**afety. HEADSSS-3.0 includes media use.	Interview	Adolescents Language of clinician	Part of interview process	Freely accessible Sources: www.bcchildrens.ca/Youth-Health-Clinic-site/Documents/headss20 assessment20guide1.pdf www.contemporarypediatrics.com/modern-medicine-feature-articles/heeadsss-30-psychosocial-interview-adolescents-updated-new-century-fueled-media
	School report cards, end-of-grade tests, Individualized Education Program (IEP), and 504 plan				

General psychosocial screening: young children aged 0–5 y				
Early Childhood Screening Assessment (ECSA)[3] *Assesses emotional and behavioral development in young children and maternal distress*	40 items, 3-point Likert scale responses and an additional option for parents to identify whether they are concerned and would like help with an item	18–60 mo English Spanish Romanian Reading level: fifth grade	10–15 min to complete Scoring time: 1–2 min Should be administered by health care professional or MHS whose training and scope of practice includes interpreting screening test results and interpreting positive or negative screening results for parents	Freely accessible Source: www.infantinstitute.org/wp-content/uploads/2013/07/ECSA-40-Child-Care1.pdf
Ages & Stages Questionnaires (ASQ): Social-Emotional, Second Edition (ASQ:SE-2)[4] *Screens for social-emotional problems in young children; used in conjunction with ASQ or another tool designed to provide information on a child's communicative, motor, problem-solving, and adaptive behaviors*	From 19 items (6 mo)–33 items (30 mo) Parent report	6–60 mo English Spanish Reading level: sixth grade	10–15 min Scoring: 1–5 min (can be scored by paraprofessionals)	Proprietary Source: http://agesandstages.com/products-services/asqse-2
Brief Infant Toddler Social Emotional Assessment (BITSEA)[5] *Screens for social-emotional problems in young children*	42 items Parent report Child care report	12–36 mo English Spanish	7–10 min	Proprietary Margaret.Briggs-Gowan@yale.edu or Alice.Carter@umb.edu

Table A2-1. Mental Health Tools for Pediatrics (continued)

Psychosocial Measure	Tools and Description	Number of Items and Format	Age-group and Any Languages Reading Level if Specified	Administration and Scoring Time Training[a]	Source
Initial Psychosocial Assessment (Algorithm Step 2): Previsit or Intra-visit Data Collection and Screening					
General psychosocial screening: young children aged 0–5 y	Survey of Well-being of Young Children (SWYC)[6-8] Consists of subscales appropriate to age **Milestones** Assesses cognitive, language, and motor development **Baby Pediatric Symptom Checklist (BPSC)** up to 18 mo Assesses irritability, inflexibility, and difficulty with routines **Preschool Pediatric Symptom Checklist (PPSC)** 18–66 mo Assesses for emotional/behavioral symptoms **Parent's Observations of Social Interactions (POSI)** 18–35 mo Screens for ASD **Family questions** Assesses stress in family environment (eg, parental depression; discord; substance use; food insecurity; parent's concerns about child's behavior, learning, or development)	Parent questionnaires with embedded subscales 34–47 questions Paper and electronic versions	2–60 mo English Spanish Burmese Nepali Portuguese (Translations not independently validated)	10–15 min	Freely accessible Source: www.floatinghospital.org/ The-Survey-of-Wellbeing-of-Young-Children/Age-Specific-Forms.aspx

General psychosocial screening: children aged 6–10 y	Pediatric Symptom Checklist—35 items (PSC-35)[9,10] *General psychosocial screening and functional assessment in the domains of attention, externalizing symptoms, and internalizing symptoms*	35 items Self-administered Parent or youth ≥11 y	4–16 y English Spanish Chinese Japanese Pictorial versions available	<5 min Scoring: 1–2 min	Freely accessible Source: Massachusetts General Hospital Web site at www.massgeneral.org/psychiatry/services/psc_home.aspx
	Pediatric Symptom Checklist—17 items (PSC-17)[11] *General psychosocial screening and functional assessment in the domains of attention, externalizing symptoms, and internalizing symptoms*	17 items Self-administered Parent or youth ≥11 y	4–16 y English Spanish Chinese Reading level: fifth grade– sixth grade	<5 min Scoring: 2 min	Freely accessible Source: https://depts.washington.edu/hcsats/FCAP/resources/PSC-17%20English.pdf
	Strengths and Difficulties Questionnaires (SDQ)[12] *Assesses 25 attributes, some positive and some negative, divided among 5 scales. Some versions have an impact scale on the second page.*	25 items Self-administered versions for parent, teacher, or youth aged 11–17 y	3–17 y >40 languages	10 min	Freely accessible Source: Youth in Mind Web site at www.sdqinfo.org
General psychosocial screening: adolescents and young adults aged 11–21 y	PSC-35[9,10] PSC-17[11] SDQ[12]				

Table A2-1. Mental Health Tools for Pediatrics (continued)

Psychosocial Measure	Tools and Description	Number of Items and Format	Age-group and Any Languages Reading Level if Specified	Administration and Scoring Time Training[a]	Source
Initial Psychosocial Assessment (Algorithm Step 2): Previsit or Intra-visit Data Collection and Screening					
General psychosocial screening: adolescents and young adults aged 11–21 y	The Rapid Assessment for Adolescent Preventive Services (RAAPS)[13,14] *Web-based screening tool developed to identify youths most at risk for school dropout, using factors such as discrimination, abuse, and access to tangible needs (eg, food, water, electricity) that contribute to morbidity, mortality, and social problems*	21 items	Age specific for older child (9–12 y), adolescent (13–18 y), and young adult (18–24 y) Includes audio and multilingual options	Approximately 5 min to self-administer. Scored automatically and pertinent information is downloaded. 30-min demonstration available (www. possibilities forchange.com/ raaps).	Proprietary. Review and download free of charge at www.raaps.org.
Targeted screening: substance use[b]	Screening to Brief Intervention (S2BI)[15] *Brief screening to determine whether further assessment is necessary*	2 items	Adolescents English	1–2 min if responses negative	Freely accessible Source: https://pubs.niaaa.nih.gov/ publications/Practitioner/ YouthGuide/YouthGuide.pdf
	Brief Screener for Tobacco, Alcohol, and Other Drugs (BSTAD)[16] *Identifies problematic tobacco, alcohol, and marijuana use in pediatric settings*	3 frequency questions (one for each substance) Interview or iPad self-administration (preferred)	12–17 y English	1–2 min if responses negative	Freely accessible Source: www.drugabuse.gov/ast/ bstad/#

	NIAAA youth alcohol screening[17] *Screens for friends' uses and own use*	2 questions	Adolescents English	1–2 min if responses negative	Freely accessible Source: www.niaaa.nih.gov/Publications/EducationTraining Materials/Pages/YouthGuide.aspx
	CRAFFT (Car, Relax, Alone, Forget, Friends, Trouble) lifetime use[18] *Screens for substance use*	3 screener questions and then 6 items Self-administered or youth report	Adolescents English	1–2 min if responses negative	Freely accessible. Use at this step or in algorithm step 11, later in this table, as brief assessment if S2B1 result is positive. Source: Center for Adolescent Substance Abuse Research Web site at www.ceasar-boston.org/CRAFFT/index.php.
Targeted screening: adolescent depression[c]	Patient Health Questionnaire-Adolescent (PHQ-A) depression screening[19] *Consists of questions on depression from full PHQ-A (See full PHQ-A tool later in this table.)*	Abbreviated 9-item screening specifically for depression	11–17 y English	<5 min to complete and score	Free with permission Source: www.aacap.org/App_Themes/AACAP/docs/member_resources/toolbox_for_clinical_practice_and_outcomes/symptoms/GLAD-PC_PHQ-9.pdf
	Kutcher Adolescent Depression Scale (KADS)[20] *Screens for depression*	6, 11, or 16 items	12–17 y English	5 min Scoring: 1 min	Freely accessible. 6-Item Kutcher Adolescent Depression Scale (KADS-6). http://lphi.org/CMSuploads/Kutcher-Adolescent-Depression-Scale-47583.pdf.
Parent/family general screening	Pediatric Intake Form (Family Psychosocial Screen)[21] *Screens for parental depression, substance use, domestic violence, parental history of being abused, and social supports*	22 items	0–21 y English	Variable	Freely accessible Source: www.pedstest.com/Portals/0/TheBook/FPSinEnglish.pdf
	SWYC[c-8]				

Table A2-1. Mental Health Tools for Pediatrics (continued)

Psychosocial Measure	Tools and Description	Number of Items and Format	Age-group and Any Languages Reading Level if Specified	Administration and Scoring Time Training[a]	Source
Initial Psychosocial Assessment (Algorithm Step 2): Previsit or Intra-visit Data Collection and Screening					
Parent/family general screening	A Safe Environment for Every Kid (SEEK) Parent Questionnaire - R (PQ-R)[22] *Includes questions about smoking, guns, food availability, depression, substance use, discipline, and domestic violence*	15 yes-or-no questions	0–5 y English Spanish	3 min Scoring: <3 min	Proprietary Source: www.seekwellbeing.org/the-seek-parent-questionnaire-
	Parents' Assessment of Protective Factors[23] *Self-assessment of parents' resilience, their social connections, concrete support they receive in times of need, and their social-emotional competence of children*	46 questions, including 10 background questions	Parents of children from birth–8 y English Spanish	20 min	Freely accessible Source: www.cssp.org/reform/child-welfare/pregnant-and-parenting-youth/Parents-Assessment-of-Protective-Factors.pdf
	Health Leads Screening[24] *Assesses food insecurity, housing instability, utility needs, strained financial resources, transportation difficulty, exposure to violence, and sociodemographic information*	10 questions In each category, alternative questions, plus follow-up questions as indicated	Parents of children of all ages. Multiple languages. Reading level varies by question.	5 min	Freely accessible Source: toolkit available at https://healthleadsusa.org/wp-content/uploads/2016/07/Health-Leads-Screening-Toolkit-July-2016.pdf

Tool	Items/format	Population/language	Time	Availability
McMaster Family Functioning Scale[25] *Assesses family functioning*	12 items Self-report	Adolescents and adults Translated into 24 languages	<5 min	Freely accessible Source: www.clintools.com/victims/resources/assessment/interpersonal/mcmaster.html
Parent Stress Index (PSI), Third Edition[26] *Elicits indicators of stress and identifies parent-child problem areas in parents of children aged 1 mo–12 y* PSI-Short Form	120 items plus 19 optional items Parent self-report PSI-Short Form: 36 items Version for parenting adolescents	Parents of children aged 1 mo–12 y English	20–30 min	Proprietary Source: PAR Web site at www.parinc.com/Products/Pkey/337
Stress Index for Parents of Adolescents (SIPA)[27] *Elicits indicators of stress in parents of adolescents*	112 items	Parents of pre-adolescents and adolescents aged 11–19 y English	20 min Scoring: 10 min	Proprietary Source: www.parinc.com/Products/Pkey/412
Caregiver Strain Questionnaire (CGSQ) and CGSQ Short Form 7 (CGSQ-SF7)[28] *Assesses strain experienced by caregivers and families of youths with emotional problems*	21 items 7 items (CGSQ-SF7) Self-report by parents or caregivers	Parents/caregivers of adolescents with emotional problems English Spanish	Variable	Freely accessible Source: www.hospicepatients.org/caregiver-strain-questionaire-robinson.pdf
Multidimensional Scale of Perceived Social Support Parent Stress Inventory (MSPSS)[29] *Assesses social support*	12 items Parent report	Adult Multiple languages	2–5 min	Freely accessible Source: www.yorku.ca/rokada/psyctest/socsupp.pdf

Table A2-1. Mental Health Tools for Pediatrics (*continued*)

Psychosocial Measure	Tools and Description	Number of Items and Format	Age-group and Any Languages Reading Level if Specified	Administration and Scoring Time Training[a]	Source
Initial Psychosocial Assessment (Algorithm Step 2): Previsit or Intra-visit Data Collection and Screening					
Parent/family targeted screening	Patient Health Questionnaire-2 (PHQ-2)—first 2 items from PHQ-9[30] *Screens adults for depression*	2 items Parent self-report	Adult English	1 min	Freely accessible Source: www.cqaimh.org/pdf/tool_phq2.pdf
	Patient Health Questionnaire-9 (PHQ-9)[31] *Screens adults for depression*	9 items Parent self-report	Adult English	<5 min to administer Scoring: <3 min	Freely accessible Source: www.phqscreeners.com/sites/g/files/g1016261/f/201412/PHQ-9_English.pdf
	Edinburgh Postnatal Depression Scale (EPDS)[32] *Screens women for depression*	10 items Parent self-report	Peripartum women Multiple languages	<5 min to administer Scoring: 5 min	Freely accessible Source: www.perinatalservicesbc.ca/health-professionals/professional-resources/health-promo/edinburgh-postnatal-depression-scale-(epds)
	Abuse Assessment Screen (AAS)[33] *Screens for domestic violence*	5–6 items Parent report	Adolescent girls and adult women English	About 45 s if all answers are no	Freely accessible Source: http://peaceathome.com/wordpress/wp-content/uploads/2014/10/Abuse_Assessment_Screen_AAS.pdf

	Hunger Vital Sign[34] *Identifies food insecurity and its associated social determinants*	2 questions	Parents of children—birth–3 y English Russian Somalian Vietnamese Korean Chinese Spanish Arabic Swahili French Nepali	≤5 min	Freely accessible Source: http://childrenshealthwatch.org/public-policy/hunger-vital-sign
Trauma exposure[d]	The Acute Stress Checklist for Children (ASC-Kids)[35] *Assesses acute stress reactions within the first month after exposure to a potentially traumatic event*	29 items (25 DSM-related; 4 additional items for clinical use: subjective life threat, family context, and coping) Self-report or may be read aloud to child	8–17 y English Spanish	5 min	Proprietary Source: www.istss.org/assessing-trauma/acute-stress-checklist-for-children.aspx
	Children's Revised Impact of Event Scale (CRIES)-8[36] *Assesses impact of traumatic events*	8 items Self-report	≥8 y who can read Multiple languages	<5 min	Freely accessible Instructions and forms available at Children and War Foundation Web site at www.childrenandwar.org/measures/children's-revised-impact-of-event-scale-8—cries-8

Table A2-1. Mental Health Tools for Pediatrics (*continued*)

Psychosocial Measure	Tools and Description	Number of Items and Format	Age-group and Any Languages Reading Level if Specified	Administration and Scoring Time Training[a]	Source
Initial Psychosocial Assessment (Algorithm Step 2): Previsit or Intra-visit Data Collection and Screening					
Global functioning	Brief Impairment Scale (BIS) multidimensional[37] *Assesses global functioning in domains of interpersonal relations, school/work, and self-care/self-fulfillment*	23 items Parent report	4–17 y English Spanish	10 min	Freely accessible Source: www.heardalliance.org/wp-content/uploads/2011/04/Brief-Impairment-Scale-English.pdf
	Columbia Impairment Scale (CIS)—part of Child/Adolescent Wellness Assessment (CAWA)[38] *Assesses global functioning in domains of interpersonal relations, psychopathology, school performance, and use of leisure time; monitors progress after 6 mo of treatment*	13 items administered by clinician. "Nonclinical version" can be administered directly by lay or clinical interviewers to parents or youth.	Children and adolescents English	5 min	Freely accessible Sources: Youth version at www.hrcec.org/images/PDF/CIS-Y.pdf Parent version at www.hrcec.org/images/PDF/CIS-P.pdf
	SDQ Impact Scale[12] *Assesses global functioning in domains of home life, friendships, learning, and play*	5 items Parent Teacher Youth ≥11 y	3–17 y >40 languages	<5 min	Freely accessible Source: www.sdqinfo.com

Brief MH Update (Algorithm Step 6)

Brief screenings	AAP brief MH update[39,40]	Questions selected from a list and sorted by age-group	Birth–21 y English	1–5 min, depending on provider's preference	Freely accessible Source: http://pediatrics. aappublications.org/content/ 125/Supplement_3/S159
	SDQ Impact Scale[12]				
Screen for somatization symptom disorder and related disorders	Children's Somatization Inventory (CSI)-24 (CSI-24)[41] *Shortened version of original CSI assesses for the presence of multiple somatic symptoms.*	24 items. Interviewer administers orally; child selects response from cards.	Multiple languages	<10 min	Freely accessible Source (parent and child versions): www.childrenshospital.vanderbilt. org/uploads/documents/CSI-24_ English_parent_and_child.pdf

Assessing Emergencies (Algorithm Step 9)

Suicide assessment	Ask Suicide-Screening Questions (ASQ)[42] Note: This tool is not to be confused with the ASQ, a developmental screening tool, or the ASQ:SE-2, described earlier in this table. *Assesses for suicide risk among youths with psychiatric concerns in emergency department settings*	4 screening items	10–24 y English	20 sec	Toolkit freely accessible at www.nimh. nih.gov/labs-at-nimh/asq-toolkit-materials/index.shtml

Table A2-1. Mental Health Tools for Pediatrics (*continued*)

Psychosocial Measure	Tools and Description	Number of Items and Format	Age-group and Any Languages Reading Level if Specified	Administration and Scoring Time Training[a]	Source
Assessing Emergencies (Algorithm Step 9)					
Suicide assessment	Suicide Assessment Five-step Evaluation and Triage (SAFE-T)[43] *Process includes identifying risk factors, identifying protective factors, conducting suicide inquiry, determining risk level/ intervention, and documenting.*	Protocol with prompts for each step to guide clinical process	Children and adolescents English	Variable	Source: www.shiacmh.org/docs/ safe-t.pdf
	Suicide Behaviors Questionnaire-Revised (SBQ-R)[44] *Assesses 4 dimensions of suicidality*	4 items	Adolescents English	5 min	Source: www.cqaimh.org/pdf/tool_ sbq-r.pdf
	Columbia-Suicide Severity Rating Scale (C-SSRS)[45] *Supports suicide risk assessment through a series of questions; answers help users both identify whether someone is at risk for suicide and assess the severity and immediacy of that risk.*	6 items within a 2-page form	Adolescents English	5 min Requires training to administer	Freely available Source: http://cssrs.columbia.edu/ wp-content/uploads/C-SSRS_ Pediatric-SLC_11.14.16.pdf

	Suicidal Ideation Questionnaire (SIQ) and SIQ-Junior (SIQ-Jr)[46] *Appropriate for individual or group administration in clinical or school settings*	SIQ: 30 items SIQ-Jr: 15 items	Adolescents and young adults aged 13–18 y SIQ: grades 10–12 SIQ-Jr: grades 7–9 English	10 min	Proprietary Source: www.parinc.com/Products/Pkey/413
	Child-Adolescent Suicidal Potential Index (CASPI)[47] *Assesses multiple aspects of suicidal behavior: total score plus 3 subscales*	30 yes-or-no items in self-report format	Children and youths 6–18 y English	10 min	Source: Author's contact information available at http://books.google.com/books?id=-r309lLpxTkC&pg=PA95
	PHQ-A[19] or PHQ-9[31] severity items on suicide				
Delirium assessment	Delirium Rating Scale (DRS) and Revised-98 (DRS-R-98)[48] *Differentiates between delirium, dementia, depression, schizophrenia, and other conditions*	DRS 10 items DRS-R-98 16 clinician-rated items, 13 of which assess the severity of symptoms and 3 of which have diagnostic significance	Children and adolescents English, French, Italian, Spanish, Dutch, Mandarin, Chinese, Korean, Swedish, Japanese, German, and Indian	Both scales >2 h Scoring: 20–30 min	Freely accessible Source: https://neuro.psychiatryonline.org/doi/pdf/10.1176/jnp.13.2.229?code=neuro-site

Table A2-1. Mental Health Tools for Pediatrics (*continued*)

Psychosocial Measure	Tools and Description	Number of Items and Format	Age-group and Any Languages / Reading Level if Specified	Administration and Scoring Time / Training[a]	Source
Assessing Emergencies (Algorithm Step 9)					
Illness severity	Childhood Severity of Psychiatric Illness (CSPI-2)[49] *Assesses severity by eliciting risk factors, behavioral/emotional symptoms, functioning problems, involvement with juvenile justice and child protection, and caregiver needs and strengths*	34 items Individual report	3–21 y English Spanish	3–5 min after a routine crisis assessment. 25–30 min to complete if nothing is known of the child/family. Training is generally recommended and so is demonstration of reliability (ie, certification) before use (by office staff in particular). There are many trainers available and some Web-based training options.	Freely accessible Available at www.praedfoundation.org

Brief Primary Care Intervention, Secondary Screening, Collateral Data Collection (Algorithm Step 11)

Secondary screening: general[e]	ECSA[3]			
	ASQ:SE-2[4]			
	BITSEA[5]			
	SWYC[6-8]			
	PSC-35[9,10]			
	PSC-17[11]			
	SDQ[12]			
	School or child care reports			
	Behavior Assessment System for Children (BASC)[50] *Assesses adaptive and problem behaviors*	Parent version: 134–160 items Teacher version: 100–139 items Youth version	2–21 y English Spanish	Parent version: 10–20 min Teacher version: 10–20 min Youth version: 30 min Electronic scoring available Must be administered by qualified personnel	Proprietary. Source: Behavior Assessment System for Children, Second Edition (BASC-2). Pearson PsychCorp Web site. Available at http://pearsonassess.com/HAIWEB/Cultures/en-us/Productdetail.htm?Pid=PAa30000.

Table A2-1. Mental Health Tools for Pediatrics (continued)

Psychosocial Measure	Tools and Description	Number of Items and Format	Age-group and Any Languages Reading Level if Specified	Administration and Scoring Time Training[a]	Source
Brief Primary Care Intervention, Secondary Screening, Collateral Data Collection (Algorithm Step 11)					
Secondary screening: general[e]	Columbia Diagnostic Interview Schedule for Children (DISC) diagnostic predictive scales[51] *Computerized structure interview (yes-or-no) elicits symptoms of 36 mental disorders, applying DSM criteria.*	22 items (Last item is not scored.) Youth self-administered, 8-item, abbreviated version available through TeenScreen	9–17 y English	Depends on items endorsed Training needed	Free with permission Manual available at www.cdc.gov/nchs/data/nhanes/limited_access/interviewer_manual.pdf
	Patient Health Questionnaire-Adolescents (PHQ-A)[52] *Screens for anxiety, eating problems, mood problems, and substance use. Note: PHQ-A depression screening[19] is a subsection of this comprehensive questionnaire.*	83 items Self-report	13–18 y English	Variable scoring: <5 min	Freely accessible Source: www.uacap.org/uploads/3/2/5/0/3250432/phq-a.pdf

	Caregiver Teacher Report Form (C-TRF)[53]—part of CBCL (See CBCL tool later in this table.) *Assesses for emotionally reactive behavior, anxious/depressed mood, somatic concerns, withdrawn behavior, attention problems, and aggressive behavior*	99 items Child care providers Teachers	1½–5 y Multiple languages	Variable hand and computer scoring	Proprietary Source: PAR Web site at www.parinc.com/Products/Pkey/49
Secondary screening: inattention and impulsivity	National Institute for Children's Health Quality (NICHQ) Vanderbilt Diagnostic Rating Scales[54] *Elicits symptoms in domains of inattention, disruptive behavior, anxiety, and depression; separate scale assesses functioning in school performance.*	Parent: 55 items Teacher: 43 items Parent/teacher follow-up: 26 items plus items on medication side effects	6–12 y English Spanish	10 min	Freely accessible. Source: NICHQ Vanderbilt Assessment Scales. NICHQ Web site. Available at www.nichq.org/childrens-health/adhd/resources/vanderbilt-assessment-scales.
	Conners' Rating Scales-Revised[55] *Elicits symptoms in domains of oppositionality, cognitive problems/inattention, hyperactivity, anxiety-shyness, perfectionism, social problems, and psychosomatic problems*	Parent: 80 items Teacher: 59 items Self: 87 items	3–17 y for parent/teacher 12–17 y for self English Spanish	20 min	Proprietary. Conners 3rd Edition. MHS Assessments Web site. Available at www.mhs.com/product.aspx?gr=cli&prod=conners3&id=overview.

Table A2-1. Mental Health Tools for Pediatrics (*continued*)

Psychosocial Measure	Tools and Description	Number of Items and Format	Age-group and Any Languages Reading Level if Specified	Administration and Scoring Time Training[a]	Source
Brief Primary Care Intervention, Secondary Screening, Collateral Data Collection (Algorithm Step 11)					
Secondary screening: learning difficulty	Vision and hearing screening if not done previously				
	Collateral reports from school such as				
	• Teacher version of SDQ and Pediatric Symptom Checklist				
	• NICHQ Vanderbilt Diagnostic Rating Scales teacher form				
	• Psychological test results, if any				
	• Kaufman Test of Educational Achievement (KTEA)				
	• Kaufman Brief Intelligence Test (KBIT)				
	• Report cards				
	• End-of-grade tests				
	• IEP				
	• 504 plan				

Secondary screening: aggression and disruptive behavior	NICHQ Vanderbilt Diagnostic Rating Scales[54]				
	Conners' Rating Scales-Revised[55]				
	Modified Overt Aggression Scale (MOAS)[56] *Rates symptoms in domain of disruptive behavior/aggression*	4 items Clinician rating of aggression	Adults but has been used for adolescents English	Administered as a semi-structured interview asking adolescent to report on aggressive behavior 10–15 min	Freely accessible Source: https://depts.washington.edu/dbpeds/Screening%20Tools/Modified-Overt-Aggression-Scale-MOAS.pdf
	Eyberg Child Behavior Inventory (ECBI)[57] *Assesses conduct problems*	7-point Intensity scale and yes-or-no Problem scale	Parents of children and adolescents aged 2–16 y Companion tool available for teachers English	5-min administration 5-min scoring	Proprietary Source: www.parinc.com/Products/Pkey/97
	Conduct Disorder Scale (CDS)[58] *Rates symptoms in domain of disruptive behavior*	40 items Parent Teachers Siblings	5–22 y English	5–10 min	Proprietary Source: www.proedinc.com/Products/10355/conduct-disorder-scale-cds-complete-kit.aspx
Secondary screening: low mood and depressive symptoms	Preschool Feelings Checklist[59] *Assesses for depression in young children*	20-item parent checklist	36–66 mo English	10 min	Freely accessible Source: http://studylib.net/doc/7442685/preschool-feelings-checklist
	PHQ-A depression screening[19]				
	KADS[20]				

Table A2-1. Mental Health Tools for Pediatrics (continued)

Psychosocial Measure	Tools and Description	Number of Items and Format	Age-group and Any Languages Reading Level if Specified	Administration and Scoring Time Training[a]	Source
Brief Primary Care Intervention, Secondary Screening, Collateral Data Collection (Algorithm Step 11)					
Secondary screening: low mood and depressive symptoms	Modified PHQ-9[60] *Screens for symptoms in domains of depression and suicidality*	9 plus severity items	Adolescent English Spanish	5 min Scoring: 1 min	Free with permission (Contact Kroenke K, Spitzer RL, Williams JB. The PHQ-9: validity of a brief depression severity measure. *J Gen Intern Med.* 2001;16(9):606–613.) Available in the toolkit at www.gladpc.org
	Center for Epidemiological Studies Depression (CES-D) Scale modified version for children and adolescents[61] *Screens for depression and emotional turmoil*	20 items	6–17 y English Spanish French Reading level: sixth grade	5–10 min	Freely accessible Available at www.brightfutures.org/mentalhealth/pdf/professionals/bridges/ces_dc.pdf
	Children's Depression Inventory (CDI)[62] *Screens for depression*	Parent: 17 items Teacher: 12 items Youth: 27 items (Youth short form: 10 items)	7–17 y English Spanish Reading level: first grade	5–10 min (27-item)	Children's Depression Inventory 2 (CDI 2). Pearson PsychCorp Web site. Available at http://pearsonassess.com/HAIWEB/Cultures/en-us/Productdetail.htm?Pid=015-8044-762.
	Short Mood and Feelings Questionnaire (SMFQ)[63] *Screens for depression*	13 items Self-report (child and parent)	8–16 y English	<5 min	Free with permission (Contact http://devepi.duhs.duke.edu/mfq.html.)

	Beck Depression Inventory (BDI)-II[64] *Assesses for depression*	21 items Self-administered or verbally administered by a trained administrator	≥14 y English Spanish Reading level: sixth grade	5–10 min Training required	Proprietary Source: form available at www.bmc. org/sites/default/files/For_Medical_ Professionals/Pediatric_Resources/ Pediatrics__MA_Center_for_ Sudden_Infant_Death_ Syndrome__SIDS_/Beck- Depression-Inventory-BDI.pdf
	Beck Depression Inventory- FastScreen (BDI-FS)[65] *Screens for depression; useful in patients with chronic pain and medical conditions*	7 items	≥13 y English	<5 min	Proprietary Source: www.pearsonclinical.com/ psychology/products/100000173/ bdi—fastscreen-for-medical- patients-bdi.html
Secondary screening: anxiety	Spence Children's Anxiety Scale[66] *Assesses for anxiety. Subscales include panic/agoraphobia, social anxiety, separation anxiety, generalized anxiety, obsessions/compulsions, and fear of physical injury.*	Parent: 35–45 Student: 34–45	Parent: 2½–6½ y Student: 8–12 y Variety of languages	5–10 min	Freely accessible Source: Spence Children's Anxiety Scale Web site at www.scaswebsite. com
	Screen for Childhood Anxiety Related Emotional Disorders (SCARED)[67] *Assesses for anxiety—but not specifically for OCD or PTSD*	41 items Parent Youth	≥8 y English	5 min Scoring: 1–2 min	Freely accessible Source: www.midss.org/content/screen- child-anxiety-related-disorders- scared
	Generalized Anxiety Disorder 7-item (GAD-7) scale[68] *Assesses for symptoms consistent with generalized anxiety disorder; may be used to identify anxiety in patients with chronic conditions such as migraine*	7 items plus impact scale (1 item) if re- sponses positive	11–17 y English	≤7 min	Freely accessible Source: www.mdcalc.com/gad-7- general-anxiety-disorder-7

Table A2-1. Mental Health Tools for Pediatrics (continued)

Psychosocial Measure	Tools and Description	Number of Items and Format	Age-group and Any Languages Reading Level if Specified	Administration and Scoring Time Training[a]	Source
Brief Primary Care Intervention, Secondary Screening, Collateral Data Collection (Algorithm Step 11)					
Secondary screening: trauma exposure[f]	ASC-Kids[35]				
	CRIES[36]				
	Trauma Symptom Checklist for Children (TSCC) and Trauma Symptom Checklist for Young Children (TSCYC)[69] *Elicits trauma-related symptoms*	54 items. (TSCC-A is a 44-item alternative version that does not contain sexual concern items.) TSCYC is a 90-item caregiver-report instrument for young children.	TSCC: 8–16 y TSCYC: 3–12 y English Spanish	15–20 min	Proprietary Sources: www.wpspublish.com/store/p/3065/tscc-trauma-symptom-checklist-for-children
	Child PTSD Symptom Scale (CPSS)[70] *Assesses severity of PTSD in children and adolescents*	24 items (17 mapped to *DSM* symptom criteria; 7, to level of impairment) Interview or self-report	8–18 y English Spanish	Interview: 20 min Self-report: 10 min	Freely accessible Source: www.aacap.org/App_Themes/AACAP/docs/resource_centers/resources/misc/child_ptsd_symptom_scale.pdf

Secondary screening: executive function	Behavior Rating Inventory of Executive Function, Second Edition (BRIEF-2)[71] *Assesses executive functioning in the home and school environments. Contributes to evaluation of learning disabilities, ADHD, traumatic brain injury, low birth weight, Tourette disorder, and pervasive developmental disorders/ASD.*	86 items Parent Teacher	5–18 y English	10–15 min Scoring: 15–20 min	Proprietary Source: www.wpspublish.com/ store/p/3347/brief-2-behavior-rating-inventory-of-executive-function-second-edition
	BITSEA[5]				
	School reports				
Secondary screening: speech/language	Hearing screening				
	Capute Scales: Clinical Adaptive Test/Clinical Linguistic and Auditory Milestone Scale (CAT/CLAMS)[72] *Quantitatively measures expressive and receptive language and nonverbal problem-solving skills*	100 items	Birth–3 y English	Variable	Proprietary Source: http://products. brookespublishing.com/The-Capute-Scales-Test-Kit-P362.aspx
	Early Language Milestone (ELM) Scale-2[73] *Assesses language development from birth–age 3 y and intelligibility 36–48 mo*	43 items	Birth–36 mo and older children whose devel-opmental level falls within that range English	Variable	Proprietary Source: www.proedinc.com/ Products/6580/early-language-milestone-scale-elm-scale2.aspx

Table A2-1. Mental Health Tools for Pediatrics (continued)

Psychosocial Measure	Tools and Description	Number of Items and Format	Age-group and Any Languages Reading Level if Specified	Administration and Scoring Time Training[a]	Source
Brief Primary Care Intervention, Secondary Screening, Collateral Data Collection (Algorithm Step 11)					
Secondary screening: speech/ language	Language Development Survey (LDS)[74] *Identifies language delay*	310 words arranged into 14 semantic categories (eg, food, animals, people, vehicles). Parents circle each word the child uses spontaneously and whether the child uses word combinations.	18–35 mo English	10 min	Proprietary Source: www.aseba.org/research/ language.html
Secondary screening: capacity for relationships/ attachment	ASQ:SE-2[4] PSI-Short Form[26] BIS[37] EPDS[32] (mother)				

Secondary screening: somatization	CSI-24[41]				
	Functional Disability Inventory (FDI)[75] *Provides classification levels for pain-related disability, applicable to a broad spectrum of pain conditions in pediatric patients*	15 items	Parent Youth ≥8 y Multiple languages	Variable	Freely accessible Source (parent and child versions): www.childrenshospital.vanderbilt. org/uploads/documents/FDI_ English_parent_and_child.pdf
Secondary screening: sleep disturbance	BEARS Sleep Screening Tool[76] *Identifies sleep problems and gathers sleep-related information*	5 items corresponding to the mnemonic: B = bedtime issues, E = excessive daytime sleepiness, A = night awakenings, R = regularity and duration of sleep, and S = snoring.	2–12 y English	5 min	Freely accessible Source: http://keltymentalhealth. ca/sites/default/files/Kelty_ ProfToolkit_M5_ BEARSSleepScreening.pdf
Secondary screening: substance use	Alcohol Use Disorders Identification Test (AUDIT)[77] *Assesses risky drinking; not a diagnostic tool*	10 items Clinician-administration and self-report options	Preadolescents and adolescents Variety of languages	2 min	Freely accessible Source: www.drugabuse.gov/sites/ default/files/files/AUDIT.pdf

Table A2-1. Mental Health Tools for Pediatrics (*continued*)

Psychosocial Measure	Tools and Description	Number of Items and Format	Age-group and Any Languages Reading Level if Specified	Administration and Scoring Time Training[a]	Source
Brief Primary Care Intervention, Secondary Screening, Collateral Data Collection (Algorithm Step 11)					
Secondary screening: substance use	Global Appraisal of Individual Needs (GAIN)–Short Screener (GAIN-SS)[78] *One of a series of measures to assess the recency, breadth, and frequency of problems and service use related to substance use. Subscales identify internalizing disorders, externalizing disorders, substance use disorders, and crime/violence.*	20 items (four 5-item subscales)	Adults Youths aged 10–17 y Self- or clinician-administered	3–5 min	Proprietary. Source: Michael Dennis, PhD, Senior Research Psychologist, Chestnut Health Systems, 720 W Chestnut St, Bloomington, IL 61701. Phone: 309/827-6026. E-mail: mdennis www.chestnut.org/li/gain. View GAIN-SS at https://dpi.wi.gov/sites/default/files/imce/sspw/pdf/gainssmanual.pdf.
Secondary screening: military families	"Cover the Bases" (military children)[79] *Tool includes PSC-35[9,10] plus questions specific to the experiences of military families.*	Pediatric Symptom Checklist plus 4 questions	Children of all ages in military families English	As for PSC-35 with variable additional time, depending on responses to 4 military-specific questions	Freely accessible Source: www.homebase.org/media/toolkit-for-providerUpdatedLogo.pdf

Secondary screening: sexual behavior or suspected sexual trauma	Child Sexual Behavior Inventory (CSBI)[80] *Assesses children who may have been or are suspected of being sexually abused. Covers 9 major content domains: Boundary Issues, Gender Role Behavior, Sexual Interest, Sexual Knowledge, Self-Stimulation, Sexual Intrusiveness, Voyeuristic Behavior, and Sexual Anxiety.*	38-item questionnaire completed by female caregiver	2–12 y Dutch English (USA) French German Latvian Lithuanian Moldovan Polish Spanish Swedish	5–10 min Scoring: 15 min	Proprietary Source: www.parinc.com/Products/Pkey/71
Secondary screening: eating/ self-regulation	SCOFF (sick, control, one, fat, food)[81] *Screens for disordered eating*	5 items	Adolescents as young as 11 y and adults English	Administration: 1 min Scoring: 1 min	No cost Developed at St. George's Hospital, London, UK Morgan JF, Reid F, Lacey JH. The SCOFF questionnaire: a new screening tool for eating disorders. *West J Med.* 2000;172(3):164–165. https://www.ncbi.nlm.nih.gov/pmc/articles/PMC1070794
Secondary screening: eating/ self-regulation	Eating Disorder Screen for Primary Care (ESP)[82] *Simple questions to screen for eating disorders*	5 items	Adolescents and adults English	Administration: 1 min Scoring: 1 min	No cost Developed at University Hospital, London, UK Form available at www. mendedwingcounseling.com/ wp-content/uploads/2014/08/ ESP.pdf

Table A2-1. Mental Health Tools for Pediatrics (*continued*)

Psychosocial Measure	Tools and Description	Number of Items and Format	Age-group and Any Languages Reading Level if Specified	Administration and Scoring Time Training[a]	Source
Diagnostic Assessment (Algorithm Step 15)					
Previous findings	Previous screening results, steps 2 and 11 (general and specific)				
	Interview				
	Observations of patient and family				
	Collateral reports				
	Parent history				
Diagnostic tools	Child Health and Development Interactive System (CHADIS)–*DSM*[83] *Assesses broadly for mental health symptoms and problems in functioning*	Electronic Variable number of items that depends on response	Birth and on English, with some tools in Spanish	18–48 min	Proprietary Source: www.chadis.com/clinicians/assessment.html

Achenbach System of Empirically Based Assessment (ASEBA) Child Behavior Checklist (CBCL)[84] DSM-oriented scales assess for • 1½–5 y: pervasive developmental problem • 6–18 y: somatic problems and conduct problems • Both groups: affective problems, anxiety problems, oppositional defiant problems, and attention-deficit/hyperactivity problems	Parent or caregiver/ teacher for 1½–5 y: 99 items Parent/teacher: 118 items direct observation Youth self-report	1½–5 y 6–18 y 74 languages	15–20 min (both age-groups)	Proprietary Source: www.aseba.org
UCLA PTSD Reaction Index for DSM-5[85] Assesses exposure to traumatic experiences and impact of traumatic events	Child: 20 items Parent: 21 items Youth: 22 items	Child and parent: 7–12 y Youth: ≥13 y Multiple languages	20–30 min to administer Scoring: 5–10 min	Proprietary Source: http://tdg.ucla.edu/sites/ default/files/UCLA_PTSD_Reaction_ Index_Flyer.pdf Adapted version available in AAP Feelings Need Check Ups Too CD-ROM[86] to assess trauma exposure
Functional assessment tools Child and Adolescent Functional Assessment Scale (CAFAS)[38,87] Assesses the degree of impairment in youths with emotional, behavioral, psychiatric, or substance use problems. Used to assess level of need for services in MH and other systems. Also used in evaluating outcomes for programs, evidence-based treatments and evidence-informed practices.	Clinician uses information collected during a routine clinical interview and selects items that describe the youth's problematic behaviors, as well as strengths and goals.	5–19 y English French Spanish Dutch	Based on prior clinical assessment. Scoring requires approximately 10 min.	Proprietary Source: www2.fasoutcomes.com/ Content.aspx?ContentID=12

Table A2-1. Mental Health Tools for Pediatrics (*continued*)

Psychosocial Measure	Tools and Description	Number of Items and Format	Age-group and Any Languages Reading Level if Specified	Administration and Scoring Time Training[a]	Source
Diagnostic Assessment (Algorithm Step 15)					
Functional assessment tools	Children's Global Assessment Scale (CGAS)[88] *Assesses overall severity of disturbance and impact on global functioning*	1 item Rated by clinician 100-point scale with 10-point anchors Note: A "nonclinical version" can be administered by lay interviewers.	4–16 y English	Requires no administration time for clinical version because it is based on prior clinical assessment. Time to integrate knowledge of the child into a single score is estimated to be 5–10 min.	Freely accessible Source: www.rcpsych.ac.uk/pdf/CGAS%20Ratings%20Guide.pdf
	Functional Assessment Interview Form - Young Child[89] *Elicits behavioral concerns, factors that precipitate unwanted behaviors, consequences of behaviors, and functional difficulties*	9-page questionnaire/interview with caregiver or teacher aimed at developing a hypothesis about problem behaviors	½–5 y English	45–90 min	Freely accessible
	BIS[37]				
	CIS[38]				

Family-Centered Care Plan (Algorithm Step 17)				
Transition	The Transition Readiness Assessment Questionnaire (TRAQ)[90] *Identifies areas in which a youth needs education and training to achieve independence in transition-relevant skills; used also to set goals*	20 items	Adolescents and adults aged 16–26 y with chronic conditions English	<5 min	Freely accessible Source: www.etsu.edu/com/ pediatrics/traq/registration.php
	Self-Management and Transition to Adulthood with R_x=Treatment (STAR$_x$)[91] *Collects information on self-management and health care transition skills, via self-report, in a broad population of adolescents and young adults with chronic conditions*	18 items in 3 domains	Adolescents and young adults with chronic conditions English	2–3 min 5 min to score	Freely accessible Source: www.med.unc.edu/ transition/files/2017/12/STARx-Adolescent-Version.pdf
Care Plan Implementation, Comanagement, and Monitoring (Algorithm Step 18)				
Monitoring	Periodic functional assessment compared with baseline (eg, SDQ Impact Scale,[12] BIS,[37] CIS[38])			
	PSC-35[9,10]			
	PSC-17[11]			
	SDQ[12]			
	NICHQ Vanderbilt Diagnostic Rating Scales[54]			
	ASQ:SE-2[4]			

Table A2-1. Mental Health Tools for Pediatrics (*continued*)

Psychosocial Measure	Tools and Description	Number of Items and Format	Age-group and Any Languages Reading Level if Specified	Administration and Scoring Time Training[a]	Source
Care Plan Implementation, Comanagement, and Monitoring (Algorithm Step 18)					
Monitoring	BITSEA[5]				
	ECSA[3]				
	S2BI[15]				
	Functional Disability Inventory[25]				
	Fax-back forms returned from MHS				
	Shared care plan				Resources available at https://medicalhomeinfo.aap.org/tools-resources/Documents/Shared%20Plan%20of%20Care2.pdf

Abbreviations not defined within table: AAP, American Academy of Pediatrics; ADHD, attention-deficit/hyperactivity disorder; ASD, autism spectrum disorder; *DSM*, *Diagnostic and Statistical Manual of Mental Disorders* of the American Psychiatric Association; MCHB, Maternal and Child Health Bureau; MH, mental health; MHS, mental health specialist; NIAAA, National Institute on Alcohol Abuse and Alcoholism; OCD, obsessive-compulsive disorder; PCC, primary care clinician; PTSD, post-traumatic stress disorder; UCLA, University of California, Los Angeles.

[a] None unless otherwise indicated.

[b] *Bright Futures: Guidelines for Health Supervisions of Infants, Children, and Adolescents*, 4th Edition, recommends universal screening of adolescents for substance use beginning at age 11 y.

[c] *Bright Futures*, 4th Edition, recommends universal screening of adolescents for depression.

[d] Use of these tools as part of the initial psychosocial assessment (step 2) may be appropriate when recent trauma is a presenting concern; alternatively, these tools may be used at step 11 for secondary screening.

[e] General screening and surveillance tools not used in step 2 may be used at this step. They may be administered by the PCC (or an integrated MHS) or collected from collateral sources.

[f] Tools not used at step 2 can be applied at this step.

References

1. Hagan JF Jr, Shaw JS, Duncan PM, eds. *Bright Futures: Guidelines for Health Supervision of Infants, Children, and Adolescents*. 3rd ed. Elk Grove Village, IL: American Academy of Pediatrics; 2008

2. Klein DA, Goldenring JM, Adelman WP. HEEADSSS 3.0: the psychosocial interview for adolescents updated for a new century fueled by media. *Contemp Pediatr*. 2014. http://www.contemporarypediatrics.com/modern-medicine-feature-articles/heeadsss-30-psychosocial-interview-adolescents-updated-new-century-fueled-media. Published January 1, 2014. Accessed February 26, 2018

3. Gleason MM, Zeanah CH, Dickstein S. Recognizing young children in need of mental health assessment: development and preliminary validity of the Early Childhood Screening Assessment. *Infant Ment Health J*. 2010;31(3):335–357

4. Salomonsson B, Sleed M. The Ages & Stages Questionnaire: Social-Emotional: a validation study of a mother-report questionnaire on a clinical mother-infant sample. *Infant Ment Health J*. 2010;31(4):412–431

5. Briggs-Gowan MJ, Carter AS, Irwin JR, Wachtel K, Cicchetti DV. The Brief-Infant Toddler Social and Emotional Assessment: screening for social-emotional problems and delays in competence. *J Pediatr Psychol*. 2004;29(2):143–155

6. Sheldrick RC, Perrin EC. Evidence-based milestones for surveillance of cognitive, language, and motor development. *Acad Pediatr*. 2013;13(6):577–586

7. Sheldrick RC, Henson BS, Neger EN, Merchant S, Murphy JM, Perrin EC. The Baby Pediatric Symptom Checklist (BPSC): development and initial validation of a new social/emotional screening instrument. *Acad Pediatr*. 2013;13(1):72–80

8. Sheldrick RC, Henson BS, Neger EN, Merchant S, Murphy JM, Perrin EC. The Preschool Pediatric Symptom Checklist (PPSC): development and initial validation of a new social/emotional screening instrument. *Acad Pediatr*. 2012;12(5):456–467

9. Jellinek MS, Murphy JM, Little M, Pagano ME, Comer DM, Kelleher KJ. Use of the Pediatric Symptom Checklist to screen for psychosocial problems in pediatric primary care: a national feasibility study. *Arch Pediatr Adolesc Med*. 1999;153(3):254–260

10. Hacker KA, Myagmarjav E, Harris V, Suglia SF, Weidner D, Link D. Mental health screening in pediatric practice: factors related to positive screens and the contribution of parental/personal concern. *Pediatrics*. 2006;118(5):1896–1906

11. Gardner W, Lucas A, Kolko DJ, Campo JV. Comparison of the PSC-17 and alternative mental health screens in an at-risk primary care sample. *J Am Acad Child Adolesc Psychiatry*. 2007; 46(5):611–618

12. Goodman R, Ford T, Simmons H, Gatward R, Meltzer H. Using the Strengths and Difficulties Questionnaire (SDQ) to screen for child psychiatric disorders in a community sample. *Br J Psychiatry*. 2000;177:534–539

13. Yi CH, Martyn K, Salerno J, Darling-Fisher CS. Development and clinical use of Rapid Assessment for Adolescent Preventive Services (RAAPS) Questionnaire in school-based health centers. *J Pediatr Health Care*. 2009;23(1):2–9

14. Salerno J, Barnhart S. Evaluation of the RAAPS risk screening tool for use in detecting adolescents with depression. *J Child Adolesc Psychiatr Nurs*. 2014;27(1):20–25

15. Kelly SM, Gryczynski J, Mitchell SG, Kirk A, O'Grady KE, Schwartz RP. Validity of brief screening instrument for adolescent tobacco, alcohol, and drug use. *Pediatrics*. 2014;133(5): 819–826. http://www.ncbi.nlm.nih.gov/pmc/articles/PMC4006430. Published May 2014. Accessed February 26, 2018

16. Chung T, Smith GT, Donovan JE, et al. Drinking frequency as a brief screen for adolescent alcohol problems. *Pediatrics*. 2012;129(2):205–212

17. National Institute on Alcohol Abuse and Alcoholism. *Alcohol Screening and Brief Intervention for Youth: A Practitioner's Guide.* Washington, DC: National Institutes of Health; 2015. https://pubs.niaaa.nih.gov/publications/Practitioner/YouthGuide/YouthGuide.pdf. Accessed February 26, 2018

18. Knight JR, Sherritt L, Shrier LA, Harris SK, Chang G. Validity of the CRAFFT substance abuse screening test among adolescent clinic patients. *Arch Pediatr Adolesc Med.* 2002;156(6): 607–614

19. Richardson LP, McCauley E, Grossman DC, et al. Evaluation of the Patient Health Questionnaire (PHQ-9) for detecting major depression among adolescents. *Pediatrics.* 2010;126(6):1117–1123

20. Leblanc JC, Almudevar A, Brooks SJ, Kutcher S. Screening for adolescent depression: comparison of the Kutcher Adolescent Depression Scale with the Beck Depression Inventory. *J Child Adolesc Psychopharmacol.* 2002;12(2):113–126

21. Kemper KJ, Kelleher KJ. Family psychosocial screening: instruments and techniques. *Ambul Child Health.* 1996;1(4):325–339

22. Dubowitz H. The Safe Environment for Every Kid model: promotion of children's health, development, and safety, and prevention of child neglect. *Pediatr Ann.* 2014;43(11):e271–e277

23. Kiplinger VL, Browne CH. *Parents' Assessment of Protective Factors: User's Guide and Technical Report.* Washington, DC: National Quality Improvement Center on Early Childhood; 2014. https://www.cssp.org/reform/child-welfare/pregnant-and-parenting-youth/Parents-Assessment-of-Protective-Factors.pdf. Accessed February 26, 2018

24. Health Leads. *Social Needs Screening Toolkit.* Boston, MA: Health Leads; 2016. https://healthleadsusa.org/wp-content/uploads/2016/07/Health-Leads-Screening-Toolkit-July-2016.pdf. Accessed February 26, 2018

25. Kabacoff RI, Miller IW, Bishop DS, Epstein NB, Keitner GI. A psychometric study of the McMaster Family Assessment Device in psychiatric, medical, and nonclinical samples. *J Fam Psychol.* 1990;3(4):431–439

26. Loyd BH, Abidin RR. Revision of the Parenting Stress Index. *J Pediatr Psychol.* 1985;10(2): 169–177

27. Sheras PL, Abidin RR. Stress Index for Parents of Adolescents. PAR Web site. https://www.parinc.com/Products/Pkey/412. Accessed February 26, 2018

28. Brannan AM, Heflinger CA, Bickman L. The caregiver strain questionnaire: measuring the impact on the family of living with a child with serious emotional disturbance. *J Emot Behav Disord.* 1997;5(4):212–222

29. Canty-Mitchell J, Zimet GD. Psychometric properties of the Multidimensional Scale of Perceived Social Support in urban adolescents. *Am J Community Psychol.* 2000;28(3):391–400

30. Löwe B, Kroenke K, Gräfe K. Detecting and monitoring depression with a two-item questionnaire (PHQ-2). *J Psychosom Res.* 2005;58(2):163–171

31. Kroenke K, Spitzer RL, Williams JB. The PHQ-9: validity of a brief depression severity measure. *J Gen Intern Med.* 2001;16(9):606–613

32. Garcia-Esteve L, Ascaso C, Ojuel J, Navarro P. Validation of the Edinburgh Postnatal Depression Scale (EPDS) in Spanish mothers. *J Affect Disord.* 2003;75(1):71–76

33. Reichenheim ME, Moraes CL. Comparison between the abuse assessment screen and the revised conflict tactics scales for measuring physical violence during pregnancy. *J Epidemiol Community Health.* 2004;58(6):523–527

34. Gundersen C, Engelhard EE, Crumbaugh AS, Seligman HK. Brief assessment of food insecurity accurately identifies high-risk US adults. *Public Health Nutr.* 2017;20(8):1367–1371

35. Kassam-Adams N. The Acute Stress Checklist for Children (ASC-Kids): development of a child self-report measure. *J Trauma Stress.* 2006;19(1):129–139

36. Perrin S, Meiser-Stedman R, Smith P. *The Children's Revised Impact of Event Scale (CRIES): Validity as a Screening Instrument for PTSD.* London, UK: Dept of Psychology, Institute of Psychiatry/Kings College London. https://www.mrc-cbu.cam.ac.uk/wp-content/uploads/2013/02/Perrin-et-al.pdf. Accessed February 26, 2018

37. Bird HR, Canino GJ, Davies M, et al. The Brief Impairment Scale (BIS): a multidimensional scale of functional impairment for children and adolescents. *J Am Acad Child Adolesc Psychiatry.* 2005;44(7):699–707

38. Bird HR, Andrews H, Schwab-Stone M, et al. Global measures of impairment for epidemiologic and clinical use with children and adolescents. *Int J Methods Psychiatr Res.* 1997;6(4):295–307

39. Foy JM; American Academy of Pediatrics Task Force on Mental Health. Enhancing pediatric mental health care: algorithms for primary care. *Pediatrics.* 2010;125(suppl 3):S109–S125

40. *Addressing Mental Health Concerns in Primary Care: A Clinician's Toolkit.* Elk Grove Village, IL: American Academy of Pediatrics; 2010

41. Walker LS, Beck JE, Garber J, Lambert W. Children's Somatization Inventory: psychometric properties of the revised form (CSI-24). *J Pediatr Psychol.* 2009;34(4):430–440

42. Ballard ED, Cwik M, Van Eck K, et al. Identification of at-risk youth by suicide screening in a pediatric emergency department. *Prev Sci.* 2017;18(2):174–182

43. Substance Abuse and Mental Health Services Administration. *SAFE-T: Suicide Assessment Five-Step Evaluation and Triage for Clinicians* [pocket card]. Substance Abuse and Mental Health Services Administration; 2009. https://store.samhsa.gov/product/SAFE-T-Pocket-Card-Suicide-Assessment-Five-Step-Evaluation-and-Triage-for-Clinicians/SMA09-4432. Accessed February 26, 2018

44. Osman A, Bagge CL, Gutierrez PM, Konick LC, Kopper BA, Barrios FX. The Suicidal Behaviors Questionnaire-Revised (SBQ-R): validation with clinical and nonclinical samples. *Assessment.* 2001;8(4):443–454

45. Posner K, Brown GK, Stanley B, et al. The Columbia-Suicide Severity Rating Scale: initial validity and internal consistency findings from three multisite studies with adolescents and adults. *Am J Psychiatry.* 2011;168(12):1266–1277

46. Reynolds WM, Mazza JJ. Assessment of suicidal ideation in inner-city children and young adolescents: reliability and validity of the Suicidal Ideation Questionnaire. *School Psychol Rev.* 1999;28(1):17–30

47. Pfeffer CR, Jiang H, Kakuma T. Child-Adolescent Suicidal Potential Index (CASPI): a screen for risk for early onset suicidal behavior. *Psychol Assess.* 2000;12(3):304–318

48. Turkel SB, Braslow K, Tavaré CJ, Trzepacz PT. The delirium rating scale in children and adolescents. *Psychosomatics.* 2003;44(2):126–129

49. Lyons JS, Kisiel CL, Dulcan M, Cohen R, Chesler P. Crisis assessment and psychiatric hospitalization of children and adolescents in state custody. *J Child Fam Stud.* 1997;6(3):311–320

50. Sandoval J, Echandia A. Behavior assessment system for children. *J Sch Psychol.* 1994;32:419–425

51. Fisher P. Developing an epidemiological tool based on *DSM-5* criteria. Disability Research and Dissemination Center Web site. https://www.disabilityresearchcenter.com/2015/10/13/developing-epi-tool. Published October 13, 2015. Accessed February 26, 2018

52. Johnson JG, Harris ES, Spitzer RL, Williams JB. The patient health questionnaire for adolescents: validation of an instrument for the assessment of mental disorders among adolescent primary care patients. *J Adolesc Health.* 2002;30(3):196–204

53. Achenbach T, Rescorla L. *Manual for the ASEBA Preschool Forms and Profiles.* Burlington, VT: University of Vermont, Research Centre for Children, Youth, and Families; 2000

54. Wolraich ML, Lambert W, Doffing MA, Bickman L, Simmons T, Worley K. Psychometric properties of the Vanderbilt ADHD diagnostic parent rating scale in a referred population. *J Pediatr Psychol.* 2003;28(8):559–567

55. Conners CK, Wells KC, Parker JD, Sitarenios G, Diamond JM, Powell JW. A new self-report scale for assessment of adolescent psychopathology: factor structure, reliability, validity, and diagnostic sensitivity. *J Abnorm Child Psychol.* 1997;25(6):487–497

56. Chukwujekwu DC, Stanley PC. The Modified Overt Aggression Scale: how valid in this environment? *Niger J Med.* 2008;17(2):153–155

57. Boggs SR, Eyberg S, Reynolds LA. Concurrent validity of the Eyberg Child Behavior Inventory. *J Clin Child Psychol.* 1990;19(1):75–78

58. Waschbusch DA, Elgar FJ. Development and validation of the Conduct Disorder Rating Scale. *Assessment.* 2007;14(1):65–74

59. Luby JL, Heffelfinger A, Koenig-McNaught AL, Brown K, Spitznagel E. The Preschool Feelings Checklist: a brief and sensitive screening measure for depression in young children. *J Am Acad Child Adolesc Psychiatry.* 2004;43(6):708–717

60. Kroenke K, Spitzer RL. The PHQ-9: a new depression and diagnostic severity measure. *Psychiatr Ann.* 2002;32(9):509–515

61. Garrison CZ, Addy CL, Jackson KL, McKeown RE, Waller JL. The CES-D as a screen for depression and other psychiatric disorders in adolescents. *J Am Acad Child Adolesc Psychiatry.* 1991;30(4):636–641

62. Knight D, Hensley VR, Waters B. Validation of the Children's Depression Scale and the Children's Depression Inventory in a prepubertal sample. *J Child Psychol Psychiatry.* 1988;29(6):853–863

63. Rhew IC, Simpson K, Tracy M, et al. Criterion validity of the Short Mood and Feelings Questionnaire and one-and two-item depression screens in young adolescents. *Child Adolesc Psychiatry Ment Health.* 2010;4(1):8

64. Wang YP, Gorenstein C. Psychometric properties of the Beck Depression Inventory-II: a comprehensive review. *Rev Pras Psiquiatr.* 2013;35(4):416–431

65. Pietsch K, Hoyler A, Frühe B, Kruse J, Schulte-Körne G, Allgaier AK. Early detection of major depression in paediatric care: validity of the Beck Depression Inventory-Second Edition (BDI-II) and the Beck Depression Inventory-Fast Screen for Medical Patients (BDI-FS). *Psychother Psychosom Med Psychol.* 2012;62(11):418–424

66. Spence SH, Barrett PM, Turner CM. Psychometric properties of the Spence Children's Anxiety Scale with young adolescents. *J Anxiety Disord.* 2003;17(6):605–625

67. Jastrowski Mano KE, Evans JR, Tran ST, Anderson Khan K, Weisman SJ, Hainsworth KR. The psychometric properties of the Screen for Child Anxiety Related Emotional Disorders in pediatric chronic pain. *J Pediatr Psychol.* 2012;37(9):999–1011

68. Mossman SA, Luft MJ, Schroeder HK, et al. The Generalized Anxiety Disorder 7-item scale in adolescents with generalized anxiety disorder: signal detection and validation. *Ann Clin Psychiatry.* 2017;29(4):227–234A

69. Briere J, Johnson K, Bissada A, et al. The Trauma Symptom Checklist for Young Children (TSCYC): reliability and association with abuse exposure in a multi-site study. *Child Abuse Neglect.* 2001;25(8):1001–1014

70. Foa EB, Johnson KM, Feeny NC, Treadwell KR. The Child PTSD Symptom Scale: a preliminary examination of its psychometric properties. *J Clin Child Psychol.* 2001;30(3): 376–384

71. Gioia GA, Isquith PK, Retzlaff PD, Espy KA. Confirmatory factor analysis of the Behavior Rating Inventory of Executive Function (BRIEF) in a clinical sample. *Child Neuropsychol.* 2002;8(4):249–257

72. Rossman MJ, Hyman SL, Roarbaugh ML, Berlin LE, Allen MC, Modlin JF. The CAT/CLAMS assessment for early intervention services. Clinical Adaptive Test/Clinical Linguistic and Auditory Milestone Scale. *Clin Pediatr (Phila).* 1994;33(7):404–409

73. Walker D, Gugenheim S, Downs MP, Northern JL. Early Language Milestone Scale and language screening of young children. *Pediatrics.* 1989;83(2):284–288

74. Rescorla L. The Language Developmental Survey: a screening tool for delayed language in toddlers. *J Speech Hear Disord.* 1989;54(4):587–599

75. Claar RL, Walker LS. Functional assessment of pediatric pain patients: psychometric properties of the Functional Disability Inventory. *Pain.* 2006;121(1–2):77–84

76. Owens JA, Dalzell V. Use of the "BEARS" sleep screening tool in a pediatric residents' continuity clinic: a pilot study. *Sleep Med.* 2005;6(1):63–69

77. Johnson JA, Lee A, Vinson D, Seale JP. Use of AUDIT-based measures to identify unhealthy alcohol use and alcohol dependence in primary care: a validation study. *Alcohol Clin Exp Res.* 2013;37(suppl 1):E253–E259

78. Dennis ML, Chan YF, Funk RR. Development and validation of the GAIN Short Screener (GSS) for internalizing, externalizing and substance use disorders and crime/violence problems among adolescents and adults. *Am J Addict.* 2006;15(suppl 1):80–91

79. Rauch P, Ohye B, Bostic J, Masek B. *A Toolkit for the Well Child Screening of Military Children.* Boston, MA: Home Base Veteran and Family Care. http://homebase.org/media/toolkit-for-providerUpdatedLogo.pdf. Accessed February 26, 2018

80. Friedrich WN. *Child Sexual Behavioral Inventory: Professional Manual.* Odessa, FL: Psychological Assessment Resources; 1997. https://www.parinc.com/Products/Pkey/71. Accessed June 11, 2018

81. Rueda Jaimes GE, Díaz Martínez LA, Ortiz Barajas DP, Pinzón Plata C, Rodríguez Martínez J, Cadena Afanador LP. [Validation of the SCOFF questionnaire for screening the eating behavior disorders of adolescents in school.] *Aten Primaria.* 2005;35(2):89–94

82. Cotton MA, Ball C, Robinson P. Four simple questions can help screen for eating disorders. *J Gen Intern Med.* 2003;18(1):53–56

83. Howard BJ. *Developmental and Mental Health Screening.* Baltimore, MD: Johns Hopkins University School of Medicine. http://learn.pcc.com/wp/wp-content/uploads/UC2016_DevelopmentalandMentalHealthScreening.pdf. Accessed February 26, 2018

84. Reliability and validity information. ASEBA Web site. http://www.aseba.org/ordering/reliabilityvalidity.html. Accessed February 26, 2018

85. Steinberg AM, Brymer MJ, Kim S, et al. Psychometric properties of the UCLA PTSD Reaction Index: part I. *J Trauma Stress.* 2013;26(1):1–9

86. Laraque D, Jensen P, Schonfeld D. *Feelings Need Check Ups Too CD-ROM and Toolkit.* Elk Grove Village, IL: American Academy of Pediatrics; 2006. https://www.aap.org/en-us/advocacy-and-policy/aap-health-initiatives/Children-and-Disasters/Pages/Feelings-Need-Checkups-Too-CD-Page-2.aspx. Accessed February 26, 2018

87. Hodges K. Child and Adolescent Functional Assessment Scale (CAFAS): overview of reliability and validity. Functional Assessment Systems Web site. http://www2.fasoutcomes.com/RadControls/Editor/FileManager/Document/FAS611_CAFAS%20Reliability%20and%20Validity%20Rev10.pdf. Accessed February 26, 2018

88. Shaffer D, Gould MS, Brasic J, et al. A Children's Global Assessment Scale (CGAS). *Arch Gen Psychiatry.* 1983;40(11):1228–1231

89. O'Neill RE, Horner RH, Albin RW, Sprague JR. *Functional Assessment and Program Development for Problem Behavior: A Practical Handbook.* Pacific Grove, CA: Brooks/Cole Publishing; 1997

90. Wood DL, Sawicki GS, Miller MD, et al. The Transition Readiness Assessment Questionnaire (TRAQ): its factor structure, reliability, and validity. *Acad Pediatr.* 2014;14(4):415–422

91. Cohen SE, Hooper SR, Javalkar K, et al. Self-management and transition readiness assessment: concurrent, predictive and discriminant validation of the $STAR_x$ Questionnaire. *J Pediatr Nurs.* 2015;30(5):668–676

Sources of Key Mental Health Services

Table A3-1.

Specialty Services	Sources
Psychiatric emergency services	• Local mental health screening, triage, and referral service or another intake point for public specialty system • Mobile crisis unit, if available • Child psychiatrist • General psychiatrist with pediatric expertise (or consultation with child psychiatrist) • Emergency department
Medication consultation or treatment of patients with problems of high severity (MD or DO required)	• Neurodevelopmental/developmental-behavioral pediatrician • Child psychiatrist (in person or telepsychiatry) • General psychiatrist with child expertise or child psychiatry consultation • Adolescent medicine specialist • Pediatric neurologist • Local public mental health agency
Early Intervention services	• Part C agency for 0–3 y; Part B agency for 3–5 y • Developmental evaluation agency • Neurodevelopmental/developmental-behavioral pediatrician • Child psychiatrist with expertise in young children • Early Intervention specialist
Child protective services	• Department of Social Services
Grief counseling	• Licensed mental health specialist[a] • Hospice agency
Substance use disorder counseling	• Licensed substance use disorder counselor • Agency specializing in substance use disorder
Psychosocial assessment	• Licensed mental health specialist[a] with pediatric expertise
Educational assessment	• School psychologist • Child psychologist or another licensed psychologist • Neurodevelopmental/developmental-behavioral pediatrician • Educational specialist
Psychosocial treatment	• Licensed mental health specialist[a] trained in the specific intervention (eg, cognitive behavioral therapy specific to the condition, trauma-focused therapy, parent management training, mind-body therapies, family therapy)

Table A3-1. (*continued*)

Specialty Services	Sources
Specialized counseling programs (eg, domestic violence, family reunification, children of parents with alcohol use disorder, juvenile sex offender, divorce, stress management, smoking cessation)	• Licensed mental health specialist[a] with pediatric expertise • Agency specializing in that area
Parenting education	• Parent educator trained in evaluated curriculum • Family services agency • Licensed mental health specialist[a] • School system's social work services (Some have parenting education programs.) • Agricultural extension service (Some have parenting education programs.)
Care coordination/case management	• Licensed mental health specialist[a] with pediatric expertise • Local public mental health agency • Peer support program
Peer support	• Local organization of National Alliance on Mental Illness, National Federation of Families for Children's Mental Health, Family Support Network, or Children and Adults with Attention-Deficit/Hyperactivity Disorder • Local public mental health agency • Al-Anon

[a] The term *licensed mental health specialist* encompasses clinical psychologists, clinical social workers, professional counselors, and others permitted by state authority to provide the particular service. Adapted from Appendix S1: sources of specialty services for children with mental health problems and their families. *Pediatrics*. 2010;125(suppl 3):S126–S127. http://pediatrics.aappublications.org/content/125/Supplement_3/S126. Published June 2010. Accessed February 27, 2018.

PracticeWise:
Evidence-Based Child and Adolescent Psychosocial Interventions

This report is intended to guide practitioners, educators, youth, and families in developing appropriate plans using psychosocial interventions. It was created for the period October 2017 – April 2018 using the PracticeWise Evidence-Based Services (PWEBS) Database, available at www.practicewise. com. If this is not the most current version, please check the American Academy of Pediatrics (AAP) mental health Web site (www.aap.org/mentalhealth) for updates.

Please note that this chart represents an independent analysis by PracticeWise and should not be construed as endorsement by the AAP. For an explanation of PracticeWise determination of evidence/level, please see below or visit www.practicewise.com/aap.

Table A4-1.

Problem Area	Level 1 - Best Support	Level 2 - Good Support	Level 3 - Moderate Support	Level 4 - Minimal Support	Level 5 - No Support
Anxious or Avoidant Behaviors	Cognitive Behavior Therapy (CBT), CBT and Medication, CBT for Child and Parent, CBT with Parents, Education, Exposure, Modeling	Assertiveness Training, Attention, Attention Training, CBT and Music Therapy, CBT and Parent Management Training (PMT), CBT with Parents Only, Cultural Storytelling, Family Psychoeducation, Hypnosis, Mindfulness, Relaxation, Stress Inoculation	Contingency Management, Group Therapy	Behavioral Activation and Exposure, Biofeedback, Play Therapy, PMT, Psychodynamic Therapy, Rational Emotive Therapy, Social Skills	Assessment/Monitoring, Attachment Therapy, Client Centered Therapy, Eye Movement Desensitization and Reprocessing (EMDR), Peer Pairing, Psychoeducation, Relationship Counseling, Teacher Psychoeducation
Autism Spectrum Disorders	CBT, Intensive Behavioral Treatment, Intensive Communication Training, Joint Attention/Engagement, PMT, Social Skills	Imitation, Peer Pairing, Theory of Mind Training	None	Massage, Peer Pairing and Modeling, Play Therapy	Attention Training, Biofeedback, Cognitive Flexibility Training, Communication Skills, Contingent Responding, Eclectic Therapy, Executive Functioning Training, Fine Motor Training, Modeling, Parent Psychoeducation, Physical/Social/Occupational Therapy, Sensory Integration Training, Structured Listening, Working Memory Training
Delinquency and Disruptive Behavior	Anger Control, Assertiveness Training, CBT, Contingency Management, Multisystemic Therapy, PMT, PMT and Problem Solving, Problem Solving, Social Skills, Therapeutic Foster Care	CBT and PMT, CBT and Teacher Training, Communication Skills, Cooperative Problem Solving, Family Therapy, Functional Family Therapy, PMT and Classroom Management, PMT and Social Skills, Rational Emotive Therapy, Self Control Training, Transactional Analysis	Client Centered Therapy, Moral Reasoning Training, Outreach Counseling, Peer Pairing	CBT and Teacher Psychoeducation, Exposure, Physical Exercise, PMT and Classroom Management and CBT, PMT and Self-Verbalization, Stress Inoculation	Behavioral Family Therapy, Catharsis, CBT with Parents, Education, Family Empowerment and Support, Family Systems Therapy, Group Therapy, Imagery Training, Play Therapy, PMT and Peer Support, Psychodynamic Therapy, Self Verbalization, Skill Development, Wraparound

Depressive or Withdrawn Behaviors	CBT, CBT and Medication, CBT with Parents, Client Centered Therapy, Family Therapy	Attention Training, Cognitive Behavioral Psychoeducation, Expression, Interpersonal Therapy, Motivational Interviewing (MI)/Engagement and CBT, Physical Exercise, Problem Solving, Relaxation	None	Self Control Training, Self Modeling, Social Skills	CBT and Anger Control, CBT and Behavioral Sleep Intervention, CBT and PMT, Goal Setting, Life Skills, Mindfulness, Play Therapy, PMT, PMT and Emotion Regulation, Psychodynamic Therapy, Psychoeducation
Eating Disorders	CBT, Physical Exercise and Dietary Care and Behavioral Feedback	Family-Focused Therapy, Family Systems Therapy, Family Therapy with Parents Only	None	Physical Exercise and Dietary Care	Behavioral Training and Dietary Care, CBT with Parents, Client Centered Therapy, Dietary Care, Education, Family Therapy, Family Therapy with Parent Consultant, Goal Setting, Psychoeducation, Yoga
Elimination Disorders	Behavior Alert, Behavior Alert and Behavioral Training, Behavioral Training, Behavioral Training and Biofeedback and Dietary Care and Medical Care, Behavioral Training and Dietary Care and Medical Care	Behavioral Training and Dietary Care, Behavioral Training and Hypnosis and Dietary Care, CBT	Behavior Alert and Medication	None	Assessment/Monitoring, Assessment/Monitoring and Medication, Behavioral Training and Medical Care, Biofeedback, Contingency Management, Dietary Care, Dietary Care and Medical Care, Hypnosis, Medical Care, Psychoeducation
Mania	None	CBT for Child and Parent, Cognitive Behavioral Psychoeducation	None	None	Cognitive Behavioral Psychoeducation and Dietary Care, Dialectical Behavior Therapy and Medication, Family-Focused Therapy, Psychoeducation

Table A4-1. (continued)

Problem Area	Level 1- Best Support	Level 2- Good Support	Level 3- Moderate Support	Level 4- Minimal Support	Level 5- No Support
Substance Use	CBT, Community Reinforcement, Contingency Management, Family Therapy, MI/Engagement	Assertive Continuing Care, CBT and Contingency Management, CBT and Medication, CBT with Parents, Family Systems Therapy, Functional Family Therapy, Goal Setting/Monitoring, MI/Engagement and CBT, MI/Engagement and Expression, Multidimensional Family Therapy, Problem Solving, Purdue Brief Family Therapy	Drug Court, Drug Court and Multisystemic Therapy and Contingency Management, Eclectic Therapy	Goal Setting, Psychoeducation	Advice/Encouragement, Assessment/Monitoring, Behavioral Family Therapy, Case Management, CBT and Community Information Campaign, CBT and Functional Family Therapy, Client Centered Therapy, Drug Court and Multisystemic Therapy, Drug Education, Education, Family Court, Feedback, Group Therapy, Mindfulness, MI/Engagement and CBT and Family Therapy, Multisystemic Therapy, Parent Psychoeducation, PMT, Therapeutic Vocational Training
Suicidality	None	Attachment Therapy, CBT with Parents, Counselors Care, Counselors Care and Support Training, Interpersonal Therapy, Multisystemic Therapy, Parent Coping/Stress Management, Psychodynamic Therapy, Social Support	None	None	Accelerated Hospitalization, Case Management, CBT, Communication Skills, Counselors Care and Anger Management

Traumatic Stress	CBT, CBT with Parents, EMDR	Exposure		None	Play Therapy, Psychodrama, Relaxation and Expression	Advice/Encouragement, Client Centered Therapy, CBT and Medication, CBT with Parents Only, Education, Expressive Play, Interpersonal Therapy, Problem Solving, Psychodynamic Therapy, Psychoeducation, Relaxation, Structured Listening

Adapted with permission from PracticeWise.

Note: CBT = Cognitive Behavior Therapy; EMDR = Eye Movement Desensitization and Reprocessing; MI = Motivational Interviewing; PMT = Parent Management Training; Level 5 refers to treatments whose tests were unsupportive or inconclusive. This report updates and replaces the "Blue Menu" originally distributed by the Hawaii Department of Health, Child and Adolescent Mental Health Division, Evidence-Based Services Committee from 2002–2009.

The recommendations in this publication do not indicate an exclusive course of treatment or serve as a standard of medical care. Variations, taking into account individual circumstances, may be appropriate. Original document included as part of *Addressing Mental Health Concerns in Primary Care: A Clinician's Toolkit*. Copyright © 2010 American Academy of Pediatrics. All Rights Reserved. The American Academy of Pediatrics (AAP) does not review or endorse any modifications made to this document and in no event shall the AAP be liable for any such changes.

Background

The PracticeWise "Evidence-Based Child and Adolescent Psychosocial Interventions" tool is created twice each year and posted on the AAP Web site at www.aap.org/mentalhealth, using data from the PWEBS Database, available at www.practicewise.com. The table is based on an ongoing review of randomized clinical psychosocial and combined treatment trials for children and adolescents with mental health needs. The contents of the table represent the treatments that best fit a patient's characteristics, based on the primary problem (rows) and the strength of evidence behind the treatments (columns). Thus, when seeking an intervention with the best empirical support for an adolescent with depression, one might select from among cognitive behavior therapy (CBT) alone, CBT with medication, CBT with parents included, client centered therapy, or family therapy. Each clinical trial must have been published in a peer-reviewed scientific journal, and each study is coded by 2 independent raters whose discrepancies are reviewed and resolved by a third expert judge. Prior to report development, data are subject to extensive quality analyses to identify and eliminate remaining errors, inconsistencies, or formatting problems.

Strength of Evidence Definitions

The strength of evidence classification uses a 5-level system that was originally adapted from the American Psychological Association Division 12 Task Force on the Promotion and Dissemination of Psychological Procedures.[1] These definitions can be seen in the Strength of Evidence Definitions section later in this appendix. Higher strength of evidence is an indicator of the reliability of the findings behind the treatment, not an index of the expected size of the effect.

Treatment Definitions

"Evidence-Based Child and Adolescent Psychosocial Interventions" uses a broad level of analysis for defining treatments, such that interventions sharing a majority of components with similar clinical strategies and theoretical underpinnings are considered to belong to a single treatment approach. For example, rather than list each CBT protocol for depression on its own, the tool handles these as a single group that collectively has achieved a particular level of scientific support. This approach focuses more on "generic" as opposed to "brand name" treatment modalities, and it also is designed to reduce the more than 500 distinct treatments that would otherwise be represented on this tool to a more practical level of analysis.

Problem Definition

The presenting problems represented in the table rows are coded using a checklist of 25 different problem areas (e.g., anxious or avoidant behaviors, eating disorders, substance use). The problem area refers to the condition that a treatment explicitly targeted and for which clinical outcomes were measured. These problem areas are inclusive of diagnostic conditions (e.g., all randomized trials targeting separation anxiety disorder are considered collectively within the "Anxious or Avoidant Behaviors" row) but also include the much larger number of research trials that tested treatments but did not use diagnosis as a study entry criterion. For example, many studies use elevated scores on behavior or emotion checklists or problems such as arrests or suicide attempts to define participants. Mental health diagnoses are therefore nested under these broader categories.

History of This Tool

This tool has its origins with the Child and Adolescent Mental Health Division of the Hawaii Department of Health. Under the leadership of then-division chief Christina Donkervoet, work was commissioned starting in 1999 to review child mental health treatment outcome literature and produce reports that could serve the mental health system in selecting appropriate treatments for its youth.[2] Following an initial review of more than 120 randomized clinical trials,[3] the division began to issue the results of these reviews in quarterly matrix reports known as the Blue Menu (named for the blue paper on which it was originally printed and distributed). This document was designed to be user-friendly and transportable, thereby making it amenable to broad and easy dissemination. As of 2010, the AAP supports the posting of the next generation of this tool. "Evidence-Based Child and Adolescent Psychosocial Interventions" now represents over 900 randomized trials of psychosocial treatments for youth. PracticeWise continues to identify, review, and code new research trials and plans to continue providing updates to this tool to the AAP for the foreseeable future.

Strength of Evidence Definitions

Level 1: Best Support

I.   At least 2 randomized trials demonstrating efficacy in one or more of the following ways:

    a.   Superior to pill placebo, psychological placebo, or another treatment.

    b.   Equivalent to all other groups representing at least one level 1 or level 2 treatment in a study with adequate statistical power (30 participants per group on average) that showed significant pre-study to post-study change in the index group as well as the group(s) being tied. Ties of treatments that have previously qualified only through ties are ineligible.

II. Experiments must be conducted with treatment manuals.

III. Effects must have been demonstrated by at least 2 different investigator teams.

Level 2: Good Support

I.   Two experiments showing the treatment is (statistically significantly) superior to a waiting list or no-treatment control group. *Manuals, specification of sample, and independent investigators are not required.* OR

II. One between-group design experiment with clear specification of group, use of manuals, and demonstrating efficacy by either

    a.   Superior to pill placebo, psychological placebo, or another treatment

    b.   Equivalent to an established treatment (See qualifying tie definition above.)

Level 3: Moderate Support

One between-group design experiment with clear specification of group and treatment approach and demonstrating efficacy by either

    a.   Superior to pill placebo, psychological placebo, or another treatment

    b.   Equivalent to an already established treatment in experiments with adequate statistical power (30 participants per group on average)

Level 4: Minimal Support

One experiment showing the treatment is (statistically significantly) superior to a waiting list or no-treatment control group. *Manuals, specification of sample, and independent investigators are not required.*

Level 5: No Support

The treatment has been tested in at least one study but has failed to meet criteria for levels 1 through 4.

References

1. American Psychological Association Task Force on Promotion and Dissemination of Psychological Procedures, Division of Clinical Psychology. Training in and dissemination of empirically-validated psychological treatments: report and recommendations. *Clin Psychol.* 1995;48:3–23
2. Chorpita BF, Donkervoet CM. Implementation of the Felix Consent Decree in Hawaii: the implementation of the Felix Consent Decree in Hawaii. In: Steele RG, Roberts MC, eds. *Handbook of Mental Health Services for Children, Adolescents, and Families.* New York, NY: Kluwer Academic/Plenum Publishers; 2005:317–332
3. Chorpita BF, Yim LM, Donkervoet JC, et al. Toward large-scale implementation of empirically supported treatments for children: a review and observations by the Hawaii Empirical Basis to Services Task Force. *Clin Psychol Sci Pract.* 2002;9(2):165–190

See more on the PracticeWise publications page (www.practicewise.com/Community/Publications).

Appendix

Common Elements of Evidence-Based Practice Amenable to Primary Care: Indications and Sources

Table A5-1. Common Elements

Indications[a]	EBP Sources[b]	Common Elements of EBPs Amenable to Primary Care
Preparation of patient or family to address any health risk or mental health need Resistance to care seeking Barriers to care seeking	Family therapy Cognitive behavioral therapy Motivational interviewing Family engagement Family-focused pediatrics Solution-focused therapy	"Common factors" communication techniques
Pain • Acute (eg, injury, illness, procedural) • Chronic or recurrent (eg, chronic illness, disability, trauma, recurrent procedures) Stress Habit problems and disorders Behavioral problems (eg, attention problems, anger management) Medical-biobehavioral disorders (eg, asthma, migraine, Tourette syndrome, inflammatory bowel disease, warts, pruritus) Anxiety (eg, performance anxiety [eg, examinations, stage fright, sports], anxiety disorders, PTSD, phobias)	Self-regulation therapies and mind-body therapies	Teach… • Breathing techniques • Relaxation (eg, progressive muscle relaxation) • Mental imagery • Self-hypnosis Offer adjunct biofeedback.

Table A5-1. Common Elements (*continued*)

Indications[a]	EBP Sources[b]	Common Elements of EBPs Amenable to Primary Care
Psychophysiological problems (eg, enuresis, encopresis, conditioned nausea and vomiting, irritable bowel syndrome, sleep disorders) Chronic disease, multisystem disease, and terminal illness (eg, cancer, hemophilia, AIDS, cystic fibrosis, diabetes, chronic renal disease)		
Anxiety Phobias	Cognitive behavioral therapy for anxiety Young children: PCIT (See also "Self-regulation therapies and mind-body therapies" cell earlier in this table.)	Provide psychoeducation. Gradually increase exposure to feared objects or activities. Teach… • Relaxation strategies • Positive self-talk • Thought stopping or substituting • Thoughts of a safe place Reward brave behavior.
Symptoms related to a past trauma	Trauma-focused cognitive behavioral therapy Young children: • Child-Parent Psychotherapy • PCIT	Gently challenge negative thoughts about shame, guilt, and hopelessness. Encourage self-care and ways of seeking a feeling of security. When symptoms are prominent, suggest distraction, relaxation, or supportive company. Plan to manage or avoid unnecessary or extreme triggers. Provide positive attention for positive behavior. Remove attention for provocative behaviors. Provide safe, consistent consequences for unsafe/ unacceptable behaviors. Define the importance of a healthy relationship for recovery.

Table A5-1. Common Elements (*continued*)

Indications[a]	EBP Sources[b]	Common Elements of EBPs Amenable to Primary Care
Low mood Depression	Cognitive behavioral therapy for depression	Provide psychoeducation. Gently challenge negative thoughts. Use behavioral activation (ie, more of enjoyable activities ["prescribe pleasure"]). Focus on strengths, not weaknesses. Teach… • Distraction • Problem-solving skills • Rehearsal of behavior and social skills • Expressive writing Facilitate conversation between parents and youth that is focused on youth's concerns. Reinforce social supports.
Any symptoms associated with… • Inconsistent parenting • Harsh discipline • Inappropriate parental expectations Disruptive behavior Aggression Conduct problems Inattention Hyperactivity	Parenting education Examples: • The Incredible Years • Triple P – Positive Parenting Program • PCIT • "Helping the Noncompliant Child" parent training program	Teach… • Positive time with parents • Encouragement and rewards for positive behavior • Prevention of triggers • Emotional communication skills • Consistent, calm consequences for negative behavior • Reparation for negative behavior • Clear, simple commands and limit setting • Correct use of time-out • De-escalation techniques • Practice of skills
Substance use Other risky behaviors Poor adherence to therapy	Motivational interviewing Family-centered therapy	Request patient's permission to engage. Assess stage of readiness to act. Use Elicit-Provide-Elicit sequence in brief interventions. Listen for and reflect "change talk." Address barriers to change.

Table A5-1. Common Elements (*continued*)

Indications[a]	EBP Sources[b]	Common Elements of EBPs Amenable to Primary Care
Family conflict	Family-centered therapy Motivational interviewing	Apply the following techniques: • Unconditional positive regard • Active listening • Affirmation • Reflection • Open-ended questions • Professional neutrality • Reframing • Summaries
Symptoms of emotional distress in young children (eg, dysregulation, aggression, extreme tantrums, irritability, unhappy mood, extreme anxiety, lack of social reciprocity with caregiver, poor attachment)	Parenting education (See examples in the "Parenting Education" cell earlier in this table.) Promoting First Relationships Parents as Teachers Child-Parent Psychotherapy Cognitive behavioral therapy	Reframe child's perceived bad behavior. Reinforce strengths and protective factors. Teach… • Prevention of unnecessary or extreme triggers • Attention and praise for positive behavior • Clear, simple commands and limit setting • Relaxation and anxiety management • Consistent, safe responses to negative behavior Special time ("time in") with parents

Abbreviations: EBP, evidence-based practice; PCIT, Parent-Child Interaction Therapy; PTSD, post-traumatic stress disorder.

[a] Use of common elements approaches for these indications should not delay full diagnostic evaluation or definitive therapy if the patient's symptoms suggest a psychiatric emergency, severe impairment, or marked distress. Common elements approaches are well suited to the care of patients whose symptoms do not reach a diagnostic threshold, the care of patients who are resistant or otherwise not yet ready to pursue further diagnostic assessment or treatment, and the care of patients who are awaiting further diagnostic assessment and treatment.

[b] See Appendix 4, PracticeWise: Evidence-Based Child and Adolescent Psychosocial Interventions, for more information about these evidence-based practices.

Index

Page numbers followed by an *f,* a *t,* or a *b* denote a figure, a table, or a box, respectively.

Promoting Mental Health

in Children and Adolescents

PRIMARY CARE PRACTICE AND ADVOCACY

EDITOR

Jane Meschan Foy, MD, FAAP

Effectively care for children and adolescents with mental health issues!
This indispensable resource guides pediatric primary care clinicians with a framework for addressing mental health problems in the primary care practice. Handy surveillance and screening tools help identify early signs and symptoms of mental disorders and provide evidence-based interventions to care for children and adolescents with mental health issues.

Topics include

- Strength-based approach to promoting healthy child development
- Children exposed to adverse childhood experiences
- Caring for families new to the United States
- Violence prevention
- Healthy sleep, weight, use of media, and active living
- Children in foster or kinship care or involved with child welfare
- Children of divorce
- Adopted children
- Children with chronic medical conditions
- And more…

American Academy of Pediatrics

DEDICATED TO THE HEALTH OF ALL CHILDREN®

For other pediatric resources, visit the American Academy of Pediatrics at shop.aap.org

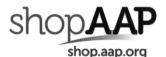
shop.aap.org

ISBN 978-1-61002-227-9

90000>

9 781610 022279